Pediatric
Examination & Board
Review

Pediatric Examination & Board Review

Robert S. Daum, MD, CM

Professor of Pediatrics
Professor, Committee on Microbiology
Professor, Committee on Molecular Medicine
Section Chief, Section of Infectious Diseases
University of Chicago
Chicago, Illinois

Jason J. Canel, MD, FAAP

Instructor of Clinical Pediatrics
Northwestern University Feinberg School of Medicine
Chicago, Illinois
Attending, Pediatrics
Evanston Hospital
Evanston, Illinois

McGRAW-HILL
Medical Publishing Division

New York Chicago San Francisco Lisbon London Madrid Mexico City Milan
New Delhi San Juan Seoul Singapore Sydney Toronto

Pediatric Examination & Board Review

1 2 3 4 5 6 7 8 9 0 QPDQPD 0 9 8 7 6

ISBN-13: 978-0-07-142378-6
ISBN-10: 0-07-142378-8

This book was set in Janson by Silverchair Science + Communications, Inc.
The editors were James T. Shanahan, Anne Sydor, Karen Edmonson, and Peter J. Boyle.
The production supervisor was Sherri Souffrance.
The index was prepared by Coughlin Indexing Services.
Quebecor World Dubuque was printer and binder.

This book is printed on acid-free paper.

Library of Congress Cataloging-in-Publication Data
Pediatric examination & board review / [edited by] Robert S. Daum, Jason J. Canel.
    p. ; cm.
    Includes bibliographical references and index.
    ISBN-13: 978-0-07-142378-6 (alk. paper)
    ISBN-10: 0-07-142378-8 (alk. paper)
    1. Pediatrics--Examinations, questions, etc. 2. Pediatrics--Case studies. I. Daum,
Robert S. II. Canel, Jason J. III. Title: Pediatric examination and board review.
    [DNLM: 1. Pediatrics--Examination Questions. WS 18.2 P36996 2007]
RJ48.2.P343 2007
18.8200076--dc26
                                                                          2006047223

Loved ones gave up quality time so that a project like this could be completed. To Susan, my beloved, and Michael, Jeremy, Abigail, Robert and Shannon, my children, I thank each for their sacrifice to make this effort possible.
—BOB

To Jennifer, my bride forever. To Leah my sweet pea and Noah my bud, both of whom make me a proud dad every day.
—JASON

Contents

COLOR PLATES APPEAR BETWEEN PAGES 434 AND 435.

Contributors

Holly Benjamin, MD, FAAP, FACSM
Assistant Professor of Pediatrics and Surgery
Director of Primary Care Sports Medicine
University of Chicago
Chicago, Illinois

Lynda Brady, MD
Director of Pediatric Gastroenterology
St. Johns Mercy
St. Louis, Missouri

Jason J. Canel, MD, FAAP
Instructor of Clinical Pediatrics
Northwestern University Feinberg School of
Medicine
Chicago, Illinois
Attending, Pediatrics
Evanston Hospital
Evanston, Illinois

Robert S. Daum, MD, CM
Professor of Pediatrics
Professor, Committee on Microbiology
Professor, Committee on Molecular Medicine
Section Chief, Section of Infectious Diseases
University of Chicago
Chicago, Illinois

Dianne Deplewski, MD
Assistant Professor of Pediatrics
Section of Pediatric Endocrinology
Committee on Molecular Metabolism and Nutrition
University of Chicago
Chicago, Illinois

H. Barrett Fromme, MD
Assistant Professor of Pediatrics
Assistant Program Director, Recruitment, Pediatric
Residency Program
University of Chicago
Chicago, Illinois

Jill Glick, MD
Associate Professor of Pediatrics
Medical Director, Child Protective Services
University of Chicago
Chicago, Illinois

Marguerite Herschel, MD (Deceased)
Associate Professor of Pediatrics
University of Chicago
Chicago, Illinois

Heather A. Johnston, MD
Clinical Associate, Department of Pediatrics
Associate Clerkship Director, Pediatrics
University of Chicago
Chicago, Illinois

Madelyn D. Kahana, MD
Professor of Pediatrics and Anesthesiology
Program Director, Pediatrics
Interim Section Chief, Pediatric Critical Care Medicine
University of Chicago
Chicago, Illinois

Marta Killner, MD
Assistant Professor of Pediatrics
Director, Adolescent Medicine Program
University of Chicago
Chicago, Illinois

Jennifer Liedel, MD
Instructor of Pediatrics
University of Chicago
Chicago, Illinois

John Marcinak, MD
Associate Professor of Pediatrics
Associate Director, University of Chicago Hospitals
Infection Control Program
University of Chicago
Chicago, Illinois

Charles J. Marcuccilli, PhD, MD
Assistant Professor of Neurology
Division of Pediatric Neurology
Medical College of Wisconsin
Milwaukee, Wisconsin

Donald I. Moel, MD, MM
Associate Professor of Pediatrics
Attending, Pediatric Nephrology
University of Chicago
Chicago, Illinois

Michael E. Msall, MD
Professor of Pediatrics
Chief, Developmental and Behavioral Pediatrics
University of Chicago
Chicago, Illinois

Izhar ul Qamar, MD, FRCPC
Assistant Professor of Pediatrics
University of Chicago
Chicago, Illinois

Jaideep K. Singh, MD
Associate Professor of Pediatrics
Clinical Director of Neonatal Intensive Care Unit
University of Chicago
Chicago, Illinois

Sarah L. Stein, MD
Assistant Professor of Medicine and Pediatrics
Section of Dermatology
University of Chicago
Chicago, Illinois

Darrel Waggoner, MD
Assistant Professor, Human Genetics and Pediatrics
University of Chicago
Chicago, Illinois

Linda Wagner-Weiner, MD
Assistant Professor of Pediatrics
Attending, Pediatric Rheumatology, LaRabida Hospital
University of Chicago
Chicago, Illinois

Peter E. Zage, PhD, MD
Assistant Professor of Pediatrics
The University of Texas, M.D. Anderson Cancer Center
Houston, Texas

Frank Zimmerman, MD
Assistant Professor of Pediatrics and Medicine
University of Chicago
Chicago, Illinois

Preface

Many medical schools and residency programs have had great success in converting learning by lecture into case-based or "vignette" style learning. Professors using vignettes when teaching students can convey important teaching points in a relevant context that forces participants to be proactive, rather than passive learners.

Tests in medical school and residency have thus migrated towards the vignette model. Testing with vignette-based questions has permeated oral exams, written exams, and interactive, computer-based exams. So too follows the mini-vignette style on many pediatric board exam questions, and we have therefore produced this book, made up entirely of vignettes, followed by question choices and discussion thereof.

We anticipate that this book will be a valuable tool for exam preparation. Of course, we expect that this book will be useful and interesting to all learners; not only to the pediatrician reviewing for board exams, but to the broader continuum of life-long learners, from medical school students in pediatric clerkships to seasoned pediatricians.

And finally to you who hopefully purchased this book in preparation for your Board examination or as an aid for your teaching efforts. To the former, welcome to our discipline of pediatric medicine. May you delight and profit from the knowledge we have tried to impart in these pages. May you also take a minute, should you disagree with any little thing, to inform us of inaccurate questions, statements, or answers. If there are to be future editions, we will make sure your advice is incorporated.

Good luck with your Board examination. May this volume make your preparations more successful.

Robert S. Daum, MD
Jason J. Canel, MD

Acknowledgments

Many images found in this book were made available by multiple sources including, without limit, the University of Chicago Department of Microbiology and the personal archives of contributors and colleagues thereof.

The amazing diligence and careful writing of current and former members of the faculty in the Department of Pediatrics here at the University of Chicago have been a wonder to behold. While some have moved on to greener pastures, our sense of community persists and I hope will be reinforced by their belonging to the distinguished group of authors comprising this book.

We are grateful for the outstanding support of Ms. LaKesha Lloyd, who put forth a friendly face to those few authors needing an extra week, month, or year to complete their contributions. We would also like to thank Kimberly Abogunrin for assisting us in starting the project.

The McGraw Hill staff has been most supportive, and in particular, we would like to thank James Shanahan, Executive Editor, and Karen Edmonson, Managing Editor. Without their support and encouragement, this project would not have been possible.

Finally, our thanks to you, our reader. For this project to be a success, we depend on both your need and enthusiasm for vignette-style learning and, ultimately, for our product. We hope to learn from you if there is any way to improve this book's utility to your practice. We thereby encourage you to send us your ideas and comments for future editions.

Robert S. Daum, MD
Jason J. Canel, MD

Cardiology

CASE 1: A NEONATE WITH A HEART MURMUR

A full-term newborn delivered without complications is noted to have a heart murmur at 1 day of age. The murmur is described as a grade 2/6 systolic ejection-type murmur heard best at the upper left sternal border. The heart sounds are normal. The blood pressure is normal. The peripheral pulses are normal. The oxygen saturation is 100% in room air. On day of life 3, the murmur has changed from a systolic murmur to a continuous murmur again heard best at the upper left sternal border. The baby appears well and is tolerating feeds without difficulties.

SELECT THE ONE BEST ANSWER

1. What is the likely cause of this heart murmur?

    (A) patent ductus arteriosus
    (B) atrial septal defect
    (C) ventricular septal defect
    (D) peripheral pulmonary stenosis

2. A continuous murmur persists for more than 72 hours. What is the most appropriate test to evaluate the etiology of this murmur?

    (A) chest radiograph
    (B) ECG
    (C) complete blood count
    (D) echocardiogram

3. The echocardiogram demonstrates a small patent ductus arteriosus with no associated cardiac lesions and no evidence of left heart volume overload. What advice would you give to the family regarding further follow-up?

    (A) no further cardiology follow-up is needed
    (B) there is a lifelong ongoing risk for endarteritis and antibiotic prophylaxis should be given as needed
    (C) immediate surgical repair is required
    (D) all of the above

4. At day of life 7, the neonate described develops increased shortness of breath, decreased feeding, and a chest radiograph shows pulmonary edema. What is the best first-line course of action?

    (A) prostaglandin E_1 infusion
    (B) indomethacin course
    (C) supplemental oxygen
    (D) nitric oxide

5. A full-term newborn delivered via normal spontaneous vaginal delivery with Apgars of 9 at 1 minute and 9 at 5 minutes, is noted to have a grade 2/6 systolic murmur at the left sternal border on day 1 of life. Upon reexamination on day 4 of life, the neonate is found to have poor perfusion, poor pulses, hypotension, and shock. What is the least likely cause of shock in this neonate?

    (A) asphyxia
    (B) sepsis
    (C) hypoglycemia
    (D) cardiogenic shock

6. Which of the following congenital heart lesions may result in cardiogenic shock following spontaneous closure of the ductus arteriosus?

   (A) atrial septal defect
   (B) hypoplastic left heart syndrome
   (C) mitral valve prolapse
   (D) ventricular septal defect

7. What test would be most helpful to diagnose the cause of shock in this neonate?

   (A) chest radiograph
   (B) arterial blood gas
   (C) blood glucose level
   (D) echocardiogram

8. What is the most appropriate acute treatment for cardiogenic shock as a result of left heart obstructive lesions?

   (A) prostaglandin E_1 infusion
   (B) indomethacin administration
   (C) supplemental oxygen administration
   (D) nitric oxide

9. What are other courses of action to be taken in patients with cardiogenic shock?

   (A) inotropic medications such as epinephrine and dopamine
   (B) ventilatory support
   (C) oxygen supplementation
   (D) all of the above

10. A neonate with a heart murmur on examination is noted to have a bluish tinge to the lips. The baby is smiling and eating well in no apparent distress. The baby is warm with good pulses. An oxygen saturation monitor was placed on the baby's finger and the saturations in room air are 80%. Which of the following is likely to account for this patient's finding of cyanosis?

   (A) cyanotic congenital heart disease
   (B) hemoglobinopathy
   (C) respiratory disease
   (D) all of the above

11. Which test would most likely help differentiate a cardiac versus pulmonary cause for cyanosis?

   (A) hyperoxia test
   (B) blood gas on room air
   (C) chest radiograph
   (D) complete blood count

12. What is the most common cyanotic heart lesion in the neonate?

   (A) transposition of the great arteries
   (B) total anomalous pulmonary venous return
   (C) tricuspid atresia
   (D) tetralogy of Fallot

13. What would be an appropriate first line treatment for the management of cyanosis as a result of heart disease?

   (A) prostaglandin E_1 infusion
   (B) indomethacin administration
   (C) nitric oxide
   (D) surfactant

14. A 4-year-old with known diagnosis of unrepaired tetralogy of Fallot becomes severely cyanotic while crying. Which of the following is not indicated for acute management of this situation?

   (A) administering of oxygen
   (B) placing the child in the knee-chest position
   (C) administering morphine sulfate
   (D) rectal stimulation

15. Which of the following is not a complication of chronic cyanosis?

   (A) polycythemia
   (B) stroke
   (C) brain abscess
   (D) cognitive abnormalities
   (E) cerebral aneurysms

Answers

1. **(A)** The most likely cause of this murmur is a patent ductus arteriosus. Atrial septal defects are unlikely to cause heart murmur at this early age and ventricular septal defects cause a holosystolic murmur that does not evolve into a continuous murmur. Peripheral pulmonary stenosis is associated with a systolic ejection murmur that radiates

to the back and to both axilla. The patent ductus arteriosus is required for fetal circulation; however, the structure usually closes within hours after delivery secondary to changes in oxygen tension as well as other circulating factors such as prostaglandin. Persistence of the ductus arteriosus occurs in approximately 0.8 per 1000 live births but is much more common in premature newborns with an incidence of as high as 20% in neonates weighing <1750 g. In patients with low oxygen tension, pulmonary hypertension, or congenital heart disease, there is delayed closure of the ductus arteriosus.

2. **(D)** The ductus arteriosus in this neonate remains patent after 72 hours. The most appropriate test to confirm this is the echocardiogram. This test will not only confirm the diagnosis of the patent ductus arteriosus but will also assess for any associated cardiac lesions. It is critical to assess for pulmonary artery hypertension or ductal-dependent cardiac lesions when planning for closure of the patent ductus arteriosus.

3. **(B)** The presence of a small patent ductus arteriosus is unlikely to lead to significant left-to-right shunting or volume overloading and therefore does not place the child at risk for development of heart failure. There is approximately 5% incidence of spontaneous closure of small patent ductus arteriosus and thus immediate surgery is usually not required in that situation. However, there is a lifelong risk for bacterial endarteritis with the presence of a patent ductus arteriosus of approximately 0.5% per year. Therefore, the family should be advised that the patient thus requires bacterial endocarditis prophylaxis as recommended. Furthermore, some have advocated that hemodynamically insignificant patent ductus arteriosus be closed at some point to avoid the lifelong risks of bacterial endarteritis.

4. **(B)** In this situation, a large patent ductus arteriosus has allowed for significant left-to-right shunting resulting in pulmonary edema, shortness of breath, and left ventricular volume overload. The treatment options at this point include administration of indomethacin in an attempt to close the patent ductus arteriosus. Indomethacin is effective in approximately 80% of cases; however, its effectiveness decreases if administered after 2 weeks of age. Other treatment options for closure of hemodynamically significant ductus arteriosus include surgery or transcatheter device closure. Both can be performed safely and effectively with minimal morbidity and mortality. Administration of oxygen in the patient with congestive heart failure because of large left-to-right shunt would be detrimental in that it may decrease pulmonary vascular resistance and increase the degree of left-to-right shunting, exacerbating the symptoms of heart failure. The same is true for administration of nitric oxide in this situation.

5. **(A)** The etiology of shock in the neonate includes the following:

Hypoglycemia
Asphyxia
Sepsis
Intracranial bleeding
Arrhythmias including tachyarrhythmias and bradycardias
Cardiogenic shock because of left-sided obstructive lesions
Myocarditis

The least likely explanation of shock in this baby is asphyxia as there is no history of perinatal asphyxia or distress based on the birth history.

6. **(B)** Cardiogenic shock may be the first presentation in the neonate with congenital heart disease. Specific heart lesions causing left ventricular outflow tract obstruction may present in this manner. These lesions include critical aortic stenosis, hypoplastic left heart syndrome, and coarctation of the aorta. A patent ductus arteriosus allows for blood to bypass left-sided obstructions thus maintaining adequate cardiac output. With closure of the ductus, cardiac output is diminished. The neonate with cardiogenic shock from ductal-dependent lesions often presents between 1 and 2 weeks of age with shock related to the spontaneous closure of the ductus arteriosus.

7. **(D)** An echocardiogram would be the most useful test in this situation to determine if there is a

ductal-dependent cardiac lesion. It is also useful to detect primary myocardial dysfunction related to other causes of shock.

8. **(A)** Acute therapy for shock as a result of ductal-dependent cardiac lesions is infusion of prostaglandin E_1 in hopes of reestablishing patency of the ductus arteriosus.

9. **(D)** The other acute management strategies for shock in the neonate include inotropic support with dopamine or epinephrine, ventilatory support in cases of respiratory compromise, and oxygen supplementation.

10. **(D)** Cyanosis can be divided into two clinical categories, central or peripheral. Central cyanosis is a result of a decrease in the oxygen saturation of blood supplying the body. Peripheral cyanosis is a benign finding because of increased oxygen extraction in distal capillary beds and is commonly seen in normal neonates. The clinical detection of cyanosis occurs when approximately 3 g/dL to 5 g/dL of desaturated hemoglobin is present in the systemic circulation. The most common causes of central cyanosis in the neonate include cyanotic heart disease, hemoglobinopathies, and respiratory distress.

11. **(A)** The test most likely to help differentiate cyanotic heart disease from respiratory disease is the hyperoxia test. In this test, 100% oxygen is administered to the patient and the partial pressure of oxygen is measured. In patients with cyanotic heart disease, the partial pressure of oxygen rarely increases above the level of 100 mm Hg while in lung disease, there is usually some change from the baseline PO_2 with administration of oxygen. The lack of response to oxygen in cyanotic heart disease is a result of fixed right-to-left shunting of desaturated blood to the systemic circulation. While the other tests mentioned may be helpful in the evaluation of the cyanotic neonate, they are not as sensitive in differentiating cardiac from respiratory etiologies.

12. **(A)** Cardiac lesions associated with cyanosis include:

Transposition of the great arteries (the most common)

Tetralogy of Fallot
Truncus arteriosus
Tricuspid atresia
Pulmonary atresia
Total anomalous pulmonary venous return

Other lesions include single-ventricle physiology such as hypoplastic left heart syndrome, or Ebstein's anomaly of the tricuspid valve with right-to-left shunting across an atrial septal defect.

13. **(A)** In patients with cyanosis because of heart disease, there is either obligate mixing of saturated and desaturated blood reaching the systemic circulation (e.g., truncus arteriosus) or decreased effective pulmonary blood flow. In either situation, promotion of increased pulmonary blood flow would increase the systemic oxygen saturation. This is acutely achieved by infusion of prostaglandin E_1 to reestablish (or maintain) patency of the ductus arteriosus. Therefore, in situations where cyanosis because of heart disease is suspected, infusion of prostaglandin E_1 should be instituted as soon as possible.

14. **(D)** Patients with tetralogy of Fallot are at risk for a hypercyanotic "tet" spell. This usually occurs in patients older than 2 years of age, although it has been reported at younger ages. The mechanism of a hypercyanotic spell is acute and progressive increase in the degree of pulmonary stenosis, with increased right-to-left shunting of desaturated blood to the systemic circulation. This is precipitated by an increase in circulating catecholamines, anxiety, hypoxia, or dehydration. Interventions to break this cycle include administration of oxygen, morphine, propranolol, or phenylephrine, placing the child in a knee-chest position and in extreme cases, muscle relaxation and intubation are required. Rectal stimulation would serve to worsen the crisis by increasing the catecholamine levels.

15. **(E)** Complications in patients with chronic cyanosis include polycythemia (compensation for decreased systemic oxygen tension), risk for strokes because of an increased propensity for forming blood clots and from an increased blood viscosity. This is particularly concerning when hematocrit levels are greater than 70%. A rela-

tive anemia may be seen in patients with cyanosis with low hemoglobin indices and some have suggested that this also increases the risk of stroke because of increased blood viscosity. Another complication is brain abscess formation because of poor venous blood flow and increased susceptibility to infection. Impaired cognitive function is associated with long-standing cyanosis. The degree of impairment is related to both the degree and period of cyanosis.

SUGGESTED READING

Emmanouilides GC, Riemenschneider TA, Allen HD, et al, eds: *Moss and Adams Heart Disease in Infants, Children and Adolescents*, 5th ed. Philadelphia: Williams and Wilkins, 1995.

Braunwald E, Zipes DP, Libbey P, eds: *Heart Disease: A Textbook of Cardiovascular Medicine*, 6th ed. Philadelphia: WB Saunders, 2001.

Fyler DC, ed: *Nadas' Pediatric Cardiology*, Philadelphia: Hanley and Belfus, 1980.

Park M, ed: *Pediatric Cardiology for Practitioners*, 4th ed. St. Louis: Mosby, 2002.

CASE 2: A 10-YEAR-OLD BOY WITH PALPITATIONS

A 10-year-old male presents to the clinic with a history of intermittent episodes of palpitations occurring one time per month. The episodes are not associated with exercise or activity, last for several minutes, and resolve spontaneously. There is no significant past medical history, no new medications, and no dizziness or syncope. A 12-lead ECG is performed while he is asymptomatic and it is normal.

SELECT THE ONE BEST ANSWER

1. Which test would best help to evaluate the etiology of this patient's palpitations?

    (A) echocardiogram
    (B) chest radiograph
    (C) event recorder monitor
    (D) exercise stress test

Match the ECG rhythm strips in questions 2 through 5 to one of the findings below.

    (A) premature atrial contractions
    (B) premature ventricular contractions

    (C) sinus tachycardia
    (D) sinus arrhythmia

2. Figure 2-1 shown below

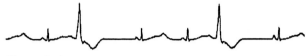

Figure 2-1.

3. Figure 2-2 shown below

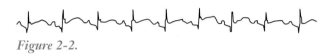

Figure 2-2.

4. Figure 2-3 shown below

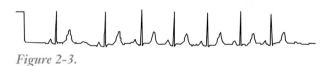

Figure 2-3.

5. Figure 2-4 shown below

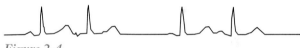

Figure 2-4.

6. What is the most likely cause of supraventricular tachycardia in this patient?

    (A) concealed accessory bypass tract causing orthodromic reciprocating tachycardia
    (B) AV node reentry tachycardia
    (C) ectopic atrial tachycardia
    (D) atrial flutter

7. What is the most appropriate acute therapy for symptomatic orthodromic reciprocating tachycardia?

    (A) DC cardioversion
    (B) IV adenosine
    (C) vagal maneuvers
    (D) all of the above

8. Which of the following agents is considered first-line therapy for chronic control of orthodromic reciprocating tachycardia?

(A) propafenone
(B) atenolol
(C) sotalol
(D) amiodarone

9. What would be the most appropriate acute therapy for symptomatic ectopic atrial tachycardia?

(A) DC cardioversion
(B) IV adenosine
(C) vagal maneuvers
(D) IV esmolol

10. A child with supraventricular tachycardia is found to have a resting ECG rhythm strip shown below in Figure 2-5. What is the diagnosis?

(A) sinus tachycardia
(B) ventricular preexcitation
(C) ventricular tachycardia
(D) sinus rhythm

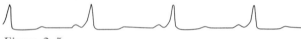

Figure 2-5.

11. Which statement is true regarding the diagnosis of Wolff-Parkinson-White (WPW) syndrome?

(A) There is an increased risk of sudden cardiac death.
(B) There is an increased risk of ectopic atrial tachycardia.
(C) There is an increased risk of tachycardia-induced cardiomyopathy.
(D) There is no risk of atrial fibrillation.

12. Which of the following agents is considered first-line therapy for chronic control of orthodromically reciprocating tachycardia associated with ventricular preexcitation (WPW syndrome)?

(A) digoxin
(B) verapamil
(C) propranolol
(D) amiodarone

13. A 10-year-old child experiences palpitations associated with dizziness when standing. He has had one episode of syncope following standing in school. What is the most common etiology of syncope in this age group?

(A) seizures
(B) cardiac disease
(C) hypoglycemia
(D) neurocardiogenic (vasovagal)

14. Which of the following features would suggest neurocardiogenic syncope?

(A) urinary incontinence during episodes of syncope
(B) auditory aura preceding episode of syncope
(C) transient right arm paralysis following episode of syncope
(D) symptoms of dizziness, blurred vision, diaphoresis preceding syncope

15. Which of the following is true regarding tilt table testing for syncope?

(A) Tilt table testing should be performed for every patient with syncope.
(B) The results of tilt table testing are highly reproducible for an individual.
(C) Tilt table testing is reserved for complicated cases where the diagnosis of syncope is uncertain.
(D) Tilt table testing is useful for predicting response to medications.

16. A newborn baby presents with a heart rate of 45 beats per minute with a normal blood pressure and good perfusion. The ECG rhythm strip is shown below in Figure 2-6. What is the diagnosis?

(A) first-degree AV block
(B) second-degree AV block (type 1)
(C) second-degree AV block (type 2)
(D) third-degree AV block

17. What is the most likely cause of congenital AV block in newborns?

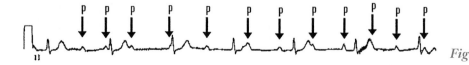

Figure 2-6.

(A) maternal lupus
(B) maternal rubella
(C) maternal use of lithium
(D) maternal diabetes mellitus

18. The patient subsequently develops signs of heart failure with poor perfusion and tachypnea. What is the most appropriate long-term therapy for this patient?

(A) pacemaker implantation
(B) digoxin
(C) theophylline
(D) atropine

19. A 10-year-old patient with history of palpitations is found to have the ECG rhythm strip shown below in Figure 2-7. What is the most likely diagnosis of his palpitations?

(A) myocardial ischemia
(B) orthodromic reentry tachycardia
(C) ventricular arrhythmias
(D) premature atrial beat

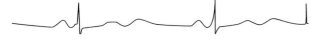

Figure 2-7.

20. What are the known modes of inheritance for congenital long QT syndrome?

(A) autosomal recessive inheritance
(B) autosomal dominant inheritance
(C) spontaneous mutation
(D) all of the above

21. Which of the following medications is associated with drug-induced long QT syndrome?

(A) propranolol
(B) amitriptyline
(C) metoclopramide
(D) amoxicillin

Answers

1. **(C)** Palpitations are a common complaint in young patients reported by 16% of patients in a survey of a large primary care clinic. Palpitations are associated with acute arrhythmias in less than 5% of cases when evaluated with long-term monitoring. Palpitations associated with symptoms of dizziness or syncope or in the setting of a family history of arrhythmias or sudden cardiac death would increase the suspicion for an underlying cardiac disorder. While the echocardiogram, stress test, and chest radiograph are often used to exclude significant cardiac disease, they are unlikely to determine the specific etiology of the palpitations. In this situation, an event recorder could be used to record an ECG rhythm strip during symptoms. An event recorder is a long-term monitoring device that is used for patients with symptoms that occur infrequently.

2. **(B)** The ECG in Figure 2-1 shows normal sinus rhythm with a premature ventricular contraction. Premature ventricular contractions are a less common finding in young patients occurring with an incidence of approximately 5% to 10%. They are usually benign; however, they may rarely be associated with significant heart disease. Therefore, the evaluation often includes an echocardiogram or stress test to assess for associated cardiac disease. Premature ventricular contractions that are not associated with significant heart disease do not require therapy unless they are associated with significant symptoms of discomfort or palpitations.

3. **(C)** The ECG in Figure 2-2 shows sinus tachycardia. The more common etiologies of sinus tachycardia at this age include anxiety or emotion, hyperthyroidism, anemia, postural orthostatic tachycardia syndrome, and dehydration. It is the most common cause of palpitations in young patients.

4. **(D)** The ECG in Figure 2-3 shows sinus arrhythmia. This is a benign finding that is associated with an irregular heart rhythm heard during auscultation. It may vary with respiration and can be pronounced in children. There is no association with significant heart disease

5. **(A)** The ECG in Figure 2-4 demonstrates normal sinus rhythm with a single premature atrial contraction. Premature atrial contractions are a common benign fining in young patients occurring with an incidence of approximately 17% to 25%. They are usually not associated with significant cardiac disease. Because of the benign na-

ture of the premature atrial contractions, they do not require further investigation.

6. **(A)** The most likely cause of supraventricular tachycardia at this age is orthodromic reciprocating tachycardia because of an accessory bypass tract ("concealed" in this case based on the normal resting ECG). AV node reentry tachycardia is less common at this age; however, this becomes the predominant mechanism of tachycardia in young adults. Ectopic atrial tachycardia and atrial flutter occur with a low incidence throughout childhood. Atrial flutter is more commonly seen in patients who have congenital heart disease.

7. **(D)** Acceptable therapy for orthodromic reciprocating tachycardia because of a concealed bypass tract includes DC cardioversion, IV adenosine, or vagal maneuvers. Other antiarrhythmic drugs such as calcium channel blockers can also be used. The determination of which therapy is used is based on the patient's clinical status at the time of presentation. In patients with stable tachycardia and stable vital signs, vagal maneuvers or IV adenosine may be first-line treatment. In patients with unstable tachycardia, DC cardioversion may be the first-line therapy. Of note, IV calcium channel blockers are not recommended for use in infants younger than 1 year of age secondary to an increased risk for hypotension.

8. **(B)** First-line medical therapy for chronic treatment of supraventricular tachycardia includes digoxin, calcium channel blockers, and beta-blockers (e.g., atenolol). Amiodarone, propafenone, and sotalol are all effective drugs for treatment of SVT but have a higher incidence of side effects (proarrhythmia) and are usually reserved for cases that are resistant to first-line medications.

9. **(D)** Ectopic atrial tachycardia is a rare tachycardia occurring with an incidence of approximately 10% throughout childhood. In some cases of automatic atrial tachycardia, the heart rates are only slightly above sinus rhythm and thus the tachycardia may go undetected for months to years. Patients with ectopic tachycardia are at risk for ventricular dysfunction and heart failure. Unlike orthodromic reciprocating tachycardia and AV node reentry tachy-cardia, ectopic atrial tachycardia arises from a single atrial focus that is not dependent on the AV node. Therefore, adenosine, vagal maneuvers, and DC cardioversion are ineffective. Appropriate acute therapy includes IV beta-blockers, calcium channel blockers, or amiodarone.

10. **(B)** The ECG in Figure 2-5 demonstrates ventricular preexcitation (short PR interval and slurred upstroke of the QRS or delta wave) because of an accessory bypass tract. When associated with tachycardia, this is known as WPW syndrome. The incidence of WPW syndrome is approximately 0.3%. This mechanism of tachycardia is orthodromic reciprocating tachycardia similar to that in patients with concealed bypass tracts.

11. **(A)** There is an increased risk of sudden cardiac death (approximately 1/1000 patient years) in WPW syndrome. Sudden cardiac death occurs because of rapid conduction over the accessory bypass tract during an atrial tachycardia resulting in ventricular compromise. Patients with WPW syndrome are not at increased risk for ectopic atrial tachycardia or tachycardia-induced cardiomyopathy but there is an increased incidence of atrial fibrillation in this population.

12. **(C)** First-line chronic medical therapy for patients with WPW syndrome includes beta-blockers or other anti-arrhythmic medications such as flecainide or amiodarone. The use of digoxin and/or verapamil is contraindicated in these patients because these agents may potentiate rapid antegrade conduction over the accessory pathway and may increase the risk for sudden death.

13. **(D)** The most common etiology of syncope in young patients is neurocardiogenic or vasovagal syncope. This occurs in up to 20% of the population. Other causes include neurologic (e.g., seizures), metabolic (e.g., anemia, dehydration), or cardiac (e.g., arrhythmia).

14. **(D)** Typical features of neurocardiogenic syncope include preceding symptoms of nausea, dizziness, diaphoresis, or blurred vision. The episodes are related to position and usually occur when sitting or standing. Loss of consciousness is brief and resolves

spontaneously. The other features mentioned are suggestive of syncope because of a seizure.

15. **(C)** Tilt table testing is a simple test used to reproduce neurocardiogenic syncope. However, the low sensitivity and specificity as well as the lack of reproducibility of the test limit its utility. It is usually reserved for difficult situations where the etiology of syncope is uncertain. It is not recommended for all patients with syncope and is not useful for predicting response to medications.

16. **(D)** The ECG rhythm strip in Figure 2-6 demonstrates third-degree AV block. This is defined as complete dissociation of the atrial and ventricular electrical activity.

17. **(A)** The most common cause of congenital complete AV block is maternal lupus. The pathogenesis is thought to be a result of maternal transfer of lupus antibodies (anti-Ro or anti-La) to the fetus and subsequent damage of the developing conduction system. In patients with congenital AV block, the chances of their mother having anti-Ro or anti-La antibodies are approximately 60% to 70%. For mothers with lupus, there is a 5% incidence of having a child with complete AV block. Other causes of AV block in the neonate include structural heart disease, myocarditis, and metabolic disease.

18. **(A)** In patients with congenital AV block and symptomatic bradycardia, the treatment of choice is pacemaker implantation. No other therapy has been shown to affect long-term outcome in these patients. Medications are not consistently effective for prevention of bradycardia and therefore are not recommended for chronic therapy. Other indications for pacemaker implantation in patients with complete heart block include a wide QRS escape rhythm, a prolonged QT interval, asymptomatic infants with a heart rate less than 55 bpm, asymptomatic children with a heart rate less than 50 bpm, and asymptomatic complete heart block with heart rate of less than 75 bpm associated with congenital heart disease.

19. **(C)** The ECG in Figure 2-7 demonstrates a prolonged QT interval. The QT interval is usually corrected for heart rate (QTc) and normal limits vary with age and gender. Palpitations associated with this ECG would most likely be a result of a polymorphic ventricular tachycardia known as torsades de pointes. The ventricular arrhythmia may be self-limited or result in symptoms of dizziness, syncope, or death. The occurrence of torsades de pointes is associated with exercise or activity; however, in some cases it may occur at rest.

20. **(D)** Congenital long QT syndrome is most commonly inherited in an autosomal dominant manner (Romano-Ward). It is a result of a defect in one of five known genes that affect potassium and sodium ion channels in the heart. A specific gene defect has been identified in 50% of patients with clinical long QT syndrome. A less common mode of inheritance is autosomal recessive (Jervell and Lange-Nielsen). In these patients, there is often associated conductive hearing loss and a higher risk for ventricular arrhythmias and sudden death. Finally, some cases of congenital long QT syndrome occur because of spontaneous mutations. The risk for sudden death in patients with long QT syndrome who present with symptoms of dizziness or syncope is approximately 20% in 1 year if untreated. The use of beta-blockers decreases the risk of sudden death to less than 5% in this population. Therefore, beta-blockers have become the mainstay of therapy as well as avoidance of strenuous activities, especially swimming. Pacemaker implantation is occasionally required for patients with either baseline bradycardia or those who develop bradycardia following treatment with beta-blockers. Implantable cardioverter defibrillators are now used more frequently in patients who are continuing to become symptomatic despite medical therapy with beta-blocker or those in whom there is a strong family history of sudden death.

21. **(B)** Acquired long QT syndrome can occur with head trauma, myocardial infarction, cardiomyopathy, or as a result of drugs or medications. This list of drugs/medications associated with acquired prolonged QT is extensive and updated regularly. Some of the more common medications on this list include amitriptyline or other tricyclic antidepressants, erythromycin, and cisapride.

SUGGESTED READING

Emmanouilides GC, Riemenschneider TA, Allen HD, et al, eds: *Moss and Adams Heart Disease in Infants, Children and Adolescents*, 5th ed. Philadelphia: Williams and Wilkins, 1995.

Braunwald E, Zipes DP, Libbey P, eds: *Braunwald: Heart Disease: A Textbook of Cardiovascular Medicine*, 6th ed. Philadelphia: WB Saunders, 2001.

Fyler DC, ed: *Nadas' Pediatric Cardiology.* Philadelphia: Hanley and Belfus, 1980.

Park M, ed: *Pediatric Cardiology for Practitioners*, 4th ed. St. Louis: Mosby, 2002.

CASE 3: A 7-YEAR-OLD CHILD WITH A HEART MURMUR

A 7-year-old boy with no significant past medical history is noted to have a heart murmur heard for the first time during a routine physical evaluation by his lifelong pediatrician. The physical examination is significant for a grade 2/6 vibratory systolic murmur heard best at the lower left sternal border with no radiation. The remainder of the physical examination was normal.

SELECT THE ONE BEST ANSWER

1. What is the most likely diagnosis of this heart murmur?

   (A) Still's murmur
   (B) ventricular septal defect
   (C) atrial septal defect
   (D) peripheral pulmonary stenosis
   (E) venous hum

2. What supporting evidence would help to confirm the diagnosis of an innocent Still's murmur?

   (A) a fixed, split second heart sound
   (B) the murmur is louder in the supine position compared to the sitting or standing position
   (C) a diastolic rumble
   (D) the murmur is associated with a precordial thrill (grade IV)

3. Which test would not be indicated for this patient at this time?

   (A) ECG
   (B) echocardiogram
   (C) chest radiograph
   (D) cardiac catheterization

4. What would be appropriate advice to the family regarding a child with this murmur?

   (A) endocarditis prophylaxis is needed
   (B) rigorous sports should be avoided
   (C) sports participation is allowable
   (D) annual echocardiograms are required

5. A 6-week-old infant presents with a heart murmur and a history of poor feeding, diaphoresis, and tachypnea. On examination, he is playful but tachypneic with a grade 2/6 systolic regurgitant murmur heard best in the mid left sternal border, hepatomegaly, rales, and intermittent wheezes, cool extremities with normal distal pulses, and an active precordium. What is the likely diagnosis of this patient?

   (A) chronic lung disease
   (B) acute upper respiratory infection
   (C) congestive heart failure
   (D) dehydration

6. What test would not be helpful in evaluating this patient?

   (A) an echocardiogram
   (B) an ECG
   (C) a chest radiograph
   (D) a throat culture

7. What heart lesion is least likely to present with congestive heart failure symptoms at age 6 weeks?

   (A) ventricular septal defect
   (B) patent ductus arteriosus
   (C) atrial septal defect
   (D) aortopulmonary window

8. Which feature may help to distinguish heart failure from an anomalous left coronary artery arising from the pulmonary artery versus heart failure from a ventricular septal defect?

   (A) extreme irritability and crying at the onset of feeding
   (B) diaphoresis
   (C) weight loss
   (D) decreased frequency of wet diapers

9. Which therapy would not be indicated for the acute management of congestive heart failure because of a left-to-right shunting lesion?

(A) digoxin
(B) oxygen supplementation
(C) dobutamine
(D) furosemide (Lasix)

10. A 2-year-old patient presents with symptoms of heart failure. An echocardiogram demonstrates no intracardiac lesion but a dilated, poorly functioning left ventricle. What is the least likely cause of the dilated cardiomyopathy in this patient?

    (A) myocarditis
    (B) metabolic disease
    (C) idiopathic
    (D) myocardial ischemia

11. Which of the following would be supportive evidence of the diagnosis of myocarditis?

    (A) an endomyocardial biopsy showing fibrosis
    (B) an endomyocardial biopsy showing fibrosis and inflammation
    (C) systolic flow murmur
    (D) an S3 gallop on cardiac exam

12. What is the most common cause of myocarditis?

    (A) *Staphylococcus aureus*
    (B) streptococcus infection
    (C) Epstein-Barr virus
    (D) enterovirus

13. Which of the following should be avoided for the treatment of acute myocarditis?

    (A) IV inotropes
    (B) IV immunoglobulins
    (C) supportive therapy with diuretics
    (D) IV digoxin

14. Which therapy would not be considered standard management for patients with chronic congestive heart failure?

    (A) beta-blockers
    (B) diuretics
    (C) ACE inhibitors
    (D) calcium channel blockers

15. A 7-year-old presents with heart murmur, chest pain, and shortness of breath. The murmur is a continuous-type murmur that varies in quality with position changes. The patient seems to have relief when sitting and leaning forward. The heart sounds are distant. What is the likely diagnosis for this patient?

    (A) pulmonary embolus
    (B) pericarditis
    (C) myocardial infarction
    (D) GE reflux

16. What is the most common cause of this 7-year-old's diagnosis in young patients in the United States?

    (A) viral infection
    (B) acute rheumatic fever
    (C) bacterial infection
    (D) collagen vascular disease

17. While in the office, the 7-year-old becomes lethargic with poor perfusion and hypotension. What is the most likely explanation?

    (A) pulmonary embolus
    (B) myocardial infarction
    (C) stroke
    (D) cardiac tamponade

Answers

1. **(A)** The patient most likely has a Still's murmur. This is described as a vibratory or musical systolic ejection murmur occurring at the left sternal border with no other associated cardiac findings. It is the most common innocent heart murmur in children and usually presents between 2 and 7 years of age. Other innocent murmurs include pulmonary outflow tract murmur, the peripheral pulmonary stenosis murmur of the newborn, and venous hum. The incidence of innocent heart murmurs in young patients after infancy is approximately 17% to 66%.

2. **(B)** Features of innocent heart murmurs include not only the quality and location of the heart murmur but also the fact that the first and second heart sounds are normal. The murmurs are usually well localized without much radiation and are usually graded between 1 and 3 with no association with a precordial thrill. The murmurs are usually described as vibratory, musical, or blowing, and are louder in the supine position

compared to the sitting or standing position. This is not the case with the innocent venous hum that is often louder in the sitting position. Venous hum can be distinguished by the great amount of variability in quality with position changes and with turning the head. Innocent murmurs are typically not associated with diastolic components. A split, fixed second heart sound is associated with an atrial septal defect.

3. **(D)** Common tests performed in evaluation of innocent heart murmurs include 12-lead ECGs, chest radiographs, and echocardiograms. The use of these tests is at discretion of the examining physician and depends on the findings on physical examination as well as the past medical history and family history. An invasive procedure such as a cardiac catheterization is usually not recommended for evaluation of an innocent heart murmur if the preceding tests have been normal.

4. **(C)** Innocent heart murmurs are not associated with any increased risk for bacterial endocarditis and thus prophylaxis is not needed. Sports participation is not restricted as there is not an increase in cardiac events associated with innocent heart murmurs. Since innocent murmurs, by definition, are not associated with structural heart disease, yearly echocardiograms are usually not recommended. Depending on the age at time of diagnosis, a follow-up visit is occasionally recommended for younger patients.

5. **(C)** The child presents with evidence of congestive heart failure. In addition to the clinical findings described, other findings associated with congestive heart failure include edema, usually of the eyelids, or dependent areas, jugular venous distention, an S3 or S4 gallop on examination, and cardiomegaly or pulmonary edema on chest radiograph.

6. **(D)** Evaluation of a young patient with congestive heart failure requires an echocardiogram to assess cardiac function and for any associated cardiac structural abnormalities. A 12-lead ECG is use to assess for any ischemic changes, arrhythmias, or bradycardia. A chest radiograph is helpful to assess for cardiomegaly or pulmonary edema as well as to assess for any obvious pri-

mary pulmonary disorders. The throat culture would not be useful at this age for evaluation of heart failure.

7. **(C)** Cardiac lesions that present with heart failure at this age are usually a result of an increase in the amount of left-to-right shunting secondary to the natural decrease in the pulmonary vascular resistance. Common left-to-right shunting lesions include ventricular septal defects, patent ductus arteriosus, and aortopulmonary windows. Atrial septal defects do not usually present with heart failure at this age mainly because the amount of left-to-right shunting is dependent on the compliance of the right ventricle rather than the drop in pulmonary vascular resistance.

8. **(A)** Anomalous left coronary artery from the pulmonary artery is a rare congenital heart defect in which the right coronary artery arises normally from the aorta but the left coronary artery arises from the pulmonary artery. A number of collateral vessels develop between the right and left coronary arteries and thus when there is a drop of pulmonary vascular resistance, a steal phenomenon occurs with coronary blood essentially flowing from the aorta to the right coronary artery across the collaterals to the left coronary artery and into the pulmonary artery. Because of this, certain areas of the myocardium are at risk for ischemia. The patients with this lesion often present at 6 to 8 weeks of age with extreme irritability (especially at the onset of feeding) that is a result of angina. Other symptoms such as diaphoresis, weight loss, and decreased frequency of wet diapers are similar in conditions associated with heart failure.

9. **(B)** Acute management of heart failure because of left-to-right shunting lesions include inotropic support with digoxin, dopamine, dobutamine, or epinephrine. Diuretics are also used to relieve symptoms of edema. Milrinone is an inotrope and afterload-reducing agent and is commonly employed for treatment of heart failure. Use of oxygen may exacerbate symptoms of heart failure in the presence of left-to-right shunting lesions by decreasing pulmonary vascular resistance and increasing the degree of left-to-right shunting. The ultimate long-term ther-

apy is to eliminate the left-to-the right shunting lesion either with surgery or interventional cardiac catheterization.

10. **(D)** Myocardial dysfunction resulting in dilated cardiomyopathy is uncommon in the pediatric population. The causes include myocarditis, metabolic diseases, idiopathic, or familial dilated cardiomyopathy. Ischemic heart disease is a rare cause of dilated cardiomyopathy at this age but becomes the most common cause in the adult population.

11. **(B)** Myocarditis is defined as inflammation of the myocardium likely because of a cell-mediated immunologic reaction. The diagnosis is confirmed by endomyocardial biopsy showing fibrosis and inflammation. A biopsy showing fibrosis alone may be seen with any form of cardiomyopathy and is not specific for acute myocarditis. Other features suggestive of myocarditis include tachycardia out of proportion to the symptoms of heart failure, cardiac dysfunction, a pericardial effusion, and a preceding history of upper respiratory illness. A systolic flow murmur and S3 gallop may occur with myocarditis but are nonspecific findings for this diagnosis.

12. **(D)** The most common cause of myocarditis is infection because of enterovirus (e.g., coxsackievirus, adenovirus, and echovirus) as demonstrated by PCR of endomyocardial biopsies. Other agents include other viruses, bacteria, rickettsia, fungi, protozoa, and parasites. Other etiologies include immune-mediated diseases, toxic myocarditis, and collagen vascular diseases.

13. **(D)** The acute management for myocarditis includes the use of steroids, IV immunoglobulins, diuretics, and inotropic support. Use of IV digoxin during the acute phase of myocarditis has been reported to be associated with increased occurrence of arrhythmias and thus is typically not recommended. There are mixed data regarding the efficacy of these therapies in that no single therapy has shown to significantly improve the long-term outcomes in patients with myocarditis. Generally, the majority of patients improve and have complete recovery although the acute mortality rate may be as high as 75% in neonates.

14. **(D)** In patients with ventricular dysfunction and chronic congestive heart failure, therapy includes the use of diuretics and digoxin. The use of afterload-reducing agents such as ACE inhibitors has been shown to reduce morbidity and mortality. The recent use of beta-blockers has been shown to decrease myocardial oxygen demand and also reduces morbidity and mortality in adults with ventricular dysfunction. The use of calcium channel blockers is not recommended because of the significant negative inotropic effect. The long-term management in patients with ventricular dysfunction and heart failure includes not only medical therapy but also routine monitoring with exercises tests in order to obtain objective data regarding cardiac performance.

15. **(B)** The most likely diagnosis of this patient is acute pericarditis. This is defined as inflammation of the parietal and visceral pericardium and results in serous, hemorrhagic, or purulent pericardial effusion. The clinical manifestations include a pericardial friction rub and the presence of a dull, substernal chest pain that improves when leaning forward. There may be a history of upper respiratory tract infection and fever.

16. **(A)** The most common cause of pericarditis in the United States is viral infection. Acute rheumatic fever is a common cause in certain parts of the world. Other causes included bacterial infection, collagen vascular disease, tuberculosis, oncologic disease, and uremia.

17. **(D)** Cardiac tamponade is the most likely cause of this patient's acute decompensation. The clinical features of cardiac tamponade include distant heart sounds, tachycardia, pulsus paradoxus, hepatomegaly, venous distention, and hypotension. The diagnosis can be confirmed with echocardiogram. Acute management would include pericardiocentesis or surgical drainage of pericardial fluid. Chronic management is directed at the cause of the pericarditis.

Pulsus paradoxus is defined as a drop of 10 mm Hg or more in the systolic blood pressure with breathing. The normal variation of systolic blood pressure with breathing (less than 10 mm Hg) is a result of fluctuation of left ventricular filling as intrapulmonary pressures vary with respiration. This phenomenon is exaggerated with cardiac tamponade and may also been seen with pulmonary embolism, obstructive respiratory disease, or hypotension.

SUGGESTED READING

Emmanouilides GC, Riemenschneider TA, Allen HD, et al, eds: *Moss and Adams Heart Disease in Infants, Children and Adolescents*, 5th ed. Philadelphia: Williams and Wilkins, 1995.

Braunwald E, Zipes DP, Libbey P, eds: *Braunwald: Heart Disease: A Textbook of Cardiovascular Medicine*, 6th ed. Philadelphia: WB Saunders, 2001.

Fyler DC, ed: *Nadas' Pediatric Cardiology*. Philadelphia: Hanley and Belfus, 1980.

Park M, ed: *Pediatric Cardiology for Practitioners*, 4th ed. St. Louis: Mosby, 2002.

CASE 4: A 5-YEAR-OLD CHILD WITH A HEART MURMUR AND FEVER

A 5-year-old child presents to the clinic with a history of fever, rash, a swollen knee and ankle, shortness of breath, and fatigue. His past medical history is significant for the fact that he had a strep throat infection 3 weeks prior to this visit but did not take the amoxicillin that was prescribed for him. On physical exam, he has a temperature of 38.9°C. He has a grade 2/6 systolic regurgitant murmur at the apex and an S3 gallop. He has hepatomegaly and good peripheral pulses.

SELECT THE ONE BEST ANSWER

1. What is the most likely diagnosis in this child?

    (A) acute rheumatic fever
    (B) infective endocarditis
    (C) Kawasaki disease
    (D) sickle cell disease

2. What is the most common cause of this disease?

    (A) group A beta hemolytic streptococcal pharyngitis
    (B) group A beta hemolytic streptococcal impetigo
    (C) *Staphylococcus aureus* skin infection
    (D) enterococcus infection

3. What is the incidence of acute rheumatic fever following untreated streptococcal pharyngitis?

    (A) 0.001%
    (B) 0.3% to 3%
    (C) 13% to 15%
    (D) 25% to 33%

4. Which heart valve is the most commonly affected with acute rheumatic fever?

    (A) mitral valve
    (B) aortic valve
    (C) tricuspid valve
    (D) pulmonary valve

5. Which of the following is not a major criterion for diagnosis of acute rheumatic fever?

    (A) erythema marginatum
    (B) carditis
    (C) chorea
    (D) arthralgias

6. Which statement is true regarding antibiotic therapy for acute rheumatic fever?

    (A) Eradication of streptococci from the pharynx is not attempted.
    (B) Penicillin prophylaxis for 1 year is required but then can be stopped.
    (C) Penicillin prophylaxis can be given either twice daily by mouth or once monthly by IM injection.
    (D) Oral sulfadiazine or tetracycline can be substituted for penicillin in patients who are penicillin allergic.

7. The heart murmur in this patient is most likely a result of which of the following?

    (A) mitral valve regurgitation
    (B) mitral valve stenosis
    (C) tricuspid valve regurgitation
    (D) pulmonary valve regurgitation

8. A 2-year-old child presents with a 10-day history of fever, a heart murmur, bilateral nonexudative conjunctivitis, swollen and erythematous lips and strawberry tongue with erythematous and edematous hands and feet and a polymorphous rash on the face, trunks, and extremities. The most likely diagnosis in this patient is:

    (A) Kawasaki disease

(B) measles

(C) viral upper respiratory tract infection

(D) group A beta hemolytic streptococcal pharyngitis

9. What acute finding would not be expected to be associated with this 2-year-old's diagnosis?

(A) sterile pyuria

(B) hydrops of the gallbladder

(C) cervical adenopathy greater than 1.5 cm

(D) thrombocytosis

10. Which of the following statements is true regarding coronary artery involvement with this 2-year-old's disease?

(A) There is a 50% incidence of coronary artery aneurysms if untreated.

(B) The peak incidence for coronary artery aneurysms is 6 to 12 months following the onset of fever.

(C) Patients with giant coronary artery aneurysms greater than 8 mm in diameter are at highest risk for late stenosis and myocardial infarction.

(D) Coronary artery rupture is the most common cause of mortality within the first 7 days of the onset of fever.

11. Name the two drugs most commonly used for acute management of this disease.

(A) aspirin and IVIG

(B) penicillin and IVIG

(C) steroids and aspirin

(D) steroids and penicillin

12. A 5-year-old boy presents with a fever of 10 days, weight loss, night sweats, a new heart murmur, splenomegaly, joint pains, and a history of having had his teeth cleaned by the dentist 1 month prior to this visit. On exam, he was found to have a grade 2/4 diastolic murmur heard best at the mid left sternal border radiating to the apex. There is an S3 gallop rhythm. What is the most likely diagnosis for this patient?

(A) infective endocarditis

(B) juvenile rheumatoid arthritis

(C) Kawasaki disease

(D) acute rheumatic fever

13. Which of the following laboratory evidence would most likely support the diagnosis of infective endocarditis?

(A) two positive blood cultures with the same organism and no other source other than the heart

(B) increased white blood cell count

(C) increased C-reactive protein

(D) throat culture positive for group A beta hemolytic streptococcus

14. Which organism would be the most common cause of infective endocarditis in this 5-year-old's situation?

(A) alpha hemolytic streptococcus

(B) *Staphylococcus aureus*

(C) *Staphylococcus epidermidis*

(D) enterococcus

15. What percent of cases of infective endocarditis are culture negative?

(A) 10%

(B) 20%

(C) 30%

(D) 40%

16. Which of the following heart lesions would not be considered at increased risk for development of infective endocarditis?

(A) mitral regurgitation

(B) aortic insufficiency

(C) aortic stenosis

(D) atrial septal defect

17. What is the most common antibiotic regimen that should be started in cases of suspected infective endocarditis prior to knowing the results of the blood culture?

(A) vancomycin or oxacillin and gentamicin

(B) ampicillin and gentamicin

(C) ampicillin and ceftriaxone

(D) vancomycin alone

18. Which of the following procedures does not require endocarditis prophylaxis?

(A) tonsillectomy

(B) urinary tract surgery
(C) professional dental cleaning
(D) endotracheal intubation

Answers

1. **(A)** The most common cause of this constellation of symptoms is acute rheumatic fever. Acute rheumatic fever is a multisystem inflammatory disease triggered by group A beta hemolytic streptococcal infection of the upper respiratory tract. The disease occurs between 5 and 15 years of age with a peak incidence of 8 years and is rarely seen in children younger than 2 years of age.

2. **(A)** Acute rheumatic fever does not occur following streptococcal skin infections, staph infections, or enterococcal infections. The pathogenesis of rheumatic fever is thought to be because of an immune response to antigens in the M protein of the capsule of the group A beta hemolytic streptococcus, which occurs in susceptible hosts and cross-reacts with similar epitopes in human joint tissue, heart, and brain tissue. Pathologic findings include inflammatory lesions in these tissues that include granulomas of perivascular infiltrates of cells and fibrin also known as Aschoff bodies.

3. **(B)** The incidence of acute rheumatic fever is approximately 0.3% to 3% in untreated patients with *Streptococcus pharyngitis*. The onset of disease occurs between 1 to 5 weeks with a mean of 18 days following the onset of pharyngitis. The typical course is that a patient with pharyngitis has improvement of symptoms and then 2 weeks later begins to develop a low-grade fever in conjunction with the inflammatory response of rheumatic fever.

4. **(A)**

5. **(D)** Although there is no specific diagnostic laboratory test for rheumatic fever, the diagnosis is based on the Jones criteria. These are separated into major and minor manifestations. Major criteria include polyarthritis, carditis, erythema marginatum, subcutaneous nodules, and chorea. The most common manifestation is polyarthritis occurring in up to 70% of patients and includes migratory arthritis involving the large joints (knees, hips, ankles, elbows), which characteristically responds dramatically to salicylate therapy. Carditis occurs in approximately 50% of cases and includes myocarditis, pericardial effusions, arrhythmias, and valvular heart disease. Erythema marginatum occurs in less than 10% of patients and is described as a nonpruritic, serpiginous rash that occurs on the torso and is almost never seen on the face. The rash is evanescent and becomes more apparent following hot baths or being wrapped in warm blankets. Subcutaneous nodules are nontender, freely mobile nodules occurring usually over the bony surfaces of the elbows, wrists, shins, knees, ankles, and spine. They occur in 2% to 10% of cases. Chorea occurs in up to 15% of cases and is a neuropsychiatric disorder that includes choreic movements, hypotonia, emotional lability, anxiety, and obsessive-compulsive disorder. Chorea usually occurs late after the initial pharyngitis with the average time to onset of approximately 6 to 7 months, and may last as long as 18 months. Recent evidence suggests that chorea is associated with the presence of antineuronal antibodies. Minor manifestations include fever, arthralgias (when polyarthritis is not present), elevated acute-phase reactants such as the C-reactive protein, and a prolonged PR interval on ECG (in the absence of other evidence of carditis). The diagnosis of acute rheumatic fever is made with either two major manifestations or with a single major manifestation and two minor manifestations. This criterion should be supported by evidence of a preceding streptococcal infection either by a positive throat culture or by rising streptococcal antibody titers (e.g., antistreptolysin O). There are three exceptions to the Jones criteria for diagnosis of acute rheumatic fever:

1. Chorea may occur as the only manifestation of rheumatic fever.
2. Indolent carditis may be the only manifestation in patients following the initial infection.
3. Recurrences often do not fulfill strict Jones criteria, therefore, presumptive diagnosis may be made with fewer than the usual number of criteria. Again, this should only be diagnosed if there is supporting evidence of a recent streptococcal infection.

6. **(C)** Treatment for acute rheumatic fever includes therapy directed at the streptococcal infection with penicillin followed by prevention of recurrences with either twice-daily oral penicillin or once-monthly IM penicillin injections. While some advocate prophylaxis to be continued at least until the patient is 21 years of age, others recommend that prophylaxis be lifelong. In patients who are penicillin allergic, prophylaxis can be substituted with either oral sulfadiazine or erythromycin. Recurrences of acute rheumatic fever usually occur within the first 5 years after the initial disease and are characterized by more severe cardiac valve involvement. It is estimated that approximately 10% to 25% of patients with heart valve involvement will have complete resolution by 10 years.

7. **(A)** The mitral valve is the most commonly affected followed by the aortic valve and rarely the tricuspid or pulmonary valves are affected. Initially, the affected valves develop regurgitation as a result of inflammation and valve dysfunction. However, with healing of the inflammation, long-term development of mitral valve stenosis can occur. This may be seen as early as 2 to 3 years following the acute episode but usually occurs 10 to 20 years later.

8. **(A)** The child described most likely has Kawasaki disease, an acute vasculitis of unknown etiology. Kawasaki disease is the leading cause of acquired heart disease in children in the United States. The incidence ranges from 2 to 6/100,000 children and is highest in Asian-American children. The peak incidence is between 1 and 2 years of age with 85% of the cases occurring in children younger than 5 years of age. The disease is uncommon in patients older than 8 years of age or younger than 3 months of age. The clinical manifestations include the presence of fever for at least 4 days and 4 of 5 of the following findings.

   1. A nonexudative conjunctivitis that is usually bilateral
   2. Erythema of the lips, oral mucosa, and pharynx, including a strawberry tongue and cracking or peeling of the lips later into the disease
   3. A polymorphous rash of the face, trunk, and extremities that later can involve the perineal area and is characterized by desquamation at 5 to 7 days
   4. Cervical adenopathy greater than 1.5 cm in diameter that is usually unilateral
   5. Changes in the extremities, including edema and erythema of the hands and feet followed by periungual desquamation at 11 to 25 days into the disease

   Incomplete Kawasaki disease can be diagnosed when fever is present for ≥5 days in the presence of two to three of the above criteria when the CRP is ≥3.0 mg/dL and/or the ESR is ≥40 mm/hr. In this instance, certain laboratory criteria must be met including hypoalbuminemia, anemia, increased serum alanine aminotransferase, thrombocytosis, leukocytosis and sterile pyuria.

9. **(D)** Other supportive findings of the acute phase of Kawasaki disease include urethritis because of sterile pyuria, aseptic meningitis, abdominal pain, hydrops of the gallbladder, and arthritis usually of the small joints but may involve the large joints 2 to 3 weeks into the disease. Also, mild carditis and arrhythmias may occur. The subacute phase occurs between 11 and 25 days following the onset of fever and is characterized by a decrease in the rash and fever with the onset of desquamation of the fingers and toes. Thrombocytosis peaks at 2 to 4 weeks into the course of the disease. It is during this phase that coronary artery aneurysms usually become evident.

10. **(C)** Coronary artery aneurysms are the most feared complication of Kawasaki disease and occur in up to 15% to 25% of untreated patients. They are a result of the panvasculitis resulting in aneurysmal transformation of the coronary arteries and may be seen as early as 7 days after the onset of the fever, but their incidence peaks at 3 to 4 weeks and they are seldom found after 8 weeks into the course of the disease. Giant aneurysms are described as having a diameter of greater than 8 mm and are associated with increased mortality and morbidity. Patients with aneurysms also have a higher incidence of developing stenoses leading to myocardial ischemia and infarction with long-term follow-up. Coronary artery rupture is the most common cause of mortality in the subacute phase while myocarditis, heart failure, and ar-

rhythmias are the most common cause of mortality in the acute phase within the first 10 days after the onset of fever. Risk factors for the development of coronary artery aneurysms include male gender, age less than 1 year, hemoglobin less than 10 g/dL, white blood cell count greater than 30,000/mm^3, ESR greater than 101 mm/hr, and prolonged fever. Echocardiogram testing is recommended for assessment of coronary artery involvement with Kawasaki disease. The most recent recommendations suggest that an echocardiogram is obtained at diagnosis, and if no coronary disease is seen, then it should be repeated 6 to 8 weeks. If coronary artery involvement is documented, then follow-up should be more frequent based on the extent of the disease.

11. **(A)** The management of Kawasaki disease includes high-dose aspirin, which is given during the acute phase, followed by low-dose aspirin for 6 to 8 weeks. This is given for antithrombotic effect while thrombocytosis is present. IVIG is administered within the first 10 days of the disease at a dose of 2 g/kg and may be repeated if fever persists following this therapy. The use of IVIG has been shown to decrease the incidence of coronary artery aneurysms to less than 5%. If aneurysms persist past 2 months, then aspirin or other anticlotting agents should be continued. The use of steroids is not indicated for uncomplicated Kawasaki disease.

12. **(A)** The most likely diagnosis in this situation is infective endocarditis. This is an inflammatory disorder of the heart resulting from an infection. The signs and symptoms of infective endocarditis include acute findings of fever, anorexia, weight loss, pallor, night sweats, myalgias, and new onset of a heart murmur, usually as a result of valve disease from infection. Later findings are a result of embolic phenomenon and include splinter hemorrhages, Roth spots (retinal hemorrhages), Janeway lesion, Osler nodes, splenomegaly, clubbing, arthralgias, arthritis, glomerulonephritis, and aseptic meningitis. The pathogenesis of infective endocarditis results from the initial setting of a jet of blood or turbulence within the heart leading to cardiac endothelial damage and formation of a sterile clot or vegetation. This serves as a nidus for bacterial infection.

13. **(A)** The diagnosis of infective endocarditis can be determined by:

    1. Pathologic evidence either by surgery or embolectomy of an infected thrombus within the heart.
    2. Two positive blood cultures with the same organism with no other source other than the heart.
    3. A clinical course compatible with infective endocarditis.

    Supportive evidence of endocarditis includes laboratory findings of anemia, increased white blood cell count, increased ESR or CRP, hematuria, decreased C3 complement component, and increased bilirubinemia. The echocardiogram is useful for detecting intracardiac vegetations. The type of echocardiogram performed, whether it be transthoracic or transesophageal, depends on the age of the patient and the ability to achieve good acoustic windows.

14. **(A)** The most common organism causing infective endocarditis following dental procedures is *Streptococcus viridans*. However, *Staphylococcus aureus* and *Staphylococcus epidermidis* have become important causes of infective endocarditis. Indeed *S. aureus* is now, overall, the leading cause. Enterococcus is the more common cause of endocarditis in adults. In patients with burns or IV drug abuses, staphylococcus is the most common organism. Infants with sepsis are also at higher risk for endocarditis with no cardiac disease.

15. **(A)** Up to 10% of cases of endocarditis are culture negative. On the other hand, in 90% of cases, the causative agent may be identified by obtaining at least three blood cultures during the first 24 hours of hospitalization.

16. **(D)** Valvular heart lesions are most commonly associated with predisposition for the development of infective endocarditis; however, other forms of congenital heart disease, including tetralogy of Fallot, ventricular septal defect, patent ductus arteriosus, coarctation of the aorta, and pulmonary valve stenosis, have also been implicated. Congenital heart defects such as atrial septal defect, peripheral pulmonary stenosis, and mitral valve prolapse without mitral regurgita-

tion are not considered to be high-risk lesions for development of infective endocarditis, and thus bacterial endocarditis prophylaxis is not indicated in these situations.

17. **(A)** In patients with suspected infective endocarditis, a course of either vancomycin or oxacillin and gentamicin is started as the most likely organisms include streptococci and staphylococci, depending on the rate of methicillin-resistant *S. aureus* in the patient's area. Once the organism is identified, the antibiotic regimen can be adjusted accordingly. Surgical intervention is occasionally required for removal of foreign bodies that are difficult to sterilize with IV antibiotics or repair of valves that have been damaged by infection. Other complications associated with endocarditis include mycotic aneurysms, localized cardiac abscesses, and autoimmune phenomena such as nephritis and arthritis.

18. **(D)** Procedures in which there is a risk for significant bacteremia would require bacterial endocarditis prophylaxis in patients who are susceptible. These procedures include dental procedures where bleeding is anticipated, tonsillectomy, cardiac surgery, incision of infected sites, urologic surgery, and Foley placement in the presence of a urinary tract infection. Endotracheal intubation is not associated with a high incidence of bacteremia and thus antibiotic prophylaxis is not required.

SUGGESTED READING

Emmanouilides GC, Riemenschneider TA, Allen HD, et al, eds: *Moss and Adams Heart Disease in Infants, Children and Adolescents*, 5th ed. Philadelphia: Williams and Wilkins, 1995.

Braunwald E, Zipes DP, Libbey P, eds: *Braunwald: Heart Disease: A Textbook of Cardiovascular Medicine*, 6th ed. Philadelphia: WB Saunders, 2001.

Fyler DC, ed: *Nadas' Pediatric Cardiology*. Philadelphia: Hanley and Belfus, 1980.

Park M, ed: *Pediatric Cardiology for Practitioners*, 4th ed. St. Louis: Mosby, 2002.

Newburger J, Takahashi M, Gerber M, et al: Diagnosis, treatment and long-term management of Kawasaki Disease. A Statement for Health Professionals From the Committee on Rheumatic Fever, Endocarditis, and Kawasaki Disease, Council on Cardiovascular Disease in the Young, American Heart Association. *Pediatrics* 114:1708–1733, 2004.

CASE 5: A 10-YEAR-OLD BOY WITH ELEVATED BLOOD PRESSURE AT A PHYSICAL

A 10-year-old boy presents for a preparticipation sports physical examination. He has previously been well with no significant past medical history. His vital signs demonstrate a heart rate of 101 bpm and a blood pressure of 130/85 mm Hg (greater than the 95th percentile for age). The remainder of his exam is normal.

SELECT THE ONE BEST ANSWER

1. What is the most appropriate next step?

   (A) Recheck the blood pressure with a smaller blood pressure cuff.
   (B) Recheck the blood pressure on at least two other separate occasions before beginning further evaluation.
   (C) Begin medical therapy with antihypertensive medications.
   (D) Order a renal ultrasound.

2. At this age, what is the most common cause of hypertension?

   (A) primary familial or idiopathic hypertension
   (B) coarctation of the aorta
   (C) renal artery thrombosis
   (D) renal parenchymal disease

3. Renal parenchymal hypertension is caused by all but which of the following mechanisms?

   (A) salt retention
   (B) water retention
   (C) increased renin levels
   (D) excess levels of catecholamines

4. On the third visit, the patient continues to demonstrate evidence of systemic hypertension with elevated blood pressure recordings. Of the following, which is the most appropriate testing at this time?

   (A) urinalysis
   (B) serum catecholamine levels.
   (C) renal CT scan
   (D) urine 17-hydroxy steroids or 17-ketosteroids

5. Which of the following interventions would not be recommended at this time?

(A) stop all exercise
(B) weight reduction
(C) stop tobacco use
(D) salt reduction

6. Beta-blockers are useful for treatment of hypertension but are contraindicated in all but which of the following?

(A) asthmatics
(B) diabetics
(C) hyperthyroidism
(D) bradycardia

7. The patient returns with a hypertensive crisis with a systolic blood pressure greater than 180 mm Hg and a diastolic blood pressure greater than 110 mm Hg associated with headache, vomiting, and pulmonary edema. What is the most commonly used medication in this setting?

(A) nitroprusside sodium (Nipride)
(B) captopril
(C) phentolamine
(D) aldactone

8. A 10-year-old child presents for a sports physical. The exam and blood pressure are completely normal. There is a family history of hypercholesterolemia in his mother. What is the most appropriate advice for this patient?

(A) Total serum cholesterol should be evaluated.
(B) Total serum cholesterol and lipoprotein analysis should be evaluated.
(C) Exercise stress test should be performed.
(D) Total serum cholesterol should be evaluated at 21 years of age.

9. At what serum cholesterol level would lipoprotein analysis be indicated?

(A) 120 mg/100 mL
(B) 140 mg/100 mL
(C) 180 mg/100 mL
(D) 220 mg/100 mL

10. Which of the following is not a common cause of secondary hypercholesteremia in children?

(A) obesity
(B) isotretinoin (Accutane)

(C) oral contraceptive pills
(D) hyperthyroidism

11. What is the most common form of inherited hyperlipidemia?

(A) familial hypercholesterolemia
(B) familial combined hyperlipidemia
(C) mild hypertriglyceridemia
(D) severe hypertriglyceridemia

12. Which of the following is a true statement regarding the treatment for hypercholesterolemia in children?

(A) A Step 1 diet is recommended for children younger than 2 years of age.
(B) Bile acid sequestrants are recommended for children older than 10 years of age when diet is not effective.
(C) Lovastatin may be used in selected cases for children younger than 2 years of age.
(D) none of the above

13. A 10-year-old child with physical features of tall stature, a long thin face, scoliosis, pectus excavatum with a family history of sudden death at a young age (an uncle who died while playing basketball) presents for a preparticipation sports physical. What is the likely diagnosis in this patient?

(A) Marfan syndrome
(B) hypertrophic cardiomyopathy
(C) Turner syndrome
(D) Down syndrome

14. What is the most common cardiac lesion associated with this 10-year-old's diagnosis?

(A) mitral valve prolapse
(B) aortic stenosis
(C) coarctation of the aorta
(D) left ventricular outflow tract obstruction

15. An echocardiogram is ordered and demonstrates mild aortic root dilatation. What is the recommendation for further management?

(A) participation in sports is unrestricted
(B) follow-up echocardiogram in 10 years
(C) return to clinic only if symptoms of chest pain occur during activities

(D) treatment with beta-blockers may decrease the risk of further aortic root dilatation

16. What findings during routine preparticipation physical examination would place a child at risk for sudden death during sports?

(A) a harsh systolic murmur at the upper right sternal border
(B) family history for diabetes
(C) respiratory sinus arrhythmia
(D) a single elevated blood pressure reading that returns to normal on subsequent visits

Answers

1. **(B)** Hypertension is defined as systolic or diastolic blood pressure recordings greater than the 95th percentile for age and gender, recorded on three separate occasions. Severe hypertension is defined as blood pressure recordings greater than the 95th percentile by 8 to 10 mm Hg. Accurate blood pressure recordings are crucial for this diagnosis and should be taken in a quiet, nonthreatening manner. The width of the blood pressure cuff should be greater than or equal to 40% to 50% of the arm circumference. Smaller blood pressure cuffs result in erroneously high blood pressure recordings. Ideally, blood pressure recordings should be taken in all four extremities. Anxiety leading to transient elevations in blood pressure (white coat hypertension) accounts for up to 40% of elevated blood pressure recordings in children. Because the diagnosis of hypertension should not be based on a single reading, medical therapy and testing for secondary causes of hypertension are not appropriate during this first visit.

2. **(A)** Hypertension is classified as either primary (essential or idiopathic) or secondary. Primary hypertension is the most common cause in older patients such as this child while secondary hypertension is common in younger patients with more severely elevated blood pressure recordings. Ninety percent of secondary causes are because of renal parenchymal disease, renal artery disease, and coarctation of the aorta.

3. **(D)** Renal parenchymal hypertension causes salt and water retention and in some cases elevated re-

nin levels leading to increase vascular resistance. Increase serum catecholamine levels causing hypertension are seen with pheochromocytomas or with the congenital adrenal hyperplasia (11-hydroxylase deficiency or 17-hydroxylase deficiency). Hypertension is also seen with use of certain drugs or medications and in cases of hypercalcemia.

4. **(A)** The initial evaluation of hypertension is guided by both the exam and the family history. The important features of the history include a past medical history of urinary tract infections, cardiovascular surgeries, weakness or cramps, medication use, and tobacco use. Important features of the family history include history of hypertension or premature heart disease. The important features of the physical exam include accurate blood pressure recordings in four extremities, assessment for heart murmurs or bruits, assessment of peripheral pulses, assessment of renal tenderness, and a thorough eye exam. The usual initial laboratory evaluation includes a urinalysis, serum electrolytes including a BUN and creatinine, and possibly a 12-lead ECG, chest radiograph, and echocardiogram. Cholesterol levels and lipoprotein analysis are indicated in select cases. If there is severe hypertension and end-organ involvement or hypertension refractory to therapy, then tests evaluating for secondary causes of hypertension can be performed.

5. **(A)** Additional management in patients with hypertension includes nonpharmacologic intervention such as exercise proscription, weight reduction, avoidance of tobacco or oral contraceptive pills, and reduction of dietary salt intake. In severe hypertension or persistent hypertension despite nonpharmacologic interventions, pharmacologic agents are often used and include diuretics, beta-blockers, and vasodilators.

6. **(C)** Beta-blockers are often used in conjunction with diuretics or in conditions where hyperthyroidism results in hypertension. However, beta-blockers are contraindicated for use in patients with asthma (can precipitate bronchospasm), diabetes (prevents manifestation of symptoms of hyperglycemia), and in patients with bradycardia.

7. **(A)** A hypertensive emergency requires immediate reduction of blood pressure usually within

minutes to hours. Hypertensive crises can be associated with neurological signs or congestive heart failure. Administration of parental medications is important for the acute treatment of hypertensive emergencies. These medications include diazoxide, nitroprusside sodium (Nipride IV), diuretics, IV nifedipine, hydralazine, or labetalol. Phentolamine is usually reserved for patients with pheochromocytomas.

8. **(A)** Hypercholesterolemia is a major risk factor for coronary artery disease. Several long-term prospective studies have shown that lowering serum cholesterol levels decreases the risk for coronary artery disease in the future. This has prompted a more aggressive approach to screening and therapy for hypercholesterolemia in young patients. The current recommendations for serum cholesterol screening include the child of a single parent with a cholesterol level greater than 240 mg/100 mL or if the history is unobtainable but there is a suspicion of hypercholesterolemia. The recommendations for performing a serum cholesterol level and lipoprotein analysis include children with parents or grandparents with a history of coronary angioplasty or coronary artery bypass surgery in men younger than 55 years of age or women younger than 65 years of age and children with parents or grandparents with a documented myocardial infarction in men younger than 55 years of age or women younger than 65 years of age.

9. **(D)** Serum cholesterol levels can be measured in the nonfasting state anytime after the age of 2 years. If serum cholesterol levels are greater than 200 mg/dL, then lipoprotein analysis is indicated. Lipoprotein analysis requires the patient to be fasting for 12 hours prior to the testing. LDL = total serum cholesterol – HDL – triglyceride/5. LDL levels less than 110 mg/dL, in the face of elevated cholesterol levels, should be repeated in 5 years. If the LDL level is 110 to 129 mg/dL, a Step 1 diet is recommended. If the LDL level is greater than 130 mg/dL, then a Step 1 or Step 2 diet is recommended with consideration of medical therapy and further evaluation for secondary causes of hyperlipidemia.

10. **(D)** Secondary causes of hyperlipidemia include:

Exogenous factors such as obesity, isotretinoin (Accutane) use, oral contraceptive use
Endocrine or metabolic diseases including hypothyroidism
Obstructive liver disease
Renal failure
Other factors including anorexia or a high-fat and high-cholesterol diet

11. **(B)** Familial combined hyperlipidemia is the most common etiology for inherited hyperlipidemias in children. It occurs with an incidence of approximately 1 in 300 individuals and is inherited in autosomal dominant fashion. Laboratory analysis reveals elevation of cholesterol and/or elevation of triglyceride levels. The etiology of familial combined hyperlipidemia is a result of an increased apoB-100 production by the liver related to multiple genetic factors. The clinical course is characterized by late onset of coronary artery disease and peripheral vascular disease. Familial hypercholesterolemia occurs in approximately 1 in 500 individuals and is inherited by an autosomal co-dominant fashion. In the heterozygous form, there are elevated serum cholesterol levels and a high risk of premature coronary artery disease. The etiology of the hypercholesterolemia is a result of a decrease in the number of LDL receptors. In the homozygous form, there is severe hypercholesterolemia with increase risk for myocardial infarction. The etiology for hypercholesterolemia is near complete absence of LDL receptors. Mild hypertriglyceridemia is associated with obesity, glucose intolerance, hyperuricemia, and increased alcohol intake. Severe hypertriglyceridemia is a result of a deficiency of lipoprotein lipase and is associated with recurrent pancreatitis, hepatosplenomegaly, and xanthomas.

12. **(B)** In patients with hypercholesterolemia, therapy is not indicated for children younger than 2 years of age. In children older than 2 years of age, initial treatment includes the Step 1 diet recommended for approximately 3 months. If the serum cholesterol levels remain elevated, then a Step 2 diet is recommended for a total of 6 to 12 months. If levels continue to be elevated and the child is older than 10 years of age with an LDL of greater than 190 or an LDL of greater than 160 and a family history of hypercholesterol-

emia, then bile acid sequestrants such as cholestyramine are the first-line choice of medical therapy. In selected cases, lovastatin has been reported to be of beneficial use. However, it is currently not recommended for routine use.

13. **(A)** The patient in this scenario most likely carries the diagnosis of Marfan syndrome. Marfan syndrome is an autosomal dominant genetic disorder because of a mutation in the fibrillin gene on chromosome 15. This leads to defective connective tissue disease. The clinical features include a long thin face, tall stature with the arm span greater than the height, pectus excavatum or carinatum, scoliosis, lens subluxation, and high arched palate. There is a family history of Marfan syndrome in 70% to 85% of cases. Patients with hypertropic cardiomyopathy do not have the physical stigmata described in this case, but it is an important diagnosis in cases where there is a family history of sudden unexpected death. Patients with Turner syndrome have physical stigmata consistent with short stature and web neck, and patients with Down syndrome also have short stature with characteristic facial features.

14. **(A)** The most common heart lesions seen in patients with Marfan syndrome include mitral valve prolapse and dilatation of the aortic root. This again is because of abnormalities in the connective tissue as a result of the mutation in the fibrillin gene. Aortic stenosis because of bicuspid aortic valve and coarctation of the aorta are commonly seen in patients with Turner syndrome, and LV outflow tract obstruction may be seen in patients with severe forms of hypertrophic cardiomyopathy. The typical exam feature in a patient with mitral valve prolapse includes a systolic ejection click that varies in timing when the patient is standing versus when he is squatting. A diastolic murmur of mitral regurgitation may be heard in conjunction with more severe cases of mitral valve prolapse.

15. **(D)** In patients with Marfan syndrome, participation in activities is limited to mild aerobic, low-impact sports. This is to avoid precipitation of further aortic root dilatation or rupture and to avoid retinal detachment. It is recommended that patients with Marfan syndrome undergo routine echocardiographic evaluation to assess aortic root dilatation as well as routine ophthalmologic exams. Beta-blockers have been shown to be effective to decrease the progression of aortic root dilatation.

16. **(A)** The American Heart Association recommendations for preparticipation physical examination screening include obtaining a family history for sudden cardiac death and a review of systems significant for dizziness or syncope. Physical findings of Marfan syndrome, hypertension, decrease peripheral pulses or pathological murmur such as a harsh systolic murmur described would indicate the need for further evaluation. The finding of family history of diabetes, respiratory, sinus arrhythmia, or a single elevated blood pressure returning to normal at subsequent visits would not place this patient at risk for sudden death during sports.

SUGGESTED READING

Emmanouilides GC, Riemenschneider TA, Allen HD, et al, eds: *Moss and Adams Heart Disease in Infants, Children and Adolescents*, 5th ed. Philadelphia: Williams and Wilkins, 1995.

Braunwald E, Zipes DP, Libbey P, eds: *Braunwald: Heart Disease: A Textbook of Cardiovascular Medicine*, 6th ed. Philadelphia: WB Saunders, 2001.

Fyler DC, ed: *Nadas' Pediatric Cardiology*. Philadelphia: Hanley and Belfus, 1980.

Park M, ed: *Pediatric Cardiology for Practitioners*, 4th ed. St. Louis: Mosby, 2002.

Critical Care

2

CASE 6: A 5-MONTH-OLD INFANT WITH APNEA AND CYANOSIS

A 5-month-old male infant is brought to the emergency room after he "stopped breathing for approximately 20 seconds and became blue around his lips." He began breathing again after the mother "blew in his face." There have been no other symptoms such as upper respiratory tract illness, fever, vomiting, diarrhea, or change in eating habits. He takes approximately 28 to 34 ounces of formula per day as well as some solids and has always eaten well although he often "spits up" after eating.

When you first see this child, he is somewhat irritable. His physical examination is completely normal except that there is dried blood in both of the child's nares. His room air oxygen saturation is 98%. It has been approximately 90 minutes since the baby "turned blue" and the mother appears to be quite frightened by these events.

The family history is remarkable for a sibling's death during sleep 2 years ago, subsequently labeled as "SIDS."

SELECT THE ONE BEST ANSWER

1. The screening test(s) that need to be performed stat include:

   (A) serum glucose and electrolytes
   (B) a CBC and differential
   (C) an erythrocyte sedimentation rate and serum CRP level
   (D) examination of CSF

2. In addition to the stat screening test performed in question number 1, the initial workup should also include:

   (A) a CT scan of the head, chest radiograph, and EEG
   (B) a pH probe, thyroid functions, and EEG
   (C) an echocardiogram, head CT, and thyroid function tests
   (D) an abdominal radiograph, head MRI, and glucose tolerance test

3. Which characteristic of this event makes it an acute life-threatening event (ALTE)?

   (A) the fear it instilled in the mother
   (B) the color change in the child
   (C) the apnea as described
   (D) all of the above

4. The family history of the previous sibling that died from "SIDS":

   (A) raises suspicion of nonaccidental trauma
   (B) is a common family history in a child with an ALTE
   (C) increases the likelihood of future ALTEs in this patient
   (D) indicates that an extensive workup in this patient for metabolic disease is needed

5. In the emergency room, the child has normal electrolytes, coagulation profile, and CBC. What is the appropriate next intervention?

(A) The child should be discharged to home with a home monitor.

(B) The child should be admitted to the hospital for a period of observation.

(C) The child should be discharged to home with scheduled workup as an outpatient for head CT and pH probe.

(D) The child should be admitted to the hospital for observation and workup including head CT, eye exam, and skeletal survey.

6. This child is admitted and the workup performed is negative except for posterior rib fractures on the right of ribs 9 and 10. Which is the most likely explanation?

(A) The rib fractures are secondary to old birth trauma and are not relevant to the current illness.

(B) The rib fractures are secondary to the resuscitation efforts of the mother in the day of admission.

(C) The rib fractures are clear signs of prior nonaccidental trauma and should lead to a social service evaluation and police report.

(D) The rib fractures are found in otherwise normal children and occur as a result of routine handing of an infant.

7. The percent of "SIDS" cases that is thought to be because of nonaccidental trauma is closest to:

(A) 1% to 5%

(B) 6% to 20%

(C) 21% to 40%

(D) >40%

8. In the child admitted with ALTE for whom a diagnosis is not made (idiopathic), the examination was normal on admission and remained normal in the hospital. Discharge plans from the hospital should include:

(A) home monitoring until there is no apnea for 6 weeks, and weekly visits to the pediatrician

(B) home monitoring for 2 years and daily home nursing visits

(C) routine health care and no monitoring as there is no evidence that home monitoring prevents later death

(D) routine health care and home monitoring for 6 months if no apnea recurs

9. In general, the siblings of a child with an ALTE with a negative workup and no suspicion of abuse as an etiology:

(A) should receive polysomnography

(B) should be placed on a home apnea monitor if <8 months old

(C) should receive immediate evaluation by an appropriate health care provider

(D) should receive routine care by an appropriate health care provider

10. In children who present with ALTE, workup most frequently results in:

(A) demonstration of no abnormality

(B) demonstration of GE reflux

(C) demonstration of seizure disorder

(D) demonstration of a prolonged QT syndrome

11. Important aspects of the history of the ALTE are:

(A) relationship to feeding

(B) respiratory effort during the event

(C) muscle tone during the event

(D) all of the above

12. All of the following are clinical features of an ALTE that point to a seizure except:

(A) relationship to feeding

(B) muscle tone during the event

(C) rhythmic movements during the event

(D) fever at the time of the event

13. In a child who presents with an ALTE, which of the following histories would be consistent with GE reflux as a diagnosis?

(A) The mother reports arching of the back during the event.

(B) The mother reports choking during the event.

(C) The mother reports that the event happened just after feeding.

(D) All of the above.

Answers

1. **(A)** A seizure is a distinct possibility in a child with an ALTE. Metabolic derangements are common causes of seizures in this age group. Although hypomagnesemia may cause seizures, hypoglycemia, hypocalcemia, and hyponatremia are the three electrolyte disturbances most frequently associated with seizures. Therefore, it is imperative to obtain a serum glucose and electrolytes upon the child's arrival in the emergency department.

2. **(A)** If the history and the initial lab work are not revealing, the initial evaluation should include a CT scan of the head, a chest radiograph, an ECG, and, perhaps, a lumbar puncture. Knowledge gained from a careful history of the event will direct the testing required and urgency of those tests. Detailed questioning should include: the duration of the event, color change in the infant, respiratory efforts made by the child, and the intervention required for the episode to cease. Further questions should assess the child's muscle tone, activity, the relationship to feeding, episodes of emesis, choking or gasping, the presence of fever, and rhythmic movement of the extremities or the eyes. An understanding of the ambient lighting available to the observer may also be helpful. The presence of dried blood in the nose of this small child should prompt the clinician to consider the possibility that this is nonaccidental trauma. Further suspicion is suggested by the family history for SIDS. An EEG and a pH probe should be done after urgent studies have been obtained. If nonaccidental trauma is high on the list of possible etiologies, the workup for other concomitant trauma should be pursued with an ophthalmologic examination for retinal hemorrhage and a radiograph skeletal survey for occult fractures.

3. **(D)** An episode of ALTE in an infant is characterized by clinical symptoms that are sufficiently frightening to the caregiver, who believes the child may have experienced cardiac arrest or may die. These events generate substantial anxiety in the family and are also costly to the health care system to fully evaluate. Although it a very common reason for admission to the hospital, the precise incidence and prevalence of ALTE in the United States are not known.

4. **(A)** SIDS has been defined by the National Institutes of Health as the sudden death of an infant or young child, that is "unexplained by history," and in whom the autopsy fails to demonstrate a cause of death. The child who presents with an ALTE is no more likely to subsequently die from SIDS than are other children. However, SIDS is an important cause of death in infants. The 1999 summary of vital statistics suggested that SIDS is the third leading cause of infant mortality following congenital abnormalities and disorders related to preterm gestation. The rate of SIDS death is now approximately 64 per 100,000 live births, representing a decline of over 40% in the United States since the "Back To Sleep" program began in 1994. The etiology of SIDS is still unknown, but dramatic decreases in the incidence of SIDS have been demonstrated across the world since warnings against prone positioning during sleep have been implemented. The peak incidence is between 3 and 5 months of age. Sleeping in the prone position clearly places infants at risk, as does young maternal age, low socioeconomic status, smoking in the house where the infant sleeps, and soft bedding. There is no association between apnea of prematurity and SIDS. Of note, fewer than 1% of children who have an ALTE go on to have any other event that is life challenging. The Back To Sleep campaign has made no impact on the incidence of ALTEs, further strengthening the assertion that these two diagnoses are not related. It is also important for the clinician to recognize that SIDS is not a familial event. Therefore, SIDS that recurs in a family should strongly suggest the possibility of abuse and homicide. The presence of dried blood in the child's nose should heighten the clinician's suspicion for nonaccidental trauma such as suffocation.

5. **(D)** Nearly all infants who experience an ALTE should be hospitalized for observation and evaluation. Polysomnography may be useful in the child with a negative initial evaluation and, thus, no identified etiology. When an etiology is discovered for the ALTE, treatment is significantly easier than for those infants in whom no identifiable

cause is found. The family history of a child with SIDS should lead the clinician down the path of a very thorough workup for nonaccidental trauma.

6. **(C)** Rib fractures are not a "normal" finding in infants. Fractures are generally not identified until callus has formed and therefore would not be seen immediately following resuscitative efforts. Posterior rib fractures found on radiography of the chest are further evidence of nonaccidental trauma, specifically a shaking injury.

7. **(A)** Estimates suggest that nonaccidental trauma is responsible for 1% to 5% of "SIDS" cases.

8. **(C)** Where no explanation for the inciting event can be found, many families will raise the issue of home monitoring. Evidence for home monitoring to prevent consequences from an ALTE is nonexistent. In preterm infants with apnea of prematurity, home monitoring appears to be helpful until 43 weeks postconceptional age. Home monitoring may be disruptive to the family and should not be recommended after an ALTE.

9. **(D)** ALTE is not thought to be familial. Siblings would only require routine care. "Familial" ALTE or SIDS should lead one to consider nonaccidental trauma as a cause.

10. **(A)** The differential diagnosis is broad and includes infection, particularly RSV and meningitis, GERD, neurologic disorders such as seizures, or nonaccidental trauma, airway abnormalities, cardiac rhythm abnormalities, such as prolonged QT, metabolic abnormalities, and Münchausen syndrome by proxy. The etiology in most ALTEs remains unknown even when exhaustively evaluated.

11. **(D)** Knowledge gained from a careful history of the event will direct the testing required and urgency of those tests. Detailed questioning should include: the duration of the event, color change in the infant, respiratory efforts made by the child, and the intervention required for the episode to cease. Further questions should assess the child's muscle tone, activity, the relationship to feeding, episodes of emesis, choking or gasping, the presence of fever, and finally, rhythmic movement of the extremities or the eyes.

12. **(A)** A child with symptoms after eating suggests a diagnosis of GERD.

13. **(D)**

SUGGESTED READING

Ferrell PA, Weiner GM, Lemons JA: SIDS, ALTE, apnea, and the use of home monitors. *Pediatr Rev* 23(1): 3–9, 2002.

CASE 7: A 4-MONTH-OLD INFANT WITH HYPOTONIA AND A WEAK CRY

A 4-month-old female infant is brought to the emergency department for poor feeding, a weak cry, and lethargy. There have been no other symptoms: no upper respiratory tract illness, no fever, no vomiting or diarrhea. In fact, she has not had a bowel movement in 4 days. She normally takes approximately 6 to 8 ounces of formula at a time but for the last few days she seems to tire after taking only 2 ounces. During the preceding 2 weeks, she has become less active. Her mother also reports that she can no longer hold her head up without support.

Her heart rate is modestly elevated at 130 bpm, while the remaining vital signs are normal. She has markedly diminished muscle tone. On physical examination, she seems alert but very quiet. The anterior fontanelle is soft. There are no murmurs. Breath sounds are normal. Abdominal exam is normal. Pupils are 3 mm in size and react to light bilaterally. She has generalized weakness with diminished gag and cough reflexes, a marked head lag, and diminished deep tendon reflexes.

SELECT THE ONE BEST ANSWER

1. The most likely cause of this child's weakness is:

   (A) Guillain-Barré syndrome
   (B) amyotrophic lateral sclerosis
   (C) polio
   (D) infant botulism

2. The action that is the most likely to lead to the appropriate diagnosis is:

   (A) serum CK and aldolase
   (B) CT scan of the head
   (C) stool studies for bacterial toxin
   (D) examination of CSF

3. An alternative diagnostic test that might be useful is:

   (A) EEG
   (B) EMG
   (C) polysomnography
   (D) SSEP

4. The clinical hallmarks of infant botulism are:

   (A) muscle weakness and constipation
   (B) muscle weakness and hypotension
   (C) muscle weakness and ptosis
   (D) muscle weakness and head lag

5. The cause of infant botulism is:

   (A) *Clostridium botulinum* bacteria
   (B) *Clostridium botulinum* toxin
   (C) *Clostridium difficile* bacteria
   (D) *Clostridium difficile* toxin

6. The manner in which most infants contract botulism is:

   (A) ingestion of *Clostridium* spores
   (B) inhalation of *Clostridium* spores
   (C) fecal-oral contamination with *Clostridium* bacteria
   (D) blood-borne infection with *Clostridium* bacteria

7. Of the following, the infant most likely to have botulism is:

   (A) a 15-month-old who was given home-canned peaches by her grandmother
   (B) a 1-month-old who was given honey-dipped pacifiers for "colic"
   (C) a 3-month-old living in Philadelphia in a subdivision under construction
   (D) a 9-month-old who is living in urban Chicago in public housing

8. The incubation period for infant botulism is:

   (A) 3 to 5 days
   (B) 7 to 10 days
   (C) 2 to 4 weeks
   (D) 6 to 8 weeks

9. The symptoms of botulism occur because:

   (A) there is generalized degeneration of the anterior horn cells in the spinal cord
   (B) there is reversible blockade of the acetylcholine receptor at the motor end plate
   (C) there is inflammation of the myofibrils of somatic muscle
   (D) there is an irreversible block of the release of acetylcholine at the motor end plate

10. Medications that might potentiate botulism include:

    (A) cephalosporins
    (B) NSAIDs
    (C) aminoglycosides
    (D) antihistamines

11. Possible in-hospital issue(s) in an infant with botulism include:

    (A) respiratory failure
    (B) autonomic instability
    (C) feeding intolerance
    (D) all of the above

12. Which of the following findings least supports an alternative diagnosis of Werdnig-Hoffman disease in this low-tone infant?

    (A) weakness
    (B) wasting
    (C) constipation
    (D) absence of tendon reflexes

13. In Werdnig-Hoffman disease, the affected anatomic structures are:

    (A) the alpha motor neurons
    (B) the motor end plates
    (C) the muscle membranes
    (D) the myelin sheaths of peripheral nerves

14. In polio, the affected anatomic structures of the nervous system are:

    (A) the alpha motor neurons
    (B) the motor end plates
    (C) the muscle membranes
    (D) the myelin sheaths of peripheral nerves

15. In Guillain-Barré disease, the affected anatomic structures on the nervous system are:

(A) the alpha motor neurons
(B) the motor end plates
(C) the muscle membranes
(D) the myelin sheaths of peripheral nerves

16. With pancuronium use, the affected anatomic structures on the nervous system are:

(A) the alpha motor neurons
(B) the motor end plates
(C) the muscle membranes
(D) the myelin sheaths of peripheral nerves

Answers

1. **(D)** This case raises the lengthy differential diagnosis of "the floppy infant" or hypotonia. This particular child presented with a concomitant prominent history of constipation, which may direct physicians toward a diagnosis of either infant botulism or hypothyroidism. Although endemic polio is absent from the United States in the 21st century, a history of foreign travel to an endemic area might suggest the diagnosis of polio. The diagnosis of Guillain-Barré syndrome must be considered as well. In a 4-month-old, Guillain-Barré is also unusual. Although congenital or infantile hypothyroidism becomes apparent at this age, it is unlikely to be missed by newborn testing in the United States. Acquired hypothyroidism is rare in this age range. Thyroid function tests certainly should be sent and the results of the child's newborn screening should be checked. Amyotrophic lateral sclerosis (Lou Gehrig's disease) is a disease of adults.

2. **(C)** The diagnosis of infant botulism is largely based on significant clinical suspicion. A presumptive diagnosis must be made based on clinical presentation while confirmatory studies are pending. Once suspected, stool samples can be sent to the Centers for Disease Control and Prevention for identification of *C. botulinum* toxin. Do remember, however, that these patients are frequently constipated so the acquisition of that stool specimen may take some time and does not always yield positive results.

3. **(B)** EMG testing can be performed on infants with suspected botulism. Classic findings include de-creased amplitude of compound muscle action potentials, tetanic facilitation, and the absence of post-tetanic exhaustion. These EMG findings, nonetheless, are not pathognomonic, and the EMG may be normal early in the course of the disease.

4. **(A)** The presentation and severity of the disease can be very variable and, for unknown reasons, it appears to be more common in breastfed babies. The initial presentation may simply involve constipation and some feeding difficulty. If left unrecognized and unsupported, the patient may progress to global hypotonia, drooling, inability to eat, and respiratory failure. Symptoms will progress for 1 to 3 weeks before a plateau is reached, at which time the clinical condition stabilizes for another 2 to 3 weeks and recovery begins. Should the child need to be hospitalized, intubated, and ventilated, the hospital stay is frequently 3 to 6 weeks.

5. **(B)** Botulism is a rare but potentially fatal neuroparalytic disease, resulting from the action of a neurotoxin synthesized by *Clostridium botulinum*. Seen in only 100 U.S. children each year, infant botulism is a disease that occurs in the first year of life. The presentation and severity of the disease is very variable and, for unknown reasons, it appears to be more common in breastfed babies.

6. **(B)** The toxin is usually acquired by ingestion of *C. botulinum* spores followed by their germination in the GI tract.

7. **(C)** Spores can be acquired from one of two sources in infants—exposure to contaminated soil or exposure to contaminated food. Although more publicized, the incidence of botulism acquired from food represents only 15% to 20% of cases of infant botulism. Notoriously contaminated food products are home-canned fruits and raw honey. More commonly, spores are acquired by inhalation from soil with high concentration of *C. botulinum* spores. States with the highest soil concentrations of spores include Utah, Pennsylvania, and California.

8. **(C)** Once germinated, *C. botulinum* bacteria release toxin over 2 to 4 weeks and symptoms begin to be noted by the family.

9. **(D)** Neuromuscular transmission begins at the anterior horn cell of the motor nerve in the spinal cord, which is directed at the part of the anatomy receiving the signal for muscular activity. Electrical signals are transmitted down the myelinated peripheral nerve. The myelin sheath is responsible for the rapidity of transmission of that neural impulse, not the nervous impulse itself. At the peripheral nerve ending there is release of acetylcholine into the synaptic cleft separating the peripheral nerve from the motor endplate, which is located on the muscle membrane. Acetylcholine attaches to receptors on the motor endplate causing depolarization of the muscle and muscle activity.

An abnormality of the myelin sheath can be seen, as well, in diseases of both children and adults. The most common demyelinating disorder is Landry-Guillain-Barré syndrome (LGB). LGB is a postinfectious destruction of the myelin such that nervous transmission is significantly slowed and ultimately functionally stops. Unlike botulism, this presents most often as an ascending weakness. However, like botulism, Guillain-Barré syndrome may result in respiratory insufficiency requiring mechanical ventilation.

In some diseases acetylcholine metabolism can be blocked or its attachment to the motor endplate can be altered. In the case of botulism, the toxin causes irreversible inhibition of the release of acetylcholine at the presynaptic nerve terminal. Complete resolution of clinical symptoms requires that new nerve terminals sprout and normal release of acetylcholine resumes.

Beyond the neuromuscular receptor lies the muscle itself. A variety of disorders affecting the myocyte might well present with generalized weakness and can be classified as either a myopathy or myositis. The differential diagnosis of myopathy is beyond the scope of this discussion but is generally marked by the elevation of muscle enzymes—creatine phosphokinase and aldolase, and muscle tenderness. Constipation is rare.

10. **(C)** When aminoglycosides are given to treat intercurrent infection, they can potentiate the muscle weakness and are, therefore, relatively contraindicated. Aminoglycosides and hypermagnesemia augment the symptoms of botulism by causing neuromuscular failure by presynaptic blockade of acetylcholine release.

11. **(D)** Treatment for infant botulism is largely supportive and includes close monitoring in an intermediate or intensive care unit setting in order to detect progressive respiratory insufficiency. Human-derived botulinum antitoxin, also known as botulinum immunoglobulin, should be administered as well. In a controlled trial from the University of Pennsylvania, administration of botulinum immunoglobulin reduced the need for mechanical ventilation and shortened the duration of hospitalization when compared with patients in the control group. Antibiotics are helpful only to treat nosocomial infections that arise in a hospitalized patient and do not change the course of botulism.

12. **(C)** Werdnig-Hoffmann disease or infantile spinal muscular atrophy can present with hypotonia in infancy. These infants would be expected to have weakness, wasting, and absence of tendon reflexes. Tongue fasciculation might also be observed. Constipation would be rare.

13. **(A)** The neurologic examination will lead you down the path of a myelopathy, neuropathy, or a myopathy. Nerve conduction and electromyographic studies can confirm your suspicion of the anatomic location of the pathology. In Werdnig-Hoffman, the interruption in neuromuscular transmission is at the anterior horn cell. In the adult patient, the most common disease affecting the anterior horn cell is amyotrophic lateral sclerosis (Lou Gehrig's disease.)

14. **(A)** In polio the interruption is also at the anterior horn cell. Beyond the anterior horn cell level, there are a variety of neuropathies that can interrupt peripheral nervous transmission. Most do not present with generalized weakness. Nor do they present in the first 4 months of life.

15. **(D)** An abnormality of the myelin sheath can be seen as well in diseases of both children and adults. The most common demyelinating disorder is LGB. Guillain-Barré syndrome is a postinfectious destruction of the myelin such that nervous transmission is significantly slowed and ultimately functionally stops. Unlike botulism, this presents most often as an ascending weakness. However, like botulism, Guillain-Barré

syndrome may result in respiratory insufficiency requiring mechanical ventilation.

16. **(B)** Normal functioning of the neuromuscular endplate may also be temporarily disrupted by medications commonly used in the operating room. Nondepolarizing muscle relaxants such as pancuronium bind reversibly to the motor endplates and prevent neuromuscular transmission for a short period of time. The reversibility of this process distinguishes it from other pathologic disease states such as myasthenia gravis. In myasthenia, antibodies directed against the acetylcholine receptor on the motor endplate result in postsynaptic inhibition of neuromuscular transmission. This inhibition results in weakness, which worsens with repetitive stimulation of the endplate.

SUGGESTED READINGS

Bartlett JC: Infant botulism in adults. *N Engl J Med* 315(4):254–255, 1986.

Nelson KE: Editorial: The clinical recognition of botulism. *JAMA* 241(5):503–504, 1979.

L'Hommedieu CL, Polin RA: Progression of clinical signs in severe infant botulism. *Clin Pediatr* 20(2):90–95, 1981.

Chia JK, Clark JB, Ryan CA, et al: Botulism in an adult associated with food-borne intestinal infection with *Clostridium botulinum*. *N Engl J Med* 315(4):239–240, 1986.

CASE 8: A 5-YEAR-OLD BOY WITH FEVER, DROOLING, AND STRIDOR

A 5-year-old boy presents to the emergency room with a 12-hour history of fever and drooling. He was well previously. His temperature is 39.5°C and he appears toxic. There have been no other symptoms and no sick contacts. He is visiting his aunt in the United States and lives in Guatemala. He has received no immunizations.

On physical exam, the heart rate is 120 bpm, the respiratory rate is 26, and the room air blood oxygen saturation is 92%. The child has marked inspiratory stridor and refuses to swallow. He is sitting, leaning forward slightly and refuses to lie down for the examination.

A chest radiograph is normal. The leukocyte count is 28,000/mm^3 with a significant left shift.

SELECT THE ONE BEST ANSWER

1. What is the best initial diagnostic procedure indicated?

(A) The best diagnostic procedure is a radiograph of the neck.
(B) The best diagnostic procedure is an evaluation of the upper airway by an otolaryngologist.
(C) The best diagnostic procedure is ultrasonography of the neck.
(D) The best diagnostic procedure is a nasopharyngeal aspirate.

2. In this case, if the diagnosis is epiglottitis, what is the likely pathogen?

(A) The likely pathogen is coagulase-negative staphylococcus.
(B) The likely pathogen is *Streptococcus pneumoniae*.
(C) The likely pathogen is *Haemophilus influenzae*.
(D) The likely pathogen is parainfluenza virus.

3. If the diagnosis of epiglottitis is confirmed in the operating room by direct visualization by an otolaryngologist, the best next step would be:

(A) a transfer to the ICU with supplemental humidified oxygen
(B) an endotracheal intubation before transfer to the ICU
(C) a tracheostomy before transfer to the ICU
(D) a transfer to the ICU with administration of corticosteroids

4. In the United States, epiglottitis is best characterized as:

(A) seasonal
(B) sporadic
(C) largely eradicated by immunization
(D) endemic

5. The differential diagnosis of the febrile illness described includes all of the following except:

(A) bacterial tracheitis
(B) retropharyngeal abscess
(C) peritonsillar abscess
(D) maxillary sinusitis

6. In bacterial tracheitis, the most likely pathogen is:

(A) *Staphylococcus aureus*
(B) *Haemophilus influenzae*
(C) *Neisseria meningitidis*
(D) *Streptococcus pneumoniae*

7. In the case of a patient with peritonsillar abscess, which of the following is true?

   (A) Operative intervention is often needed.
   (B) Intravenous antibiotics are always sufficient treatment.
   (C) Outpatient treatment with oral antibiotics is effective.
   (D) Endotracheal intubation is required for at least a week of antibiotic therapy to avoid airway obstruction.

8. In a febrile toxic-appearing patient with a maxillary sinusitis, sufficient initial treatment is:

   (A) intravenous antibiotics for 1 week
   (B) oral antibiotics for 3 weeks
   (C) scheduled outpatient endoscopic sinus surgical drainage
   (D) evaluation of CSF for possible meningitis, then a course of intravenous antibiotics

9. Differences between viral croup and epiglottitis include:

   (A) the child with viral croup is often older than the patient with epiglottitis
   (B) the child with viral croup always has a more abrupt onset of stridor than the patient with epiglottitis
   (C) the child with viral croup is more likely to present in the middle of an upper respiratory infection than the patient with epiglottitis
   (D) the child with viral croup looks identical to the child with epiglottitis

10. The classic clinical findings of viral croup are:

    (A) steeple sign, inspiratory stridor, low-grade fever, URI symptoms, barking cough
    (B) steeple sign, high fever, dysphagia, rash, staccato cough
    (C) thumb sign, inspiratory stridor, URI, dysphagia, barking cough
    (D) thumb sign, high fever, expiratory wheeze, inspiratory stridor, staccato cough

11. Treatments for viral croup requiring supportive care in a hospital setting most likely include:

    (A) antibiotic coverage for possible superinfection
    (B) humidified oxygen, racemic epinephrine, and corticosteroids

   (C) oseltamivir and humidified oxygen

12. Pick the false statement from the following:

    (A) All patients with viral croup must be hospitalized because of the risk of airway obstruction.
    (B) All patients with epiglottitis must be hospitalized because of the risk of airway obstruction.
    (C) All patients with epiglottitis benefit from antibiotic therapy.
    (D) Almost all patients with viral croup benefit from anti-inflammatory agents.

13. Pick the false statement from the following:

    (A) Patients with viral croup who have received racemic epinephrine may be discharged to home without a period of observation.
    (B) Patients with viral croup may be sent home safely after receiving parenteral corticosteroids.
    (C) Patients with epiglottitis respond little to racemic epinephrine and therefore it is not recommended for treatment.
    (D) Patients with epiglottitis do not respond to corticosteroids sufficiently to warrant their use in the disease.

14. The ominous sign of impending respiratory failure in a patient with viral croup is:

    (A) expiratory wheezes and rales
    (B) inspiratory stridor and crackles
    (C) muffled biphasic stridor
    (D) expiratory wheezes and rhonchi

Answers

1. **(B)** Making the diagnosis of epiglottitis can be difficult. A high index of suspicion by the initial evaluating physician is imperative, especially in a young child. The patient typically presents with a sudden onset of fever, sore throat, drooling, and difficulty swallowing. Classically, the child appears toxic with fevers that reach 39°C to 40°C and prefers the position of maximal airflow, sitting forward with the neck hyperextended, chin forward. An urgent referral to otolaryngology or anesthesiology is required. The patient should be taken immediately to an operating room setting and gently anesthetized. After the induction of anesthesia, an

upper airway evaluation can be performed. Routine examination of the pharynx should be deferred until anesthesia is induced as sudden, complete airway obstruction might result. In this case, time spent obtaining a neck radiograph would only delay evaluation and can increase the chance of further respiratory compromise.

2. **(C)** Epiglottitis (in the pre-Hib vaccine era) was caused almost exclusively by Hib and usually occurred between the ages of 1 and 5 years with a peak incidence in the third year of life and a slight male predominance. Since the introduction of the Hib vaccine, the epidemiology of epiglottitis has significantly shifted. In the United States, this is no longer a disease of young children but rather a disease of teenagers and young adults. In the unvaccinated patient the likely culprit may still be Hib, to which antibiotic therapy should be targeted. For patients who are vaccinated or in older patients, antibiotic therapy should cover both Hib and *S. aureus*.

3. **(B)** Anatomically, epiglottitis is not limited to the epiglottis. It is a cellulitis of all structures of the larynx, including the aryepiglottic folds and arytenoid cartilages. The large potential space between the epithelial layer and the cartilage in these tissues allows for the accumulation of inflammatory cells and edema during infection. As this potential space enlarges, the swollen epiglottis and adjacent structures begin to obstruct airflow through the laryngeal inlet during inspiration. Abrupt onset and rapid progression of airway symptoms are the hallmarks of epiglottitis. In the operating room the diagnosis can be made by direct inspection. If confirmed, an endotracheal tube should be introduced under direct vision and secured. After securing the airway and obtaining cultures in the operating room, the patient should be transferred to the intensive care unit where mechanical ventilation is often needed in order to allow the child to be adequately sedated. Reinspection of the epiglottitis using a flexible bronchoscope can be easily performed and will guide appropriate timing of removal of the endotracheal tube. In general, 48 to 72 hours of antibiotic therapy is sufficient for elimination of airway obstruction. Corticosteroids have no role in epiglottitis in small children. There may be some role for corticosteroids in opportunistic infections in older patients, especially when epiglottitis is of an uncommon etiology.

4. **(C)** Infectious diseases of the upper respiratory tract in children are common. Inflammatory disease involving the larynx in the first 6 years of life includes croup and epiglottitis. Croup is a viral infection of the larynx, trachea, and bronchi. In contrast, epiglottitis is a bacterial disease of the larynx that has been virtually eliminated in the United States by the introduction of the Hib vaccines. Since their introduction in 1991 all diseases caused by Hib have substantially decreased, from an incidence of 100/100,000 population to 0.3/100,000 population. However, in other countries where this vaccine is not available, Hib may still be a significant cause of disease.

5. **(D)** Diagnoses that may mimic acute epiglottitis include laryngotracheobronchitis, croup or spasmodic croup, bacterial tracheobronchitis, a foreign body lodged in the larynx or vallecula, retropharyngeal or peritonsillar abscess, and hereditary or drug-induced angioedema.

   Diagnosis of viral laryngotracheobronchitis is usually made on clinical grounds. The typical child with croup is about 1 to 6 years of age, is in the midst of an upper respiratory infection, has symptoms compatible with viral croup, particularly stridor and cough, and is nontoxic in appearance. Under these circumstances, confirmation of the diagnosis can be made with neck radiographs. Narrowing of the upper airway, commonly referred to as a steeple sign, is especially apparent on the AP radiograph. In epiglottitis, a lateral neck radiograph would show an enlarged epiglottis referred to as a thumb sign, if a radiograph were obtained (see answer #1).

   For children with retropharyngeal or peritonsillar abscess there may be prominent swelling and erythema of the tonsillar bed or posterior pharyngeal wall, and inspection of the mouth can be diagnostic. The clinical presentation of diphtheria can also resemble epiglottitis. However, with the widespread use of DTaP vaccination, diphtheria is rare. A child with maxillary sinusitis would present with facial pain, toothache or headache. The physical exam would reveal the presence of significant pain on pressure applied to the area of the sinus. The patient who has pu-rulent pansinusitis can appear quite toxic but does not have airway symptoms.

6. **(A)** The epidemiology of epiglottitis has changed. In the United States, this is no longer a disease of young children caused by *Haemophilus influenza* but rather a disease of teenagers and young adults. In these patients, the offending bacteriologic agent is usually *S. aureus. Streptococcus pneumoniae*, beta-hemolytic streptococci, and nontypeable *H. influenzae* and even fungi have also been impli-cated. In teens and adults with symptoms of epi-glottitis, it is important to verify HIV status as opportunistic infections of the larynx are not un-common in these patients.

7. **(A)** The primary cause of these deep neck infec-tions is either *S. aureus* or streptococcus species, particularly group A streptococcus. If there is con-cern for a diagnosis of deep neck abscess in a child, antimicrobial agents should be directed at these organisms. However, despite appropriate antibiotic therapy surgical drainage of a periton-sillar abscess is often necessary.

8. **(D)** Evaluation of spinal fluid in the toxic child with sinusitis is required prior to a course of anti-biotic therapy as meningitis is not uncommon in this setting and will alter therapy. A CT scan may help localize any possible CNS extension and is generally performed prior to lumbar puncture.

9. **(C)** Epiglottitis is distinguished from croup by the toxic appearance and the profound dysphagia seen in the child with epiglottitis. Patients with epiglot-titis are 2 to 6 years old. Children with croup are 1 to 6 years of age and usually present amidst an up-per respiratory infection with prominent airway symptoms including stridor and a "barking" cough.

10. **(A)** Infectious croup (laryngotracheobronchitis) is most often caused by parainfluenza types 1 or 2. There is currently no vaccine for the parain-fluenza virus and croup remains common in the United States and all over the world. As in epi-glottitis, croup affects young children. Initially patients with croup present with low-grade fever, rhinorrhea, stridor, and cough. If the disease progresses to significant airway obstruction, the child will have severe stridor and shortness of breath. With respiratory efforts, significant su-prasternal retractions are also observed in chil-dren with severe croup.

11. **(B)** Most parainfluenza virus disease is mild with episodes of laryngotracheobronchitis lasting for 3 to 4 days and treatment is largely symptomatic. Marked improvement in the duration of airway obstruction has been seen with the use of cortico-steroids. Parenteral dexamethasone in a dose ex-ceeding 0.3 mg/kg has been recommended for se-vere airway obstruction. For example, a single dose of 0.6 mg/kg intramuscularly may be given as an adjunctive therapy in severe croup. Oral dexa-methasone in doses of 0.15 to 0.6 mg/kg has been shown to lessen severity, duration of symptoms, and need for hospitalization in patients with less severe croup. Although for many years cold mist has been recommended to treat croup, there is lit-tle evidence that this intervention is beneficial.

12. **(A)** For the child with epiglottitis, after securing the airway and obtaining cultures in the operat-ing room, the patient should be transported to the intensive care unit where mechanical ventila-tion is often needed in order to allow the child to be adequately sedated during a period of antibi-otic treatment. Reinspection of the epiglottitis using a flexible bronchoscope can be easily per-formed and will guide appropriate timing of re-moval of the endotracheal tube. In general, 48 to 72 hours of antibiotic therapy are sufficient for eradication of airway obstruction.

13. **(A)** Once a child has received racemic epineph-rine, it is important to observe for a period of no less than 6 hours because there may be a rebound increase in airway obstruction and progressive symptoms during this time period.

14. **(C)** Should symptoms of croup progress to airway obstruction, there will be a classic series of signs demonstrated by the patient. Initially, patients with upper airway disease (extrathoracic symptoms) present with inspiratory stridor. As the extratho-racic airway obstruction progresses, both inspira-tory and expiratory stridor develop. Finally as the airway narrows critically, stridor becomes quite muffled until there is little air movement at all and

no sound. When patients develop biphasic stridor, respiratory failure can be anticipated and the patient should be placed in a monitored setting and aggressively treated, perhaps even intubated.

Physiologically, the airway is divided into two portions—an extrathoracic and an intrathoracic portion. Symptoms of airway disease depend upon the location of the pathology in the airway. Epiglottitis and croup represent diseases of the extrathoracic airway. Under these conditions, airway symptoms begin on inspiration because the extrathoracic airway narrows on inhalation, whereas the intrathoracic airway will expand with the negative intrathoracic pressure generated with inhalation. Intrathoracic airway pathology, such as a vascular ring or a mediastinal tumor, presents with symptoms on exhalation. That sound heard on exhalation as a result of airway disease is frequently misconstrued for wheezing and treated as asthma when, in fact, the clinician is dealing with expiratory stridor.

Disease that compromises the intrathoracic airway causes expiratory stridor first because the intrathoracic airway is reduced in caliber during exhalation. As airway caliber is reduced to critical levels, regardless of the location, stridor will be present on inspiration and expiration (biphasic stridor) and heralds impending respiratory failure.

SUGGESTED READING

Cohen LF: Stridor and upper airway obstruction in children. *Pediatr Rev* 21:4–5, 2000.

Malhotra A, Krilov LR: Viral croup. *Pediatr Rev* 22:5–12, 2001.

Leipzig B, Oski FA, Cummings CW, et al: A prospective randomized study to determine the efficacy of steroids in treatment of croup. *J Pediatr* 94(2):194–196, 1979.

Gallagher PG, Myer III CM: An approach to the diagnosis and treatment of membranous laryngotracheobronchitis in infants and children. *Pediatr Emerg Med* 7(6):337–334, 1991.

CASE 9: A 6-YEAR-OLD BOY FOUND AT THE BOTTOM OF THE NEIGHBOR'S POOL

A 6-year-old boy is brought to the emergency department by EMS. He was found at the bottom of his neighbor's swimming pool and rescued. At the scene, he was without vital signs initially. After 5 minutes of basic life support efforts, he had a cardiac rhythm and a pulse, but he was making no respiratory effort. The child was intubated and placed in a cervical collar.

On physical exam the child is unresponsive. His vital signs are blood pressure 110/56, pulse 100, respiratory rate while bagging 22, temperature 34.5°C, and oxygen saturation 100%. Auscultation of the chest reveals wheezing in the right hemithorax and coarse breath sounds throughout. The cardiac rhythm is sinus and there are no murmurs. The only other part of the physical examination that is abnormal is the neurologic exam. The child remains unresponsive to pain or voice. Pupils are 4 mm bilaterally and are very sluggish in response to light. The muscle tone is generally reduced and there is no rectal tone.

SELECT THE ONE BEST ANSWER

1. The condition of this child dictates the need for the following:

   (A) obtaining an AP chest film
   (B) obtaining a blood sample for toxicology
   (C) obtaining imaging studies of the head and cervical spine
   (D) obtaining left and right lateral decubitus chest films

2. The clinical scenario that best predicts poor outcome in drowning is:

   (A) CPR required at the scene of the accident
   (B) CPR required in the emergency department
   (C) failure to achieve spontaneous cardiac rhythm for 25 minutes
   (D) submersion time duration of >5 minutes

3. The clinical scenario that best predicts good outcome in drowning is:

   (A) core temperature on arrival in the emergency department of <32°C
   (B) return of spontaneous circulation in the emergency department
   (C) responsive pupils in the emergency room
   (D) spontaneous circulation at the accident scene

4. Which of the following is the common cause of morbidity and mortality in drowning?

   (A) The common cause is hypoxic encephalopathy.
   (B) The common cause is acute hypoxic respiratory failure.

(C) The common cause is renal failure.

(D) The common cause is acute hyponatremia from water absorption.

5. Which of the following statements is true?

(A) Salt water drowning is more common than drowning in fresh water.

(B) The lung injury that occurs in a fresh water drowning is more severe than the lung injury that occurs in salt water.

(C) Salt water and fresh water drowning are more alike than they are different.

(D) Drowning results in the aspiration of large volumes of water into the tracheobronchial tree and lungs, irrespective of the type of water.

6. The frequency of drowning in the United States is best described as:

(A) an uncommon cause of death

(B) the second most common cause of pediatric death in many states

(C) is more likely in girls irrespective of age

(D) is more likely in boys younger than the age of 6, but it is of equal magnitude between the genders in older children

7. The most important intervention that prevents accidental pool drowning is:

(A) swimming lessons

(B) flotation devices

(C) pool fencing

(D) pool covers

8. On the second hospital day, the child's examination was consistent with brain death. This diagnosis would not be possible to make by clinical exam if:

(A) the child's temperature is 35°C

(B) the patient's phenobarbital level is 10 mg/dL

(C) the patient has a C1-2 fracture

(D) the patient has an L4-5 fracture

9. The definition of brain death in children requires that the child be:

(A) older than 7 days of age and term at birth

(B) older than 6 months old, irrespective of gestational age

(C) older than 1 year of age, irrespective of gestational age

(D) older than 60 weeks' postconceptual age

10. Confirmatory tests for brain death include the following except:

(A) brain nuclear blood flow study

(B) MRI of the brain

(C) cerebral angiogram

(D) electroencephalogram

11. Which of the following may be present and still have the patient meet brain death criteria as of 2004 according to the American Academy of Pediatrics' guidelines?

(A) Spinal reflexes may be present.

(B) Corneal reflexes may be present.

(C) Doll's eyes (oculocephalics) may be present.

(D) Pupillary response to light may be present.

12. Which is true about the original Harvard description of "brain death"? (Note that the terminology actually used by the Harvard group was "irreversible coma" as opposed to "brain death.")

(A) The recommendations of the original Harvard group specified special criteria in children younger than 2 years of age.

(B) The recommendations of the original Harvard group did not address this issue in children.

(C) The "Harvard Criteria" required confirmatory tests be used in all children younger than 1 year of age prior to declaration of death.

(D) The "Harvard Criteria" for brain death required 2 EEGs to confirm brain death for children, but made no such requirement for adults.

13. The diagnosis of brain death in children as currently described by the leading societies of neurology and pediatrics requires that:

(A) confirmatory tests be used in all age children prior to declaration of death

(B) confirmatory tests be used in all children younger than 1 year of age prior to declaration of death

(C) a neurologist examine all children prior to the declaration of brain death

(D) the declaration of brain death can be made in all children on the first physical examination consistent with brain death

14. Which of the following children meet the definition of brain death?

   (A) a 6-day-old with birth asphyxia who has an isoelectric EEG
   (B) a 6-month-old infant found pulseless at home with agonal respirations, otherwise completely unresponsive
   (C) a 2-year-old drowning victim with no brainstem function
   (D) a 16-year-old adolescent found unresponsive at a "Rave" party and brought to the emergency room intubated by EMS

15. Which of the following children should have confirmatory diagnostic testing in radiology before declaration of brain death because the brain death physical examination is not valid?

   (A) a 3-year-old after MVA with concomitant thoracic spine trauma
   (B) a 6-year-old after MVA with concomitant cervical spine trauma
   (C) a 7-year-old after MVA with diffuse axonal injury
   (D) a 4-year-old MVA who has spina bifida occulta

Answers

1. **(C)** In the case scenario, the initial physical exam was complicated by the absence of rectal tone. Once the airway has been carefully secured and hemodynamic status stabilized, this finding should direct your initial workup to urgent imaging of the head and cervical spine. Frequently, diving accidents are followed by prolonged submersion when concomitant spinal injury is involved. As with all patients who suffer traumatic accidents, coexisting injuries need to be diligently sought. Notably, especially in the older child who suffers a submersion event, a concomitant diving injury may also be present. It is wise to image both the head and cervical spine in a victim who is unable to communicate and particularly when the accident was not witnessed. Prehospital care providers should treat patients with drowning injury as if concomitant cervical spine trauma is present unless it is clearly observed that the patient did not dive into the body of water from which he or she was rescued.

   Importantly, submersion injury may be the initial presentation for a child with prolonged QT syndrome, especially if the event was not witnessed. This mandates an ECG be performed on all submersion victims when they are normothermic and their electrolytes are normal.

2. **(C)** The ultimate determinant of the quality of a submersion victim's recovery is the duration of hypoxic injury. The most reliable predictors of poor outcome in the pediatric population are: submersion that exceeds 10 minutes in duration, resuscitation efforts to achieve spontaneous cardiac rhythm that exceed 25 minutes, and admission to a pediatric intensive care unit with a Glasgow Coma Scale score of <5 (Table 9-1). Despite this, 8% to 30% of children who require CPR at the scene of a drowning accident survive neurologically intact.

   Prompt prehospital intervention is crucial for the injured child with a potentially reversible process. Delay in the initiation of basic and/or advanced life support in this patient population augments the hypoxic insult. A great deal of discussion has occurred regarding the routine use of the Heimlich maneuver in the prehospital care of the drowning victim. The American Red Cross continues to dissuade delaying basic life support in order to perform this maneuver except in the case of a patient with an airway obstruction. The presence of water in the tracheobronchial tree does not warrant the routine performance of the Heimlich maneuver, which instead may increase the quantity of regurgitated material and hamper efforts at maintaining a patent airway. There must be no delay in instituting basic and advanced life support maneuvers for the child in full arrest after a drowning.

3. **(D)** The best predictors of a good neurological outcome are the return of spontaneous circulation at the scene of the accident and never losing spontaneous circulation at all. Eight percent to 30% of children who require CPR at the scene of a drowning accident will survive neuro-

Table 9-1. **GLASGOW COMA SCALE**

Eye Opening	Motor Response	Verbal Response
1. No response	1. No response	1. No response
2. Responds to pain	2. Abnormal extension (decerebrate)	2. Incomprehensible
3. Responds to voice	3. Abnormal flexion (decorticate)	3. Inappropriate
4. Spontaneous	4. Withdraws from pain	4. Confused
	5. Localizes pain	
	6. Obeys verbal commands	Alternatives for young/nonverbal children:
		1. No response
		2. Restless, agitated
		3. Persistently irritable
		4. Consolable crying
		5. Appropriate words, smiles, fixes, and follows

logically intact. Much has also been made of the circumstance of cold water submersion. Cold water locations are implicated in only 2% of all submersion deaths. Because of the protective effects of hypothermia on the brain and other vital organs, intact survivors of prolonged submersions are possible. It should be noted that the water needs to be cold enough to support ice on its surface in order for the protective effects of hypothermia to be seen. Water temperature must be <86°F or <30°C. Cool water does not offer the same protection. The child must cool quickly to rapidly reduce cerebral-oxygen consumption to be afforded protection by the cold. In spite of descriptions in the medical literature and lay press of dramatic recoveries from prolonged cold water submersions, these are rare. It is much more important to prevent the injury than to attempt to resuscitate the child who is already injured.

4. **(A)** Morbidity and mortality in drowning are largely the result of prolonged hypoxemia. Deaths that result from drowning events are largely the result of anoxic encephalopathy, that is, brain swelling, with subsequent herniation and ultimately brain death. Aspiration of water into the tracheobronchial tree causes lung injury that results in decreased lung compliance, ventilation perfusion mismatch, surfactant deactivation, and intrapulmonary shunting. These lead to a patient with continued hypoxemia, compli-

cating the initial neurologic injury, which also largely results from hypoxemia. Prompt prehospital intervention is crucial for the injured child with a potentially reversible process. Delay in the initiation of basic and/or advanced life support in this patient population also augments the hypoxic insult. Frequently, hypoxic encephalopathy is apparent at the time of initial examination and worsens over the first 24 to 48 hours with progressive cerebral edema. It can be stated with reasonable certainty that for a patient who makes no improvement in the first 24 to 48 hours, the outcome from a drowning is almost certainly poor.

5. **(C)** Much has been made of the difference between drowning in salt water and drowning in fresh water. Because the submersion generally causes laryngospasm, it does not result in the aspiration of more than 3 to 4 mL/kg of water. Therefore the distinction between salt water drowning and fresh water drowning is not considered clinically important. Both types of drowning result in decreased lung compliance, increased ventilation perfusion mismatch, surfactant deactivation, and increased intrapulmonary shunting. These lead to a patient with continued hypoxemia, complicating the initial injury, which also largely results from hypoxemia.

6. **(B)** Strictly speaking, drowning is defined as an immersion or submersion injury resulting in

death. The term *near drowning* implies survival for more than 24 hours following immersion injury. Drowning is the third most common cause of accidental death in the United States. In some states with access to swimming pools, beaches and lakes, drowning is the leading cause of death in children younger than 5 years of age. Submersion injury has a bimodal distribution of age. The first peak occurs in children younger than 5 years who are victims of unprotected backyard swimming pools. The second peak occurs in adolescents, who are victims of boating and/or swimming accidents in lakes and at beaches. These are frequently associated with alcohol or drugs and may be accompanied by spinal cord injury. In all age ranges, male victims outnumber female victims. For every child who is hospitalized following a submersion injury, at least 10 never seek medical attention and 8 others are evaluated in an emergency department and discharged. Among female children younger than 19 years of age, 1:3300 will drown; 1:1000 will be hospitalized following a water emergency. In male children younger than 19 years of age, 1:1100 will drown and 1:300 will require hospital stay for nonfatal submersion injury.

7. **(C)** Evidence from both epidemiologic and clinical studies suggests that the most effective means to reduce submersion injury of children should focus on prevention rather than therapy. The best method to prevent pediatric drowning is adequate supervision of a child at risk. Drowning in residential pools can be decreased substantially by the installation of complete pool fencing. This intervention has been well studied in Australia and New Zealand where pool fencing is mandated by law. To be effective, the fence must completely surround the pool with an automatic locking gate. Should the gate be disabled or propped open, the protection of the fence is eliminated. Pool covers do not provide the same protection as they frequently collapse under the weight of a child. Swimming lessons also do not provide the same protection, as a child frequently overestimates his or her ability to swim.

8. **(C)** It is imperative that the care provider identify any coexisting neurologic injury as it will change the course of therapy and the ability to perform a prognostic physical examination. Should the child have a cervical injury associated with submersion, the spinal cord insult will prevent the physician from assessing brain stem function by a careful neurologic exam. It will, therefore, be impossible to provide the family with an adequate description of the extent of neurologic insult without confirmatory testing, particularly if it is suspected that the child has progressed to brain death.

9. **(A)** The determination of brain death in children varies with the age of the child and it is important to recognize that there is no definition of brain death for a child who is younger than 7 days of age. The original Harvard description of irreversible coma required multiple examinations as well as EEG.

10. **(B)** MRI has no role in the determination of brain death.

11. **(A)** The brain death examination consists of the following:

    1. coma and apnea must coexist
    2. there must be no evidence of brainstem function
       - pupils are unreactive to light
       - no eye movement in response to turning the head (doll's eyes, oculocephalic reflex)
       - no response to cold water into the ear canal (oculovestibular reflex testing)
       - no movement of bulbar muscles (tested by checking for the presence of the corneal reflex, the gag reflex, coughing, suckling, or rooting)
       - patient is apneic off mechanical ventilation (this assumes that the patient does not have a cervical spine injury that would prevent breathing efforts even in the face of a normal functioning brainstem)
       - Apnea testing needs to be performed in a fashion that guarantees the patient neither becomes hypoxemic nor hypotensive during the period of challenge. There must also be demonstration of respiratory acidosis to a pH that is ≤ 7.25 with concomitant absence of respiratory efforts in order to declare that the patient in fact has no respiratory brainstem function.

3. absence of hypotension or hypothermia during the exam
4. muscle tone should be flaccid and there should be no spontaneous movements and no response to central painful stimuli
5. confirmatory testing requirements are defined again by age and no confirmatory test is required or recommended for children older than 1 year of age without other injury

The presence of deep tendon reflexes (DTR) does not preclude the diagnosis of brain death even though it is more common for them to be absent. DTRs are considered spinal reflexes, as is flexion of an extremity in response to painful stimuli applied to the distal part of that extremity. Those movements, with time, almost always vanish and do not negate the determination of brain death, but can be confusing to families.

An examination for brain death by a neurologist or neurosurgeon is not required by the current societies of neurology or pediatrics, although it is recommended that a physician who is familiar with this examination be asked to evaluate the patient. This physician might be a neurologist, neurosurgeon, intensivist, neonatologist, or emergency room physician. Clearly there are local requirements, both in individual academic practices or private hospitals, that define the requirements for the declaration of brain death in each venue.

12. **(B)** The notion of brain death was first described by Dr. Henry K. Beecher, a neurologist from the Harvard Medical School in 1968. This concept was introduced in an effort to identify patients with irreversible coma who could be considered for organ transplantation. These criteria for irreversible coma later became the criteria for brain death determination. However, these guidelines omitted children. It was not until the mid-1980s that the issues of hypoxic-ischemic encephalopathy progressive to brain death and the definition of brain death in children were addressed. The diagnosis of brain death in children as currently described by the leading societies of neurology and pediatrics has specific recommendations for performing a brain death exam as well as the use of confirmatory data.

13. **(B)** Modern definitions of brain death in adults and children older than 1 year of age require

only that the examination of the patient be consistent with brain death and that there not be confounding issues that will prevent the accuracy of that examination (as with a cervical spine injury). Multiple examinations are recommended in children <1 year of age. The American Academy of Pediatrics as well as the American Society of Neurology and Neurosurgery suggest that confirmatory tests of brain function be used in these children. For infants 7 days to 2 months of age, they recommend two physical examinations and two EEGs separated by 48 hours. Between 2 months and 1 year, two physical examinations and two EEGs separated by 24 hours are recommended. Beyond 1 year of age, physical exam alone is sufficient. It is suggested, but not required, that an observation period of at least 12 hours be used in the older child in whom 2 examinations are performed. Nuclear medicine study of cerebral blood flow or cerebral angiogram can replace the two EEGs in either case.

14. **(C)** See answers to questions 11 and 13.

15. **(B)** If there is an additional injury, particularly a cervical spine injury, which interferes with the apnea test, the brain death exam is not valid. Even with intact cerebral and/or brain stem function, apnea would be present in the child with the cervical spine injury above or involving C3. Diaphragmatic paralysis and thoracic weakness are found with injury to C4 and C5, also confounding the apnea test. Therefore, one cannot do a brain death exam accurately in the presence of cervical spine trauma. A test such as a cerebral angiogram or nuclear medicine study is needed to confirm the absence of cerebral blood flow. Hypothermia, excessive doses of barbiturates, or other metabolic intoxications also limit the accuracy of the brain death exam. Prior to testing, it is required that patients be normothermic with a barbiturate level sufficiently low so as not to confound the examination.

SUGGESTED READING

Quan L, Kinder D: Pediatric submersions: prehospital predictors of outcome. *Pediatrics* 90(6):909–913, 1992.
Lavelle JM, Shaw KN: Near drowning: is emergency department cardiopulmonary resuscitation or intensive

care unit cerebral resuscitation indicated? *Crit Care Med* 21(3):368–373, 1993.

Liller KD, Kent EB, Arcari C, et al: Risk factors for drowning and near-drowning among children in Hillsborough County, Florida. *Public Health Rep* 108(3):346–353, 1993.

Wintemute GJ, Drake C, Wright M: Immersion events in residential swimming pools. Evidence for an experience effect. *Am J Dis Child* 145:1200–1203, 1991.

Quan L, Gore EJ, Wentz K, et al: Ten-year study of pediatric drownings and near-drownings in King County, Washington: Lessons in injury prevention. *Pediatrics* 83(6):1035–1040, 1989.

Ashwal S, Schneider S: Brain death in children: Part I. *Pediatr Neurol* 3:5–11, 1987.

CASE 10: A 2-YEAR-OLD BOY WITH SUDDEN ONSET OF COUGHING

A 2-year-old boy is brought to the emergency department with the sudden onset of coughing. He has not had any symptoms of upper respiratory tract illness. He has no past history of reactive airway disease, nor a family history of asthma. Prior to the onset of symptoms, he was playing with his older sister in the kitchen.

On physical exam the child is nontoxic but cannot stop coughing. Results of his physical examination are normal except his room air saturation is 94% and auscultation of the chest reveals wheezing in the right hemithorax and coarse breath sounds throughout.

SELECT THE ONE BEST ANSWER

1. Which of the following would be the best way to order radiographs to maximize potential for identifying the presence of a radiolucent foreign body in a cooperative child?

    (A) The best approach would be AP and lateral chest films.
    (B) The best approach would be PA and left decubitus chest films.
    (C) The best approach would be inspiratory and expiratory films.
    (D) The best approach would be right lateral decubitus film.

2. If the child cannot cooperate with the requested CXR, what is the next appropriate diagnostic test?

    (A) A chest CT scan is the next test.
    (B) A chest MRI is the next test.
    (C) An airway fluoroscopy is the next test.
    (D) A ventilation/perfusion scan is the next test.

3. This child has a normal CXR. Which of the following statements is true?

    (A) A normal CXR rules out a foreign body in the airway.
    (B) Many children with a normal CXR have had airway foreign bodies.
    (C) A normal CXR mandates that you proceed to a CT for diagnosis if a foreign body is suspected.
    (D) The CXR must be mislabeled, as this child could not have a normal CXR.

4. The most common aspirated airway foreign body in childhood is:

    (A) a peanut
    (B) a marble
    (C) a hotdog
    (D) a balloon

5. The most common airway foreign body that is lethal is:

    (A) a peanut
    (B) a marble
    (C) a penny
    (D) a balloon

6. The most common esophageal foreign body found in children is a:

    (A) a matchstick
    (B) a marble
    (C) a penny
    (D) a quarter

7. The most appropriate therapeutic intervention when there is a suspected tracheal foreign body in a coughing child would be:

    (A) urgent thoracotomy
    (B) urgent upper GI
    (C) urgent bronchoscopy
    (D) the Heimlich maneuver

8. If the radiograph reveals an aspirated coin in the proximal esophagus, what would the appropriate intervention be?

(A) Send the child home. The coin will pass without intervention.
(B) Remove the coin in the emergency room using a balloon-tipped catheter.
(C) Schedule endoscopy in the next 12 to 24 hours to remove the coin.
(D) Push the coin into the stomach with an nasogastric tube.

9. If the radiograph reveals an aspirated watch battery, the treatment is:

(A) no different from that of an aspirated coin
(B) a more urgent situation requiring more rapid endoscopy because of the risk of tissue injury
(C) a better situation for pushing the object into the stomach because it is smaller than all U.S. coins
(D) admission to the hospital and serial abdominal radiographs documenting the passage of the battery into the stool

10. If a foreign body is causing near total tracheal obstruction in a child, you should first:

(A) perform a blind oropharyngeal finger sweep
(B) perform a Heimlich maneuver
(C) perform an emergency tracheostomy
(D) perform a needle cricothyroidotomy

11. The narrowest portion of a toddler's airway is at the level of the:

(A) vocal cords
(B) carina
(C) thyroid cartilage
(D) cricoid cartilage

12. The narrowest portion of a toddler's upper gastrointestinal tract is at the level of the:

(A) lower esophageal sphincter
(B) pylorus
(C) cricopharyngeus muscle
(D) second portion of the duodenum

13. The most hazardous items, from the perspective of childhood aspiration, that can be found in a pediatrician's office are:

(A) gauze bandages
(B) ear speculums
(C) cotton balls
(D) exam gloves

14. Should an airway aspiration event be missed, it is likely to present as:

(A) recurrent pneumonia
(B) wheezing
(C) chronic cough
(D) all of the above

Answers

1. **(C)** The clinician should be suspicious for the aspiration of some kind of foreign body. Unfortunately, many foreign bodies are radiolucent. Inspiratory and expiratory films should be attempted. Hyperinflation of the lung is seen on the chest radiograph during exhalation when a foreign body is present. The alternative approach is to request both right and left lateral decubitus radiographs. In the decubitus position, there should usually be relative pulmonary volume loss. However, when in the decubitus position on the side where the foreign body has lodged, this expected volume loss will be absent.

2. **(C)** If the child cannot cooperate with the requested CXR or the result is not helpful, airway fluoroscopy is the next test to be performed. With airway fluoroscopy, obstruction of the airway on exhalation is frequently visible; the most common abnormality to be seen is hyperinflation of the lung segment remote from the aspiration.

3. **(B)** More than 50% of children who have an airway foreign body have a normal CXR. So a normal radiograph does not exclude this diagnosis.

4. **(A)** A variety of foreign bodies have been aspirated by children. In 2004, the most commonly aspirated material were small foods such as peanuts.

5. **(D)** Lethal foreign bodies are most often balloon-like substances such as latex balloons.

6. **(C)** The most common esophageal foreign body in children is the penny. On the floor, the lost coin

is readily available for the exploring hand and mouth of a small child. Apparently the penny is not so valuable as to encourage adults to remove them from the floor when dropped. In fact, there has been discussion among pediatric political action groups to suggest that the penny be designated a public health hazard and eliminated.

7. **(C)** If one suspects a tracheal or bronchial foreign body, the prudent therapeutic intervention is a trip to the operating room. A pediatric anesthesiologist and otolaryngologist should be present. The child should be anesthetized but spontaneously breathing. A flexible or rigid bronchoscope should then be introduced into the airway. The flexible bronchoscope may allow simpler visualization of the airway but is rarely sufficient to retrieve the foreign body. Introduction of a rigid bronchoscope into a small child is almost always required for the removal of the foreign body such as a peanut.

8. **(C)** If an esophageal foreign body is suspected, the urgency to move to the operating room is significantly reduced. An esophageal foreign body often lodges at the cricopharyngeal muscle, the narrowest portion of the esophagus. An object lodged high in the esophagus may be easily aspirated into the airway. Retrieval of esophageal foreign bodies should occur in the operating room, not in the emergency room. There is no role for the use of a balloon catheter to remove an esophageal foreign body in a child. A clinician can worsen the situation if this is attempted. With inadvertent movement of the foreign body into a position obstructing the larynx, a non–life-threatening situation changes into a life-threatening event. When the trachea or larynx is completely obstructed, the Heimlich maneuver can be lifesaving even in a small child.

9. **(B)** Batteries lodged within the esophagus may rapidly produce perforation with life-threatening sequelae. The current generated from the battery and mucosal surface of the esophagus produces sodium hydroxide, which leads to liquefactive necrosis of the tissue, resulting in perforation. Therefore, this situation requires urgent endoscopy for removal.

10. **(B)** Near or total airway obstruction should be treated with a Heimlich maneuver first in older children. In infants a combination of back blows and chest thrusts is recommended. Use of finger-sweep to remove the object from the airway may cause the object to become more deeply lodged and should not be used. If a patent airway cannot be obtained, additional life support may be necessary.

11. **(D)** The anatomy of the upper airway in a small child is significantly different from that of the adult. The cartilage is much less sturdy and therefore much more compressible. The airway in its entirety is smaller, with the narrowest portion at the cricoid ring until the age of 8 years. This is distinguished from the adult airway where the narrowest portion is the vocal cords. In a small child, tracheal foreign bodies are most likely lodged at the cricoid ring. This is a life-threatening emergency. An aspirated tracheal foreign body will be below the level of the vocal cords in the child, well out of sight of an examiner performing direct laryngoscopy. In an adult, a foreign body lodged in the glottis is quite visible on plain direct laryngoscopy. Should the foreign body be small enough to move through the trachea to the mainstem bronchi, either bronchus is vulnerable. Not until the child is approximately 8 years of age, when the anatomy of the airway approximates that of an adult, does the left mainstem bronchus acquire a more acute angle. The development of the aortic knob creates this angle. Therefore in the older child and adult, an aspirated foreign body usually enters the right mainstem bronchus while in childhood, either bronchus is equally available.

12. **(C)** While the narrowest portion of a child's airway is at the level of cricoid ring, the narrowest portion of the esophagus is the level of the cricopharyngeus muscle. Therefore it is not unusual to find an esophageal foreign body fairly high in the esophagus. When a large esophageal foreign body is lodged at the level of the cricopharyngeus, significant airway compression can occur and airway symptoms may accompany dysphagia. A high esophageal foreign body is quite vulnerable to aspiration should an inappropriate attempt be made to remove that foreign body with a balloon-tipped catheter.

13. **(D)** A latex glove that has been inflated to assume the character of a balloon may be easily broken and aspirated, an event that can be lethal.

14. **(D)** Aspiration of foreign bodies by children remains a significant problem in the 21st century. Although deaths by aspiration have decreased significantly since legislation has mandated the labeling of toys appropriate for age, mechanical suffocation still accounts for 5% of all unintentional deaths among children in the United States. Almost without exception, the clinical history of a child with foreign body aspiration is marked by an acute choking episode followed by coughing, wheezing, and stridor.

Acquisition of this history mandates the clinician to pursue the possibility of a foreign body aspiration. The child frequently presents with cough and tachypnea with diminished breath sounds, wheezing, stridor, shortness of breath, and retractions. The acute onset of wheezing is the signature of an intrathoracic airway obstruction. The symptoms associated with the foreign body often hints at its location. If the aspirated foreign body is extrathoracic, stridor will predominate; if it is intrathoracic, wheezing will predominate. Once the airway has been significantly comprised, biphasic stridor will be apparent. Of note, an esophageal foreign body can also present with stridor because of compression of the extrathoracic airway. Pneumothorax and esophageal perforation have been reported with esophageal foreign body aspiration. The high likelihood of significant complications combined with the relative low morbidity and mortality associated with an intra-operative examination of the upper airway and upper esophagus mandates that the clinician proceed to the operating room when there is a significant suspicion of an aspirated foreign body. A rate of 10% to 15% for negative bronchoscopy and esophagoscopy is acceptable when compared with the risk of missing an aspirated foreign body and the consequences of recurrent pneumonia, bronchiectasis, and even death.

SUGGESTED READING

Harris CS, Baker SP, Smith GA, et al: Childhood asphyxiation by food. A national analysis and overview. *JAMA* 251(17):2231–2235, 1984.

Rimell FL, Thome A, Stool S, et al: Characteristics of objects that cause choking in children. *JAMA* 274(22): 1763–1766, 1995.

Hambidge SJ, Wong S: Index of suspicion. *Pediatr Rev* 23(3):95–100, 2002.

CASE 11: A 3-YEAR-OLD GIRL WITH HYPOXIA AND A HISTORY OF HOARSENESS

A 3-year-old girl presents to the emergency room with hypoxia and increased work of breathing. Her family has recently moved and you are seeing her for the first time. She has spastic cerebral palsy and the cognitive development of a 6-month-old. She has had regular health care and her immunizations are up to date. On presentation she clearly has a hoarse voice and cry that her mother reports have been present since the age of 1 year. The mother also reports that her child drools continually. As a young infant she "spit up" but that resolved by age 6 months. Other than two episodes of "pneumonia" she has been healthy. Neither episode of pneumonia required hospitalization. Her previous pediatrician had reassured the family that her voice was "normal."

On physical exam, she is small and appears chronically undernourished. Her heart rate is 120, respiratory rate 42. She is febrile to 39°C and has a room air O_2 saturation of 84%. The only other significant physical findings are hoarse voice, coarse bilateral breath sounds, and moderate intercostal retractions.

SELECT THE ONE BEST ANSWER

1. What is the next diagnostic procedure indicated?

   (A) a throat culture
   (B) CXR
   (C) ultrasound of the neck
   (D) nasopharyngeal aspirate for viral DFAs

2. The first therapeutic intervention appropriate for this child is:

   (A) supplemental oxygen
   (B) albuterol nebulizer treatment
   (C) intravenous antibiotics
   (D) racemic epinephrine

3. The CXR reveals a right lower lobe infiltrate. The appropriate next intervention is:

   (A) postural drainage
   (B) bronchial lavage and culture

(C) intravenous clindamycin and ceftriaxone

(D) thoracentesis for culture and Gram stain

4. The child deteriorates and requires endotracheal intubation. The best indicator of the need for mechanical ventilation in this patient is:

(A) severe increased work of breathing

(B) abnormal blood gas analysis

(C) pulse oximeter reading of 92% on simple face mask oxygen

(D) failure of the child to respond to verbal commands

5. Once on mechanical ventilation, the patient's CXR progresses to now reveal infiltrates in all lung fields. Her oxygen requirement has also increased and the ventilator is providing 100% oxygen and a PEEP of 5 to maintain a saturation of 89%. The strategy to improve oxygenation most likely to work is:

(A) increase her tidal volume

(B) increase the respiratory rate

(C) increase the PEEP

(D) administer surfactant in her endotracheal tube

6. In spite of your best efforts to improve gas exchange on mechanical ventilation, the child continues to worsen. Her ABG on 100% oxygen, PEEP 15, tidal volume 12 mL/kg is pH: 7.29, P_{CO_2}: 66, P_{O_2}: 55. The blood gas represents a:

(A) a metabolic alkalosis

(B) a metabolic acidosis

(C) a respiratory alkalosis

(D) a respiratory acidosis

7. Given the clinical scenario in question 6, your next intervention is:

(A) do nothing as the patient is stable

(B) turn the patient prone and see if you can wean the FiO_2

(C) place prophylactic chest tubes because the risk of pneumothorax is large at a PEEP of 15

(D) bronchoalveolar lavage for removal of bronchial debris

8. The lung injury from a mechanical ventilator is seen most often in which condition?

(A) the use of 50% FiO_2

(B) delivery of a tidal volume in excess of 8 mL/kg

(C) the use of 15 cm PEEP

(D) a consistent peak airway pressure of 30 cm H_2O

9. If conventional mechanical ventilation fails in acute hypoxic respiratory failure beyond the neonatal period, options include:

(A) the oscillator

(B) the Thera vest

(C) the use of BiPAP

(D) the use of extracorporeal CO_2 removal

10. Adjuncts to conventional therapy for acute hypoxic respiratory failure include all of the following except:

(A) nitric oxide

(B) surfactant

(C) ECMO

(D) heliox

11. All cultures in this child are negative. The tracheal aspirate however is positive for lipid-laden macrophages, leading you to a diagnosis of:

(A) aspiration

(B) toxic shock

(C) viral pneumonia

(D) *Mycoplasma* infection

12. The history of hoarseness in this child is:

(A) not relevant as it is a normal finding

(B) leads you to be more suspicious of aspiration and GERD

(C) makes the diagnosis of *Mycoplasma* infection more likely because of its indolent course

(D) is a distinct clinical entity that is most likely unrelated to the more acute event

13. After this child recovers, what, if anything, would the next appropriate diagnostic test be?

(A) The next appropriate test would be a pH probe.

(B) The next appropriate test would be nothing, as the child has now recovered from a viral illness.

(C) The next appropriate test would be a chest CT scan to evaluate for chronic lung disease.

(D) The next appropriate test would be a cardiac catheterization to evaluate pulmonary artery pressures.

14. The residual lung dysfunction following acute hypoxic respiratory failure is:

(A) exercise intolerance/reactive airways disease
(B) chronic cough
(C) increased diffusion capacity
(D) sleep disordered breathing

15. Untreated GERD can lead to:

(A) chronic obstructive lung disease
(B) esophageal dysplasia
(C) vocal cord nodules
(D) all of the above

Answers

1. **(B)** This child is in respiratory distress. A CXR is the initial procedure that needs to be done. The history illustrates a neurologically disabled child at high risk for reflux and aspiration of oral or GI flora. After the radiograph is performed, it would be reasonable to obtain viral or bacterial studies to determine an infectious etiology.

2. **(A)** Supplemental oxygen should be the first intervention as she has a room air O_2 saturation of 84%. Additional therapies may be administered after oxygen is started.

3. **(C)** This child presents with a history of hoarseness and respiratory distress followed by respiratory failure, likely caused by aspiration pneumonitis. Antibiotics used to treat this event should cover oral flora including gram-positive and anaerobic organisms. If this child's respiratory failure progresses and she requires intubation, a bronchial lavage may help in the diagnosis.

4. **(A)** This child progressed to acute hypoxic respiratory insufficiency (AHRF), a complex diagnosis with many etiologies. The best indicator of the need for mechanical ventilation is a marked increase work of breathing. Blood gas analysis can be useful but the need for mechanical ventilation is largely based on clinical assessment.

5. **(C)** While supported with mechanical ventilation, oxygenation is enhanced or improved by increasing the inspired concentration of oxygen (FiO_2), the PEEP, and/or the inspiratory time. Improved ventilation, i.e., enhanced removal of carbon dioxide, can be accomplished by increases in tidal volume and/or minute ventilation. This is achieved in volume mode ventilation by increasing tidal volume, and in pressure mode ventilation by increasing peak inflation pressure. In either mode, the respiratory rate can be increased to enhance minute ventilation and CO_2 removal.

6. **(D)** The blood gas presented represents a respiratory acidosis but not a profound one. In order to avoid the complications of mechanical ventilation, one could argue that in significant respiratory disease, permissive hypercapnia, or the acceptance of modest elevation of PCO_2 and acidosis, (pH ≥7.25) is acceptable.

7. **(B)** This child requires 100% oxygen to remain relatively well saturated in her current state. She is already on significant PEEP, but her inspiratory time could be increased. Additionally, the patient could be turned to the prone position to augment oxygenation and facilitate reduction of FiO_2, if that is not possible in the supine position. One hundred percent oxygen is likely to result in oxygen toxicity and is not recommended. Generally, a PaO_2 >50 mm Hg is acceptable and the FiO_2 should be reduced. If the patient has a shunt lesion, the inspired FiO_2 will have a lesser impact on oxygenation. It is likely that an acceptable arterial PaO_2 could be achieved with less inspired oxygen.

8. **(B)** The goal of mechanical ventilation should be gas exchange that is acceptable if not normal, especially when ventilatory support parameters accelerate to the point at which they are toxic themselves. Recent advances in the understanding of ventilator-associated lung injury in the adult have been applied to children with significant pulmonary disease. In these children, it is important to reduce tidal volumes to ≤6 to 8 mL/kg, to use PEEP to reduce FiO_2 to <60%, and to employ a

long inspiratory time. Although AHRF is a significant cause of morbidity in the intensive care unit, it is rarely the primary cause of mortality. In general, patients who have hypoxic respiratory failure succumb from the other failed organ system(s) that accompany this particular insult.

9. **(A)** When there is consolidation, areas of the lung are perfused but not ventilated. Despite exposure to 100% oxygen, venous admixture will persist in the unventilated lung. Although the patient remains relatively desaturated, the impact of FiO_2 will not be linear. Therefore, it is imperative to protect the patient from toxic oxygen exposure (>60% FiO_2). In the patient with persistent AHRF, high-frequency oscillatory ventilation has been useful, as have nitric oxide, surfactant, and ECMO. As a substitute for conventional mechanical ventilation, the oscillator has been perhaps the most useful of these strategies. BiPAP, or noninvasive mechanical ventilation, can also be used to supply positive pressure to support patients with less severe disease.

10. **(D)** Heliox is a mixture of helium and oxygen. Helium is less dense than oxygen and when mixed together improves the flow characteristics of gas in patients with airway obstruction. Unfortunately, to achieve the beneficial flow characteristics, the helium must be present at ≥60% and thus, the maximum FiO_2 is limited to 40%. A higher FiO_2 is usually desired in acute hypoxic respiratory failure.

11. **(A)** Lipid-laden macrophages discovered in her endotracheal aspirate confirm the suspicion of reflux disease and aspiration.

12. **(B)** This child presents to the clinician as a neurologically impaired child with respiratory insufficiency. Her initial evaluation should have led one to suspect GERD, as hoarseness in a child is not a "normal" finding. The hoarseness could be the result of vocal cord disturbances, either physiologic or anatomic. However, a more common scenario in an impaired 3-year-old who develops persistent hoarseness is undetected GERD.

13. **(A)** Following her recovery, this child will require a full evaluation. GERD is particularly

common in infants. At 4 months of age, it is present in 50% to 70% of infants, but typically resolves by 1 year of age. A minority of infants go on to develop other symptoms, including dysphagia, arching of the back during feedings, refusal to eat, and failure to thrive. GERD can also be a cause for an acute life-threatening event (ALTE), stridor, chronic cough, recurrent pneumonia, reactive airway disease, and hoarseness. In preschool children, GERD presents with intermittent vomiting and symptoms of esophagitis. In older children and adolescents, the cardinal symptom is chronic heartburn or regurgitation. Hoarseness, asthma, chronic cough, and chronic esophagitis may also occur. Significant GERD can be severe enough to waken patients from sleep, may be exacerbated by emotional stress, and usually is postprandial.

In the child with GERD, the assessment and treatment recommendations are summarized as follows:

- For the infant with recurrent vomiting, the history and physical examination are sufficient to make the diagnosis of GERD. Further testing is not necessary, particularly in children in whom growth is uninterrupted. Reassurance and thickening of feeds may be all that is necessary.
- In the neonate and infant with recurrent vomiting and poor weight gain, a comprehensive investigation for other causes of vomiting and failure to thrive is indicated. An upper GI series to rule out anatomic abnormalities that would result in vomiting and an upper endoscopy are recommended.
- In a child or adolescent with vomiting and heartburn, an upper GI series or upper tract endoscopy is indicated followed by lifestyle changes: food restrictions, weight loss, smoking cessation, and so on. This patient may also require a trial of medication to reduce acid production.
- In children with apnea or ALTE, a pH probe is the diagnostic intervention of choice. In fact, in ALL ages, a pH probe, properly done, is the "gold standard" of diagnosis.

14. **(A)** Long-term health issues in survivors of acute hypoxic respiratory failure include poor exercise

tolerance, difficulty in return to work or school, and persistent symptoms of small airway obstruction or reactive airway disease.

15. **(D)** Untreated, GERD can lead to a significant chronic obstructive lung disease, bronchiectasis, esophageal dysphasia, and ultimately esophageal carcinoma. Treatment of significant GERD begins with medical management: in a 2- to 4-week trial using H$_2$ blockers or PPIs. Should the medical management trial be unsuccessful or if the child suffers severely from GERD with respiratory insufficiency, surgical intervention may well be necessary. The most commonly performed operation is a Nissen fundoplication, which now can be done using a laproscopic approach with minimal perioperative risk. Restriction of the size of the lower esophageal sphincter can be done endoscopically using radiofrequency ablation (the Stretta system). This procedure is common in adults and is increasingly performed in children. It is particularly useful in the high–surgical risk child with GERD.

SUGGESTED READING

Hrabovsky EE, Mullett MD: Gastroesophageal reflux and the premature infant. *J Pediatr Surg* 21(7)583:587, 1986.

St. Cyr JA, Ferra TB, Thompson TR, et al: Nissen fundoplication for gastroesophageal reflux in infants. *J Cardiovascular Surg* 92(4):661–666, 1986.

Herbst JJ, Minton SD, Book LSL: Gastroesophageal reflex causing respiratory distress and apnea in newborn infants. *J Pediatr* 95(5)part 1:763–768, 1979.

Vecchia LKD, Grosfeld JL, West KW, et al: Reoperation after Nissen fundoplication in children with gastroesophageal reflux. *Annals of Surg* 226(3):315–323, 1997.

DiMarino M, Rattan S: Pathophysiology of gastroesophageal reflux disease. *Resid Staff Physician* 49(6):12–16, 2003.

CASE 12: A 16-YEAR-OLD BOY WITH VERY HIGH BODY TEMPERATURE

A 16-year-old boy is brought to the emergency room by EMS with a temperature of 42°C and seizure activity. He was transferred from a surgery center at 9 AM following dental extractions, for which he had received a brief general anesthetic and was in the recovery room when he became febrile and hemodynamically unstable. He has a cardiac rhythm with a pulse, but is making little respiratory effort. Prior to his arrival he was intubated and IV access established. He was given a dose of lorazepam before transport. The past history is remarkable for depression for which he takes phenelzine, a MAO inhibitor. Drug use was denied by his parents.

On physical exam the boy is unresponsive. His vital signs are: BP: 150/86, P: 140 RR: 22 (hand ventilation) T: 42.5°C. Auscultation of the chest revealed normal breath sounds. The rhythm is sinus tachycardia, with peaked T waves. There are no murmurs. The only other part of the physical examination that is abnormal is the neurologic exam. The boy remains unresponsive to pain or voice. His pupils are 4 mm bilaterally, symmetric, and reactive to light. Muscle tone is increased with generalized hyperreflexia and myoclonus.

SELECT THE ONE BEST ANSWER

1. The intervention least likely to be useful acutely in this setting is:

   (A) obtaining a complete blood count and differential
   (B) obtaining blood and urine samples for toxicology
   (C) obtaining an ECG
   (D) obtaining a blood gas, serum electrolytes, and a CK

2. The results of the blood gas are as follows: pH: 7.07, PCO_2: 74, PO_2: 98, BE: –8. This is best described as a:

   (A) respiratory acidosis and metabolic alkalosis
   (B) metabolic acidosis with respiratory compensation
   (C) mixed acidosis
   (D) mixed alkalosis

3. The diagnosis of malignant hyperthermia is supported by all of the following except:

   (A) hyperkalemia
   (B) CK elevation
   (C) acidosis
   (D) hypocarbia

4. Malignant hyperthermia is treated by:

   (A) external cooling
   (B) mannitol

(C) dantrolene

(D) all of the above

5. Malignant hyperthermia is best characterized as:

(A) a genetic disorder of calcium metabolism

(B) an allergic drug reaction

(C) a disorder of temperature regulation

(D) an increase of the hypothalamic temperature set point

6. The drug screen is positive for amphetamines. The street drug likely to be responsible for this is:

(A) "Crack"

(B) OxyContin

(C) Ecstasy

(D) cannabis

7. Prior to his deterioration in the recovery room, the child received an anesthetic with isoflurane, nitrous oxide, cisatracurium, and meperidine to have his teeth removed. With the drug screen positive for amphetamines, the following must be considered in the differential diagnosis:

(A) seizures and postictal state

(B) neuroleptic malignant syndrome

(C) central serotonin syndrome

(D) all of the above

8. The increased synaptic release of serotonin can be as a result of which drug in this case scenario:

(A) meperidine

(B) nitrous oxide

(C) methamphetamine

(D) lorazepam

9. The other agent in this clinical condition that affects serotonin pharmacology is:

(A) isoflurane

(B) cisatracurium

(C) phenelzine

(D) lorazepam

10. In the case of neuroleptic malignant syndrome (NMS), the neurotransmitter implicated is:

(A) epinephrine

(B) norepinephrine

(C) serotonin

(D) dopamine

11. The symptoms that are more common in the NMS than in the central serotonin syndrome include all of the following except:

(A) hyperthermia

(B) altered mental status

(C) muscle rigidity

(D) myoclonus

12. Drugs implicated in the central serotonin syndrome include the following except:

(A) dextromethorphan

(B) MAO inhibitors

(C) SSRIs

(D) acetaminophen with codeine

13. Mortality of central serotonin syndrome is:

(A) <20%

(B) 20%–40%

(C) 40%–50%

(D) >50%

14. Treatment of central serotonin syndrome includes the following except:

(A) cyproheptadine

(B) propanolol

(C) mannitol

(D) phenoxybenzamine

15. In neuroleptic malignant syndrome, treatment includes the following except:

(A) bromocriptine

(B) dantrolene

(C) chlorpromazine

(D) mannitol

Answers

1. (A) Hyperthermia is defined as an elevation of core body temperature above 37.5°C. In contrast to fever, which is a cytokine-activated inflammatory response, hyperthermia is a failure of thermoregulation. Obviously, in the child who presents with an elevated temperature, it is frequently not clear whether you are dealing with an inflammatory fever or with a hyperthermic state. Given the absence of a history of inflammatory or infectious disease of any kind, the child described in the case scenario should be presumed to have a hyperthermic state related to one of the medications he received during his medical care or, perhaps, to a medication he ingested himself. In the case described, the appropriate initial interventions as always are the ABCs of urgent care. The patient needs a patent airway, adequate respirations, and hemodynamic stability. After stabilization, there are a number of laboratory tests that are required including an ECG. In all the hyperthermic states, it is likely that the patient will have a mixed acidosis. Elevation of muscle enzymes significant enough to cause renal insufficiency, and increased serum concentrations of both potassium and phosphate are also likely present. These aberrations are largely the result of muscle membrane injury, the subsequent release of intracellular contents, and the hemodynamic challenge of significant hyperthermia. Emergency treatment must be focused on the distinct possibility of life-threatening dysrhythmias from acidosis and hyperkalemia.

2. **(C)** When there is an acute change in PCO_2 of 10, the pH will change by 0.08 in the opposite direction. In other words, the pH will fall as the PCO_2 rises. The acidosis or alkalosis present is purely respiratory if all changes are explained by changes in the PCO_2. For a change in base excess of 10 mEq/L, the pH will change by 0.15 in the same direction. If all changes are explained by a change in the base excess, then the process is entirely metabolic.

   Assuming a normal blood gas of 7.40, PCO_2 40, PO_2 100, BE 0, in the case presented, the PCO_2 is approximately 35 above the normal PCO_2. Divided by 10 and multiplied by 0.08, one would expect the pH to be 0.28 lower than the normal of 7.40, or 7.12. In this case, the pH is 7.07 with a base deficit of −10 and a metabolic acidosis is also present.

3. **(D)** Given the proximity of this event to a general anesthetic, the first cause of hyperthermia to be considered is malignant hyperthermia (MH). Early clinical findings in MH include masseter muscle spasms, generalized muscle rigidity, sinus tachycardia, increase in CO_2 production leading to hypercarbia, and elevation in body temperature. Hemodynamic instability, electrolyte abnormalities, and disseminated intravascular coagulation occur later. Appropriately treated, MH has a mortality that is <5% (see Table 12-1).

4. **(D)** Appropriate intervention in a patient with suspected or proven MH is immediate cessation of the ongoing anesthetic, aggressive external and internal cooling, and the intravenous administration of dantrolene. Dantrolene is a drug that interferes with calcium release from the sarcoplasmic reticulum and will put an end to the metabolic abnormality. Since rhabdomyolysis, which may result in acute renal failure is very common in this disorder, treatment with hydration, bicarbonate to alkalinize the urine followed by diuresis induced by mannitol is also recommended. Ultimately, after doses of dantrolene are given, the treatment of MH is supportive.

5. **(A)** MH is a rare genetic disorder associated with the administration of a variety of anesthetic agents, particularly the depolarizing muscle relaxant succinylcholine and volatile anesthetic gases. In approximately half of the cases identified, MH is inherited in an autosomal dominant fashion. In the remainder of the cases that occur, inheritance is variable. When exposed to a triggering anesthetic, susceptible patients have the uncontrolled release of calcium from their sarcoplasmic reticulum. This torrential release of calcium results in a marked increased in skeletal muscle metabolism and heat production.

   Once the episode has resolved and the patient has recovered, it is suggested that the patient and his first-degree relatives be evaluated for this diagnosis. The diagnosis requires a muscle biopsy, which should be done at a certified MH center. Abnormal augmentation of muscle contraction following treatment of the biopsy specimen with halothane or caffeine is diagnostic. A variety of MH centers are located across the country and can be accessed by calling the Malignant Hyperthermia Hotline (1-800-MH-HYPER/644-9737).

6. **(C)** In the development of this case scenario it becomes apparent that this child has a drug screen that is positive for amphetamines. The commonly used street drug responsible for this is

Table 12-1.

	Malignant Hyperthermia	Central Serotonin Syndrome	Neuroleptic Malignant Syndrome
Inducing agents			
Amphetamines (include Ecstasy)		X	
Bromocriptine		X	
Chlorpromazine			X
Clozapine			X
Cocaine		X	
Depolarizing muscle relaxants (succinylcholine)	X		
Dextromethorphan		X	
Fluphenazine			X
Haloperidol			X
Levodopa or carbidopa		X	X (withdrawal)
Lithium		X	X
LSD		X	
MAOs		X	
Meperidine		X	
Metoclopramide			X
Phenergan			X
Risperidone			X
SSRIs and SRIs		X	
TCAs		X	
Tryptophan		X	
Volatile anesthetics	X		
Symptoms			
Diarrhea		X	
Dysrhythmia	X	X	X
DIC	X	X	X
Fever	X	X	X
Hypercarbia	X		X
Hyperreflexia	X	X	X
Hypertension	X	X	X
Hypertonia/rigidity	X	X	X
Hypotension	X		X
Mental status change	X	X	X
Metabolic acidosis	X		X
Myoclonus		X	
Nausea and vomiting		X	
Rhabdomyolysis	X	X	X
Seizure		X	X
Tremor		X	X
Trismus	X	X	
Treatment			
Amantadine			X
Antipyretics	X	X	X
Bromocriptine			X*
Chlorpromazine		X*	
Cyproheptadine		X	
Dantrolene	X	±	X
Levodopa or carbidopa			X
Mannitol	X	X	X
Propranolol		±	

* These medications may predispose to another syndrome.

ecstasy. Ecstasy is a methamphetamine derivative that significantly impacts the physiology of the human nervous system by alterations in serotonin metabolism.

7. **(D)** Important causes of severe hyperthermia (>40°C temperature), not related to infectious disease, are environmental exposure, hypothalamic injury, central serotonin syndrome, MH, and neuroleptic malignant syndrome (see Table 12-1). The clinical symptoms associated with these syndromes overlap significantly. Each of these conditions can be associated with multisystem complications and each can result in death. For central serotonin syndrome to be diagnosed there needs to be an appropriate history of ingestion of medication that contributes to an increase in serotonin in the CNS. Additionally, the patient must have at least three of the following: mental status changes, agitation, myoclonus, muscle rigidity, hyperreflexia, diaphoresis, shivering or tremor, diarrhea, incoordination, and fever.

8. **(C)** In general, amphetamines increase release of serotonin at neuronal synapses in the CNS, but they also cause inhibition of serotonin reuptake and breakdown at these synapses. The resultant excess serotonin present in the CNS results in a constellation of symptoms that have come to be recognized as CSS.

9. **(C)** Complicating serotonin physiology in this child is the presence of a MAO inhibitor that the patient takes on a chronic basis for depression. MAO inhibitors also prevent the breakdown of serotonin, producing excess CNS serotonin.

10. **(D)** The neurotransmitter responsible for NMS is dopamine. Blockade of dopamine receptors within the basal ganglia is believed to precipitate symptoms. More than 25 different agents have been incriminated in the precipitation of NMS. The most commonly implicated are neuroleptic agents such as haloperidol, the withdrawal of dopamine agonists, e.g. L-dopa, other antipsychotic agents such as chlorpromazine and fluphenazine, and the narcotic agonist, meperidine.

11. **(D)** NMS is another drug-induced hyperthermic state that can be confused with central serotonin syndrome. When compared with central serotonin syndrome, patients with NMS are likely to have had gradual onset of symptoms and are less likely to have myoclonus and hyperreflexia. Rigidity found in NMS is more severe than in CSS, but the remainder of the clinical scenario may look much the same.

12. **(D)** Other agents have been reported to precipitate central serotonin syndrome and include cocaine, L-dopa, lithium, LSD, dextromethorphan, tricyclic antidepressants, serotonin reuptake inhibitors (SRIs), and SSRIs. SRIs are commonly prescribed in pediatric depression making CSS a syndrome that should be well understood by pediatric practitioners. See Answer #9.

13. **(A)** The mortality should be <20% assuming the patient arrives at a hospital and receives appropriate intervention.

14. **(D)** Although producing overlapping syndromes, treatment for these three disorders differs. For CSS, symptomatic treatment is appropriate. Dantrolene use has been reported only in isolated cases and may be useful. It also may be appropriate to consider the administration of an anti-serotonin medication. Both propanolol and cyproheptadine block serotonin activity at the postsynaptic receptor. It is possible that these drugs may be useful but this utility is supported only by case reports.

In both CSS and NMS, it is important to identify the offending agent and eliminate it from the patient's medication regimen. With respect to MH, the anesthetic will have been discontinued prior to your involvement in the case and your participation will be to help provide supportive care in an intensive care unit setting. While all of these syndromes pose a threat to life, the mortality of each of these syndromes should be well under 20% when appropriately treated. The key to successful intervention in life-threatening drug-induced hyperthermia is the prompt recognition and elimination of the drug that might have triggered such a response and careful multiorgan supportive care.

15. **(C)** Therapy for MH relies heavily on the medication dantrolene while treatment of NMS is

largely symptomatic; however, it also can improve with dantrolene and bromocriptine.

SUGGESTED READING

Arnold DH: The central serotonin syndrome: paradigm for psychotherapeutic misadventure. *Pediatr Rev* 23(12):427–432, 2002.

Rosenberg MR, Green M: Neuroleptic malignant syndrome. Review of response to therapy. *Arch Intern Med* 149:1927–1931, 1989.

CASE 13: A 4-YEAR-OLD GIRL WITH SNORING

A 4-year-old girl is brought in for a routine physical examination. Her family recently moved and this is their first visit. She has had regular health care and her immunizations are up to date. She snores with sleep and her mother allows her to sleep with her so that she can "listen to her breathe." The mother reports she worries because her daughter's breathing is often irregular with sleep and seems to pause. She is the youngest of five siblings and none of her other children breathes as this child does. Other than two episodes of "strep throat" she has not really been ill. Her previous pediatrician had reassured the family that snoring was common and normal in children.

On physical exam, she appears small for her age. She is less than the 5th percentile for height and weight. Her head circumference is 50th percentile for age. Her entire physical examination, absent the growth parameters, is normal with the exception of moderate tonsillar hypertrophy. Her developmental assessment is normal.

SELECT THE ONE BEST ANSWER

1. It is likely that the following symptom is also prominent:

   (A) encopresis
   (B) poor attention span
   (C) echolalia
   (D) dysphagia

2. Which is not true about sleep in children?

   (A) functional residual capacity falls
   (B) upper airway resistance doubles
   (C) breathing is not erratic during REM sleep, but is erratic during non-REM periods
   (D) ventilatory drive is decreased from the awake state

3. Spontaneous arousal is a potent defense against sleep-disordered breathing. Which of the following is true about sleep arousals in children?

   (A) Children have a lower threshold for arousal than adults.
   (B) Moderate hypoxia is the most potent stimulus for arousal in infants during sleep.
   (C) Hypercapnia and increased upper airway resistance is more potent than hypoxemia at stimulating sleep arousals in preschool children.
   (D) The sleep arousal index in infants is the same as it is in adolescents.

4. Central apnea in preschool children is significant if:

   (A) it exceeds 10 seconds
   (B) it exceeds 15 seconds
   (C) it exceeds 20 seconds
   (D) it exceeds 30 seconds

5. Which is true about central apnea in children?

   (A) Central apnea is common in children.
   (B) Central apnea is significant only if it is associated with bradycardia.
   (C) Obstructive apnea is more common than central apnea in normal children.
   (D) Apnea associated with transient desaturation is always pathologic in children.

6. Children with obstructive sleep apnea (OSA) differ from adults in that:

   (A) children with OSA are more likely to be obese
   (B) children with OSA are more likely to have sleep arousal and therefore have more daytime sleepiness than adults
   (C) children with OSA are more likely to have REM sleep apnea while adults have apnea with non-REM sleep
   (D) children with OSA do not suffer the cardiopulmonary insult that adults do

7. Complications of OSA in children include:

   (A) neurocognitive defects
   (B) systemic hypertension
   (C) congestive heart failure
   (D) all of the above

8. What is the next diagnostic procedure indicated?

   (A) The next step is a strep screen.
   (B) The next step is polysomnography.
   (C) The next step is an ultrasound of the neck.
   (D) The next step is a nasopharyngeal aspirate for viral DFA screens.

9. The treatment of OSA in children usually begins in children with:

   (A) nighttime oxygen supplementation
   (B) nighttime mechanical ventilation
   (C) tonsillectomy and adenoidectomy
   (D) calorie reduction diet aimed at 15% reduction in body weight

10. The child with snoring:

    (A) is always at risk for OSA
    (B) rarely has OSA
    (C) always requires surgical intervention with tonsillectomy
    (D) Should always be evaluated by polysomnography

11. A tonsillectomy in a patient with OSA is characterized by:

    (A) increased risk of postoperative respiratory failure as compared to a tonsillectomy in the same age patient with no OSA
    (B) immediate improvement of airway symptoms
    (C) increased risk of postoperative bleeding as compared to a tonsillectomy in the same age patient with no OSA
    (D) all of the above

12. Appropriate anesthetic care of a child with OSA for tonsillectomy should omit:

    (A) muscle relaxants
    (B) volatile agents
    (C) nitrous oxide
    (D) nonsteroidal anti-inflammatory agents

13. Appropriate immediate post operative care from tonsillectomy for the child younger than 2 years of age with significant OSA is:

    (A) short stay unit observation for 6 hours after surgery
    (B) discharge to home from the recovery room after the child demonstrates the ability to drink
    (C) admission to the hospital for 24 hours of cardiorespiratory monitoring
    (D) all of the above

14. The risk of postoperative bleeding is highest:

    (A) on post-op day 1 or 2
    (B) at the end of the first week post-op
    (C) on post-op day 2 or 3
    (D) for the entire first post-op week

Answers

1. **(B)** Symptoms of OSA in a child are different from those in an adult. When one compares the child with OSA with the adult, the child frequently also has failure to thrive. In children there are often other concomitant symptoms such as enuresis, behavior abnormalities, and attention deficit disorder.

2. **(C)** During sleep, functional residual capacity falls, ventilatory drive is decreased from the awake state, and resistance in the upper airway is significantly increased.

3. **(C)** When compared with adults, children are less likely to have sleep arousal triggered by hypoxia, hypercapnia, or airway resistance. Hypercapnia and airway resistance are more potent stimuli for sleep arousals in children than is hypoxemia. Because sleep arousal is uncommon in children, daytime sleepiness is unusual in children with sleep-disordered breathing.

4. **(C)** Central apnea is considered significant when it exceeds 20 seconds or is accompanied by bradycardia. Of note, central and obstructive apnea may occur in the same patient.

5. **(A)** Central apnea is more common than obstructive apnea in children.

6. **(C)** The child with OSA is rarely an obese patient in contrast to the typical adult OSA patient. A child with OSA frequently also has failure to

thrive. In children, REM sleep is the most erratic phase of sleep and most sleep disorders occur during this phase. This is different from the adult in whom OSA occurs during non-REM sleep. Untreated OSA is a severe health problem and can result in the development of heart failure unresponsive to surgical or medical treatment and ultimately can result in death.

7. **(D)** Should the symptoms of OSA in children be overlooked, complications will occur. These include neurocognitive difficulties in school, systemic hypertension, and congestive heart failure, including cor pulmonale. The systemic and pulmonary hypertension that accompanies OSA is secondary to the chronic exposure of the pulmonary arterial circulation to hypercarbia and hypoxemia.

8. **(B)** Children with a significant history of snoring and periods of apnea during sleep should be fully evaluated for OSA with polysomnography. The polysomnogram will evaluate not only central apnea but obstructive apnea as well.

Sleep disorders are very common during childhood, occurring in 20% to 30% of children. They are generally a source of stress and sleeplessness for parents, and behavior issues as well as learning difficulties for the child. These difficulties are not necessarily accompanied by obstructive sleep apnea. A careful history of breathing disorders with sleep is indicated under these circumstances. Questions about the child's sleep should be asked, including: how long it takes him to fall asleep, the child's routine bedtime every night, the child's sleep location, and how much time there is between feeding and bedtime. Should the sleep abnormality be accompanied by significant airway symptoms, polysomnography should be performed in order to delineate the contribution of airway obstruction to the disorder of sleep. More commonly, disorders of sleep are related to emotional issues and disruption of either home or school and not to OSA.

9. **(C)** In a child, should the findings on polysomnography be significant, the first treatment option in a child almost without exception is a tonsillectomy and adenoidectomy.

The lymphoid tissue of the upper airway increases in mass until approximately age 12. Simultaneously there is a growth in the size of the upper airway. Between 2 and 8 years of age, the tonsils and adenoids are the largest in relation to the underlying airway, resulting in a relatively narrow upper airway. The prominence of the lymphoid tissue in the upper airway makes a significant contribution to airway obstruction during sleep in children. The prominence of the lymphoid tissue in children may often be responsible for the symptoms of OSA. Most children significantly improve with respect to the sleep pathology following tonsillectomy and adenoidectomy.

Should tonsillectomy and adenoidectomy not result in significant improvement in sleep-disordered breathing, further surgical intervention may be necessary. Uvulopalatoplasty is an uncommon surgical intervention in the child with OSA, particularly when compared with the adult patient. In OSA refractory to other interventions, tracheostomy may be required. Nonsurgical treatment for OSA is also a viable therapeutic alternative. However, the use of nighttime constant positive airway pressure (CPAP), common for adults with obstructive sleep apnea, is not approved for children (although it is used with some frequency). Further studies in children with OSA for interventions other than tonsillectomy and adenoidectomy are needed.

Most children with OSA are not obese in contrast to most adults. Therefore, a reduced-calorie diet is not indicated.

10. **(B)** Snoring is a relatively common complaint offered to the pediatrician. Only on rare occasions is snoring a clue to the diagnosis of OSA. In the case presented, the mother describes not only snoring, but also the irregularity of her child's breathing with sleep, and even occasional periods of apnea. Should the sleep abnormality be accompanied by significant airway symptoms as described in this child, polysomnography can determine the contribution of airway obstruction.

11. **(A)** In general, marked improvement does not occur immediately after the procedure, although there is some resolution in symptoms the first night after surgery. More improvement is seen as

the residual anesthetic agent is eliminated and procedure-related edema in the immediate perioperative period resolves.

Children with significant sleep apnea in the perioperative period may well have more apnea during the first 24 hours following tonsillectomy and adenoidectomy.

12. **(D)** NSAIDs enhance bleeding risk. These medications therefore should not be administered in the perioperative period.

13. **(C)** Children should be monitored in an ICU setting where respiratory expertise is immediately available. Perioperative desaturation is common in the child with concomitant craniofacial abnormality and in the child younger than 3 years.

14. **(B)** Bleeding following a tonsillectomy and adenoidectomy occurs commonly at the end of the first postoperative week if not in the first 6 hours after surgery.

SUGGESTED READING

Helfaer MA, McColley SA, Puzik PL, et al: Polysomnography after adenotonsillectomy in mild pediatric obstructive sleep apnea. *Crit Care Med* 24(8):1323–1327, 1996.

Marcus CL: Sleep-disordered breathing in children. *Am J Res Crit Care Med* 164:16–30, 2001.

Strollo PJ, Rogers RM: Obstructive sleep apnea. *Current Concepts* 334(2):99–104, 1996.

Munford RS, Pugin J: Normal responses to injury prevent systemic inflammation and can be immunosuppressive. *Am J Respir Crit Care Med* 163:316–321, 2001.

CASE 14: A 16-MONTH-OLD BOY WITH FEVER AND COUGH

A 16-month-old African-American boy presents to the emergency room with a 3-day history of fever and cough. He was well until 3 days ago when his mother reports that he began to cough and felt warm to touch. His temperature was 38.5°C. She gave him acetaminophen and put him to bed early. For the last 2 days he has not been hungry but continues to drink well. His fever has persisted despite antipyretics and is now 39°C. There have been no other symptoms, no sick contacts, and no travel history.

On physical exam, the child appears toxic but is well hydrated. The heart rate is 140, the respiratory rate is 52, and the oxygen saturation is 82% on room air. The only significant finding on examination is markedly decreased breath sounds over the right hemithorax. There is no adenopathy or hepatosplenomegaly.

A chest radiograph reveals an opacified right hemithorax with slight mediastinal shift to the left. The CBC shows 28,000 leukocytes with a significant bandemia.

SELECT THE ONE BEST ANSWER

1. What is the next diagnostic procedure indicated?

   (A) The next procedure should be a throat culture.
   (B) The next procedure should be a review of the blood smear.
   (C) The next procedure should be an ultrasound of the right hemithorax.
   (D) The next procedure should be a nasopharyngeal aspirate for viral DFA screens.

2. The appropriate first therapeutic intervention is:

   (A) administration of supplemental oxygen
   (B) acquisition of a blood gas
   (C) placement of a thoracostomy tube
   (D) urgent bronchoscopy

3. Of the following choices, the most appropriate antibiotic choice for this child is:

   (A) ampicillin and ceftriaxone
   (B) ceftriaxone and vancomycin
   (C) oxacillin and ceftazidime
   (D) ceftazidime and gentamicin

4. A large pleural effusion is identified and aspirated from the right hemithorax. Which of the following is indicative of an empyema?

   (A) An empyema is indicated by a pH 7.0, glucose 20 mg/dL, total protein 4 g/dL, WBC 20,000/mm^3, LDH > 1000 U/L.
   (B) An empyema is indicated by a pH 7.2, glucose 80 mg/dL, total protein 4 g/dL, WBC 1000/mm^3, LDH 585 U/L.
   (C) An empyema is indicated by a pH 7.3, glucose 60 mg/dL, total protein 4 g/dL, WBC 500/mm^3, LDH 348 U/L.

(D) An empyema is indicated by a pH 7.2, glucose 80 mg/dL, total protein 4 g/dL, WBC 5000/mm^3, LDH 475 U/L.

5. If an empyema is identified, the appropriate intervention is:

   (A) instillation of antibiotics into the pleural space
   (B) daily thoracentesis for 7 days
   (C) video-assisted thoracoscopy and decortication
   (D) instillation of chlorhexidine into the pleural space

6. If, after removal of the effusion, it is apparent that there is a 2-cm lung abscess, the appropriate therapy would be:

   (A) urgent surgical drainage
   (B) elective surgical drainage after antibiotic treatment for 5 days
   (C) prolonged parenteral antibiotics
   (D) interventional radiology-directed drainage of the abscess

7. How often is pleural effusion associated with bacterial pneumonia?

   (A) <20%
   (B) 20%–30%
   (C) 35%–50%
   (D) >50%

8. Which of the following statements is true?

   (A) All patients with a parapneumonic effusion require hospitalization.
   (B) All pleural effusions require thoracoscopy for resolution.
   (C) All parapneumonic effusions, if cultured, will be positive for pathogens.
   (D) Small parapneumonic effusions are generally benign and resolve without surgical intervention.

9. In this case, the comorbidity that most needs to be considered is:

   (A) HIV
   (B) sickle cell disease
   (C) congestive heart failure
   (D) hepatitis A

10. Which pathogen on the list below is the most likely to be implicated in this 16-month-old with a lung abscess?

    (A) *Chlamydia trachomatis*
    (B) *Moraxella catarrhalis*
    (C) *Staphylococcus aureus*
    (D) *Mycoplasma pneumoniae*

11. In the neonate, the most common pathogens associated with bacterial pneumonia of the choices below are:

    (A) group B Streptococcus and *Escherichia coli*
    (B) *H. influenzae* and *Listeria monocytogenes*
    (C) *L. monocytogenes* and group D Streptococcus
    (D) group D Streptococcus and group B Streptococcus

12. In the school-age child, the most likely pathogen in bacterial pneumonia with parapneumonic effusion is:

    (A) *H. influenzae*
    (B) *Staphylococcus aureus*
    (C) *Streptococcus pneumoniae*
    (D) *Neisseria meningitidis*

13. In the perioperative period after cardiac surgery, a pleural effusion sometimes occurs. A chylothorax would be most characterized by:

    (A) pH 7.1, protein 4 g/dL, glucose 25 mg/dL, WBCs: 2,000/mm^3, triglycerides: 86 mg/dL
    (B) pH 7.3, protein 4 g/dL, glucose 75 mg/dL, WBCs: 5,000/mm^3, triglycerides: 345 mg/dL
    (C) pH 7.2, protein 3 g/dL, glucose 85 mg/dL, WBCs: 200/mm^3, triglycerides: 67 mg/dL
    (D) pH 7.4, protein 3 g/dL, glucose 210 mg/dL, WBCs: 30/mm^3, triglycerides: 95 mg/dL

14. A pleural effusion in the child that suggests malignancy is characterized by:

    (A) a pH less than 7.1
    (B) a serum glucose lower than 40 mg/dL
    (C) a blood triglyceride level of >500 mg/dL
    (D) the presence of atypical white cells

15. Malignant pleural effusion is most often seen in the child in:

(A) rhabdomyosarcoma
(B) neuroblastoma
(C) hepatoblastoma
(D) lymphoma

Answers

1. **(C)** Although a decubitus film may be obtained, ideally an ultrasound of the right hemithorax and aspiration of the fluid for diagnostic purposes would precede the administration of antibiotics. However, if the child's clinical condition appears to be rapidly deteriorating, stabilization of the child's condition and administration of appropriate antibiotics prior to thoracentesis should proceed without delay.

2. **(A)** This case represents an example of bacterial pneumonia with an associated pleural effusion. In the emergency department the most appropriate intervention is attention to the airway, adequacy of respiratory effort, and circulation. The child is desaturated on room air and should receive supplemental oxygen. After the patient is stabilized with oxygen and a CXR is acquired, an IV line should be placed and appropriate antibiotics given. Ideally, an ultrasound with aspiration of pleural fluid should be attempted in the stable child prior to antibiotics.

3. **(B)** Selection of appropriate antibiotics for this particular patient should include coverage for both *S. aureus* and *S. pneumoniae*, as well as consideration of less likely gram-negative pathogens. In 2005, community-associated methicillin-resistant *S. aureus* (MRSA) often presents with a profound, rapidly progressive, necrotizing pneumonia, so consideration should be given to an antibiotic that targets MRSA. Therefore, the initial choice of antibiotics in this child would be ceftriaxone and vancomycin.

4. **(A)** The presence of the pleural effusion in this child demands a secondary diagnostic procedure. It is imperative that fluid from this particular effusion be obtained both for diagnostic and therapeutic purposes. In children, the pleural space is a potential space defined in its boundaries by the parietal and visceral pleurae. The parietal pleura covers the inner aspect of the chest wall and the diaphragm, while the visceral pleura is strongly adherent to the surface of the lung tissue itself. A thin film of liquid separates these two spaces and creates the potential space where fluid may accumulate a number of pathologic states. In the child with an effusion, diagnostic aspiration and evaluation of pleural fluid are important and will direct further therapy.

Pleural fluid can be classified in a number of ways. One classification distinguishes between transudate, exudate, and an empyema. An alternative categorization of the fluid is the distinction between a simple parapneumonic effusion, a complex parapneumonic effusion, and an empyema. A third separates the parapneumonic effusion into a simple exudative phase, a fibrin proliferative phase, and a stage of organization

The distinction between transudate, exudate, and empyema depends upon a chemical analysis of the pleural fluid. Pleural fluid that has a fluid-to-serum LDH ratio >0.6, a pH between 7.3 and 7.4, and a pleural fluid protein concentration >3 g/dL should be considered an exudate. Most transudates have total protein concentrations <3 g/dL and have a pH >7.4. Although a positive pleural fluid culture defines an empyema, the clinician must often decide about empyema when the culture is negative. Because of the efficient clearance of organisms from the pleural space and the natural bacteriostatic host defense mechanisms of the pleural space, the pleural fluid culture may be negative even when there are organisms identified on the Gram stain. Prior antimicrobial therapy may also influence the culture results.

5. **(C)** For the child with a large parapneumonic effusion or an empyema accompanied by mediastinal shift, the management includes drainage of that fluid. Should an empyema be defined by either chemistry or the presence of organisms, video-assisted thoracostomy (VAT) and decortication early in the patient's course is recommended and may abbreviate the hospital stay. Another management strategy for a complicated parapneumonic effusion is the instillation of fibrinolytics into the pleural space if VATs cannot be done.

6. **(C)** Most children with lung abscess respond to a prolonged course of intravenous antibiotic ther-

apy and surgical intervention is rarely required. Typically the CXR reveals an air fluid level in the diseased lung field. A CT scan may be necessary to further delineate the size of the abscess and its relationship to the tracheobronchial tree. In either case, the abscess will respond to prolonged antibiotic administration. Rarely the abscess will need to be drained either surgically or by interventional radiology. Drainage may complicate the disease process as there is a significant risk for cross-contamination of unaffected pulmonary tissue as well as contamination of the pleural space at the time of surgery.

7. **(C)** Pleural effusion is a common event occurring in at least 40% of bacterial pneumonias. Generally, the effusions are uncomplicated and small. The presence of an effusion greater than 10 mm in width should be aspirated for diagnostic purposes. If the fluid is compatible with an empyema on microscopic examination, drainage is indicated.

8. **(D)** This is a case of a child with a complicated parapneumonic effusion and lung abscess. However, in the setting of a simple parapneumonic effusion, the effusion usually resolves with treatment of the underlying pneumonia. If there is a complex parapneumonic effusion that is loculated or causes mediastinal shift or if an empyema is present, more aggressive drainage of the pleural space is recommended.

9. **(B)** In general, the clinical manifestations of pneumonia in children include fever, cough, and tachypnea. Although additional signs of respiratory distress such as nasal flaring, accessory muscle use, grunting, and desaturation may be present, a respiratory rate of >50 breaths per minute at rest has a relatively high sensitivity of predicting a pneumonic process in an otherwise healthy appearing infant. Auscultatory findings associated with pneumonia include bronchial breath sounds, rales, rhonchi, wheezes, and reduction in breath sounds.

Acute chest syndrome or pneumonia associated with pleural effusion may be a first time presentation for an African-American child with sickle cell disease. It would be important to take a history for sickle cell disease and validate the child's hemoglobin type by Sickledex or hemoglobin electrophoresis. Immunodeficiencies both congenital and acquired tend to present earlier than 16 months of age but should be considered as well.

10. **(C)** In this case, after the removal of the pleural fluid, a 2-cm lung abscess is apparent. Lower respiratory tract infection illustrated in this child is most often transmitted by initial colonization of the nasopharynx with the offending organism followed by aspiration or inhalation of that organism. Invasive disease commonly occurs when a host is colonized with a new serotype of the organism. Of the pathogens listed, the most likely cause is *S. aureus* although *S. pneumoniae* is the most common cause of bacterial pneumonia. In contrast, a lung abscess in an adult usually results from aspiration of oral flora. Frequent oral aspiration often occurs in debilitated children so anaerobic organisms should be considered in these patients as well.

Associated bacteremia is present in 10% to 20% of cases of bacterial pneumonia/empyema. If the child can produce sputum, it may be a useful tool to identify the responsible organism. However, in children younger than about 9 years of age, expectoration of sputum rarely occurs and pediatricians rely on culture of the pleural fluid and the blood for "certain" microbiologic diagnosis of pneumonia.

11. **(A)** The two most common organisms causing neonatal infection including bacteremia and pneumonia are group B streptococcus and *E. coli*. Infections caused by other streptococcal species and *S. aureus* have been reported, but are less common.

12. **(C)** The abrupt onset of severe symptoms such as fever, anorexia, and tachypnea should lead the clinician to suspect a bacterial pathogen. The most common cause of bacterial pneumonia remains *S. pneumoniae*. This species is also associated with parapneumonic effusions which are sometimes complicated. At this age, additional bacterial causes of pneumonia with effusion should also be considered such as *S. aureus*, although *H. influenzae* or a variety of much less frequent organisms is rare. Common causes of pneumonia that are rarely associated with pleural

effusion include *M. pneumoniae* and *C. trachomatis*, the latter in young infants. Viral agents, particularly influenza, parainfluenza, RSV, and adenovirus, are also common causes of lower respiratory tract infection. Influenza, parainfluenza, and adenovirus may cause a high fever and all may cause a toxic-appearing child, but these viruses rarely produce a pleural effusion.

13. **(B)** Pleural effusions in children occur for reasons other than a complication of pneumonia. These effusions are associated with chest trauma, cardiac surgery, and congestive heart failure. The hemopneumothorax that occurs after chest trauma is obvious by history and by aspiration of the fluid. A transudate is commonly found in the patient with cardiac failure or following cardiac surgery and has the characteristics previously described. A chylothorax may follow trauma or thoracic surgery. It is characterized by a marked elevation in the pleural fluid triglyceride concentration reflects injury to the lymphatic system. The pH, protein, and glucose are very similar to the values found in serum.

14. **(D)** Pleural effusions in the child with a malignancy will look like a transudate or an exudate, but contain abnormal or atypical white cells suggestive of a malignancy. Notably, in malignant effusion, the glucose concentration can be as low as encountered in empyema.

15. **(D)** Malignant pleural effusion is substantially more common in the adult population. When a malignant effusion develops in a child, it is most often associated with a thoracic lymphoma.

SUGGESTED READING

Heffner JE, Brown LK, Barbieri C, et al: Pleural fluid chemical analysis in parapneumonic effusions. *Am J Respir Crit Care Med* 151:1700–1708, 1995.

Miller MA, Ben-Ami T, Daum RS: Bacterial pneumonia in neonates and older children. In: Taussig LM, Landau LI (eds), *Pediatric Respiratory Medicine*. St. Louis: Mosby, 1999, pp. 644–647.

Pistolesi M, Miniati M, Giuntini C: Pleural liquid and solute exchange. *Am Rev Respir Dis* 140:825–847, 1989.

Sahn SA: Management of complicated parapneumonic effusions. *Am Rev Respir Dis* 148:81–817, 1993.

CASE 15: A 3-MONTH-OLD INFANT WITH GENERALIZED SEIZURES

A 3-month-old male infant is brought to the emergency room by his grandmother after he began having jerking movements of his arms and legs that started approximately 20 minutes before presentation to the emergency department. The nurse reports that in triage the infant had intermittent jerking of his arms and legs and seemed sleepy. The history is uninformative. His grandmother reports that she has been feeding him only formula over the last 5 days she has been caring for him while his mother is out of town. Review of symptoms is negative for upper respiratory tract illness, fever, vomiting, diarrhea, or change in eating habits.

On physical examination, the vital signs are normal. He has no obvious jerking movements, but he has diminished muscle tone. His pupils are 3 mm and respond sluggishly to light bilaterally. The anterior fontanel is soft. His cardiorespiratory exam is normal.

SELECT THE ONE BEST ANSWER

1. If the child begins to have generalized seizures in the emergency department, the first intervention must be:

    (A) administration of phenobarbital
    (B) ensure a patent airway
    (C) obtain a stat CT scan
    (D) give 10 mL/kg 50% glucose

2. The first screening tests that need to be performed are:

    (A) serum glucose and electrolytes
    (B) a complete blood count and differential
    (C) a sedimentation rate and C reactive protein
    (D) examination of CSF

3. The patient continues to have generalized seizures even after administration of intravenous lorazepam at a dose of 0.3 mg/kg when the electrolytes return normal except for a serum sodium of 118 mEq/L. The intervention required is:

    (A) intravenous phenytoin, 5 mg/kg
    (B) intravenous 3% NaCl, 2 mEq/kg
    (C) intravenous phenobarbital, 10 mg/kg
    (D) intravenous normal saline, 2 mEq/kg

4. Additional history regarding which of the following items would most help to explain why this child had seizures:

   (A) the manner in which the grandmother is preparing food for the child
   (B) the drugs available in the grandmothers house for accidental ingestion
   (C) the family history of seizures
   (D) recent use of corticosteroids in the child

5. The child disposition after the seizures are controlled in the emergency department should be which of the following:

   (A) the child can now be safely discharged to home with close follow-up
   (B) the child should be referred to an endocrinologist
   (C) the child needs to have a genetics workup for adrenal disorders
   (D) the child should be admitted to hospital and have careful monitoring of his serum sodium

6. If trying to distinguish SIADH from water intoxication, urine electrolytes would be:

   (A) not useful
   (B) likely to show a urine sodium concentration <20mEq/L if water intoxication is to blame
   (C) likely to show excessive sodium excretion if SIADH is to blame
   (D) likely to show low urine osmolality if SIADH is to blame

7. The optimal time frame to correct the serum sodium to a normal range after the seizures are controlled in the emergency department is?

   (A) correct to normal as soon as possible
   (B) correct to normal in 6 hours
   (C) correct to normal in 24 hours
   (D) correct to normal in 4 to 5 days

8. Complications from quickly increasing a patient's serum sodium might include:

   (A) intracranial hemorrhage
   (B) hydrocephalus
   (C) pontine demyelination
   (D) occipital blindness

9. Complications from rising serum sodium most often are observed in which of the following populations?

   (A) young infants
   (B) preschool children
   (C) young adult women
   (D) teenage boys

10. The differential diagnosis of hyponatremia includes all of the following except:

    (A) diabetes insipidus
    (B) SIADH
    (C) cerebral salt wasting
    (D) congenital adrenal hyperplasia

11. The diagnostic studies that would best help narrow down the differential diagnosis of a hyponatremia would be which of the following?

    (A) The best diagnostic study would be urine sodium, serum potassium, serum calcium, urine phosphate.
    (B) The best diagnostic study would be urine sodium, serum potassium, serum glucose, serum albumin.
    (C) The best diagnostic study would be serum potassium, serum calcium, serum albumin, bilirubin.
    (D) The best diagnostic study would be urine sodium, serum sodium, serum potassium, serum glucose.

12. The routine use of hypotonic intravenous fluids in hospitalized children is:

    (A) recommended because the infant cannot manage a sodium load
    (B) recommended because the sodium requirement in ill children is the same as it is in healthy children
    (C) not recommended because the ill infant cannot excrete a sodium load
    (D) not recommended because the ill infant cannot routinely excrete excess free water

13. The quantity of fluid that can best be called "insensible loss" in a patient with normal vital signs is:

    (A) 1200 mL/m^2/day
    (B) 500 mL/m^2/day

(C) 2000 mL/m^2/day

(D) 1000 mL/m^2/day

14. The quantity of intravenous fluids that can best be called "maintenance" in a child with routine ongoing loss and normal vital signs is:

(A) 1200 mL/m^2/day

(B) 2500 mL/m^2/day

(C) 3000 mL/m^2/day

(D) 4000 mL/m^2/day

15. Of the following IV fluids listed, which would be the best choices for the child in this case to be on if admitted for observation after seizures stopped in the emergency department?

(A) The best choices would be 5% dextrose 0. 2 normal saline 1200 mL/m^2/day.

(B) The best choices would be 5% dextrose 0.45 normal saline 1200 mL/m^2/day.

(C) The best choices would be 5% dextrose 0.9 normal saline 1200 mL/m^2/day.

(D) The best choices would be 5% dextrose LR 3000 mL/m^2/day.

Answers

1. **(B)** As a general principle, it must be assured that the patient has a stable patent airway and an appropriate hemodynamic status before proceeding to the next step in management.

2. **(A)** In a patient with seizures it is imperative to obtain serum glucose and electrolytes to initiate the acute evaluation. Generalized seizure activity in an 8-month-old infant is relatively common and there are a multitude of explanations. Metabolic derangements are among the most common causes of seizures in this age group. Although hypomagnesemia may cause seizures, hypoglycemia, hypocalcemia, and hyponatremia are the three electrolyte disturbances that are most frequently associated with seizures. An examination of spinal fluid is not unreasonable, but it can wait for consideration in an afebrile and previously healthy child. Consideration should be given to intracranial pathology related either to a congenital malformation or to a traumatic event resulting in intracranial or extracranial

hemorrhage. A CT scan is appropriate to consider after the patient is stabilized and the seizure is controlled.

3. **(B)** Controlling the seizure should begin with the administration of lorazepam intravenously in a dose of 0.1 mg/kg. It is clear that at least part of the reason for this child's ictal activity is hyponatremia. Thus, it is prudent to correct the sodium. In general, if one administers 1 or 2 mEq/kg of sodium to a child with a seizure as a result of hyponatremia, the sodium will rise to a sufficient level that the seizures will be abolished. Hyponatremic seizures can be relatively resistant to anticonvulsant medications including phenytoin and phenobarbital, and intravenous sodium is often required. Although a cause for the seizure activity has been identified, the evaluation for intracranial pathology should be pursued as well. Hyponatremia might be a result of excess antidiuretic hormone resulting from intracranial malformation or injury.

4. **(A)** Patients with hyponatremia can be divided into those who present without accompanying dehydration and those who are hypovolemic. A history of fever or trauma should be sought from the caregiver. Additional important information to obtain from the caregivers are the manner in which the formula was prepared and the precise intake and urine output for the proceeding 24 hours. In this child, there is no evidence on exam or by history of any volume loss. Thus he falls into the category of euvolemia with hyponatremia. In this age range the commonest explanation for euvolemic hyponatremia is water intoxication from improper mixing of formula prior to feeding or exogenous administration of water. The alternative diagnosis in a hyponatremic child who is euvolemic is SIADH. This is generally associated with other pathology, most commonly in the CNS. For the hypovolemic child with a reliable history of volume loss and normal pre-existing health, a diagnosis of hyponatremic dehydration is usually associated with acute gastroenteritis.

5. **(D)** Children with hyponatremic seizures, even from a relatively benign cause such as water intoxication, need to be admitted to hospital and have careful monitoring of the rise of serum so-

dium. Fortunately, this entity is associated almost uniformly with full recovery.

6. **(B)** When trying to distinguish water intoxication from SIADH, if the history is unavailable or unreliable, urine studies can be quite useful. SIADH is a diagnosis that is generally associated with other pathology, most commonly in the CNS. In SIADH, urine volume is generally reduced, as the underlying pathology is the excess absorption of free water at the collecting duct of the kidney. In water intoxication, the urine osmolality is quite low, as is the urine sodium concentration (<20 mEq/L). When hyponatremia is a result of antidiuretic hormone excess, urine osmolality is elevated and the urine sodium is 50 to 75 mEq/L.

7. **(C)** Ideally, the serum sodium should be corrected no more than 0.5 to 1 mEq/L/hr to a normal value with isotonic fluid. The exception is the need to rapidly respond to epileptic activity, at which time a rapid, minimal correction of the serum sodium is indicated. In this child, should the seizures continue after anticonvulsant therapy, it would be appropriate to raise the serum sodium to about 125 mEq/L at which time the seizure activity should stop.

8. **(C)** Severe neurologic injury resulting from central pontine myelinolysis has been associated with rapid correction of serum sodium in some patients.

9. **(C)** Central pontine myelinolysis has been most associated with rapid correction of serum sodium in young women with who received excess free water in the perioperative period.

10. **(A)** In addition to SIADH, two other pathologic entities deserve to be mentioned in a pediatric discussion of hyponatremia: cerebral salt wasting and adrenal insufficiency. In diabetes insipidus, the urine is hypotonic and hypernatremia may develop.

11. **(D)** The determination of the underlying cause of hyponatremia can be made by evaluating the hydration status of the child in conjunction with electrolyte and urine studies. In cases of hyponatremia with robust urine volume and euvolemic state, water intoxication is almost always the diagnosis. Urine osmolality is quite low, as is the urine sodium (<20 mEq/L). The child is euvolemic with low urine output, a relatively high urine sodium, and high urine osmolality. When hyponatremia is a result of antidiuretic hormone excess, urine osmolality is elevated and the urine sodium is 50 to 75 mEq/L, which is clearly inappropriate in a child whose serum sodium is quite low. For the hypovolemic child with a reliable history of volume loss and a normal preexisting health status, a diagnosis of hyponatremic dehydration is usually associated with gastroenteritis.

In the case of cerebral salt wasting, the patient is likely hypovolemic, has a robust urine output, and a very high urine concentration of sodium. This occurs almost uniformly in the postoperative care of the patient with a neurosurgical procedure or after severe head trauma.

In the case of adrenal insufficiency, the patient also presents with volume loss. In addition to hyponatremia, the patient is usually hyperkalemic and hypoglycemic and may be present in shock. When the etiology of the adrenal insufficiency is congenital adrenal hyperplasia, there are often physical findings consistent with virilization.

12. **(D)** It is common in hospitalized patients or following surgical procedures to have a self-limited period of excess ADH secretion, signaling the kidney to retain free water. With the addition of hypotonic intravenous fluids in this state, hyponatremia may develop.

Isotonic fluid is often the most appropriate choice for children hospitalized for numerous conditions because the risks of giving isotonic fluid are often less than the risks of giving hypotonic fluid. Hyponatremia is found in 3% to 5% of hospitalized children. The most common cause is the administration of hypotonic intravenous fluids. If these children were restricted to water and salt that exactly met their physiologic maintenance, they would be normonatremic. It is sometimes difficult to exactly determine a child's maintenance needs for water and salt. If a clinician overestimates the volume of fluid needed and a child has increased ADH secretion, that child will retain much of the water given in IV fluids. If the fluids chosen are hypotonic, the serum sodium will be driven down over time.

13. **(B)** Insensible loss of about 500 mL/m²/day occurs in the absence of excess insensible loss, as found in fever or with radiant warmer use.

14. **(A)** The hospitalized child requires approximately 700 to 800 mL/m²/day of water to excrete a normal solute load. In addition, children require replacement of insensible losses of about 500 mL/m²/day. The sum of these requirements leads to a total IV fluid rate of approximately 1200 mL/m²/day. Additional IV fluids in excess of 1200 to 1300 mL/m²/day in a child without elevated ADH will generally result in more dilute urine. Excess hydration may be required to replace excess water losses, as occur with dehydration or ongoing losses from diarrhea, fever, or other causes.

Often it is taught that appropriate intravenous fluids for all children who are younger than 1 year of age is 0.2 N saline and those older than a year of age 0.45 N saline at a rate that approximates 2000 mL/m²/day. Weight based formulas found in text references of 100 mL/kg/day (4 mL/kg/hr) for the first 10 kg, followed by 50 mL/kg (2 mL/kg/hr) for the next 10 kilograms, and by 20 mL/kg (1 mL/kg/hr) for each kilogram greater than 20 kilograms approximate this volume of 2000 mL/m²/day for all weights. These formulas are derived from data published in the 1950s that suggested IV fluids be administered in accordance with metabolic needs of healthy children. However, many of our hospitalized patients today are not "healthy children;" they are children with increased ADH secretion.

15. **(C)** Once seizure free, the only intervention necessary in the water intoxicated child that is drinking formula would be to restrict free water. However, if intravenous fluids are required, an isotonic fluid should be chosen and given at a "maintenance" rate.

The alternative fluid regimen now proposed for the hospitalized child is the administration of isotonic fluids at a maintenance rate that more closely matches the volume required to excrete a solute load and the amount needed to replace insensible losses as discussed in Answer #14. However, this provides more than the sodium requirement of the human at any age. The consequences of the administration of excess salt are usually benign in most patients without underlying cardiovascular or renal disease and can include pulmonary edema and peripheral edema. Children who require sodium restriction, including those with renal failure, congestive heart failure, and chronic obstructive pulmonary disease such as chronic lung disease following prematurity and cystic fibrosis, are certainly exceptions and hypotonic fluids are often appropriate.

SUGGESTED READING

Sterns RH, Riggs JE, Schoechet SS, Jr: Osmotic demyelination syndrome following correction of hyponatremia. *N Engl J Med* 14(24):1335–1341, 1986.

Ayus JC, Krothapalli RK, Arieff AI: Treatment of symptomatic hyponatremia and its relation to brain damage. *N Engl J Med* 317(19):1190–1195, 1987.

Arieff AI: Hyponatremia, convulsions, respiratory arrest, and permanent brain damage after elective surgery in healthy women. *N Engl J Med* 314(24):1530–1534, 1986.

Dermatology

3

CASE 16: A NEWBORN INFANT WITH A BIRTHMARK ON THE FACE

A 30-week-gestation girl is noted shortly after birth to have a red patch on the left face. The patch involves the left forehead, extending into the scalp, and onto the left upper eyelid. Initially the lesion is flat and partially blanching. Over the subsequent 2 to 3 weeks the patch becomes more raised, with a pebbly surface. It is noted that the left eye is not as wide open as the right (Figure 16-1).

SELECT THE ONE BEST ANSWER

1. What is the most likely diagnosis?

   (A) The most likely diagnosis is hemangioma.
   (B) The most likely diagnosis is port wine stain.
   (C) The most likely diagnosis is capillary malformation.
   (D) The most likely diagnosis is angiosarcoma.

2. What syndrome might be associated with this lesion?

   (A) It is Sturge-Weber syndrome.
   (B) It is PHACES syndrome.
   (C) It is neurofibromatosis.
   (D) It is tuberous sclerosis syndrome.

3. The imaging study most likely to support a diagnosis of this syndrome?

   (A) The imaging study is an MRI of the spine.
   (B) The imaging study is an MRI of the head.
   (C) The imaging study is a renal ultrasound.
   (D) The imaging study is an ECG.

4. The most appropriate management of this lesion includes:

   (A) observation
   (B) systemic corticosteroids
   (C) phenobarbital
   (D) laser therapy

5. You educate the parents to expect that this lesion will:

   (A) be gone by 2 years of age
   (B) remain stable in size and appearance through childhood
   (C) gradually flatten and fade through childhood
   (D) require surgical excision

6. The parents report that this child's cousin has a hairless plaque in the scalp with a pebbly surface and orange hue (Figure 16-2). You are concerned that the child's cousin might have an increased risk for:

   (A) melanoma
   (B) basal cell carcinoma
   (C) tinea capitis
   (D) alopecia areata

7. An 8-year-old boy presents for evaluation of a birthmark on the abdomen (Figure 16-3). You recommend:

   (A) immediate excision
   (B) observation
   (C) radiographic examination
   (D) laser therapy

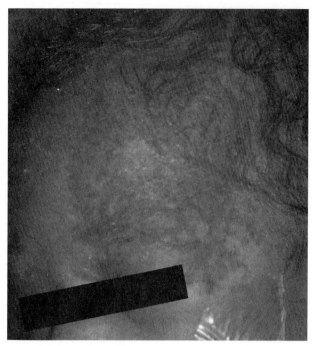

Figure 16-1. See color plates.

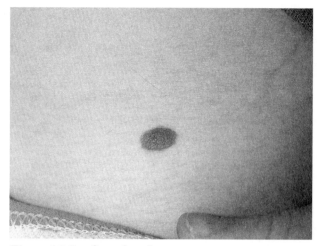

Figure 16-3. See color plates.

9. Based on your findings, you prescribe:

(A) hydrocortisone ointment
(B) hydroxyzine suspension
(C) permethrin cream
(D) excision

8. At a newborn's 1-month follow-up appointment the parents note a lesion on the child's back that has occasionally appeared raised and fluid-filled (Figure 16-4). A helpful examination technique is:

(A) firm stroking of the lesion
(B) palpation for a thrill
(C) diascopy
(D) transillumination

10. One month later, the child presents with multiple tan brown plaques, some with a thickened surface, over the trunk and extremities (Figure 16-5). You inform the parents:

(A) the child needs a bone marrow biopsy
(B) the child needs a bone marrow transplant
(C) these lesions will fade and resolve by 10 to 12 years of age
(D) the child has neurofibromatosis

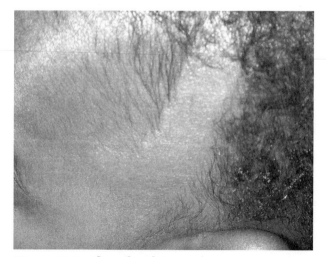

Figure 16-2. See color plates.

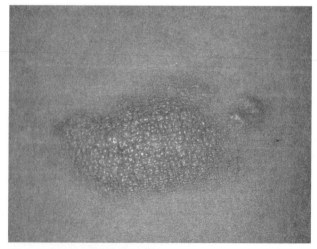

Figure 16-4. See color plates.

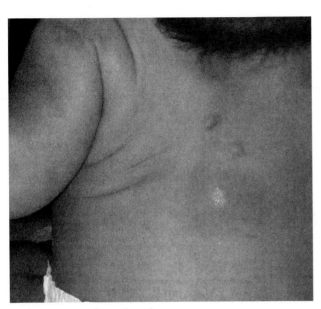

Figure 16-5. **See color plates.**

Answers

1. **(A)** This patient has a hemangioma. The description of the lesion becoming thicker and more nodular over the first couple of weeks of life is typical of the proliferative behavior of a hemangioma, as opposed to the stable nature of a port wine stain and other vascular malformations. Capillary malformation and port wine stain are synonymous. Angiosarcoma is a proliferative tumor, as is hemangioma, however extremely rare in newborns, while hemangiomas are present in up to 10% of 1-year-olds.

2. **(B)** PHACES syndrome is the association of a large plaque-type facial *h*emangioma with *p*osterior fossa defects, *a*rterial defects, *c*ardiac defects, *e*ye abnormalities, and a *s*ternal raphe. Sturge-Weber syndrome is associated with facial port wine stains in the V1 distribution most often. Neurofibromatosis and tuberous sclerosus are not typically associated with vascular birthmarks.

3. **(B)** An MRI of the head will identify the presence of a posterior fossa defect. It would also be an appropriate study to evaluate for intracranial vascular malformations seen in Sturge-Weber syndrome. An echocardiogram might also be indicated to look for the cardiac features of PHACES syndrome; however, a good cardiac exam may obviate the need for an ECG in all cases.

4. **(B)** The patient is experiencing early obstruction of the visual axis as a result of proliferation of the portion of the hemangioma involving the upper eyelid; therefore, intervention is indicated. Use of systemic corticosteroids is the best choice of the answers. It is beneficial in temporizing the growth and may expedite involution of hemangiomas during the active growth phase. It will also be critical to involve ophthalmology to follow this patient's visual development. Laser therapy does not have a role in management of hemangiomas during the acute growth phase when the function of a critical structure is compromised. Laser cannot penetrate deeply enough into a hemangioma to decrease its bulk in most cases.

5. **(C)** Hemangiomas undergo a proliferative growth phase during the first year of life. Subsequently they enter an involutional phase that may last up to 10 years or longer. Therefore, the flattening and fading observed occurs slowly and gradually over years. Port wine stains and other vascular malformations are stable, nonproliferative lesions and do not undergo involution. Surgical excision may be necessary ultimately to remove the residua of some hemangiomas, but in most cases is best undertaken once a significant portion of the spontaneous involution has occurred. Some hemangiomas may leave superficial telangiectasias; these can be treated with laser therapy to decrease residual redness on the skin surface.

6. **(B)** Nevus sebaceous is a hamartoma of sebaceous glands typically seen in the scalp. They are hairless, slightly pebbly, and yellowish plaques in childhood, which may become more raised and nodular in adolescence. There is an increased risk of basal cell carcinoma developing in these lesions over the lifetime of the individual, and typically not before young adulthood. Melanoma has not been associated with this lesion. Tinea capitis may cause hair loss, but generally there are also findings of scale, crust, broken hairs, and lymphadenopathy. Alopecia areata is a nonscarring form of alopecia that can occur at any age. Areas of hair loss are smooth without surface change.

7. **(B)** A congenital nevus is a nevomelanocytic lesion present from birth. They are classified by size as small (0–1.5 cm), medium (1.5–19 cm), and large (20 cm and larger). There is an increased risk of malignant melanoma in the large lesions, and these tumors have been reported in children before the age of 5 years. The medium and small lesions have a smaller risk of malignancy, and it is generally believed that this transformation rarely occurs before adolescence. Therefore, small and medium-sized lesions may be observed for atypical changes, or electively excised. Large congenital nevi are often technically difficult to excise. Laser procedures are not likely to remove all involved components of the lesion and therefore may not eliminate the risk of melanoma. There is no role for radiographic examination.

8. **(A)** Solitary mastocytomas are not uncommon in infants. They appear as reddish brown plaques, sometimes with a slightly pebbled surface, and can become redder and more swollen with irritation, occasionally even blistering. As a diagnostic test, the lesion may be stroked firmly and observed for the reaction of redness and swelling; this is known as a Darier's sign. Diascopy refers to applying pressure to a red lesion in an attempt to blanch it by temporarily clearing the intravascular blood locally. This technique is used to evaluate vascular lesions such as vasculitis and purpura. Transillumination and palpation for a thrill will not be revealing in the case of a mastocytoma.

9. **(B)** Systemic antihistamines are useful in mast cell disease to decrease the symptoms associated with mast cell degranulation. Histamine is the prominent mast cell mediator, and degranulation of mast cell collections in the skin may occur spontaneously, with minor trauma or friction over a lesion, with environmental stimuli such as sudden heat or cold, and with many medications. Release of histamine causes lesions to become reddened, edematous, sometimes blistered, and often itchy. Use of systemic antihistamines can block or modify this response. Topical corticosteroids may be somewhat soothing, but likely are not preventative. There is no role for permethrin in the management of mast cell disease. Excision might be curative for a single lesion, but is not generally recommended.

10. **(C)** Urticaria pigmentosa is the condition of multiple cutaneous collections of mast cells that accumulate during infancy and childhood. The number of lesions can vary from few to innumerable. Childhood urticaria pigmentosa is rarely associated with systemic manifestations. Lesions tend to accumulate during the first few years of life, then stabilize, and gradually fade and involute by early adolescence. Some patients will have complete clearance, others will demonstrate significant improvement. Adult-onset mast cell disease is associated with an increased risk of mast cell leukemia and other myelodysplasias; this has not been observed in the juvenile form.

SUGGESTED READING

Bruckner AL, Frieden IJ: Hemangiomas of infancy. *J Am Acad Dermatol* 48:477–493, 2003.

Metry DW, Hebert AA: Benign cutaneous vascular tumors of infancy: When to worry, what to do. *Arch Dermatol* 136(7):905–914, 2000.

Prose NS, Antaya RJ. Neoplastic and infiltrative diseases. In: Eichenfield LF, Frieden IJ, Esterly NB (eds), *Textbook of Neonatal Dermatology*. Philadelphia: W.B. Saunders Company, 2001, pp 442–444.

CASE 17: A NEWBORN GIRL WITH VESICLES

A 5-day-old female is brought to the ER for evaluation of a rash. The child's mother states that she has noticed small pus bumps developing on the infant's face, body, and hands and feet. This is the first child of this young mother. She is also concerned because the child is spitting up her formula and sleeps a lot during the daytime, but not at night. She is unsure whether she has had fever. She is also complaining of a new fever blister on her own lip.

On examination, there are pustules and vesicles scattered on the chin, trunk, and palms and soles. Additionally, there are hyperpigmented macules and some areas of scaling at the edge of the macules. The child is afebrile, vigorous, and has moist lips and a wet diaper.

SELECT THE ONE BEST ANSWER

1. A smear of a pustule is obtained and stained with a Wright's stain. Microscopic findings reveal:

   (A) sheets of eosinophils
   (B) sheets of neutrophils

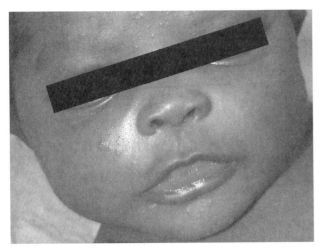

Figure 17-1.   See color plates.

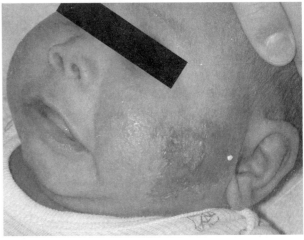

Figure 17-2.   See color plates.

(C) multinucleated giant cells

(D) hyphae and spores

2. The best course of action is to:

(A) perform a septic workup, including urinalysis, complete blood count, blood culture, and lumbar puncture

(B) admit the patient for intravenous antiviral therapy

(C) reassure the mother and discharge the patient home

(D) send a culture of the pustule fluid

3. At this infant's 1-month visit to the pediatrician, his mother is again concerned about a skin rash. She notes many red bumps on the face as well as a few pus bumps. She also is distressed by many hyperpigmented marks on the trunk (Figure 17-1). The best management is:

(A) hydrocortisone ointment to the rash twice daily

(B) benzoyl peroxide gel to the rash daily

(C) mupirocin ointment to the rash three times a day

(D) observation and reassurance

4. A 6-month-old male presents for evaluation of an erythematous plaque on the cheek, with a few small vesicles, moist surface, and yellow crust. The patient's mother reports this rash just developed in the last day and she has noticed the child scratching at it. Which of the following diagnostic tests is positive? (Figure 17-2)

(A) The positive test is a Tzanck smear.

(B) The positive test is a Gram stain.

(C) The positive test is a potassium hydroxide preparation.

(D) The positive test is a Wright's stain.

5. The best management is:

(A) mupirocin ointment to the rash three times a day

(B) acyclovir ointment 5 to 6 times a day

(C) intravenous acyclovir for 21 days

(D) clotrimazole cream twice daily

6. The next child you see is a 6-month-old presenting for routine well-child care. You notice a few comedones on the child's cheeks and upper back (Figure 17-3). The best management is:

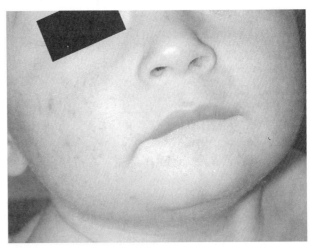

Figure 17-3.   See color plates.

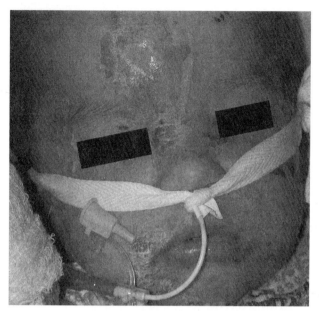

Figure 17-4. **See color plates.**

(A) tretinoin gel daily
(B) benzoyl peroxide gel daily
(C) testosterone and DHEAS levels
(D) curettage

7. One week later this patient's 3-year-old cousin presents with widespread erythema and scaling around the mouth, neck, and upper chest, revealing red moist skin under the scale. Rare fragile blisters are noted. He is clearly uncomfortable and hasn't been drinking well. His lips are dry and he is febrile (Figure 17-4). He has not been on medication. The most likely diagnosis is:

(A) toxic epidermal necrolysis
(B) Stevens-Johnson syndrome
(C) staphylococcal scalded skin syndrome
(D) toxic shock syndrome

8. What is the best diagnostic test?

(A) The best test is a culture of the blister fluid.
(B) The best test is a Gram stain of the blister fluid.
(C) The best test is a blood culture.
(D) The best test is a frozen section of sloughing skin.

9. Staphylococcal scalded skin syndrome is caused by:

(A) an allergic reaction to bacteria
(B) superantigens

(C) an exfoliatoxin
(D) a pyrogenic toxin

10. Full-thickness skin necrosis, severe mucosal involvement, and skin pain is characteristic of:

(A) scarlet fever
(B) toxic epidermal necrolysis
(C) staphylococcal scalded skin syndrome
(D) bullous impetigo

Answers

1. **(B)** The timing of this rash, the patient's otherwise good health, and the description of the lesions are all suggestive of transient neonatal pustular melanosis. This benign neonatal eruption classically presents in the first week of life, with lesions in multiple stages including vesicles, pustules, collarettes of scale, and hyperpigmented macules. It is more common in dark-skinned infants. Smear of the contents of a pustule demonstrates neutrophils and can be diagnostic. Erythema toxicum neonatorum is another common benign neonatal eruption, but tends to spare the palms and soles and demonstrates blotchy erythema with central minute pustules. A smear of the contents of the pustule demonstrates eosinophils. Multinucleated giant cells are seen on Tzanck smears of herpetic lesions. An infant with neonatal herpes infection may appear sick, with lethargy and poor feeding. The lesions are often eroded. Congenital candidiasis can present as pustules, but typically presents in the first 24 hours of life, and is more widespread with confluent-appearing lesions and scaling.

2. **(C)** Transient neonatal pustular melanosis is a benign neonatal eruption for which no treatment is necessary. New lesions cease to develop during the first week of life. The postinflammatory hyperpigmentation may linger for weeks to months. Recognition of this common neonatal rash is important in order to spare these infants from unnecessary procedures, such as a septic workup and unnecessary drugs. Cultures of these pustules are sterile.

3. **(D)** One month of age is a typical time to present with neonatal acne, which by definition

will present in the first 30 days of life. This is a common finding in both males and females. The lesions typically affect the face, and are characterized by erythematous papules and pustules without comedones. This is a self-limited eruption and no treatment is indicated. The dark patches that are noted refer to leftover hyperpigmentation from the transient neonatal pustulosis.

4. **(B)** A Gram stain will demonstrate gram-positive cocci, confirming the diagnosis of impetigo. Impetigo is a common skin infection in children, caused by both *Staphylococcus aureus* and group A streptococci. The presence of yellow crust, and the location near an orifice are suggestive of this diagnosis. More rarely, herpes simplex can present in infants and is important to recognize and rule out. The typical lesion will be grouped vesicles on a red base, without the characteristic yellow crust of impetigo. Tinea corporis might also be considered. These lesions are classically more annular with scale and not crust.

5. **(A)** Topical treatment of impetigo with an antibacterial such as mupirocin is often adequate when the lesions are localized. Treatment of HSV in patients this age is somewhat controversial. Infants younger than 3 months of age are treated aggressively with intravenous antivirals and are evaluated for CNS manifestations of herpes infection. There may still be concern at 6 months of age that a local infection can disseminate, or that the eruption represents reactivation of a congenital infection.

6. **(B)** Acneiform lesions at 6 months of age represent infantile acne, a more uncommon condition which is more common in males, is characterized by comedones, and likely is androgen-driven. However, testosterone and DHEAS levels are typically normal and do not necessarily need to be measured unless the child demonstrates other signs of virilization. Treatment with benzoyl peroxide is often helpful. Tretinoin is generally reserved for the most recalcitrant cases. Curettage is not indicated.

7. **(C)** Periorificial and flexural involvement with fragile blisters, peeling skin, and moist denuded exposed skin is typical of staphylococcal scalded skin syndrome, caused by an exfoliatoxin-producing strain of *S. aureus* phage group 2. Toxic epidermal necrolysis (TEN) and Stevens-Johnson syndrome are most commonly drug-induced hypersensitivity reactions and mucosal involvement is prominent. Toxic shock syndrome does not cause blistering.

8. **(D)** The gold standard for diagnosis of staphylococcal scalded skin syndrome is demonstration of blister formation within the stratum granulosum of the epidermis, in contrast to TEN in which full thickness epidermis is necrotic. Cultures from the blisters and denuded skin are sterile. Blood culture is only rarely positive. The highest yield of the inciting bacteria is from the nose, nasopharynx, or conjunctiva.

9. **(C)** Staphylococcal scalded skin syndrome is caused by *S. aureus* strains producing exfoliatoxin, these strains usually belong to phage group 2. Pyrogenic toxins are implicated in scarlet fever caused by streptococcus.

10. **(B)** Full-thickness skin necrosis, severe mucosal involvement, and skin pain is typical of TEN. This is usually a drug-induced hypersensitivity reaction, which is distinguished from Stevens-Johnson syndrome by the extent of surface area involvement. Ophthalmologic involvement is also common and must be addressed.

SUGGESTED READING

Lucky AW. Transient benign cutaneous lesions in the newborn. In: Eichenfield LF, Frieden IJ, Esterly NB (eds), *Textbook of Neonatal Dermatology.* Philadelphia: W.B. Saunders Co, 2001, pp 88–102.

Patel GK, Finlay AY: Staphylococcal scalded skin syndrome: Diagnosis and management. *Am J Clin Dermatol* 4(3):165–175, 2003.

CASE 18: AN 8-YEAR-OLD BOY WITH AN ITCHY RASH

An 8-year-old boy presents complaining of an itchy rash involving his whole body. His mother states that her son has been itchy and rashy "from birth." She has treated his skin with "cortisone creams" and "ringworm creams" over the years, with only inter-

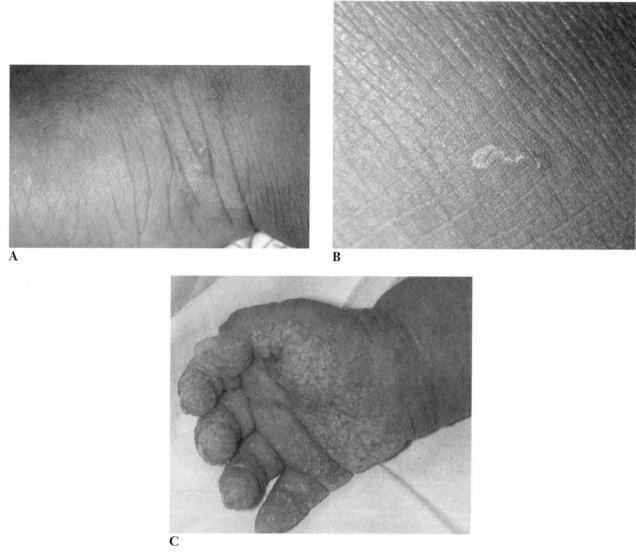

A   B

C

Figure 18-1.   See color plates.

mittent mild improvement. She admits that his itch-ing and scratching have been worse in the last couple of weeks. She has not noticed rash on her own skin, but her 6-month-old daughter also has an itchy rash (Figure 18-1).

On physical examination, there are excoriations over the upper back, abdomen, wrists, and lower legs. The antecubital fossae and popliteal fossae are clear. There are tiny papules on the fingers, and larger erythematous papules on the scrotum. The face is clear.

SELECT THE ONE BEST ANSWER

1. Examination of the patient's 6-month-old sister is likely to reveal:

(A) red scaly patches on the cheeks
(B) linear lesions within creases on the palms and soles
(C) annular scaling plaques on the buttocks
(D) grouped vesicles on an erythematous base in the diaper area

2. The patient is treated with permethrin cream and returns 1 month later without improvement. The most likely cause of treatment failure is:

(A) inadequate treatment of contacts and envi-ronment
(B) inadequate duration of treatment
(C) inappropriate choice of medication
(D) organism resistance

3. The patient's mother states that she has been applying the cream also to her baby's rash twice a day. You inform her that the treatment:

 (A) is appropriate and she needs to apply the medicine 3 times a day
 (B) should have been applied only once to the whole body
 (C) should have been applied once a week for 2 weeks to the whole body
 (D) is inappropriate and you prescribe triamcinolone ointment instead

4. Additional instructions for treatment should include:

 (A) professional extermination of the home environment
 (B) laundering all linens and clothing and vacuuming all surfaces
 (C) sealing all coats in plastic for 1 month
 (D) applying mayonnaise to the hair and then washing out

5. The finding of papules/nodules on the penis and scrotum in the setting of an itchy rash such as this child presented with is:

 (A) irrelevant to making the diagnosis
 (B) strongly suggestive of the diagnosis
 (C) pathognomonic for the diagnosis
 (D) a warning sign of sexual abuse

6. Later that day, a 6-year-old Caucasian girl presents complaining of an itchy scalp for a few weeks. Examination of the scalp and hair is most likely to reveal:

 (A) diffuse scaling of the scalp with scattered pustules and areas of broken hairs
 (B) white flecks in the hair that do not seem to come off easily
 (C) multiple round patches of smooth alopecia
 (D) greasy scale throughout the scalp

7. A common cause of treatment failure in this condition is:

 (A) resistant organisms
 (B) failure to remove all nits
 (C) incorrect use of medications
 (D) all of the above

8. Many schools advocate a "no nit" policy when evaluating whether students may return to school. The problem with this policy is:

 (A) nits represent egg sacs and never indicate active infestation
 (B) it requires all children to cut their hair short
 (C) nits that are more than 3 inches from the scalp are empty
 (D) nits that do not contain a live organism are noninfectious

9. The best place to detect body lice is:

 (A) under the nails
 (B) in the seams of clothing
 (C) in the umbilicus
 (D) in the digital web spaces

10. A 2-year-old female presents with new bumps on the skin for the last few weeks. They do not seem to itch or otherwise bother the child. On examination you notice numerous flesh-colored 2- to 3-mm smooth papules, some with a central dell, clustered behind the knee and scattered on the thigh, groin, and trunk (Figure 18-2). You inform the patient's mother that:

 (A) the patient has chickenpox and must be kept out of school
 (B) this is an allergic contact reaction and you prescribe topical hydrocortisone
 (C) the house requires fumigation by an exterminator service

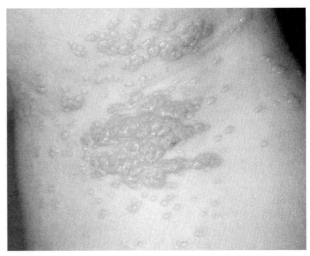

Figure 18-2. **See color plates.**

(D) this is a poxvirus infection and there is no associated systemic involvement

11. Appropriate treatment for this eruption includes:

(A) watchful waiting
(B) calamine lotion
(C) triamcinolone ointment
(D) salicylic acid solution

12. At this same visit, the patient's 12-year-old brother shows you some firm rough papules on his fingers, which he states have bled when he picks at them (Figure 18-3). On examination, these papules have a rough surface studded by pinpoint black dots. The most likely diagnosis is:

(A) callous
(B) verruca
(C) knuckle pads
(D) foreign body reaction

13. The treatment of choice for this condition is:

(A) cryotherapy
(B) surgical excision
(C) electrocautery
(D) curettage

14. Soft, flesh-colored coalescent papules in the perianal area on this patient suggest:

(A) the need for a child abuse evaluation

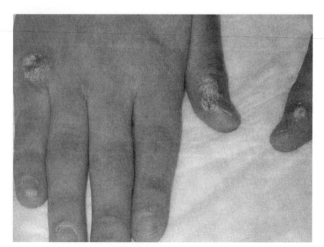

Figure 18-3. See color plates.

(B) the patient is constipated and needs to increase fiber in his diet
(C) autoinoculation of human papillomavirus
(D) A and C

15. A 9-year-old boy presents to the emergency department with a 2-day history of blisters erupting on his lower legs (Figure 18-4). He complains that his legs are itchy and somewhat sore, but he otherwise feels well and is afebrile with normal vital signs. You instruct the family:

(A) to have the family dog checked for fleas
(B) to unroof the blisters and apply antifungal cream
(C) that the child needs admission for intravenous antibiotics
(D) that the child will be admitted to the burn unit and child protective services will be called

Answers

1. (B) Infants infested with the scabies mite often manifest a very extensive rash with involvement of the palms and soles (Figure 18-1C and 18-1D). Burrows can often be found within the deep creases of these surfaces. The head can also be involved in the eruption, which is less common in older individuals, but a prominent facial rash is unusual. Annular lesions is more typical of a dermatophyte infection. Grouped vesicles on an erythematous base is the classic description of a herpetic lesion.

2. (A) The most common cause of treatment failure of scabies infestations is inadequate treatment of contacts and the environment. All individuals sharing living quarters should be treated at the same time. Treatment involves application of 5% permethrin cream from the neck to the toes, including digit web spaces, gluteal cleft, genitalia, around and under nails. Cream should be left on overnight. Symptomatic individuals should repeat this treatment 1 week later. Simultaneously, the environment should be treated: all linens and clothing must be laundered in hot water and put through the dryer;

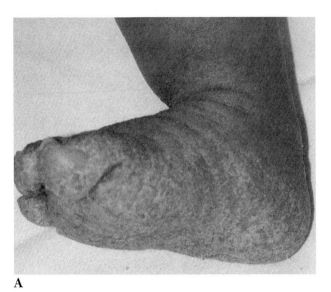

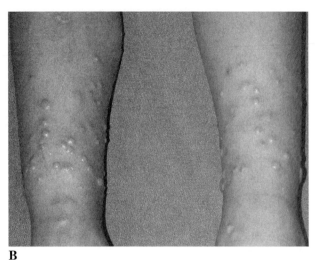

A

B

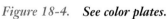

Figure 18-4. ***See color plates.***

items that cannot be laundered should be put in plastic for 1 week; floors, rugs, and furniture should be vacuumed. Permethrin-resistant scabies mites have not been reported.

3. **(C)** Appropriate use of 5% permethrin cream is a single application overnight, with repeat application in 1 week if the individual is symptomatic. This regimen applies to infants as well. The medication should be applied to the scalp of infants. Daily application is inappropriate and may lead to systemic absorption of the medication.

4. **(B)** The additional instructions for the environment are discussed in the answer to question #2. Professional extermination is not indicated. Items that cannot be laundered need to be sealed in plastic for 1 week only. Application of mayonnaise to the hair is a treatment that has been recommended for head lice.

5. **(B)** Scrotal and penile nodules are strongly suggestive of a scabies infestation. Other itchy conditions, such as atopic dermatitis, rarely cause papules or nodules in this area. Conditions such as psoriasis and lichen planus can commonly affect the genitalia, but lesions are not typically nodular. Verrucous papules and

nodules in the genital region may be a sign of sexual abuse.

6. **(B)** Head lice is common in school-age children, and is more common in races with straighter hair, and relatively uncommon in those with coarse kinky hair. It is theorized that the organism cannot attach as easily to the oval hair shafts of kinky hair. Diffuse scaling in the setting of pustules and broken hairs is more suggestive of tinea capitis, and this infection is more common in African Americans. Round patches of frank alopecia are seen in alopecia areata, and this condition is not usually itchy. Diffuse greasy scale is typical of seborrheic dermatitis and is more common in adolescents and adults.

7. **(D)** Treatment failure of head lice is common. Pyrethrin-resistant organisms are becoming increasingly common. Additionally, inadequate use of recommended treatments is common. The nonprescription cream rinse products are more effective when applied to dry hair and need to be left on the hair for several hours. Finally, removal of intact nits is critical as these represent the unhatched eggs.

8. **(D)** The "no nit" policy is controversial. In some instances, old nits may simply represent the egg-

shell, without a live organism. Therefore, some patients with old nonviable nits will be barred from school although they are in fact no longer infectious. It is thought that those nits closest to the scalp are most viable because of the necessary body temperature for hatching; however, this criterion is imprecise and should not be relied upon.

9. **(B)** Body lice are rarely spotted on the skin itself, but rather are visible to the naked eye within the seams of clothing. The skin lesions consist only of excoriations and areas of pinpoint bleeding representing sites of bites. Body lice are most commonly an ailment of the homeless and those with poor hygiene practices. Treatment consists mostly of removing infested articles of clothing and bedding.

10. **(D)** Molluscum contagiosum is a poxvirus infection that is becoming increasingly prevalent in the childhood population. It is believed to be transmitted by skin-to-skin contact; however, it is unclear whether fomites are a risk, and how much of a role is played by swimming and bathing with affected individuals. The lesions are classically found clustered in warm, moist areas such as the axillae, groin, antecubital fossae, and popliteal fossae. Patients may have few or dozens of lesions. Those with underlying skin disease such as atopic dermatitis have a higher risk of spreading the lesions because of a compromised skin barrier and baseline scratching.

11. **(A)** Watchful waiting is an acceptable treatment in uncomplicated cases. The lesions do tend to spontaneously resolve eventually, although the time course is variable from weeks to months to years. Alternate destructive treatments include curettage, cryotherapy, and cantharidin application. Salicylic acid is useful in the treatment of warts; however, it likely will not be effective for this condition and will be irritating.

12. **(B)** Verruca vulgaris refers to the common type of wart, caused by human papilloma virus. This infection is very common in children and adults. A large percentage of childhood cases will actu-

ally spontaneously resolve over months to years. Lesions are distinguished by the rough surface that disrupts skin markings and the presence of thrombosed capillaries, which account for the friability and bleeding that are often reported. Callus will always be in an area of friction and will not disrupt the skin lines nor demonstrate thrombosed capillaries. Knuckle pads are an uncommon finding on the dorsal aspect of some patients' interphalangeal and metacarpal phalangeal joints.

13. **(A)** Of the choices listed, cryotherapy is the best choice for wart therapy. Surgical excision will lead to scarring, and commonly the wart will grow back at the site because of incomplete removal. Electrocautery is also inappropriate. Curettage will not be effective for the relatively deep lesions.

14. **(D)** Soft perianal papules in this setting are likely condyloma. Condyloma in any child should raise the concern for child abuse. However, there are many cases in which no risks for abuse are found and it is believed that autoinoculation of the virus by the patient is possible in this location. Additionally, children in diapers may be at risk of acquiring the papillomavirus from the hands of caregivers. Hemorrhoids are quite rare in childhood.

15. **(A)** Bullous arthropod bites can be very exuberant and frightening. They are often because of flea bites, and one member of the family only may be affected. This individual is hypersensitive to the bite. The blisters arise on otherwise normal-appearing skin, and a punctum may be visualized centrally. The lesions occur on exposed skin predominantly, such as the lower legs and arms. Children who play on the floor or ground are particularly susceptible. Management is supportive. Blisters may be drained, but the roof should be left intact as a natural dressing. Unusual blistering reactions in unusual locations should raise suspicion for abuse as well.

SUGGESTED READING
Huynh TH, Norman RA: Scabies and pediculosis. *Dermatol Clin* 22(1):7–11, 2004.

Bodemer C. Human papillomavirus. In: Schachner LA, Hansen RC (eds), *Pediatric Dermatology*, 3rd ed. Edinburgh: Mosby, 2003, pp 1087–1092.

CASE 19: A 4-YEAR-OLD GIRL WITH AN ITCHY RASH

A 4-year-old girl presents to your office with her mother complaining of a long-standing itchy rash that has worsened over the last several days. The child's mother states that the child has had rough skin since infancy and scratches persistently. She appears exhausted and exasperated. She describes the child digging at her skin and causing open sores and bleeding. In the past week, these symptoms have worsened and the mother notes that whenever the weather changes the rash worsens.

On exam, the child is thin, notably picking and scratching at her arms and legs. She is quiet and withdrawn. There are widespread ill-defined plaques of dry, excoriated, and thickened skin with scale over the extremities predominantly, with less thickened patches on the trunk. There are areas of fissuring and erosion, and crusty exudates, particularly on the legs and near the elbows. In the folds of the elbow and knee, there are deeper erosions revealing red raw skin, also some clustered vesicles. There is widespread lymphadenopathy (Figure 19-1).

SELECT THE ONE BEST ANSWER

1. Appropriate care of this patient will include:

    (A) administration of oral corticosteroids
    (B) application of topical antibacterials
    (C) application of topical antihistamines
    (D) administration of oral antibiotics

2. The finding of clustered vesicles also raises concern for:

    (A) chickenpox infection
    (B) eczema herpeticum
    (C) allergic contact dermatitis
    (D) hand, foot, and mouth disease

3. The most helpful diagnostic test to evaluate the vesicle would be:

    (A) patch testing
    (B) bacterial culture
    (C) viral culture
    (D) direct fluorescent antibody testing

4. Initial topical therapy for this patient should include:

    (A) mid-potency topical corticosteroid ointment under wet wraps
    (B) topical antihistamine cream
    (C) topical calcineurin inhibitor cream
    (D) high-potency topical corticosteroid cream

5. Skin care recommendations in this setting should include:

    (A) regular long hot soaks in a bathtub
    (B) daily short baths in tepid water
    (C) regular use of antibiotic soaps
    (D) avoidance of topical lubricants

6. The least well-established trigger of flares of this nature is:

    (A) second-hand cigarette smoke
    (B) dust
    (C) milk protein
    (D) animal dander

7. This patient's 8-year-old brother is also complaining of an itchy rash on his belly and arms that has been present for months. On exam, you notice an ill-defined plaque of excoriated and hyperpigmented papules infraumbilically (Figure 19-2A), and flesh-colored papules over his extensor arms and legs (Figure 19-2B). You recommend that he:

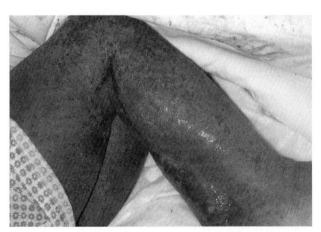

Figure 19-1. **See color plates.**

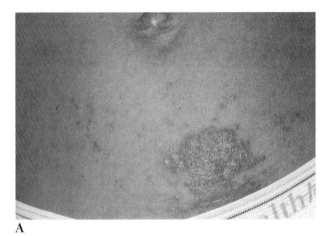

A

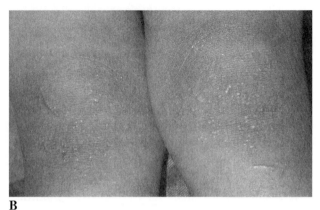

B

Figure 19-2. **See color plates.**

(A) keep his shirt tucked in at all times
(B) avoid skin contact with the metal button on his jeans and his belt buckle
(C) follow the same skin care recommendations you gave his sister
(D) be checked for scabies

8. The most common contact allergen in the United States is:

(A) laundry detergent
(B) fragrance mix
(C) nickel
(D) neomycin

9. A 5-year-old female presents to your office with a 1-week history of red scaly 1- to 3-cm plaques predominantly over her trunk and extremities. She states she has otherwise been feeling well, but her mother notes a bit more fatigue than usual. You note that the patient is afebrile, but her tongue and oropharynx are erythematous and the rash is randomly distributed on the trunk (Figure 19-3). You immediately suspect a diagnosis of:

(A) pityriasis rosea
(B) guttate psoriasis
(C) scarlet fever
(D) mononucleosis

10. The best test to do is:

(A) a throat culture
(B) a monospot
(C) a skin biopsy
(D) a KOH scraping

11. You tell the family to expect:

(A) the rash will resolve in a week followed by widespread desquamation
(B) the rash will resolve over 6 to 8 weeks with postinflammatory dyspigmentation
(C) the rash will improve with treatment, but may persist to some degree for life
(D) the patient will have to discontinue all contact sports

12. A 9-month-old infant presents with a worsening rash over the preceding month. Her mother states that the child is quite irritable and is having looser stools. She has been applying hydrocortisone with minimal improvement. On exam, there are erythematous scaling and eroded plaques on the cheeks and around the mouth, also on the lower abdomen and in the diaper area and over the hands and feet. A helpful piece of history is:

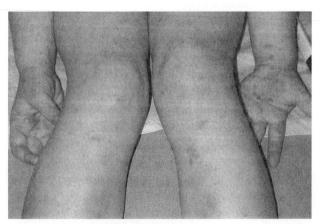

Figure 19-3. **See color plates.**

(A) whether there has been any change in diet
(B) whether there are new pets in the household
(C) whether there are any sick contacts
(D) whether the child is in daycare

Answers

1. **(D)** The patient described is presenting with an acute flare of severe atopic dermatitis. The finding of crusting exudates and erosions is strongly suggestive of secondary bacterial infection. Additionally it is known that patients with chronic atopic dermatitis are frequently colonized by bacteria such as *S. aureus*, and it is thought that the presence of the organism may drive the inflammatory reaction in the skin. Systemically administered antibiotics are much more effective for decreasing the overall carriage rate of the bacteria, and treating the secondary infection. Systemic corticosteroids are rarely indicated in the management of atopic dermatitis and should not be considered first-line treatment. Topical antihistamines are often sensitizing, leading to allergic contact dermatitis, especially in patients with a defective skin barrier; therefore, the topical agents are not recommended in this setting. Additionally, systemic absorption of these agents when applied to large surface areas in young children, especially those with a compromised skin barrier, can lead to toxic levels.

2. **(B)** Eczema herpeticum refers to a generalized eruption of herpes simplex virus infection in a patient with a compromised skin barrier, such as during a flare of atopic dermatitis. A history of cold sores within the family may be suggestive. The finding of clustered round punched-out erosions and vesicles in the setting of atopic dermatitis is also very suggestive of this potentially severe secondary infection. It is uncommon to see an active case of chickenpox in this setting. An acute allergic contact dermatitis can be very exuberant and present with vesicles, but typically will affect a limited surface area with relatively well-demarcated borders, or follow geographic patterns, such as the linear streaks from poison ivy. Hand, foot, and mouth disease typically demonstrates small shallow erosions on the hands, feet, and oropharynx.

3. **(D)** The direct fluorescent antibody test for herpes viruses can be accomplished very quickly, and provides guidance for treatment of possible cases of eczema herpeticum. The most reliable specimen is taken from the base of an intact vesicle. The vesicle should be gently unroofed, and the base then rubbed with a cotton applicator and transferred to a microscope slide. Patch testing is done to determine sensitivity to contact allergens. Bacterial and viral cultures will also be helpful in this setting, but will not provide as rapid results.

4. **(A)** Appropriate care of a patient with a widespread flare of atopic dermatitis involves very specific instructions to the family regarding skin care. The mainstay of therapy will be the use of a topical corticosteroid preparation. These agents have a long history of safety and efficacy in this setting. Choice of an appropriate-strength agent is critical. The age of the patient, extent of surface area to be covered, and sites of application will all help to determine the most appropriate potency. High-potency agents are only rarely used in children, and when used are most often used only on hands or feet and for very limited periods of time. Mid-potency agents used under occlusion with warm wet linens accomplishes hydration as well as healing. Ointment-based products provide more occlusive and emollient effects than creams and lotions, and thus are typically more effective in the setting of acute flares. Topical antihistamines, as mentioned previously, may cause sensitization. The newest agents in the armamentarium against atopic dermatitis are the topical calcineurin inhibitors. These agents are anti-inflammatory in the skin and seem to cause minimal systemic absorption and do not cause cutaneous atrophy. However, they may not be as effective as quickly as topical steroids in the setting of an acute flare. Additionally, the risks of long-term use are still unknown.

5. **(B)** Bathing in the management of atopic dermatitis has long been controversial. It is generally recognized that long soaks (>15 minutes) are detrimental to the barrier function of the skin, perhaps by compromising the lipid component of the stratum corneum. However, short baths (5 minutes) serve to hydrate the skin and are beneficial. The use of topical lubricants is also critical in the maintenance of a healthy skin barrier, and application

of these agents immediately after bathing seems to improve their penetration and efficacy. Overuse of antibacterial agents may lead to drug resistance and so are not recommended for daily use.

6. **(C)** In the majority of cases of atopic dermatitis, a single allergen is not the cause of the condition. Allergy testing in these individuals will frequently find sensitivity to many agents, only some or none of which may have any clinical relevance to the individual patient. Specific food allergies have been the hardest allergens to prove in the etiology of atopic dermatitis. Environmental agents such as dust, smoke, and dander are more often relevant.

7. **(B)** This patient's presentation is classic for nickel contact allergy with an associated hypersensitivity reaction. These patients are often atopic, or have an atopic family history. They constantly or recurrently have an active site of chronic dermatitis in the umbilical region, probably from contact with the metal buttons on many clothes, or the use of belts with metal buckles. The eruption on the extremities is probably secondary and the result of a more systemic sensitization to the local allergen. The eruption itself responds rather slowly to fairly potent topical corticosteroids, but of paramount importance is the counseling to avoid nickel metal contact. Attempting to keep a shirt tucked in as a barrier is usually inadequate. The use of nail polish lacquer on offending surfaces can be helpful.

8. **(C)** Contact allergy to nickel metal is the most common contact allergy in the United States. This allergy likely plays a significant role in the dermatitis of many atopics. When there is a localized eruption in the periumbilical region, this allergen should be strongly suspected. Other sites commonly affected are earlobes, neck, and wrist. Fragrance mix and neomycin are also common allergens for contact allergy. Laundry detergents are often suspected, but if and when they are the true offenders it is probably because of the fragrance component.

9. **(B)** The acute onset of red scaly plaques could describe pityriasis rosea or psoriasis. However, pityriasis rosea is rarely as red in color as psoriasis, and

classically there is a first larger lesion about 2 weeks before the onset of the generalized rash. Additionally the lesions are typically distributed along skin tension lines, generating the classically described "fir tree" pattern. Guttate psoriasis flares in pediatric patients are often in response to a strep pharyngitis. The lesions are small well defined red plaques with the typical adherent scale of psoriasis. There may be other stigmata of psoriasis, such as a geographic tongue or nail changes. Scarlet fever is a widespread erythematous eruptions of fine papules, without a plaque-component. Mononucleosis rarely presents with a rash, and when it does it is the more nonspecific morbilliform eruption of a viral exanthem.

10. **(A)** It is important to look for the presence of an active strep pharyngitis in the setting of guttate psoriasis. Treatment of the infection is often helpful in clearing the rash as well. A skin biopsy can be useful if the morphology of the rash makes the diagnosis less certain. A KOH is likely unnecessary, unless a diagnosis of tinea corporis is strongly suspected.

11. **(C)** Guttate psoriasis typically goes into remission with use of topical corticosteroids and occasionally the need for a limited course of phototherapy. However, these patients are at increased risk for the development of psoriasis vulgaris later in life. Pityriasis rosea generally takes 6 to 8 weeks to resolve and leaves postinflammatory changes for months. Scarlet fever fades in days, followed by significant desquamation. Limitations of physical activity are recommended in the setting of mononucleosis when splenomegaly is present.

12. **(A)** The presentation of dermatitis, irritability, and diarrhea is strongly suggestive of acrodermatitis enteropathica. A classic time for this condition to present is when the child is weaned from breast milk. One of the causes of this zinc deficient state seems to be a defect in absorption of zinc from the small intestine, perhaps because of a missing or malfunctioning transporter. The zinc in breast milk appears to be more bioavailable and therefore the condition may be masked until this source of zinc is absent. Figures 19-4 and 19-5 show examples of another child with a zinc deficient state.

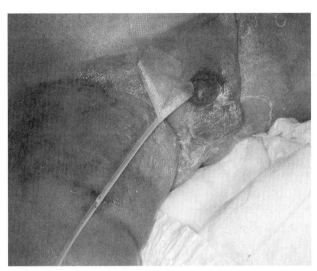

Figure 19-4. **See color plates.**

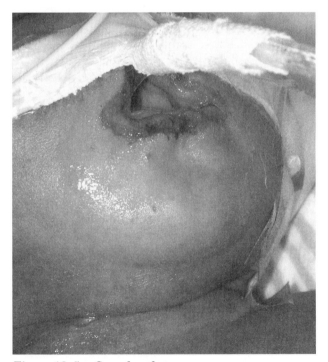

Figure 19-5. **See color plates.**

SUGGESTED READING

Hansen RC: Atopic dermatitis: Taming "The Itch that Rashes." *Contemp Pediatr* 20(7):79–87, 2003.

Hogan PA. Papulosquamous disease. In: Schachner LA, Hansen RC (eds), *Pediatric Dermatology*, 3rd ed. Edinburgh: Mosby, 2003, pp 643–656.

Silverberg NB, Licht J, Friedler S, et al: Nickel contact hypersensitivity in children. *Pediatr Dermatol* 19(2): 110–113, 2002.

CASE 20: AN 8-YEAR-OLD GIRL WITH HAIR LOSS

An 8-year-old white female presents to your office reporting a 2-month history of hair loss and breakage, accompanied by itching and flaking in the scalp. Her mother notes that there have been rashes that have come and gone repeatedly on the skin of the arms and upper back as well. These rashes have improved with topical antifungal creams, but continue to recur. Application of the antifungal cream to the scalp has not provided any relief. The child is otherwise healthy. No family members have been affected with similar rashes. The family has a dog and a cat at home. The child participates in a gymnastics school.

On physical examination, the child is well-appearing and in no distress. On the crown of the scalp there is an area of hair loss about 1- to 2-cm in diameter, with hairs broken off at the scalp and scaling. There are several pustules in the region and a tender erythematous nodule. There are two palpable occipital lymph nodes, which are nontender and nonfluctuant. On the upper back there are ill-defined, somewhat faint erythematous plaques with minimal scale.

SELECT THE ONE BEST ANSWER

1. The most appropriate treatment for this patient is:

   (A) mupirocin ointment twice daily
   (B) griseofulvin suspension twice daily
   (C) cephalexin suspension three times a day
   (D) ketoconazole shampoo daily

2. Duration of treatment should be:

   (A) 1 month
   (B) 2 months
   (C) 3 months
   (D) 2 weeks

3. The most suggestive risk factor for this condition in this patient is:

   (A) presence of a family cat and dog
   (B) past use of hair permanents
   (C) participation in gymnastics school
   (D) the patient's ethnic background

4. Failure of past treatments has likely been a result of:

   (A) noncompliance
   (B) organism resistance

   (C) immunodeficiency

   (D) endothrix infection

5. Tinea capitis infections are most common in:

   (A) teenagers

   (B) African Americans

   (C) Caucasians

   (D) immigrants

6. A helpful diagnostic test in this patient would be:

   (A) Wood's lamp examination of the scalp

   (B) Tzanck smear

   (C) hair mount

   (D) fungal culture

7. One year later, the patient returns, again complaining of hair loss. She states that "a clump of hair fell out 2 weeks ago." She denies any flaking, itching, or soreness within the scalp. She has otherwise been feeling well, but she and her mother are extremely anxious about this new development. On examination, there is a quarter-sized round patch of hair loss in the right frontal scalp. The skin in the area is smooth and devoid of all hairs. Hairs are easily pulled out at the periphery of the patch. There is no lymphadenopathy (Figure 20-1). The most likely diagnosis is:

   (A) tinea capitis

   (B) trichotillomania

   (C) alopecia areata

   (D) telogen effluvium

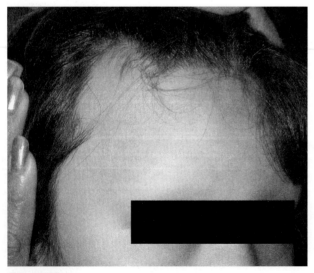

Figure 20-1.

8. The family asks if this condition is caused by stress. The most appropriate reply is:

   (A) Yes

   (B) No

   (C) Maybe

9. A diagnostic sign to look for to help confirm the diagnosis is:

   (A) exclamation point hairs

   (B) question mark hairs

   (C) trichoschisis

   (D) bubble hair

10. The best form of treatment to recommend at this stage is:

   (A) intralesional injections of corticosteroid

   (B) topical application of class I corticosteroid

   (C) observation

   (D) hair transplants

11. Which of the following tests should be considered in this patient?

   (A) The test to be considered is a complete blood count.

   (B) The test to be considered is a ferritin level.

   (C) The test to be considered is a thyroid function test.

   (D) The test to be considered is an antinuclear antibody test.

12. A 10-year-old girl presents with her parents for evaluation of hair loss. The child seems unconcerned. Her parents state that they have noticed an area on the top of the scalp where the hair seems thin and the scalp appears dirty. They have noticed these changes gradually. The child is otherwise healthy and takes no medications.

    On examination, there is a widening of the part with decreased hair density and a "spangled" appearance of the hairs in this area. The hairs appear to be of varying length and the hair feels coarse in this area. The scalp demonstrates brownish fine scaling. No hairs are obtained on a gentle pull test. There are no papules or pustules and no lymphadenopathy. The eyelashes are present, but also appear to be of varying lengths. The nails are short and ragged (Figure 20-2).

    What question should be asked?

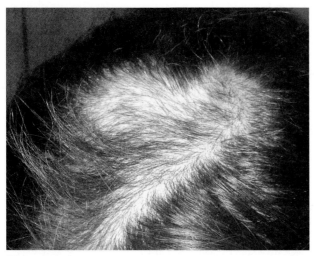

Figure 20-2.

    (A) Do you perm your hair?
    (B) Do you color your hair?
    (C) Do you use a blow dryer?
    (D) Do you pull or twirl your hair?

13. Important workup includes:

    (A) complete blood count
    (B) thyroid function tests
    (C) ferritin level
    (D) none of the above

14. Successful treatment may involve:

    (A) discontinuing all processing practices
    (B) styling the hair in looser styles
    (C) behavioral modification techniques
    (D) topical corticosteroids

15. Additional treatment options may include:

    (A) SSRIs
    (B) intralesional corticosteroid injections
    (C) permethrin-containing crème rinse
    (D) ivermectin

16. A 16-year-old girl presents complaining that her hair is thinning. She notices that her ponytail is smaller than previously and that she sees large amounts of hair in the drain and on her pillow.

    Upon examination, there are no bald patches on her scalp, the scalp appears normal without erythema or scale, and the amount of hair seems within normal limits. However, 20 to 30 hairs are easily pulled out. Instruct the patient:

    (A) it is normal to lose up to 250 hairs a day
    (B) to collect the hair she is losing at home and to bring it back for evaluation
    (C) she should decrease her frequency of hair washing to once a week
    (D) this is early-onset "female pattern" hair loss

17. An important blood test to obtain in an otherwise asymptomatic individual is:

    (A) thyroid-stimulating hormone
    (B) antinuclear antibody
    (C) ferritin level
    (D) erythrocyte sedimentation rate

18. Ask the patient if she takes any medications. The most significant medication that she reports is:

    (A) multivitamin pill
    (B) sumatriptan
    (C) estrogen and progestin (Desogen)
    (D) ibuprofen

Answers

1. **(B)** The case is most suggestive of a tinea capitis infection. Such infections are caused by dermatophytes, which are often spread from person to person, possibly via fomites. It is not uncommon to see lesions of tinea corporis in the setting of tinea capitis. The organism most often isolated in cases of tinea capitis in the United States is *Trichophyton tonsurans*. First-line treatment is generally with griseofulvin. Although the newer antifungal agents are likely as effective, duration of treatment is controversial. Topical therapies cannot penetrate the hair shafts where the organism is found. Secondary bacterial infection is occasionally present and is treated with oral antibiotics when significant. Patients should be educated regarding the transmission and infectivity of this condition, emphasizing the importance of not sharing hair implements, hats, pillows, etc. All affected individuals in a family should be treated simultaneously to avoid reinfection.

2. **(B)** The optimal length of treatment of tinea capitis with griseofulvin is 6 to 8 weeks. Optimal duration of treatment with the newer antifungal agents has not been well documented to date.

3. **(C)** Tinea capitis in the United States is generally an anthropophilic infection. This organism is preferentially pathogenic for humans and is therefore passed from human to human, rather than from animal to human (zoophilic) or from soil to human (geophilic).

4. **(D)** Tinea capitis due to *T. tonsurans* is an endothrix infection. In other words, the hair shaft itself is invaded by the fungus. Some element of the hair follicle is affected in all forms of tinea capitis and it is for this reason that systemic therapy is necessary for clearance. Topical agents cannot penetrate the hair follicle and shaft adequately.

5. **(B)** Data have shown that tinea capitis infection is more common in African American children than in other ethnic groups in the United States, though it is a worldwide problem affecting all children. One theory to explain this observation is that the shape of the hair shaft in African Americans is such that invasion by the fungus is facilitated. Hair care practices such as styling, frequency of washing, and use of greases have also been speculated as increasing risk of this infection. Postpubertal individuals appear to be at less risk, possibly because of antifungal properties of sebum.

6. **(D)** Fungal culture is the gold standard for the documentation of tinea capitis. Potassium hydroxide preparations can be helpful; however, many of these infections are within the hair shaft and may be difficult to visualize, especially if only scale is obtained. *Microsporum canis* is another dermatophyte that may be the cause of tinea capitis, but it is a relatively rare cause in the United States. This organism causes an ectothrix infection (invasion remains outside of the hair shaft) and this organism fluoresces under the Wood's lamp. Therefore, positive fluorescence can be helpful, but a negative test will not rule out a *T. tonsurans* infection. Tzanck smears are sometimes performed to look for herpes virus infections.

7. **(C)** Sudden onset of a discrete area of frank alopecia is most suggestive of alopecia areata. This autoimmune condition is relatively common, and can occur at any age. The most common presentation is of round patches of alopecia throughout the scalp. There are generally no associated symptoms and the scalp appears healthy and nonscarred. The finding of surrounding hairs that are easily pulled out suggests that the process is still active and the patch may continue to enlarge. Progression to loss of the full scalp hair (alopecia totalis) or loss of all body hair (alopecia universalis) is rare. However the condition tends to wax and wane with new patches occurring periodically.

8. **(C)** It is unclear how significant stress is in the activity of this condition. Affected individuals do report flares during periods of stress. This is generally one of the most difficult variables to control, however, so it is usually not very helpful to the patient to focus on this factor.

9. **(A)** Exclamation point hairs are short hairs found at the periphery of the areas of alopecia that are very narrow at their base and wider at the distal end. It is thought that these changes may be the effect of the dense perifollicular lymphocytic infiltrate that is observed microscopically on biopsies from active areas of scalp. Question mark hairs do not exist. Trichoschisis refers to hairs that are split because of trauma, and bubble hair refers to hair shafts that develop bubbles as the result of trauma from heat (blow dryers, curling irons).

10. **(B)** Alopecia areata is a waxing and waning condition that may improve spontaneously; therefore, the direct effect of treatment is hard to document. Likewise then, observation is an acceptable option. Intralesional administration of corticosteroids has been very effective for some individuals, and may work when the areas involved are limited in size and extent. However, most young children do not react favorably to this option. Potent topical steroids have been effective for some people and are more acceptable to children, especially early in the course of the disease.

11. **(C)** It is believed that autoimmune conditions tend to cluster in families and individuals. Therefore, in the setting of alopecia areata, it is important to consider the possibility of coexistent autoimmune diseases. Thyroid function tests are often ordered because this is such a common autoimmune disease. An ANA is not recommended as a screening test in this setting. Iron deficiency has been associated with global

hair thinning, but is not likely a factor in alopecia areata. A CBC is not necessary for screening unless other symptoms are present.

12. **(D)** The findings are most suggestive of trichotillomania. One is obligated to ask the patient and her parents about any habits involving hair pulling or twisting, though very often no one will admit to having observed this behavior. The hair manipulation may be occurring in private, or during sleep, so very often the family is truly unaware of it. The patient often is not fully cognizant of what is occurring. It often takes multiple visits to convince families of this difficult to accept diagnosis.

13. **(D)** No further workup is indicated when the findings are diagnostic.

14. **(C)** The most successful management of trichotillomania involves behavior modification techniques, which are probably most effective in conjunction with a therapist. There are self-help books written for children to help them to break this habit if they are motivated and have the insight to recognize the problem. The condition is classified as an obsessive-compulsive disorder.

15. **(A)** SSRIs have been used in the management of trichotillomania, but most authors suggest that this is most successful in conjunction with behavior modification techniques. Treatment is similar to other obsessive-compulsive disorders and patients may have periods of improvement and periods of regression. Intralesional corticosteroid injections are a treatment for alopecia areata. Permethrin crème rinses are used in the treatment of head lice. Ivermectin has been advocated for the treatment of scabies in some settings.

16. **(B)** The patient is describing a telogen effluvium—a sudden loss of more telogen hairs than is typical. It is normal to lose up to 100 telogen hairs daily. Telogen effluvium can occur for numerous reasons, including following a significant illness, surgery, postpartum, following a significant psychological stress, such as a death in the family, secondary to medications, in the setting of lupus or thyroid disease, as a result of iron deficiency, or in the setting of nutritional deficiency resulting from erratic dieting. It is sometimes

difficult for a clinician to appreciate the degree of hair loss that concerns the patient. Gentle hair pull tests in the office can be helpful. Additionally, asking patients to collect the hair lost in the normal course of hair styling can provide objective evidence of the degree of loss.

17. **(C)** Ferritin levels may be low in women who otherwise have a normal hemoglobin level. It has been observed that ferritin levels less than 40, though often reported by labs as normal, may still have an effect on hair shedding and therefore iron supplementation may be indicated. Some authors advocate screening thyroid studies and ANA for all patients with hair loss, but unless the patient is additionally symptomatic it is unclear what one would do with an abnormal value in this setting.

18. **(C)** Birth control pills are well-known causes of hair loss, and often this is a temporary phenomenon and does not indicate changing the type of birth control pill until the condition has been followed for about 6 months. Other common medications causing hair loss are beta-blockers, ACE inhibitors, some anticonvulsants, lithium, and retinoids.

SUGGESTED READING

Friedlander SF. Fungal infections. In: Schachner LA, Hansen RC (eds), *Pediatric Dermatology*, 3rd ed. Edinburgh: Mosby, 2003, pp 1093–1100.

Harrison S, Sinclair RL: Optimal management of hair loss (alopecia) in children. *Am J Clin Dermatol* 4(11): 757–770, 2003.

Norris D: Alopecia areata: Current state of knowledge. *J Am Acad Dermatol* 51(1 Suppl):S16–17, 2004.

Tay YK, Levy ML, Metry DW: Trichotillomania in childhood: Case series and review. *Pediatrics* 113(5):e494–498, 2004.

CASE 21: A 6-MONTH-OLD BOY WITH BIRTHMARKS

A 6-month-old Hispanic boy presents for routine child care. His parents report no concerns, but do note that they are becoming more aware of birthmarks on the child's skin. They feel that the spots were present at birth, but are getting larger and perhaps more numerous. They believe they are asymptomatic for the child.

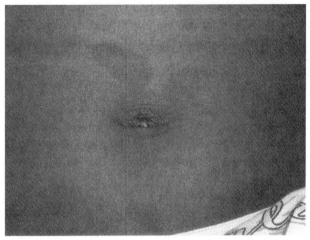

Figure 21-1. **See color plates.**

On examination, the child is well-appearing and vigorous, not able to sit independently. Over the trunk and extremities there are about eight tan-brown well-demarcated patches measuring 5 to 10 mm in diameter (Figure 21-1).

1. This patient is most likely at increased risk for:

   (A) melanoma
   (B) optic glioma
   (C) retinal phakomas
   (D) periungual fibromas

2. Multiple café-au-lait macules may be seen in all of the following except:

   (A) Bloom syndrome
   (B) neurofibromatosis
   (C) McCune-Albright syndrome
   (D) Sturge-Weber syndrome

3. Further skin evaluation of this patient is most likely to reveal:

   (A) axillary freckling
   (B) shagreen patch
   (C) ash leaf spots
   (D) periungual fibromas

4. Additional workup at this stage should include:

   (A) renal ultrasound
   (B) head MRI
   (C) cutaneous examination of family members
   (D) echocardiogram

Figure 21-2. **See color plates.**

5. Additional diagnostic criteria might be confirmed by a consultative visit to:

   (A) an ophthalmologist
   (B) a nephrologist
   (C) a cardiologist
   (D) a gastroenterologist

6. Examination of older patients with this disorder often reveals scattered soft, flesh-colored papules (Figure 21-2). This finding most likely represents:

   (A) nevi
   (B) epidermal cysts
   (C) angiofibromas
   (D) neurofibromas

7. The patient's mother reports that her mother had similar skin changes and died of a tumor. The most likely malignancy she had was:

   (A) malignant neurofibroma
   (B) malignant plexiform neurofibroma
   (C) melanoma
   (D) leiomyosarcoma

8. Another 6-month-old Hispanic male presents for well-child care. His parents note that they have become increasingly aware of light patches of skin. They are unsure whether they were present at birth since the child had much fairer skin at that time. Examination reveals six hypopigmented oval patches on the trunk and extremities measuring 1

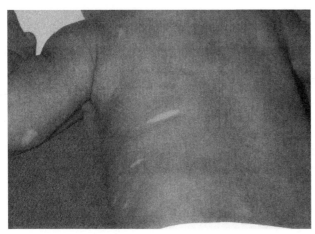

Figure 21-3. ***See color plates.***

to 5 cm in diameter (Figure 21-3). The presence of three hypopigmented macules in infancy is:

(A) a diagnostic criterion of tuberous sclerosis
(B) common in the general population
(C) a risk factor for the development of vitiligo
(D) typical of Klippel-Trenaunay syndrome

9. The mutated gene associated with tuberous sclerosus is:

(A) neurofibromin
(B) hamartin
(C) fibrillin
(D) profilaggrin

10. The following skin lesion of tuberous sclerosus is usually present at birth:

(A) angiofibroma
(B) shagreen patch
(C) confetti macules
(D) none of the above

11. The following lesion is considered pathognomonic of tuberous sclerosus:

(A) periungual fibroma
(B) forehead fibrous plaque
(C) molluscum fibrosum pendulum
(D) shagreen patch

12. The most common early seizure type observed in tuberous sclerosis is:

(A) partial
(B) infantile spasm

(C) absence
(D) febrile

13. The mutated gene of tuberous sclerosus normally functions as:

(A) a tumor suppressor
(B) epidermal growth factor
(C) gap junction protein
(D) cell cycle inhibitor

14. The cardiac lesion most closely associated with tuberous sclerosus is:

(A) coarctation of the aorta
(B) patent ductus arteriosus
(C) rhabdomyoma
(D) congenital heart block

15. An 11-year-old boy with reddish shiny papules of the face, seizures, mental retardation, and newly noted hypertension should be evaluated for:

(A) pheochromocytoma
(B) renal artery stenosis
(C) hyperthyroidism
(D) renal cyst

16. Cortical tubers associated with tuberous sclerosis:

(A) are lesions of bone
(B) may correlate with the occurrence of seizures and mental retardation
(C) are astrocytomas
(D) have malignant potential

17. A 9-month-old female presents for routine well-child care and you note a red purple patch on the left forehead, extending onto the upper eyelid, and posteriorly into the hairline (Figure 21-4).
    This lesion most likely represents a:

(A) hemangioma
(B) port wine stain
(C) café-au-lait macule
(D) congenital nevus

18. The patient is noted to have delayed developmental milestones. You inform the parents that further evaluation should include a:

(A) head MRI
(B) head ultrasound

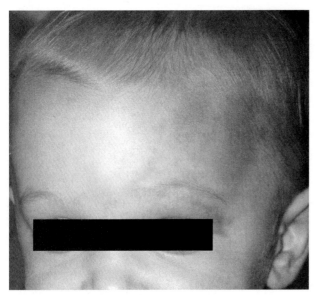

*Figure 21-4. **See color plates.***

(C) skin biopsy
(D) echocardiogram

19. Additionally, it is critical that the patient be seen by a:

    (A) pediatric orthopedist
    (B) pediatric cardiologist
    (C) pediatric ophthalmologist
    (D) geneticist

Answers

1. **(B)** The most common diagnosis in the setting of multiple café-au-lait macules is neurofibromatosis. Optic gliomas peak in incidence between 4 and 6 years of age in patients with neurofibromatosis type I. The description of tan-brown well-demarcated patches is most suggestive of café-au-lait macules and not congenital nevi as nevi are usually more irregularly colored and often have a raised or infiltrative component. Retinal phakomas and periungual fibromas are associated with tuberous sclerosus.

2. **(D)** Multiple café-au-lait macules may be seen in numerous conditions, and sometimes in isolation without other findings. The diagnostic criteria for neurofibromatosis state that the café-au-lait macules must be greater than 5 mm in diameter in children (greater than 15 mm after puberty)

and greater than 5 in number. Sturge-Weber syndrome involves a facial port wine stain and intracranial vascular malformations, café-au-lait macules are not seen more frequently in this condition.

3. **(A)** Axillary and inguinal freckling (Crowe's sign) is another diagnostic criterion for neurofibromatosis type I. These findings may not appear until 3 to 5 years of age. Shagreen patch, ash leaf spot, and periungual fibromas are seen in tuberous sclerosis.

4. **(C)** A first-degree relative with findings consistent with neurofibromatosis can confirm the diagnosis in a situation of a child with only multiple café-au-lait macules at the time of evaluation. Neurofibromatosis may run a very benign course and individuals may not be aware of their diagnosis; therefore, a careful examination of first-degree relatives can be a very important diagnostic procedure.

5. **(A)** A slit-lamp exam can facilitate visualization of Lisch nodules on the iris and this constitutes another diagnostic criterion to aid in the diagnosis of neurofibromatosis. Lisch nodules may not be present in infancy, however, and therefore a negative exam will not rule out the diagnosis.

6. **(D)** Neurofibromas develop in individuals with neurofibromatosis over time. The presence of two or more satisfies one of the diagnostic criteria. These growths are typically soft and spongy and may be flesh-colored to tan-brown or violaceous in color. They are typically asymptomatic, though sometimes patients report tenderness. Neurofibromas represent growth of nerve sheaths.

7. **(B)** The presence of one plexiform neurofibroma is a diagnostic criteria of neurofibromatosis type I. Plexiform neurofibromas are growths of nerve sheath that extend along the length of a nerve and include multiple fascicles. These lesions may be located superficially in the dermis, or more deeply in the soft tissue. There may be associated soft tissue and bony overgrowth. Malignant change may occur within these tumors. Some plexiform neurofibromas are noted to have an overlying giant café-au-lait macule and there

seems to be a higher incidence of malignant change within these lesions.

8. **(B)** Hypopigmented macules are common in the general population, reported with a prevalence as high as 4.7% in a Caucasian population. Higher incidences are typically reported in darker-skinned populations. There are not strict diagnostic criteria regarding skin lesions in tuberous sclerosus. It is generally stated that up to three hypopigmented macules in an otherwise healthy individual without a family history of tuberous sclerosus should not necessitate further workup.

9. **(B)** Hamartin and tuberin are tumor suppressor genes associated with tuberous sclerosus. Neurofibromin is the mutated gene of neurofibromatosis type I. Fibrillin is the mutated gene of Marfan syndrome. Profilaggrin is the mutated gene of ichthyosis vulgaris.

10. **(D)** All three of the listed findings increase in frequency with the age of the patient. Occasionally the lesions may be present in infancy, but more frequently are noted later in childhood or even adolescence. Angiofibromas are pink to red nodules with a smooth shiny surface most commonly distributed over the central face, especially around the nose in the malar region. The shagreen patch is a yellowish-brown or pink plaque most commonly found in the lumbosacral area of the back and having a pebbly surface. Confetti macules are hypopigmented small 1- to 3-mm patches usually distributed in large numbers over the forearms and lower legs.

11. **(A)** Periungual fibromas typically appear around puberty and therefore are less useful in the diagnosis of tuberous sclerosus in young children. Histologically, these lesions are regarded as angiofibromas, the same as the facial lesions. Clinically, they are located around or under the finger or toenails and appear as firm papules, often with a pointed keratotic surface. Some authors do report periungual fibromas in otherwise healthy adults. The forehead fibrous plaque is also histologically an angiofibroma. Molluscum fibrosum pendulum are solitary or multiple soft pedunculated growths, particularly in skin folds such as the neck or axilla.

12. **(B)** Infantile spasms are characterized by a brief contraction of the neck, trunk , and arm muscles, followed by a phase of sustained muscle contraction lasting from 2 to 10 seconds. The initial phase of contraction may consist of flexion or extension in various combinations. The seizures appear in clusters of unpredictable and variable duration. Hundreds of these seizures may occur daily. The peak age of onset of these seizures is 3 to 8 months of age, with the majority having onset before 1 year of age. Tuberous sclerosis is only one of several etiologies associated with this seizure type. There is a high incidence of mental retardation in patients with infantile spasms.

13. **(A)** As mentioned, hamartin and tuberin are gene products that have been implicated in the development of tuberous sclerosis and the genes encoding them function as tumor suppressor genes.

14. **(C)** Cardiac rhabdomyomas have been detected on fetal ultrasounds in the setting of tuberous sclerosis. These are hamartomas that can occur anywhere in the heart and may lead to conduction defects or outflow obstruction. It is estimated that 8% to 90% of infants with cardiac rhabdomyomas have tuberous sclerosis. They are found in 30% to 40% of infants with tuberous sclerosis. The lesions can regress spontaneously and may be asymptomatic.

15. **(D)** Renal cysts are very common in tuberous sclerosis, with up to one quarter of children with tuberous sclerosis younger than 5 years old noted to have renal cysts. Additionally, renal angiomyolipomas are detected in up to 8% of cases.

16. **(B)** Cortical tubers are areas of increased firmness on the cortical surface of the brain where there is loss of the gray-white matter junction. There is loss of normal cellular architecture in these areas. The number and size of these lesions correlate with the occurrence of seizures and mental retardation. "Giant cell astrocytoma" is a term used to describe large subependymal nodules that are another characteristic intracranial lesion associated with tuberous sclerosis. Some subependymal nodules may enlarge and obstruct flow of CSF, resulting in hydrocephalus. These astrocytomas are dis-

tinctly different than typical astrocytomas with rare malignant transformation.

17. **(B)** A red purple patch on the forehead in what is described as a V1 distribution is most likely a port wine stain. Hemangiomas may appear flat initially, but more often will have a pebbly texture and may not be very noticeable until 2 or 3 weeks of life. Café-au-lait macules and congenital nevi are brown and pigmented lesions and should be distinguishable from a vascular lesion at this age.

18. **(A)** A port wine stain in the V1 distribution is associated with Sturge-Weber syndrome in up to 10% of patients. The classic triad of Sturge-Weber syndrome is an ipsilateral facial port wine stain that always involves at least V1, eye abnormalities, and brain abnormalities. The brain abnormalities may include leptomeningeal vascular malformations, calcifications, cerebral atrophy, enlarged choroid plexus, and developmental venous anomalies of the brain. There is a risk for seizures, brain hypoxia, neuronal loss, and hemiplegia. The results of early neuroimaging may not demonstrate the most typical findings, but show only subtle changes such as an enlarged choroid plexus or local accelerated myelination.

19. **(C)** Sturge-Weber syndrome is associated with ocular abnormalities in up to a third of patients. The abnormalities include choroidal vascular anomalies, increased ocular pressure, buphthalmos, and glaucoma. Any facial port wine stain involving an eyelid should elicit prompt referral to an ophthalmologist for careful evaluation as there is an increased incidence of ocular anomalies in this setting.

SUGGESTED READING

Korf B. Tuberous sclerosis and neurofibromatosis. In: Schachner LA, Hansen RC (eds), *Pediatric Dermatology*, 3rd ed. Edinburgh: Mosby, 2003, pp 273–280.

Sybert VP. Selected hereditary diseases. In: Eichenfield LF, Frieden IJ, Esterly NB (eds), *Textbook of Neonatal Dermatology*. Philadelphia: W.B. Saunders Company, 2001, p 451–457.

Fitzpatrick T, Freedberg I, Eisen A, et al: *Fitzpatrick's Dermatology in General Medicine*, 5th ed. New York: McGraw-Hill, 1999. p 2150.

Vanderhooft SL, Francis JS, Pagon RA, et al: Prevalence of hypopigmented macules in a health population. *J Pediatr* 129(3):355–361, 1996.

Jozwiak S, Schwartz RA, Janniger CK, et al: Skin lesions in children with tuberous sclerosis complex: Their prevalence, natural course, and diagnostic significance. *Int J Dermatol* 37:911–917, 1998.

4

Development

CASE 22: A 2-MONTH-OLD WITH COLIC AND SUBSEQUENT DEVELOPMENT DELAY

A 2-month-old named Sarah presents for a well-child check-up. Parents report that she is having very difficult evenings. She has periods of crying that last for more than 3 hours. They have occurred in 5 of the last 6 days. Mother is exhausted and wonders if there is something wrong with the infant formula you recommended.

Sarah was adopted from an international orphanage in early childhood. She weighed 2.14 kg and her gestational age was 34 weeks. It is unknown if she had any complications in utero or at delivery. The mother was cautioned that Sarah might have "development problems."

The physical examination is normal.

SELECT THE ONE BEST ANSWER

1. All of the following statements about colic are true except:

   (A) It often begins at 41 to 42 weeks gestation.
   (B) Fussiness occurs between 5 to 8 PM.
   (C) If it occurs only in the evening, it is probably related to food intolerance.
   (D) Colic stops in 90% of children by 4 months.
   (E) Some infants may be hyperirritable and have signs of hyperarousal.

2. Which of the following are not helpful and possibly harmful in the management of colic?

   (A) a thorough physical examination to rule out a cause for pain or discomfort
   (B) extensive laboratory testing
   (C) feeding in an upright position with more frequent burping
   (D) swaddling
   (E) use of a pacifier

3. Which strategy is not useful in managing colic?

   (A) provision of close and consistent follow-up
   (B) education of the family about crying and discussion of how stressful it is
   (C) careful history and physical examinations
   (D) social services involvement to evaluate for evidence of neglect or abuse
   (E) reassuring parents that there is nothing physically wrong with their child

4. Among the following factors, which is a major risk factor for cerebral palsy?

   (A) cleft palate
   (B) breech presentation
   (C) small for gestational age
   (D) emergency C-section for fetal distress
   (E) APGAR of 5 at 1 minute and 6 at 5 minutes

5. Which of the following cranial sonographic abnormalities does not increase the risk for cerebral palsy in preterm infants?

   (A) intraventricular hemorrhage (IVH) grade 3
   (B) IVH grade 4
   (C) periventricular leukomalacia
   (D) IVH grade 1 or grade 2

6. At 9 months of age, Sarah has difficulty with rolling. During the pull-to-sit maneuver she comes to a stand. She tries to bat at rings. There are no obvious posture or tone changes when the Moro reflex and the asymmetric tonic neck reflex (fencer's response) is elicited. Her head circumference is at the 25th percentile. All of the following would likely be found on Sarah's examination except:

   (A) brisk lower extremity reflexes
   (B) clonus at ankles
   (C) ease of moving her foot toward her ear
   (D) decreased range of motion at hips
   (E) strabismus

7. At 12 months of age, motor delay continues. Sarah cannot get to sit or consistently roll both ways. There is hip abduction to 40 degrees. At what initial routine examination age would difficulty with sitting reflect a delay?

   (A) 4 months
   (B) 5 months
   (C) 6 months
   (D) 9 months
   (E) 12 months

8. At 12 months there is intermittent fisting, right greater than left. What fine motor skills are most likely to be observed?

   (A) transferring objects between hands
   (B) batting at objects
   (C) finger feeding
   (D) pincer grasping
   (E) releasing blocks

9. An audiogram, hip radiograph, cranial MRI, and Bayley Developmental Scales are obtained. If the audiogram reveals a hearing loss of greater than 60 db, what might you discover?

   (A) delays in cooing
   (B) difficulty localizing a fire siren directly
   (C) previous exposure to high levels of aminoglycosides
   (D) parents reporting she does not smile when they call her name
   (E) she was too young to test hearing

10. What potential abnormalities that may explain this child's motor disability are least likely to be found on cranial MRI?

    (A) CNS calcification
    (B) craniosynostoses
    (C) periventricular leukomalacia
    (D) ventriculomegaly
    (E) all of the above are likely to be found

11. Sarah's developmental skills on the Bayley Scales reveal an MDI of 70 and a PDI of <50. The normal range is 100 ± 15. What do these scores most likely predict?

    (A) transient motor delays
    (B) delays that qualify her for Early Intervention
    (C) delays that do not qualify her for SSI
    (D) delays that will make it difficult to learn any skills beyond these possessed by a normal 1-year-old

12. At 15 months of age, Sarah was assessed on the Battelle Developmental Scales. Her gross motor and fine motor skills are at a 6-month developmental age, her receptive language skills are at 12 months, her expressive language skills are at 9 months, and her social and emotional skills are at 15 months. Sarah would be expected to do all of the following except:

    (A) roll
    (B) maintain sitting in tripod
    (C) have head control
    (D) crawl
    (E) roll front to back

13. If Sarah's fine motor skills are at a 6-month level, which skill should be most challenging for her?

    (A) batting at objects
    (B) picking up a block
    (C) demonstrating a mature pincer when offered a pellet
    (D) holding a bottle
    (E) none of the above skills should be difficult for her

14. If her social and emotional skills are at a 15-month level, what would be most difficult for Sarah?

(A) physically separating from her mother
(B) recognizing her mother
(C) recognizing her father
(D) sharing toys with her younger cousin
(E) playing peek-a-boo

15. At 18 months of age, Sarah has anterior props and can be placed sitting in her playpen. She fully extends both arms during the parachute maneuver. There is no fisting. She can combat crawl. Her lower extremities adopt a scissoring posture when you check her ability to bear weight. Sarah's type of cerebral palsy is best characterized as:

(A) hemiplegic
(B) diplegic
(C) triplegic
(D) quadriplegic

16. At the age of 2 years, Sarah can say phrases ("mommy, cookie"), point at five pictures, point at body parts, maintain sitting balance, pull to a stand, finger feed, drink from a sippy cup, remove socks, and use a spoon. Which skill will be most difficult for Sarah to learn in her preschool years?

(A) communicating in sentences
(B) using the toilet
(C) walking with the assistance of braces and rollator
(D) running as fast as peers
(E) pedaling a tricycle

Answers

1. **(C)** Wessel has listed criteria for colic as crying for >3 hours per day, for ≥3 days a week, and for >3 weeks. Colic typically begins at 41 to 42 weeks' gestational age even in preterm infants. Thus a 34-week infant at who comes for a checkup at 8 weeks is at the peak age for beginning colic. There are two clinical patterns: 1) paroxysmal fussing, which typically occurs between 5:00 PM and 8:00 PM and the infant is content at other times; 2) hyperirritability, which occurs at all hours in response to either external or internal stimuli that are hard for adults to decipher.

2. **(B)** The key to colic is history and careful physical examination. Any problem that causes pain can also cause irritability, but rarely paroxysmal irritability.

3. **(D)** Major management tools are to empathize, give parents permission to describe the impact of crying on the family's sense of well-being, and support for feelings of anxiety, guilt, isolation, and fear. In trying various management options, such as formula changes, it is important to emphasize to a parent that this will be a clinical trial that might not work and does not mean that the child has an ongoing illness.

4. **(C)** Both small for gestational age (SGA) and moderate low-birth-weight status increase the risks for spastic diplegia. Children with SGA can have a range of colic and temperament differences as well as GE reflux and growth delays.

5. **(D)** Associated factors with CP include congenital CMV, placental abnormalities, or CNS abnormalities originating between 24 and 32 weeks. Ultrasound findings associated with CP can include IVH 3, IVH 4, and periventricular leukomalacia.

6. **(C)** Sarah is demonstrating increased tone; thus, bringing her foot to her ear is difficult.

7. **(D)** Piper and colleagues demonstrated that 1% of infants are not sitting by 8 months; thus, not sitting at 9 months reflects a delay.

8. **(B)** As children develop more mature motor skills, they become unfisted. This permits batting at objects. However, persistent hand openness is required for transferring both ways, finger feeding, pincer grasping, and releasing blocks.

9. **(C)** Children with 60-db hearing loss can respond to sirens (>100-db sound source). They also smile and coo. In an era of transient otoacoustic emissions and automated auditory brainstem response, no child is too young to be tested. Children who receive aminoglycosides may experience auditory nerve toxicity. However, both

Table 22-1. CEREBRAL PALSY SYNDROMES

Type of Cerebral Palsy	Major Risk Groups	Characteristic Features	Ambulation Potential	Associated Sensory and Developmental Impairments	Activity of Daily Living Functioning
Diplegia	VLBW with IVH 3–4, PVL, or ventriculo-megaly.	Legs involved more than arms. 50% preterm. Increased lower extremity tone is clue.	90% walk. Those not walking at 3 are high risk for deformity.	Strabismus, learning, attention, and communicative disorders are common.	Independent in self-care and sphincter control. Major academic challenges in elementary school.
Triplegia	Etiologies overlap with diplegia and hemiplegia.	Combination of diplegia and hemiplegia.	50% walk. High rates of deformities.	Strabismus, cognitive, communicative, learning, and attention disorders are common.	Difficulty with manual dressing tasks, climbing stairs, and perineal hygiene.
Hemiplegia	50% congenital. Intrauterine co-twin demise. Congenital heart surgery.	One side of body, arm more involved than leg. Early hand preference is a clue.	100% walk. Extent of parenchymal brain abnormalities related to cognition.	Visual field cut, cognitive and communicative disorders. High rate of partial seizures.	Difficulty with fasteners for dressing, independent in basic self-care and sphincter control tasks.
Quadriplegia	CNS dysgenesis, meningitis, prolonged cardiopulmonary arrest.	Significant involvement of all 4 limbs. Usually has mixed tone including spastic, and dystonic.	25% walk, however, 100% walk who have sitting balance by 2 years.	Epilepsy and significant mental retardation in 50% (IQ <50). Deafness and severe visual impairment in 50%.	High rate of self-care, communicative, and continency limitations. Benefits from assistive technologies.

genetic testing for common causes of nonsyndromic sensorineural hearing loss and evaluation for genetic vulnerabilities to ototoxicity need to be considered.

10. **(B)** Craniosynostosis is not associated with cerebral palsy. Both periventricular leukomalacia and ventriculomegaly reflect white matter injury that contributes to spastic motor disability. Children with CNS calcifications secondary to CMV, toxoplasmosis, or rubella have multiple neurodevelopment impairments including neurosensory, developmental, and motor disabilities. Children with craniosynostosis (Apert, Crouzon, Pfeiffer) have a range of cognitive and learning disorders but not cerebral palsy.

11. **(B)** Most state Early Intervention regulations require a delay of two standard deviations in one area for program eligibility. Sarah meets these criteria on both motor tasks and developmental tasks.

12. **(D)** Crawling is a 9- to 10-month developmental motor skill. This would be too difficult for Sarah.

13. **(C)** Children develop a mature pincer between 9 and 11 months. This would be difficult for Sarah at this time.

14. **(D)** Sharing with others does not become common until after the second birthday.

15. **(B)** See Table 22-1: Cerebral Palsy Syndromes.

16. **(D)** Children with diplegia have a 90% probability of becoming ambulatory. They are able to learn self-care skills. They have higher rates of learning disorders and attentional disorders. Though Sarah will have some gait differences, she should be viewed as a child who will continue to develop learning and adaptive skills.

SUGGESTED READING

Parker S, Zuckerman B: Colic. In: Parker S, Zuckerman B, Augustyn M (eds): *Development and Behavioral Pediatrics: A Handbook for Primary Care*. Philadelphia: Lippincott, Williams & Wilkins, 2005, pp 158–162.

Palmer FB, Hoon AH: Cerebral Palsy. In: Parker S, Zuckerman B, Augustyn M (eds): *Development and Behavioral Pediatrics: A Handbook for Primary Care*. Philadelphia: Lippincott, Williams & Wilkins, 2005, pp 145–151.

Piper MC, Darrah J: *Motor Assessment of the Developing Infant*. Philadelphia: WB Saunders, 1994, pp 114–139.

CASE 23: A 4-YEAR-OLD BOY WITH MOTOR DISABILITY PREPARING TO TRANSITION TO PUBLIC SCHOOL KINDERGARTEN

Casey is a 4-year-old boy getting ready for transition to public school. He has been diagnosed with cerebral palsy.

Birth history: Pregnancy was complicated by a placenta abruption at 36 weeks' gestation. This occurred during a sailing party in a rural area. It took approximately 6 hours to reach an emergency room and an additional 3 hours to bring together anesthesiology and obstetrics for a cesarean section. Casey weighed 7 pounds at birth. The neurologist informed the parents that Casey did suffer brain damage; however, there was a chance that future disability could be minimal.

Developmental history: At 5 months, Casey entered an Early Intervention program. As an infant, he was alert and responsive to social interactions, but his motor control and coordination were poor. By the age of 4 years he could use a touch talker to communicate basic needs and could use a switch to direct his powered wheelchair. His parents, particularly his mother, are very involved with his learning and have a positive partnership with his preschool. An intelligent and well-educated person, his mother communicates and listens to the professionals and provides useful input regarding Casey's learning styles and ways to promote his development.

Physical examination reveals an alert, social boy in a wheelchair. He laughed when you told him that your favorite summer food was ice cream. His growth is at the 25th percentile. His neurological examination reveals full extraocular movements, difficulty with putting his tongue to lips, chin, or cheeks on request, and inability to repeat common sounds or words. He can indicate his needs with a picture board. His lower extremity reflexes are 3+ at the knees, and sustained clonus is elicited at the ankles. With eye gaze, he identifies shapes and colors and has prepositional concepts and counting skills.

As Casey prepares his transition to a public school setting, his mother has requested a team meeting with the physical therapist, teacher, and psychologist. She says that Casey has many more capabilities than are shown by his motor skills. She is dissatisfied with timed assessments of Casey and wants the staff to use modifications that will accurately reflect Casey's abilities. She states that Casey should be mainstreamed with a same age kindergarten class.

SELECT THE ONE BEST ANSWER

1. What characteristic features are not necessary for considering the diagnosis of hypoxemic ischemic encephalopathy?

   (A) cord pH less than 7.1
   (B) severe respiratory depression
   (C) neonatal seizures
   (D) multisystem organ failure
   (E) serially abnormal neurological examination performed in the first 72 hours

2. What types of associated neurodevelopmental disorders rarely accompany cerebral palsy attributed to hypoxemic ischemic encephalopathy?

   (A) epilepsy
   (B) mental retardation
   (C) learning disability
   (D) hearing impairment
   (E) feeding disability

3. If a child with cerebral palsy has a hearing impairment, what is least likely to contribute to etiology?

   (A) peak bilirubin of 15 mg/dL in the newborn period requiring phototherapy for 24 hours
   (B) family history of early childhood hearing loss
   (C) gray forelock in his grandmother
   (D) use of ECMO for persistent fetal circulation after meconium aspiration syndrome
   (E) all of the above are likely to contribute to the hearing impairment

4. If audiological testing at 10 months revealed a severe and possibly profound bilateral hearing loss with mild abnormalities on tympanometry

and the child had no motor or developmental delays, all of the following developmental communication outcomes are likely except:

(A) inability to learn sign language
(B) difficulty in learning oral language compared with non-hearing impaired peers
(C) none, if the middle ear abnormality is corrected
(D) recognition of spoken words if cochlear implantation surgery takes place
(E) all of the above developmental-communication outcomes are likely

5. When aided binaurally by hearing aids and when given intensive speech/language therapy and audiological training, increased attention to sound is noted. Follow-up audiogram reveals aided responses in the mild range at 250 Hz and moderate at 500 to 4000 Hz. What might the consequences be of improved speech recognition?

(A) turning to loud sounds
(B) immediately beginning to talk in words
(C) learning to say some single word approximations
(D) imitating the sounds that animals make
(E) beginning to like the music in "Barney"

6. Each of the following first-trimester illnesses are commonly associated with hearing loss in the newborn except:

(A) toxoplasmosis
(B) CMV
(C) syphilis
(D) rubella
(E) influenza A

7. All of the following syndromes are associated with severe sensorineural hearing loss except:

(A) Klinefelter's syndrome
(B) Waardenburg syndrome
(C) Hurler's syndrome
(D) Usher's syndrome
(E) prolonged QT syndrome

8. All of the following diagnostic tools may be helpful in identifying the etiology of hearing loss except:

(A) CT scan of temporal bones
(B) molecular test of connexin-26 mutations
(C) dilated funduscopic examination
(D) EKG
(E) pituitary function tests

9. Of the following family actions, which is least likely to be helpful?

(A) having all family members learn sign language
(B) sending child to an out of state residential school
(C) enrolling child in Early Intervention
(D) testing other adult family members
(E) exploring options for cochlear implants

10. When using a touch talker, what output by Casey might indicate that he is above average in developmental skills?

(A) correctly identifying colors
(B) correctly naming shapes
(C) knowing the next word in a song
(D) typing his full name and phone number

11. What are the appropriate support services for Casey at kindergarten entry that are included in IDEA 1997 (Individual with Disability Education Act), the federal law specifying evaluation and supports for children with disabilities?

(A) wheelchair bus transportation
(B) augmentative communication services
(C) adapted physical education
(D) classroom aide
(E) all of the above

12. All of the following are key features of IDEA 1997 except:

(A) free public education
(B) least restrictive environment
(C) rehabilitation services that increase a child's ability to learn
(D) no modifications during standardized testing
(E) all of the above are key features

13. At the age of 5 years, Casey can count to 20, knows the alphabet, can match sounds with letters, and loves books like *The Cat in the Hat*. All of the following are reasonable short-term goals for Casey except:

(A) learning to read
(B) learning addition and subtraction
(C) learning to walk
(D) going to adaptive aquatics

14. The least important goals for Casey in kindergarten include:

(A) learning to take turns in groups
(B) following the teacher's directions
(C) making friends
(D) learning how to write with a pencil in cursive
(E) all of the above are key features

Answers

1. **(A)** Casey survived an unanticipated catastrophic event. It is important to realize that both the lay public and the American legal system often think that all at-risk obstetric events can be known and effectively prevented, and that all neurologic sequelae result in total disability. In order to clinically attribute cerebral palsy to hypoxemia and ischemia, there must be a clustering of neonatal indicators, such as blood pH <7.0 and neonatal respiratory depression, as well as associated disorders, such as neonatal seizures and organ dysfunction (cardiac, renal, bone marrow, hepatic) accompanied by sequentially abnormal neurologic examinations.

2. **(C)** Although Casey had severe motor sequelae, he was spared major cognitive, visual, auditory, and learning sequelae.

3. **(A)** Family history, ECMO, and Mendelian disorders like Waardenburg syndrome (partial albinism, medial displacement of inner canthi, and deafness in 25% follows autosomal dominant inheritance) are known etiologies for congenital hearing loss.

4. **(C)** Mild tympanographic abnormalities do not cause hearing loss of >70 db. Children with severe to profound hearing loss can learn signs or recognize some speech with cochlear implants. They have delays in learning oral language. Although a 25-db hearing loss can occur with persistent middle ear effusion, middle ear surgery alone will not correct the audiogram to normal.

5. **(C)** Improved speech recognition is initially associated with learning to make speech sounds, especially single words or single-word approximations. A child with moderate hearing loss will turn to loud sounds, imitate sounds of animals, and begin to like children's songs.

6. **(E)** Significant sensorineural hearing impairment could be etiologically related to congenital infections such as rubella, CMV, toxoplasmosis, and syphilis. The peak vulnerability for viral teratogenesis occurs during the first trimester. Embryologically this occurs for the eighth nerve ganglion at 30 days, and cochlear duct and superior colliculus at 16 weeks.

7. **(A)** Significant sensorineural hearing impairment could be etiologically related to a genetic disorder (prolonged QT, Waardenburg, Usher's, hypothyroidism, malformations of the cochlea), genetic-metabolic disorders (Hurler's, Cockayne's, osteogenesis imperfecta), and molecular disorders (connexin-26 mutations).

8. **(E)** Pituitary function tests are not indicated for the workup of deafness. However, if growth failure and/or septo-optic dysplasia is present, appropriate endocrine studies are indicated.

9. **(B)** Infants and toddlers benefit from sign language, Early Intervention, medical and genetic evaluation, and discussions with a pediatric neurotologist regarding cochlear implantation.

10. **(D)** Although 4-year-olds know colors, shapes, and words of songs and rhymes, they do not typically print their names or remember phone numbers until age 5 years.

11. **(E)** IDEA 97 provides an array of supports for children with disability, including transportation, augmentative communication aids, and both supports and modifications of the curriculum.

12. **(D)** The Americans with Disability Act provides for appropriate accommodations during testing. IDEA provides for free appropriate public education in the least restrictive environment with supports necessary to access learning.

13. **(C)** Children who are unable to sit, crawl, or pull to stand at age 5 years are unlikely to walk. All children who can sit at age 2 years can walk. Many children who sit at 4 years can ultimately walk. Casey did not sit at ages 2 or 4 years.

14. **(D)** Casey's motor control allows him to access switches but not manipulate objects. He will not be able to manipulate crayons if he cannot manipulate common objects like spoons.

Current public school law provides modifications and supports so that Casey can optimize his participation in learning activities with peers. His mother is appropriately ahead of the school system in her request for appropriate learning and educational supports.

The key developmental issue is whether or not the child can hear some speech with amplification. If he cannot, then total communication or coordination of cochlear implantations with intense aural rehabilitation is required.

SUGGESTED READING

Palmer FB, Hoon AH: Cerebral palsy. In: Parker S, Zuckerman B, Augustyn M (eds): *Development and Behavioral Pediatrics: A Handbook for Primary Care*. Philadelphia: Lippincott, Williams & Wilkins, 2005, pp 145–151.

Roizen NJ, Deifendorf AO, eds: *Hearing Loss in Children. The Pediatric Clinics of North America*, Vol. 46, no. 1. Philadelphia: W.B. Saunders, 1999.

Cheney PD, Palmer FB: Cerebral palsy. *Ment Retard Dev Disabil Res Rev* 3:109–219, 1997.

Nelson KB: The epidemiology of cerebral palsy in term infants. *Ment Retard Dev Disabil Res Rev* 8:146–150, 2002.

Wills LM, Wills KE: Hearing impairment. In: Parker S, Zuckerman B, Augustyn M (eds): *Development and Behavioral Pediatrics: A Handbook for Primary Care*. Philadelphia: Lippincott, Williams & Wilkins, 2005, pp 215–221.

CASE 24: A 1-YEAR-OLD WITH EARLY HANDEDNESS

A 1-year-old boy named Adam presents with motor delay at a physical examination with a new doctor. The mother reports that he has been "left-handed" since 6 months of age. The mother worries that Adam is not able to do the things his older brother was able to do at a similar age.

Adam weighed 6 pounds at birth and was born at 38 weeks' gestational age. There were no prenatal, perinatal, or postnatal concerns except for his motor delays. Records from his previous doctor note that a strong startle reflex (Moro) was elicited on several occasions in the first 2 months of life.

On physical examination, among other things, you note that his right hand is slightly smaller than his left. He smiles symmetrically. He is able to sit, but when pushed to his right, he falls. When prone, his right arm cannot do a marine pushup. In vertical suspension, he weight bears on his legs. His lower extremity reflexes and tone are normal. There are no birth marks.

SELECT THE ONE BEST ANSWER

1. What other examination findings might be present?

   (A) ease with pronation and supination of the right arm
   (B) ease transferring across the midline to take an object from the left hand
   (C) difficulty doing a pincer with the right hand
   (D) inability to finger feed with his left hand

2. What type of motor disorder might this be?

   (A) diplegic cerebral palsy
   (B) brachial plexus palsy
   (C) hemiplegic cerebral palsy
   (D) Sturge-Weber syndrome
   (E) none of the above

3. All of the following supportive tests are indicated except?

   (A) MRI of brain
   (B) EEG
   (C) Wood's lamp examination
   (D) urine culture for CMV
   (E) plasma amino acid

4. Adam's mother asks you if the MRI and EEG are being ordered to make sure that Adam doesn't have a brain tumor. What should you tell her?

   (A) The reason we are ordering the MRI is to make sure there is no brain tumor.
   (B) The reason we are ordering an MRI is to understand if there are differences between the right and left sides of Adam's brain.

(C) We are trying to find a brain lesion that could benefit from neurosurgery.

(D) If the EEG reveals a focal discharge, then we can treat with anticonvulsants and not worry about motor delay.

5. Diagnostic studies are done. Adam's MRI reveals a small left frontal porencephalic cyst. EEG reveals no seizure activity. Plasma amino acids are normal. Urine shows no growth of CMV. Wood's lamp reveals no depigmented macules. An adult neurologist who is a family friend states that there has been brain damage that is permanent and nothing can be done. Adam's mother calls your office in crisis. Which of the following is true?

(A) All children with hemiplegic cerebral palsy learn to walk.

(B) If the lesion involves the left hemisphere, there is poor prognosis for speech.

(C) If seizures occur, they are severe.

(D) There may be difficulty with both visual fields.

(E) Adam will require residential placement.

6. Adam's mother read that hyperbaric oxygen treatments could help children with brain injury. She asks you to write a letter justifying this treatment to the insurance company. The responsibilities of primary care physicians to families with children with hemiplegic cerebral palsy include:

(A) early intervention referral

(B) intensive PT to ensure walking

(C) orthopedic referral for consideration of inhibitive casting of the right upper extremity

(D) writing letters to the insurance companies/public aid to obtain authorization for hyperbaric oxygen treatments

(E) A and C

7. At the age of 8 years, Adam's intelligence was re-evaluated using the Stanford-Binet Intelligence Scale IV Edition. The test resulted in an IQ of 42 (normal 100 ± 15). On the Vineland Adaptive Behavior Scales, he is at a 3- to 4-year developmental level. His articulation skills were at a $3\frac{1}{2}$-year level. His receptive language skills were at a $4\frac{1}{2}$-year level and his expressive language skills were at a $3\frac{1}{2}$-year level. What is Adam's developmental diagnosis?

(A) mild mental retardation
(B) moderate mental retardation
(C) severe mental retardation
(D) learning disabilities
(E) none of the above

Questions 8 through 34. Prognostic Belief Scale. Based on the information provided in question 7, use the following probabilities to indicate the degree to which Adam will be able to perform the skills listed below when he matures into adulthood.

(A) 10% or less
(B) 25%
(C) 50%
(D) 90%
(E) 100%

8. Dress and use the toilet independently

9. Enter into a marriage contract

10. Drink from a cup independently

11. Cook a meal unsupervised

12. Raise children

13. Find his own way in unfamiliar surroundings

14. Use a lock and key

15. Indicate symptoms verbally to a physician

16. Budget for monthly expenses

17. Eat with utensils

18. Do his own laundry

19. Make change for a dollar

20. Tell time

21. Have an intimate sexual relationship

22. Fill out a job application

23. Participate in a simple conversation

24. Use public transportation independently

25. Recognize traffic and exit signs

26. Schedule daily activities independently

27. Use a pay telephone

28. Choose appropriate clothes to wear

29. Follow a national news event

30. Act appropriately toward strangers

31. Sustain a friendship with another person

32. Anticipate hazards appropriately

33. Follow a one-stage command

34. Address two people by name

35. Based on the information in question 7, by adult-hood, where would Adam most likely live?

    (A) in an unsupervised apartment
    (B) in a supervised apartment
    (C) in a group home
    (D) in an institution
    (E) in a nursing home

36. Based on the information in question 7, by adult-hood, where would Adam most likely work?

    (A) in a skilled, competitive employment
    (B) in an unskilled, competitive employment
    (C) in a supervised, full-time employment
    (D) in a supervised, part-time employment
    (E) Adam will be incapable of any productive employment

Answers

1. **(C)** Children with preference for one hand early in childhood are often indicating significant motor control abnormalities. This child would not be doing a pincer (a 9- to 11-month developmental skill) with his right hand.

2. **(C)** Children with brachial plexus palsy do not have a symmetric Moro reflex. Children with diplegic cerebral palsy have indicators of lower ex-tremity spasticity. Children with Sturge-Weber syndrome have facial vascular abnormalities (fa-cial nevus flammeus). Strong hand preference with motor delay on the uninvolved side indi-cates hemiplegic cerebral palsy.

3. **(D)** More than 50% of congenital hemiplegia is of prenatal onset. MRI will often reveal CNS dysgenesis or a porencephalic cyst. EEG might yield evidence of a partial paroxysmal abnormal-ity. A Wood's lamp examination will help rule out tuberous sclerosis complex. Plasma amino acids might indicate increased methionine, which can be part of homocystinuria. In homocystinuria there are increased risks of vascular events, in-cluding stroke, dislocated lens, osteoporosis, and mental retardation. Urine for CMV would not be helpful at 1 year as it would not necessarily in-dicate congenital CMV.

4. **(B)** Adam has congenital hemiplegic cerebral palsy. This may be associated with an intrauter-ine vascular event, especially the death of a co-twin. The purpose of neuroimaging is to assess if his CNS structures might be asymmetric.

5. **(A)** The outcome for children with hemiplegic ce-rebral palsy in sequential studies involving large cohorts is 100% for ambulation. There is a range of cognitive outcomes based on the extent of the hemispheric lesion. There is enough hemispheric plasticity that language emerges consistent with cognitive skills. Seizures, if they occur, are readily controllable. If there are visual field problems, they are unilateral. Residential placement is nei-ther in Adam's best interest nor available.

6. **(E)** Given Adam's lesion, he will benefit from Early Intervention and quality early childhood educational experiences. Hyperbaric oxygen has not improved motor or functional outcomes in children in randomized clinical trials. Complica-tions included perforated ear drums, middle ear effusions, and parental expense. Adam will walk regardless of the intensity of PT. Hyperbaric ox-ygen is not medically indicated.

7. **(B)** Adam's scores are >3 standard deviations be-low the mean, which indicates moderate mental retardation. The table (see Table 24-1 below) in-

Table 24-1. COGNITIVE ADAPTIVE INTELLECTUAL DISABILITY

Degree of Cognitive Impairment	Prevalence and Characteristic Features	Communication and Activities of Daily Living (ADL)
Mild: IQ 55–69 with concurrent adaptive disability and need for intermittent/limited supports.	20–30/1,000. Detected most often in kindergarten and early elementary school years. Major risk factors include poverty and low maternal educational achievement.	Independent in communication and all ADL. Capable of reading and writing to 4th or 5th grade level. Some resources required to maximize employment options and independent living.
Moderate: IQ 40–54 with concurrent adaptive disability and need for limited/extensive supports.	5/1,000. Detected most often in preschool years as language delay. Major known etiologies include chromosome disorders and genetic syndrome.	Independent in all ADL. Communicative of basic needs; able to learn functional-survival academic skills. Will have a spectrum of housing and employment options requiring some supervision.
Severe: IQ 25–39 with concurrent adaptive disability and need for extensive/pervasive supports.	3/1,000. Identified prior to age 3 years. High rates of genetic, bio-medical, and neurological etiologies.	Able to walk. Limited communication. Difficulty with independence in all ADL, though can master many basics. Range of behavior difficulties includes terrible twos, autistic spectrum, hyperactivity. Requires much family support, respite, and creative caretaking. Benefits from day treatment and recreational programs.
Profound: IQ <25 with concurrent adaptive disability and need for pervasive supports and specialized health services.	1–2/1,000. Identified prior to age 2 years. Highest rates of genetic, bio-medical, and neurological etiologies.	Majority without CP walk. Some can be toilet trained. Need supervision or assistance for most ADL. May be medically frail (e.g., epilepsy, aspiration). May require both nursing and humanistic interventions.

ADL, activities of daily living; CP, cerebral palsy.

dicates developmental levels of mental retardation, supports required, and outcomes at key ages.

8. (**E**) 100% to dress and use the toilet independently

9. (**A**) <10% to enter into a marriage contract

10. (**E**) 100% to drink from a cup independently

11. (**C**) 50% to cook a meal unsupervised

12. (**A**) <10% to raise children

13. (**A**) <10% to find his own way in unfamiliar surroundings

14. (**C**) 50% to use a lock and key

15. (**C**) 50% to indicate symptoms verbally to a physician

16. (**A**) <10% to budget for monthly expenses

17. (**E**) 100% to eat with utensils

18. (**C**) 50% to do own laundry

19. (**A**) <10% to make change for a dollar

20. (**B**) 25% to tell time

21. (**B**) 25% to have an intimate sexual relationship

22. (**A**) <10% to fill out a job application

23. (**E**) 100% to participate in a simple conversation

24. (**D**) 90% to use public transportation independently

25. (**C**) 50% to recognize traffic and exit signs

26. (**B**) 25% to schedule daily activities independently

27. (**B**) 25% to use a pay telephone

28. (**D**) 90% to choose appropriate clothes to wear

29. (**C**) 50% to follow a national news event

30. (**D**) 90% to act appropriately toward strangers

31. (**E**) 100% to sustain a friendship with another person

32. (**C**) 50% to anticipate hazards appropriately

33. (**E**) 100% to follow a one-stage command

34. (**E**) 100% to address two people by name
    Adam's developmental diagnosis over time became one of moderate mental retardation. He has a <10% chance of attaining functional literacy but will be independent in self-care, such as eating, dressing, bathing, and continency. Adam will be challenged by adult responsibilities, including marriage, child rearing, budgeting, and driving (see Table 24-1).

35. (**B**) Adam does not require a nursing home. Current social policy has resulted in no new admissions to institutions. Adam's most probable living arrangement will be in a supervised apartment.

36. (**D**) Adam's most likely employment will be supervised and part time.

SUGGESTED READING

Coulter DL: Mental retardation: Diagnostic evaluation. In: Parker S, Zuckerman B, Augustyn M. *Development and Behavioral Pediatrics: A Handbook for Primary Care*, 2nd ed. Philadelphia: Lippincott, Williams & Wilkins, 2005, pp 238–241.

Accardo PJ, Capute AJ: Mental retardation. In: Capute AJ, Accardo PJ (eds): *Developmental Disabilities in Infancy and Childhood*, 2nd ed, Vol. 2. Baltimore: Paul H. Brookes Publishing, 1996.

Batshaw ML, Shapiro B: Mental retardation. In: Batshaw ML (ed): *Children with Disabilities*, 5th ed. Baltimore: Paul H. Brookes Publishing, 2002, pp 287–305.

Hoon AH, Palmer FB. Cerebral palsy. In: Parker S, Zuckerman B, Augustyn M (eds): *Development and Behavioral Pediatrics: A Handbook for Primary Care*, 2nd ed. Philadelphia: Lippincott, Williams & Wilkins, 2005.

CASE 25: A CHILD WITH SPINA BIFIDA

A newborn girl named Anita presents with a lumbar meningomyelocele, noted in the delivery room of a community hospital. Mom is a 29-year-old woman with two normal children. The pregnancy was uneventful. Because of failure of labor to progress after 24 hours, a cesarean section was performed using general anesthesia. You are summoned by your emergency beeper and arrive 15 minutes later to the hospital obstetrical operative delivery room. The father is in the delivery room looking pale and tearful.

On physical examination, Anita is 6 pounds, robust and has a vigorous cry, a good urine stream, spontaneous knee flexion and extension, and club feet. The delivery room nurses have applied a sterile dressing to Anita's back.

SELECT THE ONE BEST ANSWER

1. How will you communicate your initial concerns to Anita's father?

   (A) I am concerned that there must be something seriously wrong with Anita's brain.
   (B) If Anita's mother had not run out of prenatal vitamins, this would not have happened.
   (C) Anita seems to have had a disorder impacting on her spinal cord. Even though it looks very different, specialists in pediatric neurosurgery can assist us in management.
   (D) We should make Anita comfortable but not do anything heroic.
   (E) You do not communicate any initial concerns. Allow the neurosurgeon to evaluate and talk to Anita's father.

2. Major known etiologies of neural tube disorders include all of the following except:

   (A) taking prenatal vitamins prior to conception
   (B) chromosomal disorders
   (C) maternal anticonvulsants
   (D) first-trimester hyperthermia
   (E) multiple malformation syndromes

3. You inform both parents together of your concerns. Which is the most appropriate statement?

   (A) "Anita has spina bifida and will be severely handicapped."
   (B) "I don't know how to fix this."
   (C) "The mother might have drunk too much alcohol in early pregnancy."
   (D) "The mother must have had unrecognized diabetes in pregnancy."

(E) "We are going to transfer Anita to a tertiary care center where specialists will help."

4. All of the following pertinent initial findings are reassuring except:

(A) the anterior fontanelle is flat
(B) nystagmus is present
(C) there is a vigorous Moro
(D) there is decreased movement of the feet
(E) B and D

5. Complications of spina bifida include all of the following except:

(A) hydrocephalus
(B) neurogenic bowel and bladder
(C) severe mental retardation
(D) kyphoscoliosis
(E) difficulty with lower extremity sensation

6. At age 4½, Anita arrives in your office with an aluminum lightweight wheelchair, which she expertly self-propels down the hall. She locks her brakes and, with lightweight braces and crutches, she walks to a small table.

Which of the following is true?

(A) Anita will not need a wheelchair as a teenager.
(B) Anita will learn to do her own bladder catheterization.
(C) Anita has no risk for a shunt malfunction.
(D) Anita is severely retarded.
(E) Anita does not need to take special latex precautions if she has not had a latex allergic reaction.

7. In kindergarten, Anita is able to walk with braces and a walker. She sings songs, speaks clearly in five- or six-word sentences, and knows colors, the alphabet, and counting. She is able to draw a circle and a cross, but not a triangle. She is left-handed. She can construct a three-piece bridge and a five-piece gate with blocks. Her drawing of a person consists of a head with two stick legs. She is not yet toilet trained. Anita's developmental diagnosis is:

(A) severe mental retardation
(B) severe reading disability
(C) mild perceptual delays

(D) pathologic left-handedness
(E) poor self-image

8. All of the following are signs of developmental readiness for daytime toilet training except:

(A) can pull pants off
(B) shows awareness of wetness
(C) when the parent sits the child on the toilet every 2 hours, will urinate ≥ 25% of the time.
(D) understands cause and effect
(E) can follow two-step commands and speaks in two-word phrases

9. All of the following statements about toileting are true except:

(A) stools should be treated with disgust
(B) the most important outcome is the child's sense of self-esteem and task-mastery
(C) it is wrong to fight, punish, shame, or nag
(D) girls achieve toileting earlier than boys
(E) imitating parents and siblings is helpful

10. In children, which of the following statements is true?

(A) All children with Down syndrome require diapers in kindergarten.
(B) Children with spina bifida cannot learn independent catheterization until adolescence.
(C) Nocturnal enuresis occurs in 25% of 4-year-olds.
(D) The lowest rate of success for nocturnal enuresis is with alarms.
(E) Enuresis does not run in families.

11. In preadolescents with chronic illness, indicators of low self-esteem include all of the following except:

(A) completing a board game even if one is losing
(B) not trying something for fear of failure
(C) acting silly to minimize feeling like a failure
(D) saying "I can't do anything right."

Answers

1. (**C**) Anita has a lower lumbar meningomyelocele. Initial management includes keeping the wound sterile and careful closure by an experienced pediatric neurosurgeon.

Major advances include recognition that neonatal folate decreases primary risks in populations and recurrent risk in subsequent pregnancies. The goal of pediatrics is to be supportive of the family while arranging for consultative experience. Too many fears are raised by not systematically describing spina bifida, its developmental impact, and its management. It is inappropriate to blame the mother for spina bifida.

2. **(A)** Prenatal vitamins do not cause spina bifida but are preventive for the disorder in a substantial number of individuals. Maternal anticonvulsants (e.g., valproate), chromosomal disorders, first-trimester maternal hyperthermia, and Meckel syndrome (cleft, polydactyly, cystic liver and kidneys) are associated with spina bifida.

3. **(E)** 90% of children with meningomyelocele have hydrocephalus secondary to Arnold Chiari malformations. Hydrocephalus is currently managed with ventriculo-peritoneal shunts.

4. **(E)** Although a vigorous Moro reflex and a flat anterior fontanelle are reassuring, nystagmus and decreased pedal movement reflect brainstem and spinal cord dysfunction.

5. **(C)** Unless complications such as increased intracranial pressure or ventriculitis occur, cognitive impairments are subtle and mild (i.e., learning disabilities, slow learner, mild cognitive impairment).

6. **(B)** Anita is already demonstrating the problem-solving skills of alternative mobility. With training and support, she will learn clean, intermittent catheterization techniques. Anita will need a wheelchair as a teenager. She is always at risk for a shunt malfunction. She is not severely retarded. More than one-third of children with spina bifida have latex sensitivity. There have been reports of latex anaphylaxis. Latex-free practice is currently recommended for children with spina bifida.

7. **(C)** Anita has mild perceptual delays reflected in her difficulty drawing a triangle and not completing more details during her attempt to draw a person.

8. **(C)** Although having some successes on the toilet is comforting, there should be more than 25% successes when put on the toilet every 2 hours.

9. **(A)** Given children's imaginations and easily provoked fears, stools should not be demeaned, but treated in a matter-of-fact manner.

10. **(C)** Nocturnal enuresis occurs in 25% of 4-year-olds, 10% of 8-year-olds, and 2% of 13-year-olds.

11. **(A)** Children with low self-esteem, like Anita, often avoid trying something new, act silly, and are self-derogatory. Finishing a game when one is losing reflects a maturity of learning from one's mistakes.

SUGGESTED READING

Sandler A: *Living with Spina Bifida: A Guide for Families and Professionals*. University of North Carolina Press: Chapel Hill, 1997.

Jacobs RA. Spina bifida. In: Rubin IL, Crocker AC, (eds): *Medical Care for Children and Adults with Developmental Disabilities*, 2nd ed. Baltimore, MD: Paul H Brookes Publishing, 2006, pp 139–152.

Jacobs RA: *Myelodysplasia (spina bifida-myelomeningocele)*. In: Wolraich ML (ed): *Disorders of Development and Learning*, 3rd ed. Hamilton, Ontario: BC Decker, 2003, pp 137–174.

CASE 26: 3-YEAR-OLD WITH SPEECH DELAY

A 36-month-old boy named Max presents for a 3-year-old physical examination with developmental delay. His mother, Madeleine, is 28 years old. The family has just moved into this area. She reports that Max sat at 9 months and walked at 18 months. He can walk up and down steps, and he kicks and throws a ball. A psychologist's examination indicated that Max can build a tower of eight blocks, string four beads, and scribble on paper with crayons. He can draw a vertical line but fails to copy a circle. Max began saying single words at 2 years but still has significant immature jargon use and has not yet combined two words into phrases. Max can identify three body parts, point to familiar objects in books (cat, ball, car), and follow simple commands such as "sit down," "get the doll," and "come here." He likes to roll a ball back and forth with his dad, can remove all his clothes, tries to imitate what adults do in chores, and is not toilet trained.

The psychologist who evaluated Max 3 months ago told the mother his IQ equivalent was 72 ± 5.

SELECT THE ONE BEST ANSWER

1. The developmental areas most delayed for Max are:

    (A) motor
    (B) speech
    (C) language and development
    (D) social-emotional
    (E) A and D

2. Max's developmental skills are like those of a:

    (A) 12-month-old
    (B) 18-month-old
    (C) 24-month-old
    (D) 27-month-old
    (E) 30-month-old

3. If a child has a preschool IQ of 67, what will he be like at age 7?

    (A) unable to talk in sentences
    (B) in diapers
    (C) not able to count
    (D) just starting school because he was too slow at ages 5 and 6
    (E) attending second grade in his community with special education and resource supports

4. Children with mild mental retardation:

    (A) have an IQ score of >2 standard deviations below the mean
    (B) do not have adaptive delays
    (C) cannot learn to read
    (D) cannot participate in mainstream education
    (E) are ineligible for Special Olympics

5. Children with severe language disorders (standard scores <60, normal 100 ± 15):

    (A) never learn to speak in sentences
    (B) cannot learn to read
    (C) never have ADHD
    (D) may have 10-point IQ changes if language skills increase
    (E) A and B

6. Children with classical autism:

    (A) do not walk until age 4
    (B) cannot learn any self-care skills
    (C) have difficulty communicating in sentences and carrying on a conversation
    (D) always have challenging behavior
    (E) have excellent joint attention at age 12 months

7. The goals of Early Intervention for children with preschool developmental and language delay include all of the following except:

    (A) family supports
    (B) promotion of communication skills
    (C) prevention of cognitive decline
    (D) promotion of self-care and social skills

8. At age 11, Max's interval history is significant for his mother bringing his previous school evaluations:

    Psychological: At the age of 6 years, 2 months, he was administered the Stanford-Binet Intelligence Scale. The test resulted in a mental age of 4 years, 8 months, which is equivalent to an IQ of 75.

    Speech-Language: At the age of 7 years, 10 months, he was evaluated for speech and language revealing mildly to moderately delayed articulation skills at an approximate 4-year mental age. His receptive skills were at a 5-year mental age. At the same time, his hearing was evaluated and the results indicated that his hearing was within normal limits bilaterally.

    Medical History: His history reveals no evidence of seizures, convulsions, or other significant illnesses. His vision is normal. His physical growth has been more than the 95th percentile.

    Academic Functioning: At the age of 7 years, 8 months, he was evaluated in school, where he had been placed in a special education class for children with academic difficulties. His teacher reported that he interacted well with peers, which was evidenced by his ability to share and work in groups. He could count to 50 but had difficulty in remembering sounds associated with letters. In reading, it was reported that he could recognize 15 letters of the alphabet. An assessment of his handwriting skills stated that he could print his first name neatly.

    Social History: Max lives with both natural parents and two brothers, age 6 and 8, both of whom have normal intellectual capabilities. His father is employed as a maintenance worker with the highway commission. His mother is not employed outside the home.

What is Max's developmental diagnosis?

(A) slow learner with borderline intelligence
(B) attention deficit disorder
(C) mild mental retardation
(D) learning disabilities
(E) moderate mental retardation

9. If, at the age of 10, Max reads at a third-grade level, what is his capability for becoming literate (fifth-grade reading level)?

(A) 0%
(B) 50%
(C) 90%
(D) 100%

Questions 10 through 29: Young adult prognoses. Use the following probabilities to indicate the degree to which Max will be able to perform the skills listed below when he matures into adulthood.

(A) <10%
(B) 25%
(C) 50%
(D) 90%
(E) 100%

10. Enter into a marriage contract

11. Cook a meal unsupervised

12. Raise children

13. Use a lock and key

14. Indicate symptoms verbally to a physician

15. Budget for monthly expenses

16. Do own laundry

17. Make change for a dollar

18. Tell time

19. Have an intimate sexual relationship

20. Fill out a job application

21. Use public transportation independently

22. Recognize traffic and exit signs

23. Schedule daily activities independently

24. Use a pay telephone

25. Choose appropriate clothes to wear

26. Follow a national news event

27. Act appropriately toward strangers

28. Sustain a friendship with another person

29. Anticipate hazards appropriately

30. Vocational Placement: By adulthood, where would Max most likely work?

(A) in skilled, competitive employment
(B) in unskilled, competitive employment
(C) in supervised, full-time employment
(D) in supervised, part-time employment
(E) he would be incapable of any productive employment

Answers

1. (**C**) Max presented with motor delay followed by challenges in language understanding and use as well as delays in problem-solving and adaptive skills. Children with preschool global developmental delay have standard scores of 2 standard deviations below the mean in two or more areas. They also have delays in communication skills.

2. (**C**) Twenty-four-month-olds string beads, imitate strokes, and know body parts.

3. (**E**) Children with mild mental retardation are toilet trained, talk in sentences, and can count at age 7. All children, whatever the severity of their developmental delays, can attend school from ages 3 to 21. Max will be attending second grade, but he will require supports.

4. **(A)** Children with mild mental retardation have IQ scores 2 standard deviations below the mean, with concurrent adaptive delays. They learn to read, and they can participate in both mainstream education services and Special Olympics.

5. **(D)** Children with severe language disorder can learn to talk in sentences. They also may learn to read. They can have ADHD. Since IQ tests are strongly verbally mediated, as children's language output improves, their IQ may rise.

6. **(C)** Children with autism may walk on time, but struggle with joint attention. They learn self-care. They may not have severe behavior challenges (aggression, self-injuries). They do have difficulty with language pragmatics—carrying on conversations appropriately.

7. **(C)** The goals of Early Intervention are to provide quality early child educational experiences that emphasize learning through play, opportunities that promote self-care and adaptive skills, modeling of social skills (circle time, sharing, listening in groups), and promoting communication skills (modeling activities with words, songs, rhymes).

8. **(A)** A child who was previously tested with an IQ of 75 does not have mild mental retardation (IQ 55 to 69) or moderate mental retardation (IQ 40 to 54). He is making progress and does not have a discrepancy between his cognitive, communicative, perceptual, and academic skill areas that are part of the federal definition for learning disability. His teacher and parents have not endorsed classroom or home difficulty with inattention, impulsivity, or motor hyperactivity, thus ruling out an attention deficit disorder. Max's developmental diagnosis is "slow learner with borderline intelligence (IQ 70 to 84)."

9. **(C)** When Max was tested by a school psychologist in first grade, he had below-average intelligence. Subsequent testing revealed both an articulation disorder and difficulty with complex language skills. Many schools using antiquated discrepancy formulas will treat a child with an IQ of 75 as one who cannot achieve basic functional literacy of grade 5 reading skills. Although language-related skills are a challenge for Max, the ability to orally read and comprehend third-grade material when he is 10 suggests a high probability for basic literacy.

10. **(C)** 50% to enter into a marriage contract

11. **(E)** 100% to cook a meal unsupervised

12. **(C)** 50% to raise children

13. **(D)** 90% to use a lock and key

14. **(E)** 100% to indicate symptoms verbally to a physician

15. **(D)** 90% to budget for monthly expenses

16. **(E)** 100% to do his own laundry

17. **(E)** 100% to make change for a dollar

18. **(E)** 100% to tell time

19. **(E)**100% to have an intimate sexual relationship

20. **(E)** 100% to fill out a job application

21. **(E)** 100% to use public transportation independently

22. **(E)** 100% to recognize traffic and exit signs

23. **(E)** 100% to schedule daily activities independently

24. **(E)** 100% to use a pay telephone

25. **(E)** 100% to choose appropriate clothes to wear

26. **(E)** 100% to follow a national news event

27. **(E)** 100% to act appropriately toward strangers

28. **(E)** 100% to sustain a friendship with another person

29. **(E)** 100% to anticipate hazards appropriately

As an adult, Max will be in competitive employment; however, his chances of meeting all current requirements for high school will be compromised. He will be able to marry and have children.

30. **(B)** He will be able to work many jobs not requiring college experience

SUGGESTED READING

Aylward GP: Overview of school performance problems. In: Aylward GP (ed): *Practitioner's Guide to Developmental and Psychological Testing.* New York: Plenum Medical Book Company, 1994, pp 91–103.

Palmer F, Capute A: Mental retardation. *Pediatr Rev* 15 473–479, 1994.

Roberts KB: Development and developmental disabilities. In: Roberts KB (ed): *Manual of Clinical Problems in Pediatrics.* Philadelphia: Lippincott, Williams & Wilkins, 2001, pp 96–101

Wolraich ML: Disorders of mental development: General issues. In: Wolraich ML (ed): *Disorders of Development and Learning,* 3rd ed. Hamilton, Ontario: BC Decker, 2003, pp 195–205.

Dixon SD, Stein MT: Encounters with children, 2000. In: Dixon SD, Stein MT (eds): *Encounters with Children: Pediatric Behavior and Development.* St. Louis, MO: Mosby, 2000.

Illingworth RS: The examination of the older infant and child. In: Illingworth RS (ed): *The Development of the Infant and Young Child: Normal and Abnormal.* Edinburgh: Churchill Livingstone, 1987, pp 205–230.

CASE 27: A NEWBORN GIRL WITH FLOPPY TONE AND UPWARD-SLANTING EYES

A newborn girl named Amy presents to the evening nurse in the general care nursery with floppy tone and dysmorphic features. She is born full term to a 28-year-old G2 P1 whose first pregnancy resulted in a healthy daughter. She has delivered a full-term 3-kg girl. Pregnancy, labor, and delivery were all uncomplicated except for a winter flu episode of 48 hours in the first trimester. The obstetrician has told the parents that all went well.

1. What are the medical examination findings that occur in 50% but not in 90% of individuals with Down syndrome?

   (A) mid-face hypoplasia
   (B) excess nuchal skin
   (C) small ears
   (D) central hypotonia
   (E) wide space between first and second toes

2. Your examination reveals a clustering of craniofacial dysmorphism, central hypotonia, and a strong Moro. When you come in to discuss your concerns with the family, you should:

   (A) talk to the father alone
   (B) tell the nurse what to say to mother
   (C) talk to both parents and describe what the process will involve
   (D) talk to both parents and say that you do not know what to do for children with Down syndrome
   (E) describe in detail all that children with Down syndrome cannot do

3. What medical concern listed below is not associated with GI malformations?

   (A) oligohydramnios
   (B) vomiting after first feed
   (C) delayed passage of meconium
   (D) choking during feedings
   (E) double bubble on abdominal radiograph

4. Which of the following cardiac malformations does not commonly occur in infants with Down syndrome?

   (A) atrioventricular canal
   (B) tetralogy of Fallot
   (C) hypoplastic left heart syndrome
   (D) atrial septal defects
   (E) ventricular septal defects

5. Atrioventricular canal symptoms frequently include all the following except:

   (A) constipation
   (B) feeding difficulties
   (C) difficulty gaining weight
   (D) congestive heart failure
   (E) excessive sweating

6. The karyotype report is 47XX+21. Cardiology consultation revealed an AV canal on echocardiogram. Amy is having difficulty gaining weight. The cardiovascular surgical consultant informed the parents that definitive surgical correction would take place when the child weighs at least 15 pounds. All of the following are acceptable strategies for addressing Amy's feeding difficulties except:

(A) observe breast-feeding and weigh child before and after 20 minutes of feeding

(B) tell mother that children with Down syndrome are difficult to breast-feed

(C) monitor weight using growth charts specific for Down syndrome and have dad offer pumped breast milk by bottle

(D) add nasogastric feeds at night

7. Amy gained weight slowly, but feeding difficulties continued. At age 2 months, she was hospitalized for RSV pneumonitis with congestive heart failure. At age 4 months, pulmonary artery banding took place. Now, at age 6 months, Amy weighs 10 pounds. She has continuous nasal discharge. It takes her 40 minutes to drink 4 ounces of formula with Polycose. Significant head lag is noted. In prone, Amy does not roll. She likes to put two hands on her bottle during feeding. Amy is in Early Intervention. What is the primary goal of Early Intervention?

(A) vigorous physical therapy to strengthen Amy's neck muscles

(B) developmental feeding interventions with regular feedback to physicians

(C) hospitalization of Amy so that mom might get some rest

(D) enrollment in a day care program outside of home

(E) facilitate starting solid foods to maximize weight gain velocity

8. At age 2, Amy is status post-surgical repair of her AV canal at 18 months. Since surgery, she has made rapid progress in motor skills with attainment of independent ambulation, more fine motor manipulative play, and increased verbal production of single words and jargon use. She awakes at 1:00 AM and 3:00 AM nightly. She returns to sleep if given a bottle of milk or taken into her parents' bed. Night awakening often occurs in a toddler with all of the following issues except:

(A) difficulty self-soothing

(B) nightmares

(C) sleep-onset disorder

(D) circadian rhythm disorder

(E) seizures secondary to open heart surgery

9. In the daytime, frequent temper tantrums occur, especially during feeding time of her newborn brother. Temper tantrums should be managed by:

(A) discussing in detail what Amy is doing wrong

(B) trying to figure out an exact trigger

(C) putting Amy in her room with the door closed for 30 minutes

(D) giving Amy candy to stop

(E) ignoring them

10. By age 5, Amy successfully completed 3 years of a special preschool attendance. She speaks in short sentences with 50% intelligibility to strangers. She is toilet trained during the day. She can dress with simple pullovers, but cannot handle buttons, snaps, or zippers independently. She cannot do her own Velcro sneakers. She is 10% for height and 75% for weight on the Down syndrome growth charts. Her favorite activity is watching "Sesame Street" and cartoons. All are appropriate goals for mainstreaming in kindergarten except:

(A) promoting communication

(B) promoting interaction with typical peers

(C) normalizing IQ

(D) enhancing adaptive skills

(E) providing supports for functional skills

11. At age 5, Amy pushes and bites her brother's playmates. What suggestions would you make for behavioral interventions for dealing with Amy's misbehavior around her brother's friends?

(A) Tell Amy no and put her in time-out.

(B) Explain in detail why it is wrong to bite.

(C) Praise her when she does not bite.

(D) Teach brother how to bite her back.

(E) A and C

12. At age 5, Amy rips up art work and topples over board games when her older sister is entertaining friends. What is the best approach for dealing with Amy's problem behaviors with her older sister and older sister's friends?

(A) loss of television privileges

(B) time-outs of 15 minutes alone in her room

(C) loss of dinner

(D) model appropriate behavior and read *Beren-stein Bears*

(E) overcorrect behavior

13. At age 9, Amy reads and performs math at an early second-grade level. She struggles with learning to write a short book report and she seems to have less energy after school. Her teachers are concerned that both her speech and handwriting have deteriorated. Of the following list, what is the most likely finding on evaluation in the office?

(A) hoarse voice and a mild microcytic anemia

(B) vitamin B_{12} deficiency and a mild macro-cytic anemia

(C) diabetes

(D) early puberty

(E) hearing loss

14. All of the following interventions might enhance Amy's language and communication skills except:

(A) singing songs with rhyming words

(B) teaching conversational scripts

(C) using talking books

(D) surgery to reduce her tongue size

(E) all of above would enhance language and communication

15. Which of the following functional skills is a priority in Amy's educational curriculum?

(A) enhance knowledge and understanding of warning signs and labels

(B) teach telling time

(C) teach money management skills for making basic purchases

(D) encourage responsibility for household chores

(E) promote participation in year-long Special Olympics activities

16. At age 16, Amy has become more withdrawn since her older sister left for college. She does not seem to listen when she is called into another room. During menses, she has more hygiene accidents and she seems more hostile. Her mother has observed her crying alone in her bedroom after her brother went out with friends to a movie. What are some potential medical causes of Amy's sadness and mood embodied by her crying?

(A) depression

(B) dysmenorrhea

(C) lack of exercise

(D) not having friends

(E) obstructive sleep apnea

17. What are the issues that need to be considered and discussed involving Amy's menses and menstrual hygiene?

(A) suggest sterilization

(B) find out how she handles personal hygiene

(C) discuss dating

(D) discuss contraception

(E) B, C, and D

18. At age 25, Amy lives in a L'arche home. She is employed by a hotel for room cleaning. She has begun to have frequent falls when walking longer distances. She also has had new onset of daytime encopresis. Her father recently died of pancreatic cancer. Her grandmother was recently diagnosed at age 85 with Alzheimer's disease.

What are the common treatable medical conditions in adults with Down syndrome that can be associated with motor and continency problems?

(A) hypothyroid

(B) B_{12} deficiency anemia

(C) hearing loss

(D) depression

(E) cervical spine instability

19. What are the support goals for Amy at this time?

(A) explain death and establish spiritual routines

(B) establish mentors

(C) access recreational activities

(D) have another person accompany her during medical encounters to explain Amy's decline of skills

(E) all of the above

20. Who advocates for Amy if complex medical-diagnostic or surgical interventions are considered?

(A) family

(B) guardian

(C) state

(D) older sister

(E) Amy

21. All of the following are key issues that should be discussed routinely during health care visits in young adulthood except:

    (A) risky behaviors
    (B) healthy weight and regular exercise
    (C) symptoms of Alzheimer's disease
    (D) mood
    (E) community participation and friendships

Answers

1. **(B)** Eighty percent of children with trisomy 21 are born to women younger than 35 years. Prenatal advances have included maternal prenatal serum markers (low α-fetoprotein, unconjugated estriol, human chorionic gonadotropin, inhibin A, PAPP), ultrasound markers such as excess nuchal skin, absent nasal bone, femur length, and chorionic villus or early amniocentesis prenatal chromosome testing. Key findings in 90% of children with Down syndrome are midface hypoplasia (depressed nasal bridge, epicanthal folds, small palate with relative macroglossia), small ears, wide space between first and second toes, and central hypotonia. Children with central hypotonia have low tone but not flaccid weakness. The low tone contributes to oral motor deficiencies and delays in postured skills. It does not preclude walking.

2. **(C)** The role of the pediatrician is to express concerns, begin the process of clarifying the diagnosis, and share information with families.

3. **(A)** Polyhydramnios, not oligohydramnios, is associated with GI malformations.

4. **(C)** The most common congenital heart malformations in trisomy 21 are VSD, ASD, AV canal, persistent PDA, and tetralogy of Fallot. HLHS is rare.

5. **(A)** Children with symptoms of AV canal may have feeding difficulties, difficulty gaining weight, CHF, or excessive sweating. Their constipation is part of their hypotonia, not part of the AV canal.

6. **(A)** Many children with congenital heart disorders have difficulty with feeding skills. Among children with Down syndrome this may occur whether the child is breast or bottle fed. Involvement of a developmental feeding program that is supportive and communication among all parties (pediatrician, cardiologist, developmental therapist) is helpful.

7. **(B)** Amy is having complex feeding challenges. Involvement of a pediatric developmental feeding team is in order.

8. **(E)** Night awakening can be a result of difficulty in self-soothing, nightmares, sleep onset disorder, and circadian rhythm disorder (often associated with long daytime naps). Seizures after open heart surgery often delay development.

9. **(E)** Children with Down syndrome may have sleep problems, sibling rivalry, and other typical behaviors of childhood. They benefit from management protocols used in typical kids.

10. **(C)** Children with Down syndrome benefit from developmental and educational strategies that promote communication, as well as social, adaptive, and educational skills. The literature does not support the normalization of IQ by medical or educational interventions. However, all children with Down syndrome learn.

11. **(E)** The best management of challenging behaviors is time-out and positive reinforcement.

12. **(D)** All social skills can be taught.

13. **(A)** Hoarse voice and a mild macrocytic anemia are both findings of hypothyroidism. Hypothyroidism is common in Down syndrome and children with Down syndrome should have routine thyroid function tests.

14. **(D)** Lingual reduction does not enhance speech in Down syndrome.

15. **(A)** Some knowledge of basic signs helps with community participation.

16. **(A)** Mood disorders are common in all adolescents, especially adolescents with developmental disabilities.

17. **(E)** Sterilization is not an option for handling menses and menstrual hygiene.

18. **(E)** Cervical spine instability can present with changes in bowel and bladder function.

19. **(E)** In young adults with developmental disabilities, loss of a family member requires all of the above.

20. **(B)** Though Amy may participate in these decisions, a designated guardian is the best solution.

21. **(C)** As adults, obesity, mood disorders, hearing impairment, thyroid disorders, and atlantoid-axial instability may contribute to changing performances in functional skills. Symptoms of Alzheimer's begin to manifest after age 50 years in approximately one-third of adults with trisomy 21.

SUGGESTED READING

McBries DM: Disorders of mental development: Down syndrome. In: Wolraich ML (ed): *Disorders of Development and Learning*, 3rd ed. Hamilton, Ontario: BC Decker, 2003.

Pueschel SM: Down syndrome. In: Parker S, Zuckerman B, Augustyn M (eds): *Development and Behavioral Pediatrics: A Handbook for Primary Care*. Philadelphia: Lippincott, Williams & Wilkins, 2005, pp 167–171.

Roizen NJ: Down syndrome. In: Batshaw ML (ed): *Children with Disabilities*, 5th ed. Baltimore: Paul H. Brookes Publishing, 2002, pp 307–320.

Kaplan-Sanoff M: School readiness. In: Parker S. Zuckerman B, Augustyn M (eds): *Development and Behavioral Pediatrics: A Handbook for Primary Care*. Philadelphia: Lippincott, Williams & Wilkins, 2005, pp 285–288.

CASE 28: AN 8-YEAR-OLD BOY WITH AUTISTIC BEHAVIORS THAT ARE DIFFICULT TO CONTROL

An 8-year-old boy named Joey presents to the office for behavior management problems. He is nonverbal and likes to screech and twirl. He is very active, loves to run on the playground, and rides a two-wheel bike without training wheels on a safe bike path. He attends a special school and receives speech, OT, and behavioral management services. He can be redirected from prolonged twirling but likes to put assorted nonfood items in his mouth and suck his thumb. Joey's parents come to you requesting suggestions for interventions that might help him behave more appropriately, slow down, and not be so active.

SELECT THE ONE BEST ANSWER

1. Joey's developmental diagnoses include all of the following except:

   (A) classical autism
   (B) mental retardation
   (C) pica
   (D) cerebral palsy
   (E) all of the above diagnoses

2. Key medical areas to monitor in nonverbal children include all of the following except:

   (A) dental caries
   (B) blood sugar
   (C) sleep disorders
   (D) lead levels
   (E) nonaccidental injury

3. Which of the following is/are true about thumb sucking?

   (A) Eighty percent of infants, 40% of preschoolers, and 10% of children over 5 years of age suck their thumbs or fingers.
   (B) Thumb sucking can be self-calming; it may occur when the child is tired, frustrated, hungry, or unhappy.
   (C) If thumb sucking occurs beyond age 4 years, there is increased risk of malocclusion.
   (D) Positive reinforcement techniques (e.g., treats, extra story time, stickers, and replacing thumb sucking with squeezing a foam ball) can help manage the behavior.
   (E) All of the above.

4. The mother states that Joey only sleeps 2 hours per night. Useful approaches include which of the following:

   (A) melatonin and structured behavioral management of sleep hygiene
   (B) chloral hydrate and structured sleep routines
   (C) daytime naps
   (D) long-term use of a benzodiazepine
   (E) A and B

5. Joey begins to watch wrestling after school. One day the principal calls because Joey has shoved a smaller first grader in the cafeteria and she hit

her chin on the edge of the table. The injury required sutures. Which of the following statements about TV is/are true?

(A) Hundreds of studies have demonstrated a link between exposure to TV violence and aggressive behavior.
(B) TV viewing increases the risk of obesity.
(C) TV should not be used as an electronic baby-sitter.
(D) Children who are nonverbal and at a preschool mental age may not distinguish the consequences of aggression seen on TV.
(E) All of the above.

6. One year previously, Joey's grandfather, who used to take him for long walks after school with a dog and let him choose songs from a jukebox at the drug store, died. His mother wonders if this is the reason for his nightmares and night terrors. All the following are true about night terrors except:

(A) children with night terrors bolt upright from their sleep, are glassy eyed, and may have autonomic signs
(B) night terrors occur during an abrupt transition from stage 4 non-REM sleep to REM sleep
(C) children are really awake during night terrors
(D) at the end of 5 to 20 minutes of night terrors, the child returns to sleep

7. All the following are true about nightmares except:

(A) nightmares are upsetting dreams
(B) nightmares do not occur during REM sleep
(C) parents should empathize with the child's fright
(D) parents should comfort the child and stay with him/her while there is distress
(E) transitional objects may be helpful

8. Joey continues to wake at night, strip naked, and smear stools on the walls. All of the following are helpful management strategies except:

(A) enforcing a toileting regimen during the day
(B) severe punishment
(C) restraining Joey's hands
(D) emergency behavioral consultation
(E) all of the above are helpful strategies

9. Which of the following specific behavioral interventions may be helpful?

(A) applied positive behavioral analysis
(B) placement in foster care
(C) administration of enemas after school
(D) sleeping with Joey

Answers

1. **(D)** Joey has autistic spectrum disorder, moderate mental retardation, and pica.

2. **(B)** Children who are nonverbal and children with cognitive disabilities are at risk for elevated lead levels from pica and hand-to-mouth behaviors. Because he is not always cooperative and often acts like a younger child, Joey is at risk for dental caries, sleep disorders, and nonaccidental injuries.

3. **(E)** Eighty percent of infants suck their thumb. In preschool children, thumb-sucking can be used for self-calming, or when a child is frustrated, unhappy, hungry, or tired. After age 4 years, it is associated with malocclusion. Positive reinforcement is a key management technique.

4. **(E)** Management of Joey's sleep requires establishing sleep hygiene as well as judicious use of medications with wide safety margins. These include chloral hydrate and melatonin, as well as a short-term trial of a benzodiazepine. Eliminating daytime naps and getting up at the same time every morning are also important.

5. **(E)** Increased aggression is seen in preschoolers, school-aged children, or teens exposed to TV violence. TV watching is associated with decreased physical activity and poor food choices. This results in obesity. TV should not be used as an electronic baby-sitter. Parental vigilance and proactive rule-setting are required in all ages.

6. **(C)** During night terrors, the child is in rapid eye movement sleep and not actually awake. Children do not remember the events.

7. **(B)** Nightmares do occur during REM sleep.

8. **(B)** Time-ins and time-outs are more appropriate than punishment for decreasing negative behaviors. In applied behavioral analyses, very specific targets are chosen and then shaped through use of discrete trials using appropriate reinforcers.

9. **(A)** Management of challenging behaviors includes applied behavioral analysis, family supports, and emergency respite services.

SUGGESTED READING

Towbin K, Mauk J, Batshaw ML: Pervasive developmental disorders. In: Batshaw ML (ed): *Children with Disabilities*, 5th ed. Baltimore: Paul H. Brookes Publishing, 2002, pp 365–388.

Coronna EB: Autism. In: Parker S, Zuckerman B, Augustyn M (ed): *Development and Behavioral Pediatrics: A Handbook for Primary Care*. Philadelphia: Lippincott, Williams & Wilkins, 2005, pp 124–129.

Howard B: Managing behavior. In: Parker S, Zuckerman B, Augustyn M (eds): *Development and Behavioral Pediatrics: A Handbook for Primary Care*. Philadelphia: Lippincott, Williams & Wilkins, 2005, pp 65–69.

Mindell JA, Owens JA: *A Clinical Guide to Pediatric Sleep: Diagnosis and Management of Sleep Problems*. Philadelphia: WB Saunders, 2003.

CASE 29: A 4-YEAR-OLD WHO WAS BORN PREMATURELY

David is a 4½-year-old boy who attends a Head Start preschool where staff members have requested a comprehensive assessment because they are very concerned about delayed speech, clumsiness, and kindergarten readiness. Specifically, he has poorly articulated sentences and can only be understood by strangers 50% of the time. He is very clingy and very reluctant to interact with other children, preferring to be by adults. When in the backyard, he trips frequently. His mother states that he knows his name, age, and colors. He has difficulty following verbal requests, remembering the alphabet, and counting past 10. He has difficulty with dressing, using a fork, and drawing pictures.

David was born prematurely at 32 weeks' gestation with a birth weight of 1800 grams. Apgar scores were 3 and 7. David's mother and father did not finish high school.

SELECT THE ONE BEST ANSWER

1. David may not go to kindergarten if:

   (A) his parents elect not to send him

   (B) he cannot talk clearly
   (C) he walks down steps, two feet on each
   (D) he occasionally needs to be reminded to use the bathroom
   (E) he is considered immature

2. Developmental disorders common after prematurity include all the following except:

   (A) perceptual delays
   (B) language delays
   (C) learning disabilities
   (D) attention deficit disorder
   (E) autistic spectrum disorder

3. The least common reason for children to repeat kindergarten is:

   (A) developmental delays
   (B) ADHD inattentive type in girls
   (C) treatment for lead poisoning
   (D) parent with difficulty learning to read
   (E) frequent tardiness or absences because of asthma

4. Major reasons boys have difficulty in reading are:

   (A) they have high rates of mental retardation
   (B) they have high rates of language, learning, and attention difficulties
   (C) they like sports
   (D) they misbehave and get into fights
   (E) A, B, and D

5. David's grandmother has wondered whether David might have ADHD or be mildly retarded like her brother who also was premature. Additional family pedigree history will all be helpful except:

   (A) learning, behavioral, and school performance of David's parents
   (B) learning, behavioral, and school performance of David's uncles and aunts
   (C) learning, behavioral and school performance of David's grandparents
   (D) learning, behavioral, and school performance of David's adopted cousin
   (E) all of the above will be helpful

6. David has an uncle and two cousins who experienced delayed language development. Your developmental assessment finds that David runs clumsily,

does not describe what he would do if he were tired or thirsty, has speech that is understandable to you 50% of the time, pedals a tricycle, balances briefly on one foot, follows two-step directions quickly but needs to have the second step repeated, knows three of five colors, counts to 5, makes some mistakes when reciting the alphabet, and can draw a picture of a boy that includes a head and legs but not face, trunk, or arms. David feeds himself independently, needs assistance with zippers, and reminders to use the bathroom. Based on this information, what is most likely David's type of developmental disorder?

(A) mental retardation
(B) cerebral palsy
(C) severe hearing loss
(D) oppositional defiant disorder
(E) developmental language disorder

7. During his kindergarten year David is considered very active and unable to sit still. His parents report that his favorite activities are to watch cartoons and play video games. Components of your initial assessment might include all of the following except:

(A) having his mother fill out a behavioral rating scale for attention deficit, hyperactivity, and conduct
(B) having his classroom teacher fill out a rating scale for attention deficit, hyperactivity, and conduct
(C) having the parents read a brochure about attention and learning problems
(D) ordering an EEG to rule out a seizure disorder
(E) having his full time baby-sitter fill out a behavioral rating scale for attention deficit, hyperactivity, and conduct

8. Both his mother and classroom teacher endorse that David is hyperactive and oppositional and that this is systematically impacting his classroom and home successes. Management options now include all of the following except:

(A) trial of stimulant medications
(B) 504 school plan for behavior supports
(C) teacher instituting an appropriate behavior management plan
(D) expulsion from school until he can control his behaviors
(E) all of the above are good management options

9. David is better able to sit still and pay attention, but he continues to have difficulties on the playground and gets into frequent fights. The school requests that the family discuss with you whether a different medicine should be used. Important information to obtain includes which of the following?

(A) frequency of fights
(B) presence of aggression toward parents
(C) presence of aggression toward brother
(D) David's description of the events
(E) all of the above

10. David states that he gets into fights with only one other child on the playground. That child is considered a bully by several other classmates. David has several friends in the neighborhood, attends church regularly, and sings in the choir. He is kind to the dog. He has never been accused of stealing. Indicators of conduct disorder include all of the following except:

(A) lying
(B) stealing
(C) having a sense of remorse
(D) torturing animals
(E) A and B

11. David struggles with learning sounds associated with letters and recognizing words. At the end of first grade, his teacher says he is a non-reader and cannot learn in the regular classroom. You should do all of the following except:

(A) insist on a psycho-educational assessment of strengths, difficulties, and academic achievement
(B) agree to repeating a grade
(C) observe David's attempt to read a picture book
(D) make sure tutoring supports are implemented at school and home
(E) B and D

Answers

1. **(A)** Developmental delays in speech, motor coordination, toileting accidents, or immaturity are not reasons to delay kindergarten. Schools must accommodate children with these impairments both through individual educational supports and

accommodations such as an aide, reminders, and more time. In many states it is not mandatory to attend kindergarten. Both speech therapy and developmental supports will help promote speech intelligibility and developmental maturity. Unless quality, comprehensive, affordable daycare is available, it is better not to wait another year without some focused developmental interventions.

2. **(E)** Approximately 50% of survivors of preterm birth have minor neurodevelopmental impairments, including perceptual, language, learning, and attention disorders. These disorders are more common than cerebral palsy and warrant both surveillance and proactive management by pediatricians. Autistic spectrum disorders have not been associated with prematurity unless there has been a congenital malformation (e.g., Charge, Moebius), congenital infection (rubella), or severe retinopathy of prematurity with unfavorable visual outcome.

3. **(B)** ADHD inattentive type often presents after age 8 years, and, thus, is not a reason for repeating kindergarten. Developmental delays are often inappropriately managed by grade repetition instead of receiving a comprehensive assessment and appropriate management plan. Children with elevated lead levels may have both developmental delay and ADHD. These should be managed with appropriate educational supports and interventions to lower the lead level and prevent re-exposure. Children whose parents have had difficulty learning to read require appropriate in-school and after-school supports for reading. In addition, adult literacy supports can help both parent and child. An asthma action plan should have as its goals control of nocturnal symptoms, including those that disrupt sleep, and a school-based management plan that does not lead to loss of classroom time.

4. **(E)** Males have higher rates of mild mental retardation and higher rates of language, attentional, and behavioral difficulties. Some of this is because of X-linked vulnerabilities. Some is because more disruptive behaviors result in suspension and loss of classroom time. Some is also a result of having ADHD with comorbidities in language processing and executive functioning skills helpful for school

success. Recent data, however, suggest that children with early identified reading disorders can be helped with interventions that enhance phonological awareness.

5. **(D)** If immediate family members have not completed high school, this increases David's risk for not having academic success. Maternal education is strongly correlated with educational success. If there is a pattern of male educational underachievement, then aggressive early learning strategies are required. David's adopted cousin does not increase David's genetic and multifactorial risk for educational underachievement.

6. **(E)** David has some mild delays in language, coordination, and sequencing. He is at risk for learning disabilities and ADHD. David does not have cerebral palsy as he is running and pedaling a trike. He does not have mental retardation because his core developmental skills suggest that he is functioning at a 3.5- to 4-year developmental level. David's language performance does not suggest a severe hearing loss (>70 db), but audiologic assessment is required to rule out a mild to moderate loss. David's behaviors are active, not oppositional. His rate of language performance is consistent with a developmental language disorder.

7. **(D)** EEGs are not routinely indicated for children with ADHD. Children with staring spells, automatisms, and a family history of absence seizures are at increased risk for petit-mal seizures. In children not sitting still, both parents and teachers should provide the physician with behavioral ratings for attention deficit, hyperactivity, conduct, and learning. More than one caregiver (teacher for school, after-care adults for after school) should give feedback using an instrument like the Vanderbilt or Connor Scales.

8. **(D)** Children with ADHD and behavioral challenges require a behavioral management strategy for difficult behaviors. Both his mother and classroom teacher provide evidence that David is hyperactive and oppositional and that this is systematically impacting his classroom and home successes. Management options for children with ADHD and ODD include a combination of stimulant medication, behavioral management

plan at school and at home, and a 504 plan for appropriate accommodations of David's impulsive behavior. These should be proactively implemented and if there continue to be concerns, both an IEP intervention and counseling interventions are required. David can be expelled from school if he brings a weapon or sells drugs. Pushing, shoving, noncompliance, and mouthing off are not indications for expulsion.

9. **(E)** Aggression at frequent intervals and toward multiple parties with no sense of remorse indicates a need for more sophisticated management strategies than expulsion. David is better able to sit still and pay attention, but he continues to have difficulties on the playground and gets into frequent fights. Hearing David's description of the events, explicitly probing the presence of bullying at home and at school, and determining behavioral contracting that leads to performance of school work but loss of privileges is required. Stimulant medications should continue to be used but not expected to cure David of all behavioral problems.

10. **(C)** Children with conduct disorders break rules in multiple settings, including lying, stealing, and mistreating animals. They often do not have a sense of remorse. David's history is not consistent with conduct disorders but is consistent with ADHD and being bullied. Specific school-wide interventions on the playground, bus, cafeteria, and gym need to be implemented as well as a mechanism to ensure David's safety.

11. **(B)** Most children with learning, attention, and behavioral challenges require extra supports and resources. Repeating a grade is not sufficient. The pediatrician should observe David read. He should put in writing immediately to the school a request that David requires a complete psycho-educational assessment of strengths, difficulties, and academic achievement. The pediatrician should be aware of both educational advocacy and tutoring supports that can be available to David and help the family access tutoring supports after school.

SUGGESTED READING

Coplan J: Language delays. In: Parker S, Zuckerman B, Augustyn M (eds): *Development and Behavioral Pediat-*

rics: A Handbook for Primary Care. Philadelphia: Lippincott, Williams & Wilkins, 2005, pp 222–226.
Goldson E: Developmental consequences of prematurity. In: Wolraich ML (ed): *Disorders of Development and Learning*, 3rd ed. Hamilton, Ontario: BC Decker, 2003, pp 345–360.
Parker S: Attention deficit hyperactivity disorder. In: Parker S, Zuckerman B, Augustyn M (eds): *Development and Behavioral Pediatrics: A Handbook for Primary Care*. Philadelphia: Lippincott, Williams & Wilkins, 2005, pp 114–123.
Wodey KA, Wolraich ML: Attention deficit hyperactivity disorder. In: Wolraich ML (ed): *Disorders of Development and Learning*, 3rd ed. Hamilton, Ontario: BC Decker, 2003, pp 311–328.
Aylward GP: Overview of evaluation considerations. In: Aylward GP (ed): *Practitioner's Guide to Developmental and Psychological Testing*. New York: Plenum Medical Book Company, 1994, pp 15–50.
Kaplan-Sanoff M: School readiness. In: Parker S, Zuckerman B, Augustyn M (eds): *Development and Behavioral Pediatrics: A Handbook for Primary Care*. Philadelphia: Lippincott, Williams & Wilkins, 2005, pp 285–288.
Owens JA: Sleep problems. In: Parker S, Zuckerman B, Augustyn M (eds): *Development and Behavioral Pediatrics: A Handbook for Primary Care*. Philadelphia: Lippincott, Williams & Wilkins, 2005, pp 317–321.

CASE 30: AN 8-YEAR-OLD BOY WITH LOSS OF MILESTONES

TJ is an 8-year-old male who, until the age of 2 years, was developing normally. At the age of 2 years, however, he stopped talking and began to separate himself socially, preferring to play by himself. TJ's pediatrician diagnosed the condition as autism. At age 5, TJ began experiencing seizures. He was treated with anticonvulsants including valproate and carbamazepine (Tegretol). He began to have difficulty with his gait, feeding himself, and dressing himself. Neurologic examination revealed diffuse spasticity, gait ataxia, and tremor during fine motor tasks. Urgent pediatric neurological and genetic consultation took place. A cranial MRI showed leukodystrophy with extensive white matter abnormalities. Genetic, molecular, and biochemical analyses revealed adrenal leukodystrophy.

SELECT THE ONE BEST ANSWER

1. All of the following are key indicators of a more serious problem for TJ except:

   (A) previous normal development
   (B) gain of language skills

(C) new onset of seizures

(D) difficulty with new learning

(E) all of the above are indicators of a more serious problem

2. All of the following are indicated except:

(A) skin fibroblasts for specialized genetic studies

(B) genetic testing of sister

(C) search for a bone marrow match

(D) very long chain fatty acids

(E) referral for genetic consultation

3. His parents wonder when TJ can return to school. Which of the following is a reasonable disability accommodation by school staff for TJ's health condition?

(A) require that he be seizure-free

(B) encourage the parents to sign a DNR

(C) encourage the parents to participate in pediatric hospice

(D) require that he be able to eat orally in the school cafeteria

(E) require that the parents hire a private duty nurse

Answers

1. (B) Because of his regression, TJ has more than just a developmental disorder. Loss of skills may indicate a CNS structural lesion, a complex epilepsy syndrome (for example, Landau-Kleffner syndrome) or a genetic leukodystrophy. Gain of language skills and preservation of motor skills with well-controlled seizures would be reassuring.

2. (B) A combination of expert neurologic and genetic consultations, as well as quality family supports, is required. Once TJ's diagnosis is clarified, appropriate genetic testing can be offered to other family members. Leading causes for leukodystrophy include very long chain fatty acids to rule out X-linked adrenal leukodystrophy, urine arylsulfatase for metachromatic leukodystrophy, and genetic consultation for systematic and comprehensive biochemical and molecular studies to determine the exact nature of the process. Once a diagnosis is made, specialized genetic studies on family members and discussion of management options in-

cluding appropriateness, if available, of enzyme replacement can take place.

3. (C) The support of a pediatric hospice would help family members and school professionals. Schools are required by the Americans with Disabilities Act to serve children with seizures, feeding tubes, and nursing supports. As children with these disorders may live a decade or more, a combination of school and community supports is required.

SUGGESTED READING

Fenichel GM: Psychomotor retardation and regression. In: Fenichel GM, (ed): *Clinical Pediatric Neurology: A Signs and Symptoms Approach*. Philadelphia: WB Saunders, 2001, pp 117–148.

Palfrey JS, Rodman JS: Legislation for the education of children with disabilities. In: Levine MD, Carey Wb, Crocker AC (eds): 1999. *Developmental-Behavioral Pediatrics*, 3rd ed. Philadelphia: WB Saunders, 1999, pp 869–872.

Siegel BS, Trozz M: Bereavement and loss. In: Parker S, Zuckerman B, Augustyn M (eds): *Development and Behavioral Pediatrics: A Handbook for Primary Care*. Philadelphia: Lippincott, Williams & Wilkins, 2005, pp 379–384.

Roberts KB: Death, dying, and mourning. In: Roberts KB (ed): *Manual of Clinical Problems in Pediatrics*. Philadelphia: Lippincott, Williams & Wilkins, 2001, pp 149–158.

CASE 31: A 3-YEAR-OLD BOY WITH POOR LANGUAGE AND SOCIAL SKILLS

Jason is a 3-year-old male brought to the doctor for a comprehensive assessment because of lack of language and social development. Specifically, he has only four or five poorly articulated words and no two-word combinations. He indicates his wants by pointing and grunting. The parents think he understands much more than he expresses. He is very reluctant to interact with other children, preferring to play by himself.

Jason has never traveled outside the United States. He has been in good health.

The mother and father are both college graduates. Jason has an uncle and two cousins who experienced delayed language development and had to attend special residential schools. The cousins had received extensive genetic and metabolic testing with normal results.

On developmental assessment, Jason runs well, pedals a tricycle, balances on one foot, follows directions quickly, points to a variety of body parts on request, copies a circle, builds a tower of 8 cubes easily, and feeds and partially dresses himself.

SELECT THE ONE BEST ANSWER

1. Jason's differential diagnosis includes:

   (A) cerebral palsy
   (B) Tourette's disorder
   (C) blindness from ROP
   (D) autistic spectrum disorder
   (E) a developmental adjustment because of his mom's return to work

2. What key developmental disorder is least likely to be part of Jason's developmental disability?

   (A) translocation chromosomal disorder
   (B) velocardiofacial syndrome
   (C) tuberous sclerosis complex
   (D) fragile X syndrome
   (E) untreated PKU

3. At school, a picture exchange system is started. Jason is able to express his needs and begins to take turns. Educational practices that may not be helpful for children with autism include which of the following:

   (A) structured experiences that promote communication and social skills
   (B) intensive patterning
   (C) psychotherapy
   (D) large group activities without any demanding tasks
   (E) B, C, and D

4. Jason's mother wonders if special dietary interventions might be helpful. Which of the following statements is/are true?

   (A) There is indisputable evidence that in countries where vegetarianism is the dominant practice, there is no autism.
   (B) Children with celiac disease have high rates of autism.
   (C) Children with untreated PKU never get autism.
   (D) Children with autistic behavior and recurrent diarrhea should be evaluated for malabsorption.
   (E) A and B

5. Jason's mother is concerned about the effect of immunizations on her son. Which of the following statements is/are true?

   (A) Children with congenital rubella have high rates of neuro-disability including autism.
   (B) Measles encephalitis does not cause any adverse developmental sequelae.
   (C) Children who experience mild measles do not get subacute sclerosing panencephalitis.
   (D) Mumps does not cause deafness.
   (E) C and D

6. Jason's mother wonders if he might benefit from secretin, a GI hormone that she learned about in a TV special. Choose the true statement.

   (A) Secretin has been approved for use in treating autism.
   (B) Several randomized scientific trials have shown that secretin is not superior to placebo.
   (C) Secretin is only available as a compassionate use medication.
   (D) The cost of secretin should be covered by Medicaid or private insurance.
   (E) A and D

7. Jason has difficulty going shopping or to a relative's home. He will scream, bite, and kick. Useful supports for parents include which of the following?

   (A) making no demands on Jason
   (B) implementing a behavioral management program
   (C) instituting a major tranquilizer
   (D) telling the parents he will outgrow it
   (E) A and D

8. Jason began to participate in Special Olympics. Potential benefits include all of the following:

   (A) regular physical activity
   (B) dental screening through Healthy Smiles
   (C) being able to skip gym in high school
   (D) mentoring
   (E) A, B, and D

9. Key management areas for long-term success for people with autism include which of the following?

(A) increasing positive behaviors
(B) decreasing negative behaviors
(C) teaching social skills
(D) promoting communication and functional skills
(E) all of the above

Answers

1. **(D)** Jason's difficulty in communication and social skills may indicate an autistic spectrum disorder. Manifestations of cerebral palsy include motor delay with abnormal neurological signs of spasticity, motor control, and posture. Manifestations of Tourette's disorder include tics and attentional difficulties. Neither mother's behavior in returning to work nor immunizations cause autism. Children with severe visual disabilities can have an autistic spectrum disorder. Jason did not have a severe visual impairment.

2. **(E)** Major known etiologies for autistic spectrum disorder include fragile X, untreated PKU, sequelae of congenital rubella, chromosomal disorders, genetic malformation disorders, and tuberous sclerosis. If Jason, born in the United States, underwent newborn screening for PKU, it is unlikely that he has PKU. There is a range of developmental and communicative disorders in children with velocardiofacial syndrome (22q-deletion) including autistic spectrum disorders.

3. **(E)** Key principles of management include special education, family supports, interventions that enhance communication and adaptive skills, and behavioral interventions. Educational practices that are not helpful for children with autistic spectrum disorders include patterning, psychotherapy and large group activities without any demands. A comprehensive IEP as well as recreation and after-school supports are the best ways to optimize outcomes.

4. **(D)** There is autism in India. The overwhelming majority of children with celiac disease do not have autism. More than 50% of children with untreated PKU develop autism. If there are symptoms of growth delay, bloating, retching, diarrhea, or other GI disturbances, then appropriate tests for celiac disease are indicated.

5. **(A)** Avoidance of vaccines does not eliminate autism and has other untoward consequences, i.e., risk of vaccine-preventable disease. Measles can cause both encephalitis and SSPE. Mumps can cause deafness and a spectrum of disabilities.

6. **(B)** Secretin in several randomized clinical trials has been shown to not benefit children with autism. Secretin has not been approved for use in treating autism. Neither Medicaid nor private insurance needs to cover secretin. A trip to Disneyland or a stay at a special overnight camp would be compassionate for a child with autism.

7. **(B)** Children with autism can benefit from behavioral management. There are several explicit strategies to enhance management outside the home. If these behavioral difficulties are more widespread, then consideration of judicious psychopharmacology and behavioral management is required. In order for the patient's family to access certain events, in-home respite services are required.

8. **(E)** Children in special education can receive both adaptive physical education and after-school Special Olympics training. Individuals in Special Olympics receive health, dental, vision, and hearing screening as well as mentoring and regular physical activity. This does not excuse them from participation in gym or adapted physical education in high school.

9. **(E)** Behavior management, communication enhancement, including picture exchange communication system (PECS), and social skill training can help children who have autistic spectrum disorders learn. Key management areas for long-term success for people with autism include increasing positive behaviors, decreasing negative behaviors, and teaching social skills. After-school recreation including swimming, bowling, and horseback riding can be helpful. Hobbies such as animal husbandry, horticulture, and music are also potential resources. Promoting communication and functional skills across home, education, and community settings is important in ongoing management.

SUGGESTED READING

Ruble LA, Brown S: Pervasive developmental disorders: Autism. In: Wolraich ML (ed): *Disorders of Development and Learning*, 3rd ed. Hamilton, Ontario: BC Decker, 2003, pp 249–266.

Parish JM: Promoting adaptive behavior while addressing challenging behavior. In: Batshaw ML (ed): *Children with Disabilities*, 5th ed. Baltimore: Paul H. Brookes Publishing, 2002, pp 607–628.

Meyer GA, Batshaw ML: Fragile X. In: Wolraich ML (ed): *Disorders of Development and Learning*, 3rd ed. Hamilton, Ontario: BC Decker, 2003, pp 321–332.

CASE 32: A 7-YEAR-OLD BOY WITH ADHD FAILS FIRST GRADE

Arnold is a 7-year-old male who presents with his mother after being told by his school that he needs to repeat first grade. The teacher said that he seemed bright but had not learned to read and that he was out of his seat all the time. The school psychologist saw him and reported that his IQ was 112 but that he might have "organic" problems. His mother says she trusts you, knows you are interested in school problems, and is willing to pay for you to spend extra time with Arnold. Further discussion reveals that the mother is angry that school problems were not anticipated when you did your 5-year school entry checkup. You note that your nurse had done a Denver Development Screening Test, 2nd ed (DDST-2), which Arnold passed.

There were no complications of pregnancy, labor, or delivery. You have been following Arnold since infancy with no significant illnesses. In infancy, he had several bouts of otitis media, which responded to medication. His hearing tests have been normal.

SELECT THE ONE BEST ANSWER

1. What developmental screening tests are not indicated prior to kindergarten entry?

   (A) vision
   (B) hearing
   (C) draw a person
   (D) DDST-2
   (E) timed running

2. What developmental assessment for children with concerns about kindergarten might be used by a pediatrician?

   (A) Capute Scales
   (B) Brigance Diagnostic Inventory of Early Development
   (C) Pediatric Evaluation of Developmental Skills
   (D) Bayley Scales
   (E) Kaufman Scales of Early Learning Skills

3. All of the following behavior inventories are helpful for 7-year-olds with concerns about attention and learning at school except:

   (A) Vanderbilt Behavioral Rating Scales
   (B) CBCL
   (C) Connors Rating Scales
   (D) tests of attachment
   (E) all of the above are helpful

4. Which of the following are the most important signs that Arnold may have a learning disability?

   (A) the teacher's concerns about behavior
   (B) the discrepancy between IQ and achievement
   (C) his difficulty in learning to read in first grade
   (D) a family history of reading difficulty
   (E) C and D

5. Which of the following interventions is/are helpful for children with learning disabilities?

   (A) repeating grades
   (B) phonological awareness training
   (C) avoiding talking books
   (D) optometric training
   (E) A and D

6. After your initial discussion with Arnold's mother, history, and general physical examination, Arnold returns for an additional half hour. During this time, which of the following developmental and functional areas related to school achievement is least helpful in your evaluation?

   (A) auditory memory skills
   (B) visual perceptual skills
   (C) developmental coordination skills
   (D) oral reading
   (E) reading comprehension

7. The mother says she believes sugar and food additives are causing his problem. What would be least helpful?

(A) referral to CHADD

(B) decreased intake of sugar-containing beverages

(C) consultation with an endocrinologist

(D) replacing junk food with more healthful snacks

(E) educational materials for parents

8. Arnold's mother says his teacher has suggested that medication might help his activity level. What type of medication might you first consider for Arnold?

(A) diphenhydramine

(B) stimulants

(C) clonidine

(D) lorazepam

(E) hydroxyzine

9. All but which one of the following can enhance objectivity during a trial of stimulants?

(A) choose target behaviors

(B) tell the school you are putting him on natural vitamins

(C) educate the mother about ADHD goals and side effects

(D) ask the mother to record weekly ratings

(E) ask the teacher to record weekly ratings

10. Which of the following statements about stimulants is true?

(A) They work in 80% of children with ADHD.

(B) They are addictive.

(C) They cause tics.

(D) They should always be stopped on weekends and holidays.

(E) They can all be crushed and sprinkled on apple sauce.

11. Which of the following conditions promote(s) long-term success in children with learning and attention disorders?

(A) avoiding extracurricular activities

(B) positive experiences in community-based activities, such as scouts, sports, and religious-related after-school activities

(C) having as friends peers who engage in high risk behaviors

(D) family disagreement on the value of education

(E) none of the above promotes long-term success

Answers

1. (E) Vision, hearing, perceptual, and developmental screening tests are indicated. Timed running is indicated for high school students on the track team.

2. (C) The Capute Scales assess language and problem-solving skills in children ages 0 to 3 years. Special training and testing materials used by psychologists are required for the Briggance, Bayley, and Kaufman tests. The PEDS can be used by pediatricians as a query for parents for their children's developmental and behavioral concerns.

3. (D) Connors and Vanderbilt behavior scales, as well as the Child Behavior Checklist, are appropriate behavior rating instruments. Tests of attachment are not indicated.

4. (E) Of the choices listed, the patient's difficulty learning to read in the first grade and the family history of reading difficulties should most raise the index of suspicion for a learning disability. The teacher's concern about behavior needs to be coupled with what the child is learning at school. Though many states require that there be a gap between IQ and achievement, recent research indicates that this criterion does not have adequate sensitivity and specificity.

5. (B) Phonologic awareness training, which involves learning the sounds associated with letters, is the key to learning to read. Repeating grades and optometric training have not been helpful. Talking books are important resources to help facilitate accommodations. Talking books do not interfere with learning to read.

6. (C) Developmental coordination skills are not as important as memory, perceptual, and reading skills in assessing school achievement.

7. (C) Consultation with an endocrinologist is not indicated. There have been several reviews including randomized controlled studies that do not support the notion that sugar is responsible

for the behavior of ADHD. All children and adults benefit from restricted access to sugar-containing beverages and high caloric density (junk) foods. Provision of written materials as well as referral to the organization for Children and Adults with Hyperactivity and Attention Deficit Disorders (CHADD) would be helpful.

8. **(B)** Arnold has ADHD and dyslexia. Key indicators are difficulties putting sequences together, difficulties mastering phonological skills, and difficulties with activity level and attention. He would benefit from a biopsychological strategy emphasizing behavior management, stimulants, and quality academic supports. Stimulant medications, methylphenidate, dextroamphetamine, and others, are the first-line agents in conjunction with educational accommodations, behavioral supports, and family supports. Benadryl, lorazepam, and hydroxyzine are not indicated. Clonidine is a second-line agent.

9. **(B)** Telling the school that Arnold is on vitamin therapy is not helpful. Choosing target behaviors of impulsivity, attention, and hyperactivity is helpful. Initially educating the mother about ADHD goals and side effects is critical as well as subsequently de-mythologizing the disorder for the child. Feedback from both parent and teacher and self report from older children is also useful in ongoing management and in titrating the medication.

10. **(A)** Stimulants work in 80% of children with ADHD. They are not addictive. They decrease the risk of substance misuse when properly used. They do not cause tics. One cannot crush all delivery systems. Most children benefit by staying on them on weekends and holidays as ADHD is an ongoing, not intermittent, disorder.

11. **(B)** Community successes enhance self-confidence in children with ADHD. These include sports, scouts, church, music, and clubs. Having friends who are appropriately grounded is critical. Family consensus and problem-solving communication is important to ongoing management.

SUGGESTED READING

Ramey CT, Ramey SL: Early intervention: Optimizing development of children with disabilities and risk conditions. In: Wolraich ML (ed): *Disorders of Development and Learning*, 3rd ed. Hamilton, Ontario: BC Decker, 2003, pp 89–104.

Glascol FP: Developmental screening. In: Parker S, Zuckerman B, Augustyn M (eds): *Development and Behavioral Pediatrics: A Handbook for Primary Care*. Philadelphia: Lippincott, Williams & Wilkins, 2005, pp 41–50.

Aylward G: Additional considerations. In: Aylward GP (ed): *Practitioner's Guide to Developmental and Psychological Testing*. New York: Plenum Medical Book Company, 1994, pp 221–232.

CASE 33: AN 18-MONTH-OLD WHO HAS NOT SAID ONE WORD.

Juan is an 18-month-old boy, who presents to you for well-child care and is found to not be walking yet. His mother became worried when he was not sitting at 8 months, but her pediatrician at that time said that he would grow out of this. He first rolled over at 5 months, sat alone at 10 months, crept at 12 months, and pulled to stand and cruised at 15 months. He has just started to walk with his hand held, but does not walk alone. He prefers to W-sit. He likes to play with toys, especially a busy box, which occupies him for long periods. His mother says he understands what she says but is willful and often noncompliant. He babbles occasionally, but has never said "mama."

Past medical history is remarkable for an uneventful pregnancy except that fetal movements were later and less vigorous per mom than when she was carrying his older sister. He was delivered uneventfully at term and weighed 3.85 kg. He went home with his mother on the second day and fed well. He has had all of his age-appropriate immunizations and has had no hospitalizations. He has an older sister who is doing well in second grade, but he has an uncle and two cousins with mental retardation.

Juan moved to Chicago from New York City. His mother is single and works at night.

On physical examination, his height, weight, and head circumference are at the 75th percentile. He is not noticeably dysmorphic. His skin has two 2- × 2-cm smooth hyperpigmentations, one on the abdomen and the other on his back. Otherwise, his general physical examination is normal. When you or his mother tries to engage him in play, he tries to crawl away. He seems aloof and difficult to engage. He rings a bell you show him and doesn't want to give it back. You give him some blocks and he puts them all into a cup. You hide a block under a cup and he has no problem finding it. When presented a crayon, he immediately starts scribbling. He heads toward your ophthalmoscope; you softly tell him "no," causing him to stop briefly but then continue toward it. He picks it up and you hold out your hand and say, "Give it to me" twice. On the second repetition, he hands it over. You ask him to give the cup from among the pile of cubes and he picks up a cube and holds it out to his mother. All of this time, he hasn't said anything.

SELECT THE ONE BEST ANSWER

1. What areas are most delayed for Juan?

    (A) understanding and using language
    (B) fine motor skills
    (C) play skills
    (D) gross motor skills
    (E) social-emotional skills

2. What tests might be indicated to determine etiology?

    (A) transient otoacoustic emissions and/or automated ABR
    (B) MRI of brain
    (C) molecular tests
    (D) renal sonogram
    (E) all of the above

3. Juan's hearing loss is least likely to include:

    (A) sensorineural hearing loss of 80 db
    (B) mild conductive hearing loss of 25 db
    (C) unilateral hearing loss of 40 db
    (D) mixed conductive and sensorineural hearing loss of 60 db
    (E) normal hearing

4. If Juan has bilateral hearing loss, what test is least likely to be helpful?

    (A) thyroid
    (B) connexin molecular studies
    (C) EEG
    (D) NF 1 studies
    (E) EKG

5. Management options for children with 90-db hearing loss include all of the following except:

    (A) amplification

    (B) total communication
    (C) cochlear implants
    (D) oral speech therapy if he has not talked by kindergarten entry
    (E) all of the above are good options

6. When Juan's mother goes to work, he is left with an uncle who drinks alcohol and becomes aggressive. Which of the following statements is/are true?

    (A) Since Juan is deaf, he will not be affected by his uncle's cursing.
    (B) Since Juan has no bruises, he is not being abused.
    (C) When Juan is aggressive on the playground, it may be related to having his uncle as a caregiver.
    (D) If Juan is withdrawn in school, it is only because he is beginning to understand he's deaf.
    (E) C and D

7. Helpful strategies when a relative or caregiver has a drinking problem include which of the following?

    (A) children's support groups through Alcoholics Anonymous
    (B) ignoring the problem unless there is overt physical abuse
    (C) if the caregiver is male, ensure that he is only caring for a male child to alleviate concerns of sexual abuse
    (D) foster placement until the mother can arrange for another caregiver
    (E) A and D

8. Supports for successful single-parenting include which of the following?

    (A) mentoring for the children
    (B) ignoring out-of-home behaviors
    (C) expecting the teachers to set the best educational goals
    (D) respecting a teen's privacy by never bringing up topics that might make the parent or teen uncomfortable
    (E) A and C

9. Major supports for college education for hearing-impaired teens include which of the following?

    (A) Americans with Disabilities Act

(B) National Technical Institute for the Deaf
(C) Gallaudet University
(D) sign language services only available in science classes
(E) A, B, and C

10. Which of the following statements is true about adults with deafness?

(A) They can only work at workplaces run by deaf individuals.
(B) They should not have children unless they marry a hearing adult.
(C) They can receive Supplemental Security Disability Income (SSDI) only if they cannot work.
(D) If they adopt children, they can only adopt deaf children.
(E) None of the above are true.

Answers

1. **(A)** Juan's understanding and use of language is delayed. Though he had some difficulty in learning to balance when upright, he successfully learned how to walk and run prior to age 2 years.

2. **(A)** Hearing tests are indicated. Even if a child is too active or immature for play audiometry, transient otoacoustic emission testing or auditory brainstem responses will determine if auditory mechanisms are intact. Without microcephaly, global developmental delay, macrocephaly, neurologic asymmetry, spasticity, or a movement disorder, MRI is not initially indicated. If there were unexplained global developmental delay in a male molecular testing for fragile X syndrome is indicated. Juan does not have global developmental delay. A renal sonogram would be indicated if there were craniofacial dysmorphism as part of a brachial-oto-renal syndrome.

3. **(C)** A unilateral hearing loss of 40 db would not cause delay in language. This is because intact hearing in the good ear would be adequate for picking up environmental sounds and conversations.

4. **(C)** EEG is least likely to be helpful unless there was a history suggestive of a seizure disorder. Pendred's syndrome is associated with hearing loss and hypothyroidism. An EKG is indicated to rule out long Q-T syndrome. Connexin mutations are responsible for an increasing number of nonsyndromic hearing losses.

5. **(D)** Amplification, total communication, and cochlear implants are management options to maximize communication in children with 90-db hearing loss. The critical need is to ensure a communication system so that the child can develop language skills. The choice of what language system (aural or sign) should be discussed with both medical and educational professionals. Speech therapy at kindergarten entry is indicated for children with articulation disorders. If the child has a cochlear implant, a program of aural rehabilitation that includes helping the child understand sound and communicate in words is indicated.

6. **(C)** Children with hearing impairment can learn aggressive behaviors from others. Children with hearing impairment are at risk for abuse, especially if caretakers do not understand that yelling at deaf children is counterproductive. Children with hearing impairment can be bullied by peers. It is critical to assess the safety of the home, school, and community environment. In addition, all children with disruptive behaviors should have a strategy that includes expression of feelings, appropriate social skills, and appropriate consequences for violating social rules.

7. **(A)** Alcoholics Anonymous has support groups for children in families where there are drinking problems. The impact of problem drinking is more than physical abuse. The critical issue is the need for quality adult caregivers and after-school experiences. An important resource would be some of the community organizations providing support after school that would accommodate a child with a hearing disorder.

8. **(A)** Mentoring is a key management strategy for vulnerable children. Resources include YMCA, Scouts, sports teams, and church leaders. Longitudinal studies and population-based adolescent health surveys have demonstrated the critical role of family and mentors in decreasing risk-taking behavior of teens. In large urban school systems, there are gaps in the capacity of educational pro-

fessionals alone to meet the needs of at-risk children. Though respecting a teen's privacy is essential for developing trust, parents must undertake the difficult task of communicating both values, expectations, and concerns of problem behaviors even if they cause some discomfort in the teen.

9. **(E)** Interpreter services are available for all classes. The Americans with Disabilities Act requires schools to provide reasonable accommodation to individuals with hearing disorders. Both the National Technical Institute for the Deaf and Gallaudet University are post–high school college programs of excellence for individuals who are deaf or hearing impaired.

10. **(C)** Hearing-impaired individuals can receive social security disability income (SSDI) if they cannot work. The major requirement for SSDI is disability causing an inability to work. The Americans with Disability Act requires accommodations in all workplaces whatever the boss's hearing status. Individuals who are deaf are free to marry any individual whether hearing impaired or not. Hearing-impaired individuals can adopt any child provided they are able to meet that child's health, safety, and educational needs. Given the diverse nature of deafness, it should not be assumed that two hearing impaired parents will have a hearing impaired child or only choose to have a child without a hearing disorder.

SUGGESTED READING

Kelly DP, Teplin SW: Disorders of sensation: Hearing and visual impairment. In: Wolraich ML (ed): *Disorders of Development and Learning*, 3rd ed. Hamilton, Ontario: BC Decker, 2003, pp 329–344.

Roizen NJ, Deifendorf AO: Hearing loss in children. In: Roizen NJ, Deifendorf AO (eds): *The Pediatric Clinics of North America*, Vol. 46, no. 1. Philadelphia: WB Saunders, 1999.

Wills LM, Wills KE: Hearing impairment. In: Parker S, Zuckerman B, Augustyn M (eds): *Development and Behavioral Pediatrics: A Handbook for Primary Care*. Philadelphia: Lippincott, Williams & Wilkins, 2005, pp 215–221.

Aylward GP: Additional considerations. In: Aylward GP (ed): *Practitioner's Guide to Developmental and Psychological Testing*. New York: Plenum Medical Book Company, 1994, pp 221–232.

Endocrinology

5

CASE 34: A 10-YEAR-OLD BOY WITH SHORT STATURE

A 10-year-old boy comes into your office for a routine physical examination. His only complaint is that he is shorter than all of his friends, and that he can't ride the mega roller coaster at the local amusement park because he is shorter than the requirement. You have followed this child for many years, but most visits have been for illness, and his height has not been measured for the last few years. He is on no medications. He reports occasional fatigue and occasional constipation. On physical examination, his height is less than the 3rd percentile and he is prepubertal.

SELECT THE ONE BEST ANSWER

1. Of the following, which is the least likely to help with his diagnosis?

    (A) parental heights
    (B) growth velocity
    (C) actual height
    (D) bone age

2. What is the most likely diagnosis if his growth rate is 5 cm/year, height age is 8 years, and bone age is 10 years?

    (A) constitutional delay of growth and puberty
    (B) intrinsic short stature
    (C) hypothyroidism
    (D) growth hormone deficiency

3. What is the most likely diagnosis if his growth rate is 5 cm/year, height age is 8 years, and bone age is 8 years?

    (A) intrinsic short stature
    (B) growth hormone deficiency
    (C) Cushing's syndrome
    (D) constitutional delay of growth and puberty

4. What is the most likely diagnosis if his growth rate is 3 cm/year, height age is 8 years and bone age is 8 years?

    (A) exogenous obesity
    (B) constitutional delay of growth and puberty
    (C) growth hormone deficiency
    (D) intrinsic short stature

5. What is the most likely diagnosis if he has abnormal body proportions and a narrow interpedicular distance in the lower lumbosacral area?

    (A) Noonan's syndrome
    (B) achondroplasia
    (C) hypochondroplasia
    (D) Klinefelter's syndrome

6. Which of the following is one of the most common causes of short stature in children?

    (A) familial intrinsic short stature
    (B) growth hormone deficiency
    (C) poor nutrition
    (D) chronic illness

7. Which of the following tests would you recommend as an initial screen for a 10-year-old boy with an attenuated growth rate?

   (A) complete blood count, karyotype
   (B) sedimentation rate, thyroid function tests
   (C) complete blood count, growth hormone level
   (D) sedimentation rate, gonadotropin levels

8. Your initial screening tests are negative and you advise that the child return for follow-up so you can assess his growth velocity. When would you advise follow-up?

   (A) 1 to 2 months
   (B) 2 to 3 months
   (C) 4 to 6 months
   (D) 1 year

9. What is the normal growth velocity of a child between the ages of 3 and 10?

   (A) 2.5 cm/year
   (B) 5 cm/year
   (C) 7.5 cm/year
   (D) 10 cm/year

10. Which of the following is the least accurate way to measure a child?

   (A) on a scale equipped with a flexible height arm
   (B) standing against a wall
   (C) with a stadiometer
   (D) lying supine on a flat surface

11. What is this patient's genetic height potential if his father is 5'10" and his mother 5'5"?

   (A) 5'5"
   (B) 5'7"
   (C) 5'10"
   (D) 6'0"

12. You would be most concerned about a potential growth problem in a child who crossed from the 50th to the 25th percentile for height at what age?

   (A) 8 months of age
   (B) 2 years of age
   (C) 7 years of age
   (D) 13 years of age

13. Which of the following would help you the least to differentiate between intrinsic short stature and constitutional delay of growth and puberty?

   (A) growth rate from 0 to 3 years
   (B) growth rate from 3 to 10 years
   (C) growth rate from 11 to 14 years
   (D) final stature

14. Which of the following is not a classic feature of growth hormone deficiency?

   (A) hypoglycemia during infancy
   (B) delayed bone maturation
   (C) decreased arm span
   (D) low serum IGF-1

15. Your patient eventually gets diagnosed with growth hormone deficiency and is started on growth hormone replacement therapy. He starts complaining of severe headaches. A pretreatment head MRI was normal. What would you be most concerned about?

   (A) migraine headaches
   (B) pseudotumor cerebri
   (C) brain tumor
   (D) tension headaches

16. Which of the following conditions presents with an attenuated growth pattern?

   (A) constitutional delay of puberty
   (B) intrinsic short familial stature
   (C) hypothyroidism
   (D) B and C

17. If this child were a 10-year-old girl, what test would you consider checking to help in your evaluation?

   (A) karyotype
   (B) estradiol
   (C) gonadotropin levels
   (D) chest radiograph

18. Which of the following is not a feature of Turner's syndrome?

   (A) renal anomalies
   (B) right-sided cardiac anomalies
   (C) lymphedema
   (D) cubitus valgus

19. Your patient's weight is greater than the 97th percentile and he has striae on the abdomen. What would be at the top of your differential diagnosis?

(A) genetic obesity syndrome
(B) hypothyroidism
(C) growth hormone deficiency
(D) Cushing's syndrome

20. Which of the following is not associated with tall stature as a child?

(A) Klinefelter's syndrome
(B) exogenous obesity
(C) hyperthyroidism
(D) excess exogenous corticosteroids

Answers

1. **(C)** Actual height. The actual height of a patient is least likely to help with the diagnosis since the only information it provides is that the patient is short for age. Statistically, 3% of the population will be below the normal growth curve. Data on parental heights offers information regarding the genetic height potential of the child. The growth velocity allows you to determine if the child is growing at a normal rate for his age. A predictable pattern of bone maturation occurs during bone growth, and a bone age radiograph is useful to determine the bone maturation and the growth potential of a child. Other parts of the history which are important include family growth and pubertal history, birth length and weight, current weight for height (to rule out a nutritional component to poor growth), and overall health history to rule out chronic disease as a cause of short stature.

2. **(B)** Intrinsic short stature. Children with intrinsic short stature typically grow at a normal rate, but below the normal growth chart. Their bone age is usually equivalent to their chronologic age, which are both greater than the height age (height age is the age at which the child's height falls at the 50th percentile). They go through puberty at a normal time and end up on the shorter side of normal as an adult.

3. **(D)** Constitutional delay of growth and puberty. Children with constitutional delay of growth and puberty have normal growth rates during childhood, delayed puberty with a delayed pubertal growth spurt, and attainment of normal adult height. Their bone age is usually equivalent to their height age, and both are less than their chronological age. Children with intrinsic short stature also have a normal growth rate, but their bone age would approximate their chronological age. Both growth hormone deficiency and Cushing's syndrome would have an attenuated growth pattern.

4. **(C)** Growth hormone deficiency. A growth rate of only 3 cm/year would be considered an attenuated growth rate, which is seen in endocrine causes of growth failure such as growth hormone deficiency, hypothyroidism, and Cushing's syndrome. Severe chronic disease and malnutrition can also cause an attenuated growth pattern. Children with exogenous obesity tend to be tall with a normal growth rate.

5. **(C)** Hypochondroplasia. Hypochondroplasia is often described as a milder form of achondroplasia. However, although they are both transmitted via autosomal dominant transmission, they have not been reported to occur in the same family. Hypochondroplasia is as a result of a mutation in the fibroblast growth factor receptor 3 gene. Patients present with short stature and dysmorphic features that are milder than seen in achondroplasia. They do not have the typical facial features of achondroplasia. These patients have radiological evidence of a narrow interpedicular distance in the lower lumbosacral area.

6. **(A)** Familial intrinsic short stature. The most frequent causes of short stature in children are the genetic normal variants, including familial intrinsic short stature and constitutional delay of growth and puberty.

7. **(B)** Sedimentation rate, thyroid function tests. General screening tests of overall health including a CBC to rule out anemia, a comprehensive metabolic panel to rule out kidney or liver problems, and a sedimentation rate to rule out underlying inflammation are an important first step in detecting a medical cause of short stature. Hormonal causes of short stature include hypothyroidism, which can be ruled out with thyroid function tests,

and growth hormone deficiency. Growth hormone is secreted in a pulsatile fashion, thus a random growth hormone level would not be helpful. Measurements of IGF-1 and insulin-like growth factor binding protein-3 (IGFBP-3) are often used to screen for growth hormone deficiency. Gonadotropin levels would not be helpful in a prepubertal 10-year-old child.

8. **(C)** 4 to 6 months. A minimum interval of 4 to 6 months is typically needed for an accurate determination of growth velocity, as seasonal variations in growth velocity have been reported. Although follow-up at 1 year would give the most accurate data on growth velocity, if this child had an attenuated growth pattern, valuable time would be lost in diagnosis and treatment of the growth disorder.

9. **(B)** 5 cm/year. Between the ages of 3 and 10, children tend to grow at a constant growth velocity, which averages 5 cm or 2 inches per year.

10. **(A)** On a scale equipped with a flexible height arm. The most reproducible way to measure children is using a wall-mounted stadiometer. In younger children, a supine stadiometer should be used that provides a stationary board at their head and a movable footboard. If a stadiometer is unavailable, the next best way to measure a child would be standing flat against a wall. The flexible height arm on a scale tends to be very unreliable.

11. **(C)** 5'10". A child's genetic height potential can be estimated by calculating mid-parental height. For boys, 5 inches is added to the mother's height and averaged with the father's height, and for girls, 5 inches is subtracted from the father's height and averaged with the mother's height.

12. **(C)** 7 years of age. Typically between 3 and 10 years of age, children will grow along a certain percentile for height. Any deviation from this percentile is a warning sign of a potential growth problem. During the first 3 years of life, it is not unusual for children to move upward or downward across growth channels toward their mid-parental height range. In addition, children who will go on to have constitutional delay of growth and puberty will often cross percentiles downward within the first 3 years of life. During puberty, children may again cross growth percentiles because the pubertal growth spurt of individuals is often out of phase. Thus, a 13-year-old who has delayed puberty may cross percentiles downward even though they have a normal prepubertal growth rate.

13. **(B)** Growth rate from 3 to 10 years. Children with constitutional delay of growth and puberty and intrinsic short stature grow at normal rates between the ages of 3 and 10 years; thus growth velocity alone at these ages will not help to differentiate between the causes of short stature. Children with constitutional delay in growth and puberty tend to fall off the normal growth curve between 0 and 3 years of age, grow slower than normal between the ages of 11 and 14 years because they are not yet in puberty, and end up a normal stature as an adult. In contrast, children with intrinsic short stature tend to follow parallel but below the normal growth chart, and end up shorter as adults. A bone age radiograph would help differentiate these two genetic variants.

14. **(C)** Decreased arm span. Arm span typically approximates height. Decreased arm span can be seen in conditions such as achondroplasia and hypochondroplasia, but it is not typically seen in growth hormone deficiency. Classic features of growth hormone deficiency include an attenuated growth pattern, short stature, hypoglycemia in infancy in cases of congenital growth hormone deficiency, delayed bone age, and low IGF-1 levels.

15. **(B)** Pseudotumor cerebri. A potential adverse effect of growth hormone is fluid retention which can lead to pseudotumor cerebri. This complication is typically reversed with a discontinuation of the growth hormone. Most children can be restarted on growth hormone at a lower dose without problems. Development of tumors in children without other predisposing factors has not been demonstrated.

16. **(C)** Hypothyroidism. Patients with constitutional delay of puberty and intrinsic short stature grow at a normal rate.

17. **(A)** Karyotype. Turner's syndrome is the most common pathologic cause of short stature in

girls. The incidence of Turner's syndrome is approximately 1 in 2500 newborn girls. Turner's syndrome is caused by deletion of X chromosomal material. The most characteristic features of Turner's syndrome are short stature and gonadal dysgenesis. In older girls, checking gonadotropin levels and estradiol is often used as a screen as these girls will have menopausal levels of gonadotropins and low estradiol as a result of primary ovarian failure.

18. **(B)** Right-sided cardiac anomalies. Left-sided cardiac anomalies such as coarctation of the aorta are more common in Turner's syndrome, while right-sided anomalies are more often seen in Noonan's syndrome (in which patients present with a Turner-like phenotype but normal sex chromosomes). Other features of Turner's syndrome include webbing of the neck, broad chest, widely spaced nipples, low posterior hairline, spooning of the nails, lymphedema, cubitus valgus, and renal anomalies such as horseshoe kidney. Data have shown that growth hormone treatment increases growth velocity and final adult height in girls with Turner's syndrome.

19. **(D)** Cushing's syndrome. Children with Cushing's syndrome present with short stature, excessive weight gain, and striae because of an increase in fragility of the skin as a result of excess cortisol.

20. **(D)** Excess exogenous corticosteroids. Supraphysiologic levels of exogenous steroids can attenuate growth, and cause short stature and obesity in children. This contrasts with exogenous obesity in which children tend to be tall. Klinefelter's syndrome is associated with tall stature. The most common cause of tall stature in a child is intrinsic familial tall stature.

SUGGESTED READING

Rosenfield, RL, Cuttler L: Somatic growth and maturation. In: DeGroot LJ (ed): *Endocrinology*, 4th ed. Philadelphia: WB Saunders Company, 2001, p 477.

Rosenfeld RG, Cohen P: Disorders of growth hormone/insulin-like growth factor secretion and action. In: Sperling MA (ed): *Pediatric Endocrinology*, 2nd ed. Philadelphia: WB Saunders, 2002, p 211.

Botero D, Evliyaoglu O, Cohen LE: Hypopituitarism. In: Radovick S, MacGillivray MH (eds): *Pediatric Endocrinology, A Practical Clinical Guide*. Totowa, New Jersey: Humana Press, 2003, p 383.

CASE 35: AN 8½-YEAR-OLD WITH PUBERTAL DEVELOPMENT

An 8½-year-old patient is brought into your office because of concerns of early pubertal development. The mother noted the development of breast buds approximately 2 months prior to the visit. There is no report of pubic hair development or acne. The child is otherwise healthy and has been on no medications. On physical examination, the child is friendly, and in no distress. Height and weight are at the 50th percentile. The child has Tanner stage 2 breast development, and stage 1 pubic and axillary hair.

SELECT THE ONE BEST ANSWER

1. If this child is a girl, the most likely diagnosis would be which of the following?

    (A) precocious puberty
    (B) normal puberty
    (C) premature thelarche
    (D) premature pubarche

2. On physical examination of the girl, you note that her breast development is asymmetric. What would you do next?

    (A) breast ultrasound
    (B) consult a surgeon
    (C) assure her that it is normal
    (D) mammogram

3. If this child is an 8½-year-old girl who instead has Tanner stage 2 pubic hair development with Tanner stage 1 breast development, the most likely diagnosis would be which of the following?

    (A) precocious puberty
    (B) normal puberty
    (C) premature thelarche
    (D) premature pubarche.

4. If this were a 6-year-old girl, which of the following would be the most important history to ask to narrow your differential diagnosis?

    (A) history of medications in the house
    (B) developmental history

(C) birth history
(D) parental heights

5. If this child were a boy with testicles measuring 2 cm in long diameter, the most likely diagnosis would be which of the following?

(A) precocious puberty
(B) pubertal gynecomastia
(C) premature thelarche
(D) prepubertal gynecomastia

6. The first sign of puberty in a girl is which of the following?

(A) menarche
(B) axillary hair development
(C) growth spurt
(D) appearance of breast buds

7. The first sign of puberty in boys is which of the following?

(A) growth spurt
(B) testicular enlargement
(C) appearance of pubic hair
(D) appearance of facial hair

8. If this child is a 4-year-old girl, the differential diagnosis includes which of the following?

(A) precocious puberty
(B) normal puberty
(C) premature thelarche
(D) A and C

9. A 6-year-old boy with precocious puberty is more likely to have which of the following than a 6-year-old girl with precocious puberty?

(A) neurologic disorder
(B) idiopathic precocious puberty
(C) congenital adrenal hyperplasia
(D) gonadal tumor

10. At which Tanner stage of breast development in girls does the areola and papilla form a secondary mound above the level of the breast?

(A) Tanner stage 2
(B) Tanner stage 3
(C) Tanner stage 4
(D) Tanner stage 5

11. The Tanner stage of breast development at which a girl is most likely to get menarche is which of the following?

(A) Tanner 2
(B) Tanner 3
(C) Tanner 4
(D) Tanner 5

12. The normal time range in girls from breast budding until the appearance of menarche is which of the following?

(A) 2 to 2.5 years
(B) 0.5 to 1 year
(C) 3 to 3.5 years
(D) 1 to 1.5 years

13. The average age of menarche for North American girls is which of the following?

(A) 10.7 years
(B) 11.7 years
(C) 12.7 years
(D) 13.7 years

14. The average growth remaining once a girl has experienced menarche is which of the following?

(A) 1 inch
(B) 2 inches
(C) 3 inches
(D) 4 inches

15. A boy experiences his maximal pubertal growth spurt at which of the following times?

(A) prior to testicular enlargement
(B) shortly after pubic hair development
(C) prior to penile enlargement
(D) in late puberty

16. Which of the following is a gonadotropin-dependent process?

(A) premature thelarche
(B) central precocious puberty
(C) premature adrenarche
(D) premature pubarche

17. Which of the following would you expect in a girl with premature thelarche?

(A) growth spurt
(B) pubic hair
(C) advanced bone age
(D) normal growth velocity

18. Which of the following would you not expect in a child with premature pubarche?

(A) signs of virilization
(B) normal bone age
(C) pubic hair development
(D) normal growth velocity

19. Which of the following would not be expected as a consequence of untreated, rapidly progressive central precocious puberty?

(A) tall stature as a child
(B) tall stature as an adult
(C) short stature as an adult
(D) psychologic difficulties

20. Pubertal gynecomastia occurs in what percentage of boys?

(A) <5%
(B) 20%
(C) 25%
(D) >40%

Answers

1. (**B**) Normal puberty. The appearance of any signs of puberty before the age of 8 years in a girl is considered precocious. Thus an 8½-year-old girl with breast development would be in the early range of normal for pubertal onset. Recent studies suggest that girls may be going into puberty at a younger age. Premature thelarche is the early appearance of breast development without any other signs of early puberty, and premature pubarche is the early appearance of pubic hair alone. The term premature adrenarche is utilized when there is isolated pubic hair development and biochemical evidence of maturation of the adrenal gland (increase in DHEA-sulfate level).

2. (**C**) Assure her that it is normal. It is not unusual for breast development to begin unilaterally in both boys and girls. In addition, the majority of woman have asymmetry to the breasts. If the breast anlage (breast bud) is removed surgically, no breast will form on that side. Simple assurance that this is a normal process is the proper way to proceed.

3. (**B**) Normal puberty. The appearance of pubic hair after the age of 8 in girls would not be considered precocious.

4. (**A**) History of medications in the house. Estrogen-containing creams and contraceptive pills can cause isolated thelarche in girls. Thus, it is important to determine if the child could have been exposed to these as a cause of the breast development.

5. (**D**) Prepubertal gynecomastia. A boy with 2-cm testicles is not yet in puberty, thus this would not be considered precocious puberty or pubertal gynecomastia. Prepubertal gynecomastia is rare and almost always abnormal. Etiologies include testicular, adrenal, and hCG-secreting tumors, exogenous estrogen exposure, familial aromatase excess syndrome, or idiopathic gynecomastia.

6. (**D**) Appearance of breast buds. The typical sequence of development of secondary sexual characteristics in girls is breast budding, appearance of pubic hair, peak height velocity, and menarche. Pubic or axillary hair can occur before breast budding as a normal variant.

7. (**B**) Testicular enlargement. Enlargement of the testicles in boys to 2.5 cm in long diameter (or 4 mL in volume) is the first sign of puberty. Testicular enlargement is largely because of an increase in Sertoli cells and seminiferous tubular volume with a small contribution by Leydig cells. Pubic hair typically develops approximately 1 year after testicular enlargement. The growth spurt and appearance of facial hair occur later in puberty in boys.

8. (**D**) A and C. Both precocious puberty and premature thelarche can present with isolated breast development. Thus, this child would need to be followed closely for the appearance of other signs of puberty.

9. (**A**) Neurologic disorder. Boys are more likely to have a neurologic disorder leading to precocious

puberty than girls. Approximately 95% of true precocity in girls is idiopathic. However, it is important to rule out a neurologic disorder as a cause of precocious puberty in both sexes.

10. **(C)** Tanner stage 4. The Tanner staging system consists of five categories describing the sequence of puberty, from a prepubertal child to adult development. Tanner staging of breast development in girls is shown in Table 35-1.

11. **(C)** Tanner 4. Girls typically are at stage 4 for breast development (areolar mounding) when they experience menarche.

12. **(A)** 2 to 2.5 years. Although the timing of pubertal onset is variable, the timing from breast budding to menarche in girls is typically between 2 and 2.5 years.

13. **(C)** 12.7 years.

14. **(B)** 2 inches.

15. **(D)** In late puberty. The difference between the mean height of men and women is related to the timing and peak of the pubertal growth spurt in boys and girls. Because the pubertal growth spurt is later for boys, they are taller on average once they start the growth spurt in late puberty. In addition, boys experience a greater peak height velocity than girls, leading to their greater adult stature. The typical sequence of development of secondary sexual characteristics in boys is testicular growth, pubarche, penile growth, and peak height velocity.

16. **(B)** Central precocious puberty. Central precocious puberty results from early activation of the hypothalamic-pituitary-gonadal axis.

17. **(D)** Normal growth velocity. Premature thelarche is the isolated appearance of breast development with a peak prevalence in the first 2 years of life. It is not associated with any other signs of puberty, such as a growth spurt, pubic hair development, or advanced bone maturation. The early breast development usually spontaneously regresses. These girls need to be followed closely for evidence of early puberty as breast development is the first sign of puberty in girls.

Table 35-1. TANNER STAGES OF BREAST DEVELOPMENT

Tanner Stage	Clinical Appearance
1	Prepubertal
2	Appearance of a palpable (but not always visible) breast bud
3	Enlargement and elevation of the breast with no separation of the contour of the breast and areola
4	Areola forms a separate mound above the breast
5	Adult breast

18. **(A)** Signs of virilization. Premature pubarche describes the isolated appearance of pubic hair prior to the age of 8 in girls and 9 in boys in the absence of other signs of puberty or virilization. Although this is thought of as a benign problem which does not need treatment, more recent studies suggest that many girls with a history of early pubic hair development go on to have problems with hirsutism, acne, and irregular menstrual periods during adolescence.

19. **(B)** Tall stature as an adult. One of the most significant consequences of untreated, rapidly progressive precocious puberty is rapid advancement of bone maturation with early epiphyseal fusion and short stature as an adult. Predicted adult height is a major factor in the decision as to which children will need therapy for precocious puberty.

20. **(D)** >40%. Pubertal gynecomastia occurs in greater than 40% of boys in mid-puberty. It can vary from breast buds to significant breast tissue. It will typically resolve within 2 to 3 years. The cause of pubertal gynecomastia has been studied for decades, with conflicting results. It may be because of an imbalance of testosterone to estrogen. It is more prevalent in obese boys, likely related to increased aromatase in adipose tissue. Aromatase converts testosterone to estradiol, thus leading to increased estradiol in peripheral tissues. Other pathologic etiologies include acquired testicular failure, biosynthetic defects in testosterone production, testicular or liver tumors, and hyperthyroidism. Gynecomas-

tia can also be a consequence of several drugs, including spironolactone, cimetidine, digitalis, phenothiazine, and marijuana. Treatment usually consists of reassurance and psychosocial support, with weight loss in obese boys. Surgical removal of excess breast tissue is indicated in those boys in whom the gynecomastia does not regress in 3 years. Medical therapy is usually not indicated.

SUGGESTED READING

Rosenfield RL: Puberty in the female and its disorders. In: Sperling MA (ed): *Pediatric Endocrinology*, 2nd ed. Philadelphia, WB Saunders, 2002, p 455.

Styne DM: The testes. In: Sperling MA (ed): *Pediatric Endocrinology*, 2nd ed. Philadelphia, WB Saunders, 2002, p 565.

Rodriguez H, Pescovitz OH: Precocious puberty: Clinical management. In: Radovick S, MacGillivray MH (eds): *Pediatric Endocrinology, A Practical Clinical Guide*. Totowa, New Jersey, Humana Press, 2003, p 399.

CASE 36: A 14-YEAR-OLD CHILD WITHOUT ANY SIGNS OF PUBERTY

A 14-year-old child is brought into your office because of concerns of lack of pubertal development. The parents report that the child has otherwise been healthy, but the child has been complaining that all of his/her friends seem to be getting much taller than him/her. The child's father is 6 feet tall and could not recall when he went through puberty, but did remember being shorter than all of his friends in high school. The mother is 5'6" and had menarche at age 14 years. On physical examination, the child's height is less than the 5th percentile, and weight for height is at the 30th percentile. The child is entirely prepubertal.

SELECT THE ONE BEST ANSWER

1. What is the most likely diagnosis if this is a boy with a bone age of 11 years, and his father grew 4 inches after high school?

   (A) hypergonadotropic hypogonadism
   (B) constitutional delay of puberty
   (C) hypogonadotropic hypogonadism
   (D) Klinefelter's syndrome

2. What is the most likely diagnosis if this is a boy with a bone age of 14 years, who reports that he can't smell well?

   (A) Kallmann syndrome
   (B) Noonan syndrome
   (C) Klinefelter's syndrome
   (D) panhypopituitarism

3. What would be in your differential diagnosis if this were a boy with a bone age of 10 years and prepubertal gonadotropin levels?

   (A) constitutional delay of puberty
   (B) hypergonadotropic hypogonadism
   (C) hypogonadotropic hypogonadism
   (D) all of the above

4. If this were a girl with a bone age of 13 years, which diagnosis would be least likely?

   (A) constitutional delay of puberty
   (B) hypergonadotropic hypogonadism
   (C) Turner syndrome
   (D) hypogonadotropic hypogonadism

5. Which of the following would be ruled out as a diagnosis if this child had pubic hair?

   (A) constitutional delay in puberty
   (B) hypergonadotropic hypogonadism
   (C) hypogonadotropic hypogonadism
   (D) none of the above

6. Which of the following issues in the medical history will help most with your diagnosis of delayed puberty?

   (A) nutritional habits
   (B) exercise intensity
   (C) prior medical history
   (D) all of the above

7. Which of the following is the most common cause of delayed puberty in boys?

   (A) Kallmann syndrome
   (B) constitutional delay of puberty
   (C) Klinefelter's syndrome
   (D) panhypopituitarism

8. You want to order a bone age radiograph to assess skeletal maturation. What would you order?

   (A) a radiograph of the right foot and ankle
   (B) a radiograph of the left hand and wrist

(C) a radiograph of the right hand and wrist

(D) a radiograph of the left foot and ankle

9. At what age in a boy would you be concerned about delayed puberty?

(A) 12-year-old

(B) 13-year-old

(C) 14-year-old

(D) 15-year-old

10. At what age in a girl would you be most concerned about delayed puberty?

(A) 11-year-old

(B) 12-year-old

(C) 13-year-old

(D) 14-year-old

11. The first biochemical sign of maturation of the hypothalamic-pituitary-gonadal axis is which of the following?

(A) sleep-associated rise of LH secretion

(B) early morning rise of LH secretion

(C) late morning rise of LH secretion

(D) late afternoon rise of LH secretion

12. What should be included in your work-up of delayed puberty?

(A) early morning gonadotropin levels

(B) afternoon testosterone (boy) or estradiol (girl) levels

(C) early evening gonadotropin levels

(D) early evening testosterone (boy) or estradiol (girl) levels

13. Which of the following is a cause of primary hypogonadism?

(A) Turner syndrome

(B) craniopharyngioma

(C) Kallmann syndrome

(D) anorexia nervosa

14. Which of the following is not a cause of secondary hypogonadism?

(A) hypothyroidism

(B) hypothalamic dysfunction

(C) gonadal abnormality

(D) hypopituitarism

15. Which of the following is not a feature of Turner syndrome?

(A) webbed neck

(B) low posterior hairline

(C) right-sided cardiac defects

(D) left-sided cardiac defects

16. Which of the following is not a feature of Klinefelter's syndrome?

(A) short stature

(B) seminiferous tubule dysgenesis

(C) 47,XXY

(D) normal onset of puberty

17. The age at which a child goes into puberty is most dependent on which of the following?

(A) bone age

(B) chronological age

(C) height age

(D) weight age

18. Which of the following is not a goal of therapy for lack of sexual development?

(A) age-appropriate secondary sex characteristics

(B) advancement of bone maturation

(C) growth spurt

(D) relieve concerns of immature appearance

Answers

1. **(B)** Constitutional delay of puberty. This represents the extreme of normal physiologic variation in timing of onset of puberty. Typically the patient is shorter than the mean with a delay in bone maturation (which is usually equal to the height age). They have a normal growth velocity. There is usually a family history of delayed puberty and late growth spurt. Patients will eventually go into puberty and progress through puberty normally. Treatment usually consists of reassurance. Boys can be treated with a short course of low-dose testosterone to give them pubic hair, and a slight growth spurt if there is significant psychological distress about their lack of puberty. They need to be monitored closely on treatment to avoid significant advancement of their bone maturation, which could limit their

growth potential because of premature epiphyseal closure.

2. (**A**) Kallmann syndrome. In Kallmann syndrome, hyposmia or anosmia is associated with gonadotropin deficiency. It is caused by improper migration of the GnRH neurons and olfactory bulb across the cribriform plate. It is frequently inherited as an X-linked recessive trait, but occasionally can be caused by autosomal dominant or recessive inheritance with variable penetrance. There can be significant heterogeneity within the same family with this condition. Associated anomalies may include renal agenesis, midline facial defects, cryptorchidism, microphallus, sensorineural deafness, and visual abnormalities.

3. (**D**) All of the above. Onset of puberty is typically more dependent on the bone age than the chronological age. A boy with a bone age of 10 would not be expected to be in puberty, thus his gonadotropin levels would be in the prepubertal range in all conditions listed. Once the bone age advances to a pubertal age, gonadotropin levels in boys with hypergonadotropic hypogonadism will become elevated.

4. (**A**) Constitutional delay of puberty. As puberty corresponds more closely with bone age than with chronological age, a girl with a bone age of 13 years should be in puberty, and lack of puberty at this bone age would suggest hypogonadism. The correlation between bone age and pubertal onset is less clear in obese children, as overnutrition often causes an increase in bone age.

5. (**D**) None of the above. Gonadarche (maturation of the hypothalamic-pituitary gonadal axis) and adrenarche (maturation of the adrenal gland) are two separate processes. Therefore, adrenarche leading to the development of pubic hair, can occur without gonadarche.

6. (**D**) All of the above. Nutritional disorders, intense exercise, and occult chronic illness can all affect the hypothalamic GnRH pulse generator and cause delayed puberty.

7. (**B**) Constitutional delay of puberty. Constitutional delay in puberty is the most common cause of delayed puberty in boys. Children with panhypopituitarism causing delayed puberty will usually come to attention because of other hormonal deficiencies.

8. (**B**) A radiograph of the left hand and wrist. There are several accepted techniques of assessing bone maturation including the Tanner-Whitehouse method and the method of Greulich and Pyle. Both methods focus on the left hand and wrist.

9. (**C**) 14-year-old. Delayed puberty is defined as the absence of signs of puberty in a child at a chronological age greater than two standard deviations above the mean of pubertal development for a given population. In boys, this age is 14 years. This is also the age at which most boys will be starting high school where communal showering is common, thus their concerns regarding lack of puberty increase.

10. (**C**) 13-year-old.

11. (**A**) Sleep-associated rise of LH secretion. The first biochemical sign of puberty is a sleep-associated rise in LH secretion. Puberty begins with pulsatile GnRH secretion, which is followed by pulsatile gonadotropin secretion, which is eventually followed by maturation of the gonads with a gradual increase in sex hormones. The pulsatile GnRH and gonadotropin secretion begins at night, and eventually extends throughout the day in later puberty.

12. (**A**) Early morning gonadotropin levels. In very early puberty, levels of gonadotropins and sex steroids are first detectable at night. Thus the best time to check outpatient laboratory tests would be early morning. Gonadotropin levels and sex steroid levels should be checked in a laboratory with very sensitive assays appropriate for children.

13. (**A**) Turner syndrome. Turner syndrome in girls presents with primary ovarian failure because of atresia of the ovaries in fetal life. Many girls with Turner syndrome first present in early adolescence because of short stature and delayed puberty. In Kallmann syndrome, isolated gonado-

tropin deficiency and anosmia is found because of failure of the GnRH neurons and olfactory bulb to migrate properly. Craniopharyngioma and the subsequent treatment can lead to panhypopituitarism, and anorexia nervosa can lead to hypothalamic hypogonadism.

14. **(C)** Gonadal abnormality. Secondary hypogonadism is a result of disorders that decrease gonadotropin secretion. Lack of thyroid hormone has been shown to interfere with gonadotropin secretion. An abnormality in the gonad would lead to elevated gonadotropin levels.

15. **(C)** Right-sided cardiac defects. Girls with Turner syndrome usually present with short stature and delayed puberty because of primary ovarian failure. Occasionally, girls are diagnosed at birth because of puffy hands and feet, and a webbed neck because of lymphedema. They have a 45,XO karyotype (or a mosaic karyotype, i.e., 45,XO/46,XX). Associated features include webbed neck, low posterior hairline, cubitus valgus, spooned nails, renal anomalies, and left-sided cardiac defects including coarctation of the aorta. Right-sided cardiac defects are found in Noonan's syndrome, which has similar phenotypic findings as Turner syndrome with a normal karyotype. Girls with Noonan's syndrome have normal ovarian function, but boys typically have cryptorchidism and abnormal Leydig cell function.

16. **(A)** Short stature. Klinefelter's syndrome is the most frequent form of hypogonadism in males with an incidence of 1 in 500 to 1000 males. In all cases, seminiferous tubule function is impaired. Patients have variable Leydig cell function, and thus can have testosterone levels from low to normal. Patients often have the onset of puberty at a normal age, but secondary sexual changes do not progress to the adult stage. Karyotype is 47,XXY, or variants including 48,XXXY, 49,XXXXY and male 46,XX. The typical phenotype includes tall stature with long arms and legs, small firm testes, small phallus, poor muscular development, language difficulties, and poor social adaptation.

17. **(A)** Bone age. The age at which children go into puberty varies widely. Bone age has been shown to be a better predictor of pubertal milestones than chronological age. Thus an 8-year-old girl with a bone age of 12 would be expected to be in puberty. Conditions that cause an advancement of bone maturation (such as undertreated congenital adrenal hyperplasia) can lead to precocious puberty.

18. **(B)** Advancement of bone maturation. The goals of therapy for delayed puberty include inducing the development of age-appropriate secondary sex characteristics, a growth spurt, and psychosocial benefits. Psychosocial concerns tend to be more pronounced in boys than girls because of societal pressures and can lead to low-self esteem and poor body image. If the therapy advances the bone maturation too quickly, children can have premature epiphyseal fusion and end up short as an adult.

SUGGESTED READING
Rosenfield RL: Puberty in the female and its disorders. In: Sperling MA (ed): *Pediatric Endocrinology*, 2nd ed. Philadelphia, WB Saunders, 2002, p 455.

Styne DM: The testes. In: Sperling MA (ed): *Pediatric Endocrinology*, 2nd ed. Philadelphia, WB Saunders, 2002, p 565.

Stafford DEJ: Delayed puberty. In: Radovick S, MacGillivray MH (eds): *Pediatric Endocrinology, A Practical Clinical Guide.* Totowa, New Jersey: Humana Press, 2003, p 383.

Rosen DS, Foster C: Delayed puberty. *Pediatr Rev* 22: 309–315, 2001.

CASE 37: A 10-YEAR-OLD CHILD WITH A GOITER

A 10-year-old child is brought into your office for a routine school physical. On review of systems, the child has been complaining of fatigue, but is doing okay at school. The child is on no medications. The child has otherwise been healthy. There is a history of some type of thyroid problem in the maternal grandmother and paternal aunt. On physical examination you notice that the child has a goiter with no palpable nodules (see Figure 37-1).

SELECT THE ONE BEST ANSWER

1. What other information would be most helpful to narrow your differential diagnosis?

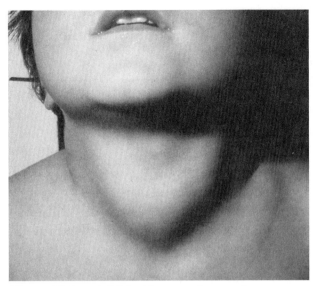

Figure 37-1. **A child with a prominent goiter.**

(A) birth history
(B) developmental history
(C) growth pattern
(D) pubertal history

2. Which of the following tests would you order first?

(A) total thyroxine (TT4), free thyroxine index (FTI), thyrotropin (TSH), and thyroid antibodies
(B) total triiodothyronine (T3), reverse T3, TSH
(C) TT4, reverse T3, TSH, thyroid antibodies
(D) thyroid ultrasound

3. The thyroid gland is tender to palpation, and the child reports that they have had an upper respiratory tract infection the last few days. What would be at the top of your differential diagnosis?

(A) Hashimoto thyroiditis
(B) Graves disease
(C) subacute thyroiditis
(D) euthyroid sick syndrome

4. What would the most likely diagnosis be if the TT4 was 4.5 µg/dL (normal, 5 to 11.5) and FTI 3 (normal, 6.0 to 10.5)?

(A) Hashimoto thyroiditis
(B) Graves disease
(C) low thyroid-binding globulin
(D) subacute thyroiditis

5. What would you expect the TSH to be for the child described in question 4? (Normal, TSH 0.4 to 6.4 mU/L)

(A) 0.01 mU/L
(B) 1.0 mU/L
(C) 6.0 mU/L
(D) 15 mU/L

6. What would the most likely diagnosis be if the TT4 was 3 µg/dL, FTI 7, and the child did not have a goiter?

(A) Hashimoto thyroiditis
(B) Graves disease
(C) low thyroid-binding globulin
(D) subacute thyroiditis

7. What would be the most likely diagnosis if the TT4 was 10 µg/dL, FTI 10, TT3 180 ng/dL (normal, 80 to 195) and thyroid antibodies were positive?

(A) Hashimoto thyroiditis
(B) Graves disease

(C) high thyroid-binding globulin

(D) none of the above

8. Which of the following is not a symptom or sign of hypothyroidism in children?

(A) growth retardation

(B) bradycardia

(C) polyphagia

(D) pubertal disorder

9. Which of the following is dependent on thyroid hormone?

(A) somatic growth

(B) bone growth

(C) tooth eruption

(D) all of the above

10. Which of the following is not a cause of acquired hypothyroidism?

(A) autoimmune thyroiditis

(B) late-onset thyroid dysgenesis

(C) TSH deficiency

(D) subacute thyroiditis

11. The majority of circulating triiodothyronine is derived from where?

(A) peripheral conversion from thyroxine

(B) thyroid gland

(C) pituitary gland

(D) parathyroid glands

12. Which of the following is the biologically active form of thyroid hormone?

(A) TSH

(B) T4

(C) T3

(D) Reverse T3

13. Which of the following is true regarding newborn screening for congenital hypothyroidism?

(A) Programs that use TT4 can miss central hypothyroidism.

(B) The optimum time to collect the sample is within the initial 24 hours of life.

(C) Transient hypothyroidism can be missed.

(D) Programs that use TSH can miss central hypothyroidism.

14. Which of the following is the leading cause of congenital hypothyroidism in iodine sufficient areas?

(A) TSH deficiency

(B) thyroid dyshormonogenesis

(C) transient hypothyroidism

(D) thyroid dysgenesis

15. What is the most worrisome consequence of untreated congenital hypothyroidism?

(A) prolonged physiologic jaundice

(B) retarded central nervous system development

(C) delayed bone maturation

(D) soft tissue myxedema

16. You notice that the patient has exophthalmos. What diagnosis would be most likely?

(A) Hashimoto thyroiditis

(B) Graves disease

(C) iodine deficiency

(D) TSH secreting pituitary tumor

17. All of the following are signs or symptoms of hyperthyroidism except which?

(A) delayed deep tendon reflexes

(B) nervousness

(C) fatigue

(D) palpitations

18. Which of the following statements is true regarding the treatment of Graves disease?

(A) Antithyroid drugs can cause granulocytopenia.

(B) Radioactive iodine should only be used in thyroid storm.

(C) Subtotal surgical thyroidectomy is the preferred initial treatment in children.

(D) Corticosteroids inhibit release of T4 from the thyroid gland.

19. Which of the following is true regarding neonatal Graves disease?

(A) Neonatal Graves occurs in 30% of neonates born to mothers with Graves.

(B) The onset of signs and symptoms can be delayed for 8 to 9 days.

(C) No treatment is necessary since it tends to be self-limited.

(D) The disease is caused by transplacental passage of thyroid hormone.

20. What would the most likely diagnosis be if this child was in the intensive care unit following cardiac surgery, and had a TT4 of 4 μg/dL, FTI 4, TT3 of 50 ng/dL, reverse T3 450 ng/dL and TSH 4 mU/L (normal, 0.4 to 6.4)?

(A) TSH deficiency

(B) TBG deficiency

(C) Hashimoto thyroiditis

(D) euthyroid sick syndrome

Answers

1. **(C)** Growth pattern. Children with hypothyroidism will often manifest slowing of their growth, while children with hyperthyroidism will eventually have accelerated growth if the disorder is not detected and treated appropriately.

2. **(A)** Total thyroxine (TT4), free thyroxine index (FTI), thyrotropin (TSH), and thyroid antibodies. Serum TT4 is the major thyroid hormone in the blood and laboratory tests measure both bound and unbound T4. As the majority of T4 is bound to thyroid-binding globulin (TBG), transthyretin or albumin, levels of binding proteins will affect the TT4 concentration. Thus, the levels of free and total thyroid hormone may not be concordant. Free thyroxin index is a calculation that reflects bioavailable thyroid hormone because it takes into account the amount of binding protein. TSH is secreted from the pituitary under the control of thyroid-releasing hormone (TRH) from the hypothalamus, and through negative feedback from thyroid hormones. Several antibodies against thyroid antigens have been demonstrated in chronic autoimmune thyroiditis, and these levels should be determined in a child with a goiter. TT3 is the active form of thyroid hormone, but it is usually not measured with the initial screen. Reverse T3 is an inactive metabolite of TT4, and measurement is important in the diagnosis of eu-

thyroid sick syndrome. Thyroid ultrasound would be indicated if nodules were detected.

3. **(C)** Subacute thyroiditis. Subacute thyroiditis is a self-limited inflammation of the thyroid gland that usually follows an upper respiratory tract infection. The thyroid gland can be very tender to palpation. There is often a pattern of hyperthyroidism secondary to inappropriate release of thyroid hormone. Signs and symptoms of hyperthyroidism can persist for 1 to 4 weeks, after which transient hypothyroidism typically develops with recovery of the gland. The total course of illness can last 2 to 9 months. Treatment is typically with anti-inflammatory drugs. Children with euthyroid sick syndrome do not present with a goiter, and this usually does not follow a mild illness.

4. **(A)** Hashimoto thyroiditis. The most common abnormality of thyroid function in children is hypothyroidism, usually caused by autoimmune (Hashimoto) thyroiditis. Hashimoto thyroiditis is characterized by circulating thyroid antibodies and varying degrees of thyroid dysfunction. It can present with or without a goiter. It is more prevalent in girls, and many patients have a family history of autoimmune thyroid disease. Spontaneous remission has been reported. Other causes of acquired hypothyroidism include late-onset thyroid dysgenesis or dyshormonogenesis, TSH deficiency, thyroid damage, and iodine deficiency. T4 replacement is the treatment of choice for hypothyroidism.

5. **(D)** 15 mU/L. In hypothyroidism secondary to Hashimoto thyroiditis, the TSH will be elevated.

6. **(C)** Low thyroid-binding globulin. TT4 measures both bound and free T4. In cases where the TBG is low, measured T4 levels will be low, even though free thyroid hormone levels are normal. High-dose glucocorticoids can lower TBG levels, and low TBG levels can also run in families. In contrast, pregnancy or estrogen administration is a common cause of high TBG levels.

7. **(A)** Hashimoto thyroiditis. There is a spectrum of presentation for Hashimoto thyroiditis. Patients can present with a picture of hyperthyroid-

ism (hashitoxicosis), euthyroidism, or hypothyroidism. Patients will typically have a nontender goiter and evidence of thyroid antibodies.

8. **(C)** Polyphagia. Polyphagia is a symptom of hyperthyroidism. The most common manifestation of hypothyroidism in children is subnormal growth velocity leading to short stature. The growth retardation can be present for many years before other symptoms occur. Other manifestations of hypothyroidism that are specific to children include delayed bone maturation and sexual disorders, including both delayed and precocious puberty. Other symptoms of hypothyroidism include bradycardia, cold intolerance, fatigue, constipation, muscle aches, and dry skin.

9. **(D)** All of the above.

10. **(D)** Subacute thyroiditis. Patients with subacute thyroiditis may present initially with hyperthyroidism, which is followed by transient hypothyroidism associated with recovery. Thyroid function then typically returns to normal with resolution of the inflammation.

11. **(A)** Peripheral conversion from thyroxine (T4). Seventy percent to 90% of circulating T3 is derived from monodeiodination of T4 in peripheral tissues, with the remainder being derived from the thyroid gland. Thus, the activity of the deiodination enzymes is critical to the production of intracellular T3 and critical for the maintenance of normal cellular activity. In contrast, the majority of T4 is made in the thyroid gland.

12. **(C)** T3. T3 is the active form of thyroid hormone. T4 is the major thyroid hormone in the blood and is metabolized to T3 and reverse T3 which is not biologically active. TSH is secreted from the pituitary gland under the control of TRH from the hypothalamus and controls thyroid hormone production and release from the thyroid gland.

13. **(D)** Programs that use TSH can miss central hypothyroidism. Most children with central hypothyroidism have normal to low normal serum TSH concentrations, and thus they will be missed if only TSH is measured. Neonates with congenital hypothyroidism typically have no specific signs at birth. The possibility of central hypothyroidism needs to be considered in any infants with other signs of pituitary deficiency such as hypoglycemia, prolonged neonatal jaundice, micropenis, midline facial defects, or poor growth.

14. **(D)** Thyroid dysgenesis. Congenital hypothyroidism occurs in approximately 1 in 4000 newborns and is the most preventable cause of mental retardation if detected and treated early. Neonates with congenital hypothyroidism usually have very few signs and symptoms, thus underlining the importance of the neonatal screen for diagnosis. Thyroid dysgenesis (agenesis, hypoplasia, or ectopic thyroid) is the leading cause of congenital hypothyroidism in iodine-sufficient areas, followed in order of decreasing incidence: transient hypothyroidism, thyroid dyshormonogenesis, and TSH deficiency.

15. **(B)** Retarded central nervous system development. Thyroid hormones exert effects that are most obvious during infancy and early childhood. Brain development is dependent on thyroid function in the first 3 years of life. The early detection of congenital hypothyroidism and early treatment prevents the development of mental retardation that would occur in untreated cases. The initial goal of treatment of congenital hypothyroidism is to restore the T4 concentration to the upper half of the normal range as rapidly as possible.

16. **(B)** Graves disease. Virtually all children with Graves disease have a goiter, and 50% to 75% have mild ophthalmopathy. Severe ophthalmopathy is much less common in children than in adults. Eye findings may include lid lag, infrequent blinking, appearance of a stare because of retraction of the upper lid, exophthalmos and ophthalmoplegia. Graves disease occurs most commonly in the 11- to 15-year age group, and girls are affected more frequently than boys.

17. **(A)** Delayed deep tendon reflexes. The development of hyperthyroidism in children can be insidious. Typical symptoms include nervousness and jitteriness, sleep disorders leading to fatigue, heat intolerance, tachycardia and palpitations,

and a decline in school performance. Children with Graves disease tend to have greater emotional lability and behavioral disturbances than adults. In prolonged hyperthyroidism in children, accelerated linear growth and advanced bone maturation can be seen. Delayed deep tendon reflexes are seen in hypothyroidism.

18. **(A)** Antithyroid drugs can cause granulocytopenia. Blocking thyroid hormone synthesis with methimazole or propylthiouracil is typically the initial therapy of hyperthyroidism in a young child. Most children will need to be on these antithyroid drugs for many years, and close supervision is necessary to monitor thyroid function tests. Side effects of these drugs include rash, granulocytopenia, and liver failure. Ablation of the thyroid gland with radioactive iodine is another treatment option for Graves disease, but this is usually not the preferred initial treatment in children. This treatment option is used extensively in adults. Subtotal surgical thyroidectomy is another treatment option but is usually reserved for children who fail medical therapy or experience serious side effects of antithyroid medications. The availability of an experienced thyroid surgeon is an important criterion for the success of this treatment option. Serious complications of subtotal thyroidectomy include hypoparathyroidism and recurrent laryngeal nerve damage. Corticosteroids can be used in thyroid storm to prevent the peripheral conversion of T4 to T3.

19. **(B)** The onset of signs and symptoms can be delayed for 8 to 9 days. Neonatal Graves disease occurs in approximately 2% of neonates born to mothers with Graves hyperthyroidism. It can be severe, and even life-threatening if not treated properly. It occurs following the transplacental passage of TSH receptor-stimulating antibody. The time of onset and severity of symptoms is variable and depends on the transplacental passage of blocking antibodies and antithyroid drugs. The characteristic manifestations of neonatal Graves disease include irritability, tachycardia, poor weight gain, diarrhea, thyromegaly, and exophthalmus. The treatment consists of iodine or antithyroid drugs, corticosteroids, and propranolol. Neonatal Graves typically resolves spontaneously in 3 to 12 weeks.

20. **(D)** Euthyroid sick syndrome. Euthyroid sick syndrome is an alteration of thyroid hormone levels seen in severe illness. Patients have a decrease in T3 because of an increased metabolism of TT4 to the bioinactive reverse T3, which is characteristically elevated. The lowest levels of T3 and T4 have been associated with increased mortality. It is controversial whether euthyroid sick syndrome is an adaptive phenomenon to decrease metabolic rate, an important contributor of the disease process, or just an associated marker of disease severity. It is controversial whether treatment with thyroid hormone is beneficial or harmful.

SUGGESTED READING

Foley TP Jr: Hypothyroidism. *Pediatr Rev* 25:94–100, 2004.

Fisher DA: Disorders of the thyroid in the newborn and infant. In: Sperling MA (ed): *Pediatric Endocrinology*, 2nd ed. Philadelphia: WB Saunders, 2002, p 161.

Fisher DA: Thyroid disorders in childhood and adolescence. In: Sperling MA (ed): *Pediatric Endocrinology*, 2nd ed. Philadelphia: WB Saunders, 2002, p 187.

Huang SA, Larsen PR: Autoimmune thyroid disease. In: Radovick S, MacGillivray MH (eds): *Pediatric Endocrinology, A Practical Clinical Guide*. Totowa, New Jersey: Humana Press, 2003, p 291.

Larsen CA: Congenital hypothyroidism. In: Radovick S, MacGillivray MH (eds): *Pediatric Endocrinology, A Practical Clinical Guide*. Totowa, New Jersey: Humana Press, 2003, p 275.

CASE 38: A 14-MONTH-OLD CHILD WITH A SEIZURE

A 14-month-old child presents to the emergency department following a brief tonic-clonic seizure. The child has no previous history of seizures. He has not been ill recently, and has had a normal appetite. He was exclusively breastfed until 6 months of age, when his mother added in cereal (mixed with breast milk), and some jar baby foods. He continues to breast-feed. It is early spring, and it has been a particularly dark and dreary winter. His mother has concerns that the child is not yet walking. He is afebrile on physical examination, and is normal size for both height and weight.

SELECT THE ONE BEST ANSWER

1. On physical examination, the patient has a positive Chvostek sign. This is typical in which of the following circumstances?

(A) hypophosphatasia
(B) hypoglycemia
(C) hypocalcemia
(D) hypophosphatemia

2. Which of the following are clinical features of hypocalcemia?

(A) laryngospasm, shortened QT interval on EKG, and a positive Trousseau's sign
(B) laryngospasm, prolonged QT interval on EKG, and a positive Trousseau's sign
(C) paresthesias, prolonged QT interval on EKG, and a negative Trousseau's sign
(D) paresthesias, normal QT interval on EKG, and a positive Trousseau's sign

3. The patient's total calcium is low at 6 mg/dL, with a low ionized calcium of 3 mg/dL. What is the most likely diagnosis if the serum phosphate is 2.5 mg/dL?

(A) nutritional rickets
(B) hypoparathyroidism
(C) X-linked hypophosphatemic rickets
(D) pseudopseudohypoparathyroidism

4. What is the most likely diagnosis if the total calcium is 6 mg/dL, ionized calcium of 3 mg/dL, and serum phosphate 8 mg/dL?

(A) nutritional rickets
(B) hypoparathyroidism
(C) X-linked hypophosphatemic rickets
(D) pseudopseudohypoparathyroidism

5. What is the most likely diagnosis if the total calcium is 6 mg/dL, ionized calcium of 3 mg/dL, serum phosphate 8 mg/dL, and PTH 130 pg/mL (normal, 9 to 52)?

(A) nutritional rickets
(B) hypoparathyroidism
(C) X-linked hypophosphatemic rickets
(D) pseudohypoparathyroidism

6. In nutritional rickets, which of the following laboratory values would you expect to be low?

(A) PTH
(B) 1,25-dihydroxyvitamin D
(C) 25-hydroxyvitamin D
(D) alkaline phosphatase

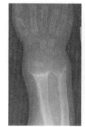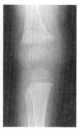

*Figure 38-1. **Radiograph of the wrist (left) and knee (right) in a 14-month-old child with a seizure.***

7. The radiograph shown in Figure 38-1 is most representative of which of the following?

(A) hypoparathyroidism
(B) pseudohypoparathyroidism
(C) nutritional rickets
(D) pseudopseudohypoparathyroidism.

8. Rachitic bone deformities include which of the following?

(A) craniotabes
(B) rachitic rosary
(C) Harrison's grooves
(D) all of the above

9. You start the child on intravenous calcium replacement, but the serum calcium does not normalize. Which of the following should you look for?

(A) hypokalemia
(B) hypoglycemia
(C) hypomagnesemia
(D) hypophosphatasia

10. PTH controls serum calcium levels through its action on all of the following organs except which of the following?

(A) bone
(B) kidney
(C) liver
(D) intestinal tract

11. The active form of vitamin D is which of the following?

(A) 25-hydroxyvitamin D
(B) 24,25-dihydroxyvitamin D
(C) vitamin D$_3$
(D) 1,25-dihydroxyvitamin D

12. The major impact of the active form of vitamin D is on which organ?

    (A) kidney
    (B) intestinal tract
    (C) bone
    (D) liver

13. Which of the following is not a typical cause of early neonatal hypocalcemia (within the first 72 hours of life)?

    (A) prematurity
    (B) infant of a diabetic mother
    (C) congenital hypoparathyroidism
    (D) asphyxia

14. Late neonatal hypocalcemia (between 5 and 10 days of life) is most likely caused by each of the following except:

    (A) asphyxia
    (B) transient hypoparathyroidism
    (C) hyperphosphatemia
    (D) infant of a mother with marginal vitamin D intake

15. You diagnose your patient with nutritional rickets because of vitamin D deficiency. You would likely use all of the following except which in your management of the patient?

    (A) calcium supplementation
    (B) phosphate supplementation
    (C) calcitriol (1,25-dihydroxy vitamin D)
    (D) ergocalciferol (Vitamin D2)

16. Your patient has a low calcium, low phosphate, and elevated alkaline phosphatase. You acutely start the child on intravenous calcium, calcitriol (1,25-dihydroxyvitamin D), and oral ergocalciferol. The calcium normalizes quickly with your therapy. After several days, you stop the calcitriol, and to your surprise, the calcium level falls. What is the most likely cause?

    (A) Laboratory error
    (B) Patient has 1-α-hydroxylase deficiency.
    (C) Patient remains hypophosphatemic.
    (D) The patient received too much calcium.

17. You diagnose your patient with hypoparathyroidism, and once the serum calcium is stabi-

lized, you discharge him home on calcitriol and supplemental calcium. The mother calls in 1 week complaining that she is changing her child's urine-soaked diaper every 2 hours. What should you be most concerned about?

    (A) hypermagnesemia
    (B) hypocalcemia
    (C) hypercalcemia
    (D) hyperphosphatemia

18. What test(s) would help in the diagnosis if your patient was an infant with hypocalcemia and cardiac defects?

    (A) chest radiograph
    (B) analysis of chromosome 15q11
    (C) analysis of chromosome 22q11
    (D) A and C

Answers

1. **(C)** Hypocalcemia. Chvostek's sign is a twitching of the circumoral muscles in response to gentle tapping on the facial nerve just anterior to the ear. It is a sign of hypocalcemia; however, up to 10% of normal individuals will have a slight twitch in response to this maneuver.

2. **(B)** Laryngospasm, prolonged QT interval on EKG, and a positive Trousseau's sign. The signs and symptoms of acute hypocalcemia typically result from increased neuromuscular irritability. This can be elicited by checking for a positive Chvostek or Trousseau's sign. Trousseau's sign is carpal spasm seen with hypoxia. To test for Trousseau's sign, a blood pressure cuff should be inflated to 20 mm Hg above the patient's systolic blood pressure for 3 minutes. Figure 38-2 shows the classic response of a positive Trousseau's sign. Unlike Chvostek's sign, which can be seen in patients with normal calcium levels, a positive Trousseau's sign is rare in the absence of hypocalcemia. Patients often complain of paresthesias of the fingers, toes, and circumoral region. Muscle cramps are also seen and may progress to tetany (spontaneous carpopedal spasm). Laryngospasm and bronchospasm can be seen. Other signs and symptoms include seizures, irritability, impaired school performance, and behavioral changes. With severe hypocalce-

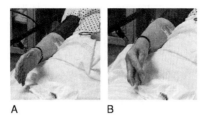

A   B

Figure 38-2.   An example of Trousseau's sign. The photo on the right demonstrates flexion of the wrist and meta-carpophalangeal joints, with extension of the interpha-langeal joints and adduction of the finger after insuffla-tion of the blood pressure cuff. (Reprinted with permission from Meininger ME, Kendler JS: Trousseau's sign. N Engl J Med 343:1855, 2000.)

mia, patients can have prolongation of their QT interval, and can be prone to arrhythmias.

3. **(A)** Nutritional rickets. Children with nutritional rickets usually present with both low serum calcium and phosphate because of a deficiency of vitamin D, leading to a decrease of both calcium and phosphate absorption in the gut. Rickets can also develop with a deficiency of either calcium or phosphate, especially in the rapidly growing premature infant. Hypoparathyroidism usually presents with hyperphosphatemia because of a lack of PTH action on the kidney where PTH typically stimulates excretion of phosphate. Children with pseudopseudohypoparathyroidism have the phenotypic features of Albright's hereditary osteodystrophy (pseudohypoparathyroidism type 1a) without the biochemical abnormalities. X-linked hypophosphatemic rickets is because of a defect in the kidney causing a loss of phosphate, but these children do not present with hypocalcemia.

4. **(B)** Hypoparathyroidism. Hypoparathyroidism occurs when the PTH produced by the parathyroid glands is insufficient to maintain the serum calcium in the normal range. As PTH causes renal calcium absorption and renal phosphate excretion, insufficient PTH will cause both hypocalcemia and hyperphosphatemia. Serum PTH is low, serum 1,25-dihydroxyvitamin D is usually low to low normal (PTH enhances the conversion of 25-hydroxy- to 1,25-dihydroxyvitamin D), and alkaline phosphatase is usually normal.

5. **(D)** Pseudohypoparathyroidism. Pseudohypoparathyroidism (PHP) is a syndrome characterized by

target tissue unresponsiveness to the actions of PTH. Biochemical abnormalities of hypoparathyroidism are seen including hypocalcemia and hyperphosphatemia in the face of elevated PTH levels. PHP type 1a is also called Albright's hereditary osteodystrophy, which presents with PTH resistance with other somatic defects including short stature, round facies, obesity, and developmental delay.

6. **(C)** 25-Hydroxyvitamin D. In nutritional rickets, hypocalcemia will cause a secondary hyperparathyroidism, and thus PTH levels will be elevated. As PTH and hypophosphatemia stimulate renal production of 1,25-dihydroxyvitamin D, levels of this hormone will be normal to high. Alkaline phosphatase is a marker of bone turnover that tends to be elevated in nutritional rickets. 25-Hydroxyvitamin D reflects the nutritional component of vitamin D, and these levels would be low in vitamin D deficient rickets.

7. **(C)** Nutritional rickets. The radiograph demonstrates typical findings of nutritional rickets including widening with cupping and fraying of the metaphyses. The bones are often demineralized in general. In general, no bone changes are seen in hypoparathyroidism and pseudopseudohypoparathyroidism. Occasionally, bone changes consistent with hyperparathyroidism are seen in PHP because of the bones not being resistant to PTH.

8. **(D)** All of the above. Craniotabes is a generalized softening of the calvaria that can be seen in younger infants with rickets, along with frontal bossing and parietal flattening. Rachitic rosary is caused by prominence of the costochondral junction of the ribs. This is typically palpable on the lateral aspect of the chest in a young child as the ribs are not fully formed. Harrison's groves are indentations of the lower ribs from the vessels that run under the ribs and indent the soft bone. Genu varum (bowleg deformity) is also a common rachitic bone deformity, which becomes more pronounced with weight bearing. Children will also present with thickening of the wrists and ankles. There is an increased risk of fracture in children with rickets.

9. **(C)** Hypomagnesemia. Low magnesium levels inhibit both PTH secretion and action of PTH at bone and kidney, which will hinder the correc-

tion of serum calcium. Serum magnesium should be corrected.

10. **(C)** Liver. PTH promotes calcium mobilization from bone by osteoblast-mediated activation of bone resorbing osteoclasts. In the proximal tubule of the kidney, PTH increases the reabsorption of calcium while inhibiting phosphate reabsorption, and activates the enzyme 1-α-hydroxylase, which catalyzes the conversion of 25-hydroxyvitamin D to 1,25-dihydroxyvitamin D. PTH indirectly promotes the absorption of calcium and phosphate in the intestinal tract through the action of 1,25-dihydroxyvitamin D. PTH does not control calcium through effects on the liver.

11. **(D)** 1,25-Dihydroxyvitamin D. The skin produces vitamin D$_3$ from 7-deoxycholesterol after exposure to the sun. People with increased skin melanin pigmentation have decreased photosynthesis of vitamin D, and thus require more time in the sun to make the same amount of vitamin D as those with lighter skin color. Season of the year and geographic latitude can greatly effect the production of vitamin D in the skin. The natural sources of vitamin D include fatty fish such as salmon, and fatty fish oils such as cod liver oil. Most vitamin D obtained from the diet comes from fortified foods such as milk and bread. Vitamin D$_3$ is biologically inert and must undergo 25-hydroxylation in the liver, with subsequent 1-α-hydroxylation in the kidney to form the biologically active form of vitamin D, 1,25-dihydroxyvitamin D. 24,25-Dihydroxyvitamin D is biologically inert, and one of the first steps of vitamin D degradation.

12. **(B)** Intestinal tract. 1,25-Dihydroxy vitamin D has its major impact in the gut, as it promotes the reabsorption of calcium and phosphate in the duodenum and jejunum.

13. **(C)** Congenital hypoparathyroidism. Early neonatal hypocalcemia is characteristically seen in premature infants, infants with asphyxia at birth, and infants of diabetic mothers. Premature infants often have an exaggerated postnatal depression of serum calcium. In addition, both premature infants and asphyxiated infants tend to have an exaggerated rise in calcitonin,

which antagonizes the effect of PTH on bone and kidney, and may provoke hypocalcemia. Infants of diabetic mothers may also have an exaggerated postnatal depression of serum calcium, and maternal glycosuria is accompanied by significant losses of magnesium, which predisposes the infant to total body magnesium losses. Hypomagnesemia in turn inhibits both PTH secretion and action.

14. **(A)** Asphyxia. An asphyxiated infant is more likely to present with early neonatal hypocalcemia, rather than late neonatal hypocalcemia.

15. **(B)** Phosphate supplementation. Children with rickets because of vitamin D deficiency typically require calcium supplementation and calcitriol acutely to raise their calcium into the normal range. Ergocalciferol is used to replenish the vitamin D stores, but its effects are typically not seen for 4 to 7 days, hence the use of the biologically active calcitriol acutely. Phosphate supplementation is typically not used unless the rickets is caused by phosphate depletion (as is sometimes seen in premature infants or patients on total parenteral nutrition), or if your patient has hypophosphatemic rickets (in which case they would not have hypocalcemia).

16. **(B)** Patient has 1-α-hydroxylase deficiency. In 1-α-hydroxylase deficiency, or what is also termed vitamin D dependent rickets type I (VDDR type I), 25-hydroxyvitamin D is not converted into the biologically active 1,25-dihydroxyvitamin D in the kidney because of a deficiency of 1-α-hydroxylase. These patients cannot make biologically active vitamin D when treated with ergocalciferol, and they must be maintained on calcitriol. This disorder usually presents between 3 and 12 months of life, and children have similar symptoms and signs as children with nutritional rickets. Vitamin D resistant rickets or vitamin D dependent rickets type II (VDDR type II) is caused by a defect in the vitamin D receptor, leading to resistance to vitamin D. They can present with both hypocalcemia and hypophosphatemia.

17. **(C)** Hypercalcemia. Mild hypercalcemia can present with generalized weakness, anorexia, constipation, and polyuria. More severe hypercalcemia

can present with nausea, vomiting, dehydration, seizures, and coma. Patients who are hypercalcemic can also present with significant psychological changes such as depression or paranoia.

18. (**D**) A and C. Children with DiGeorge syndrome typically present with transient or permanent hypocalcemia because of hypoplasia of the parathyroid glands, hypoplasia or aplasia of the thymus leading to impaired cell-mediated immunity, and anomalies of the outflow tract of the heart. Abnormalities in the chest radiograph are common, and absence of the thymic shadow should be looked for. Mutations in chromosome 22q11 have been described in DiGeorge syndrome. Other clinical characteristics include facial malformations, short stature, and developmental delay. Mutations in chromosome 15q11 are seen in Prader-Willi syndrome.

SUGGESTED READING

Favus MJ, ed: *Primer on the Metabolic Bone Diseases and Disorders of Mineral Metabolism*, 5th ed. New York: Raven Press, 2003.

Diamond FB, Root AW: Disorders of calcium metabolism in the child and adolescent. In: Sperling MA (ed): *Pediatric Endocrinology*, 2nd ed. Philadelphia: WB Saunders, 2002, p 629.

Root AW, Diamond FB: Disorders of calcium metabolism in the newborn and infant. In: Sperling MA (ed): *Pediatric Endocrinology*, 2nd ed. Philadelphia: WB Saunders, 2002, p 97.

Diaz R: Abnormalities in calcium homeostasis. In: Radovick S, MacGillivray MH (eds): *Pediatric Endocrinology, A Practical Clinical Guide*. Totowa, New Jersey: Humana Press, 2003, p 343.

Levine B-S, Carpenter TO: Rickets: The skeletal disorders of impaired calcium or phosphate availability. In: Radovick S, MacGillivray MH (eds): *Pediatric Endocrinology, A Practical Clinical Guide*. Totowa, New Jersey: Humana Press, 2003, p 365.

CASE 39: A 12-YEAR-OLD GIRL WITH NAUSEA, ABDOMINAL PAIN, AND VOMITING

A 12-year-old girl comes to your office with complaints of nausea, abdominal pain, and emesis for the past 24 hours. She has previously been healthy, but her parents believe that she has lost weight over the summer despite a very good appetite. She has been drinking more water during the day, which her parents relate to it being summertime. She also com-

plains of nocturia for the last few months. She is on no medications. On examination, she appears ill, with dry mucous membranes. She is afebrile. Respirations are deep and rapid.

SELECT THE ONE BEST ANSWER

1. What diagnosis would be at the top of your differential?

   (A) appendicitis
   (B) gastroenteritis
   (C) diabetes insipidus
   (D) diabetes mellitus

2. What test would you do first?

   (A) serum amylase
   (B) abdominal ultrasound
   (C) urinalysis
   (D) hemoglobin A1c

3. Diabetic ketoacidosis (DKA) is typically characterized by all of the following except:

   (A) hyperkalemia
   (B) hyperglycemia
   (C) ketosis
   (D) acidosis

4. The following hormones play a role in DKA except?

   (A) cortisol
   (B) growth hormone
   (C) epinephrine
   (D) prolactin

5. Your patient has a serum blood glucose of 900 mg/dL, pH 7.0, serum ketones large, sodium 126, potassium 4.2, chloride 102, bicarbonate <5, and phosphate 4.2 mEq/L. Which of the following is true?

   (A) She should be treated for hyponatremia.
   (B) She should receive an ampule of sodium bicarbonate.
   (C) She should have additional potassium in the IV fluids.
   (D) Further monitoring of phosphate is not necessary.

6. Which of the following is not a potential drawback to the use of sodium bicarbonate in DKA?

(A) cerebral edema
(B) rebound alkalosis
(C) sodium overload
(D) rise in CSF pH

7. What would the most appropriate initial management be if her serum blood sugar was 800 mg/dL, serum and urine ketones were large, and pH was 7.12?

(A) bolus of normal saline
(B) bolus of IV insulin
(C) bolus of IV bicarbonate
(D) a subcutaneous dose of insulin

8. What would the most appropriate initial management be if her serum blood sugar was 250 mg/dL, serum ketones small, pH 7.38, and she appeared well hydrated?

(A) a subcutaneous dose of insulin
(B) bolus of IV insulin
(C) start an oral hypoglycemic medication
(D) watch and repeat serum glucose in 6 to 24 hours.

9. What would the most appropriate initial management be if her serum blood sugar was 180 mg/dL, ketones negative, pH 7.38, and the child has had an illness with a fever for the last week?

(A) a subcutaneous dose of insulin
(B) bolus of IV insulin
(C) start an oral hypoglycemic medication
(D) watch and repeat serum glucose in 6 hours

10. Her mother, maternal aunt, maternal grandmother, and maternal great-grandmother all have a history of diabetes. This family history would worry you most about what type of diabetes?

(A) type 1 diabetes
(B) type 2 diabetes
(C) atypical diabetes
(D) maturity-onset diabetes of youth

11. In a child in DKA, when would you worry most about the development of cerebral edema?

(A) prior to any treatment
(B) immediately after the initial bolus of normal saline

(C) several hours after the institution of therapy
(D) once the ketosis clears

12. Which of the following is not a manifestation of cerebral edema?

(A) tachycardia
(B) papilledema
(C) widened pulse pressure
(D) headache

13. Which of the following would not be an appropriate initial treatment for cerebral edema associated with DKA?

(A) decrease IV fluids
(B) stop insulin therapy
(C) hyperventilation
(D) mannitol

14. You diagnose your patient with type 1 diabetes and start her on subcutaneous insulin. Several months later the mother calls you to inform you that her daughter is ill and has vomited four times in the last 2 hours. She has not been eating well, and her mother is unsure of what to do. You would advise she do which of the following first?

(A) hold the insulin since she is not eating
(B) check urine ketones
(C) come directly to the emergency department
(D) push fluids and call you back in 4 hours

15. Several months later you get a page at 6 AM from the child's mother because the child is having a seizure. You would advise the mother to do which of the following first?

(A) administer glucose tablets
(B) give orange juice
(C) administer glucagon
(D) hold the insulin dose

16. On a routine follow-up 2 years later, your patient reports that she checks her blood sugars four times daily (they range from 80 to 120), and she follows her meal plan consistently. She does all of her own care. You note on examination that she has lost 10 lbs in the past 3 months, and is now below the 5th percentile for weight. Her hemoglobin A1c is elevated at 12%. What should be your main concern at this time?

(A) anorexia
(B) poor compliance
(C) insulin resistance
(D) celiac disease

17. On your initial examination, you notice that the patient is obese and has acanthosis nigricans. This can be a marker for which of the following?

(A) hyperglycemia
(B) type 1 diabetes
(C) autoimmunity
(D) hyperinsulinism

18. On hospital follow-up in 3 months, your patient has gained 10 kg and now has a BMI of 36. Which of the following would be most helpful with distinguishing between type 1 and type 2 diabetes in your patient?

(A) reported blood glucose
(B) hemoglobin A1c level
(C) C-peptide
(D) family history

Answers

1. **(D)** Diabetes mellitus. Typical clinical symptoms of diabetes mellitus include polyuria, polydipsia, and polyphagia. Vomiting is often seen in diabetic ketoacidosis (DKA) associated with ketosis. Abdominal pain is also present in many cases and may mimic appendicitis or pancreatitis. The abdominal pain usually resolves within a few hours of fluid and insulin therapy. Cerebral obtundation can be present, and is usually related to the degree of hyperosmolarity. Kussmaul respirations (deep, sighing and rapid) are often seen with profound acidosis.

2. **(C)** Urinalysis. A urinalysis is an important first step to detect glucosuria. A serum amylase and abdominal ultrasound would only be required if the patient's abdominal pain did not subside after several hours of fluid resuscitation and improvement of the patient's metabolic state. A hemoglobin A1c is important to confirm the presence of hyperglycemia over the last several months and is important in long-term follow-up of the patient, but this does not usually help in the acute management of the patient.

3. **(A)** Hyperkalemia. Measured serum potassium is usually normal to high; however, patients are usually depleted of total body potassium for the following reasons: insulin deficiency causes decreased Na/K ATPase activity, and decreased Na/K exchange leading to increased extracellular K, acidosis causes exchange of K from intracellular to extracellular compartment in exchange for H+ ions, which move into the cell along a concentration gradient, and K+ is then lost in part via osmotic diuresis and vomiting, and in part via the actions of aldosterone, which is elevated secondary to volume depletion. Blood glucose in DKA is typically greater than 300 mg/dL. However, the blood glucose can be <300 mg/dL in known diabetics because of vomiting with decreased carbohydrate intake and continued insulin administration. The primary mode of ketoacid production in DKA is from free fatty acid. The ketoacids relative to DKA are β-hydroxybutyric acid and acetoacetic acid. Acetone has no effect on blood pH but is clinically important because of its characteristic odor. Most laboratories measure acetoacetate in blood and urine. However, the ratio of acetoacetate to β-hydroxybutyrate is 1:3 in the fasted state and 1:7 to 1:15 in DKA. Thus the degree of ketosis in DKA is typically underestimated. Acidosis is defined as a blood pH <7.3, or serum bicarbonate <15 mEq/L. In DKA, acidosis is predominantly because of the accumulation of ketoacids, and thus patients will have an increased anion gap. Other mechanisms contributing to acidosis include lactic acidosis from tissue hypoperfusion and hyperchloremic acidosis during fluid replacement. In general, the degree of acidosis in DKA bears no relation to the degree of hyperglycemia.

4. **(D)** Prolactin. The cardinal hormonal alterations seen in diabetic ketoacidosis include an absolute or relative insulin deficiency, with an excess of the stress hormones epinephrine, cortisol, and growth hormone (GH). Epinephrine activates glycogenolysis, gluconeogenesis and lipolysis, and inhibits insulin release by the pancreas. Cortisol decreases glucose use in muscle and stimulates gluconeogenesis. GH increases lipolysis and impairs insulin action on muscle. The catabolic and metabolic effects of each of the stress hormones are accentuated during insulin deficiency. Prolactin plays no known role in DKA.

5. **(C)** She should have additional potassium in the IV fluids. The serum sodium is usually factitiously low because of the hyperglycemia. For every 100-mg/dL glucose increment over 100 mg/dl, there is a decrease of 1.6 mEq/L sodium. Thus this patient's true sodium is closer to 139 mEq/L. Measured serum potassium is usually normal or high, but patients are usually depleted of total body potassium (please see answer to question 3). It is therefore important to treat with 30 to 40 mEq/L K+ once the child urinates, as correction of acidosis, restoration of intravascular volume, insulin, and improvement of renal function tend to decrease extracellular K+. Approximately one-fourth to one-half of K+ administered during fluid replacement is lost in the urine. Hypokalemia is one of the avoidable causes of fatality in DKA. It is also important to monitor and replace phosphate, as these patients can have a total body depletion of phosphate as a result of extracellular shifting and subsequent loss in the urine because of the catabolic state. Furthermore, with insulin treatment and fluid replacement, phosphate shifts back into the intracellular compartment, and a hypophosphatemic state occurs if phosphate is not replaced. Hypophosphatemia impairs insulin action and results in a decrease in synthesis of ATP and other energy intermediates. Sodium bicarbonate should only be used if the serum pH is less than 7.1 and if the patient is unstable. Sodium bicarbonate should never be administered as a bolus.

6. **(D)** Rise in CSF pH. The use of sodium bicarbonate in DKA may increase the risk of cerebral edema because of osmotic shifts. Other drawbacks include hypokalemia, impaired tissue oxygenation with left shift of the oxyhemoglobin dissociation curve, rebound alkalosis, sodium overload, and the potential for a paradoxical fall in CSF pH while correcting peripheral acidosis.

7. **(A)** Bolus of normal saline. Dehydration is virtually universal in patients with DKA, and if unrecognized or mismanaged contributes significantly to morbidity and mortality of DKA. The degree of dehydration varies from patient to patient, and the extent of the losses is unpredictable in any given patient. In DKA, there is an osmotically driven shift of water from intracellular to extracellular compartments. This results in underestimation of the extent of dehydration and is responsible for the unusual laboratory finding of hyponatremia despite dehydration and hyperosmolarity. There are three main mechanisms of water and electrolyte loss in DKA, which include osmotic diuresis secondary to hyperglycemia, losses via the respiratory tract secondary to hyperventilation from metabolic acidosis, and losses from the GI tract from vomiting. Serum blood sugar will typically decrease with a normal saline bolus. To avoid rapid shifts in osmolality, the serum glucose should be lowered by 100 mg/dL an hour. Thus, a continuous insulin drip is preferred to a bolus of either IV or subcutaneous insulin as it allows titration of the insulin based on the blood glucose response. Sodium bicarbonate should be avoided as discussed in the answer to question 6.

8. **(A)** A subcutaneous dose of insulin. In this situation, the patient is not in DKA with the lack of acidosis and will respond to subcutaneous insulin.

9. **(D)** Watch and repeat serum glucose in 6 hours. In this situation, the child may have stress-induced hyperglycemia rather than diabetes mellitus, which warrants close following and treatment if worsening hyperglycemia or ketosis develops. There are no current data to suggest that children with stress-induced diabetes in the absence of islet cell and GAD-65 autoimmunity are a greater risk of developing diabetes in the future.

10. **(D)** Maturity-onset diabetes of youth. Maturity onset diabetes of youth is a rare group of disorders with characteristics of type 2 diabetes mellitus caused by monogenic defects of beta cell function. Clinical criteria include the onset of type 2 diabetes at an early age (before 25 years) and autosomal dominant inheritance.

11. **(C)** Several hours after the institution of therapy. Cerebral edema is usually not seen until the patient has been treated with fluids and insulin and laboratory data have shown improvement.

12. **(A)** Tachycardia. Manifestations of cerebral edema include headache, deepening coma, fever, bradycardia, widened pulse pressure, papilledema, and

unequal pupils. The exact cause of cerebral edema is still controversial, but it is likely related to overtreatment with hypotonic solutions and rapid changes in plasma osmolality.

13. **(B)** Stop insulin therapy. A decrease of IV fluids, mannitol administration, and hyperventilation are all appropriate measures to decrease intracranial pressure to avoid brain herniation. Insulin therapy would still be indicated to correct the metabolic state.

14. **(B)** Check urine ketones. Children with diabetes are prone to develop DKA in times of illness because of the secreted stress hormones associated with illness (see question 4 above), which makes them relatively insulin-resistant. Furthermore, the production of ketones can be the result of gastroenteritis, or can cause a child to feel ill and vomit. If the child does have ketones, holding the insulin will make the situation worse and additional insulin is required to reverse the catabolic state. Although pushing fluids is important in children who are vomiting to prevent dehydration, determination of urine ketone status is the most important first step in caring for this child.

15. **(C)** Administer glucagon. Glucagon will rapidly increase the blood sugar and get the child to a point where they are conscious enough to ingest oral glucose. Nothing should be put into the mouth of a seizing child to avoid aspiration. Depending on the cause of the hypoglycemia, the child may need an adjustment to the insulin dose.

16. **(B)** Poor compliance. Weight loss and an elevated hemoglobin A1c in a diabetic suggests foremost a deficiency of insulin. It unfortunately is not uncommon to detect poor compliance in an adolescent with diabetes. The hemoglobin A1c measures how much glucose is irreversibly bound to hemoglobin, and thus is a marker of blood sugar levels over the last 3 months (life span of red blood cells).

17. **(D)** Hyperinsulinism. Acanthosis nigricans is characterized by hyperpigmented, thick, velvety lesions that occur most commonly on the posterior neck, groin, and axilla. It is commonly seen in obese patients who have insulin resistance.

18. **(C)** C-peptide. C-peptide is generated from the cleavage of proinsulin, and one molecule of C-peptide is released into the circulation for every molecule of insulin. Thus, C-peptide can be used as an index of insulin secretion. C-peptide levels are generally low in type 1 diabetes associated with insulin deficiency, and normal to high in type 2 diabetes associated with insulin resistance.

SUGGESTED READING

Kaufman FR: Type 1 diabetes mellitus. *Pediatr Rev* 24: 291, 2003.
Rosenbloom A, et al: Type 2 diabetes in children and adolescents. *Diabetes Care* 23:381, 2000.
Sperling MA: Diabetes mellitus. In: Sperling MA (ed): *Pediatric Endocrinology*, 2nd ed. Philadelphia: WB Saunders, 2002, p 323.

CASE 40: A NEWBORN WITH AMBIGUOUS GENITALIA

You are called to the newborn nursery emergently to see a full-term baby with ambiguous genitalia. The pregnancy and delivery were unremarkable. On physical examination, the baby is in no distress. The baby has a phallus, which is 2 cm in stretched length, there is a 1-mm orifice at the base of the phallus, no obvious vaginal opening, and no palpable gonads (Figure 40-1).

SELECT THE ONE BEST ANSWER

1. If the karyotype is 46,XX, what would be the most likely diagnosis?

    (A) maternal androgen exposure
    (B) true hermaphroditism
    (C) congenital adrenal hyperplasia
    (D) 5α-reductase deficiency

2. Which of the following is the most frequent enzymatic defect in congenital adrenal hyperplasia?

    (A) 3-β-hydroxysteroid dehydrogenase deficiency
    (B) 11-β-hydroxylase deficiency
    (C) 21-hydroxylase deficiency
    (D) 17-hydroxylase deficiency

3. What would your immediate concern be for the baby in question 1?

    (A) possibility of salt-wasting crisis
    (B) surgical correction of the genital abnormality

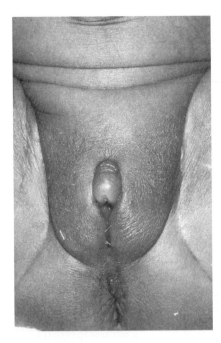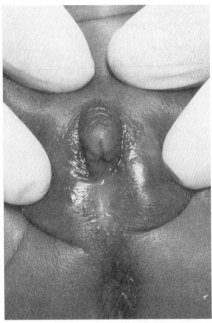

Figure 40-1.

(C) assigning a sex

(D) renal anomalies

4. You diagnose the patient with congenital adrenal hyperplasia as a result of 21-hydroxylase deficiency. What are the mother's chances of having another baby with congenital adrenal hyperplasia?

(A) <5%

(B) 25%

(C) 50%

(D) 100%

5. Which of the following is measured as part of the newborn screen to detect CAH?

(A) 17-hydroxyprogesterone

(B) 17-hydroxypregnenolone

(C) testosterone

(D) androstenedione

6. What would be the most likely diagnosis if the baby has palpable gonads, a phallic urethra, and also has other midline defects such as cleft lip and palate?

(A) congenital adrenal hyperplasia

(B) panhypopituitarism

(C) true hermaphroditism

(D) androgen insensitivity syndrome

7. The initial evaluation of an infant with ambiguous genitalia should include which of the following?

(A) karyotype, pelvic ultrasound, measurement of adrenal steroids

(B) pelvic ultrasound, measurement of adrenal steroids, biopsy of gonads

(C) karyotype, measurement of adrenal steroids, biopsy of gonads

(D) measurement of sex steroids, abdominal radiograph, karyotype

8. Which of the following disorders does not usually have associated external genital abnormalities?

(A) Smith-Lemli-Opitz syndrome

(B) Prader-Willi syndrome

(C) Turner syndrome

(D) trisomy 18

9. What is the role of the sex-determining region on the Y chromosome (SRY)?

(A) initiate external male genitalia formation

(B) initiate testis formation

(C) inhibit formation of internal female genitalia

(D) inhibit formation of external female genitalia

10. 5α-reductase has what function?

(A) converts testosterone into estradiol
(B) converts testosterone into dihydrotestoste-
rone
(C) converts dihydrotestosterone into testoster-
one
(D) converts estradiol into testosterone

11. Abnormalities in which of the following genes
lead to abnormalities in sexual differentiation?

(A) sex-determining region on the Y chromosome
(B) 5α-reductase
(C) androgen receptor
(D) all of the above

12. What structures do the Müllerian ducts form?

(A) fallopian tubes, uterus, and upper vagina
(B) ovaries, fallopian tubes, and uterus
(C) fallopian tubes, uterus, and upper and lower
vagina
(D) ovaries, uterus, and upper vagina

13. What structures do the Wolffian ducts form?

(A) epididymis, vas deferens, penile urethra
(B) testis, epididymis, vas deferens
(C) testis, epididymis, seminal vesicles
(D) epididymis, vas deferens, seminal vesicles

14. What is the role of Leydig cells in sexual differentiation?

(A) cause testicular enlargement
(B) produce testosterone which stabilizes the
Wolffian ducts
(C) enhance Sertoli cell formation
(D) cause regression of the Müllerian ducts

15. Growth and differentiation of the external genitalia in males is most dependent on which of the
following?

(A) testosterone
(B) Müllerian-inhibiting hormone
(C) SRY
(D) dihydrotestosterone

16. Infants born with 5α-reductase deficiency have
which of the following features?

(A) 46,XX, male internal genitalia, female external genitalia

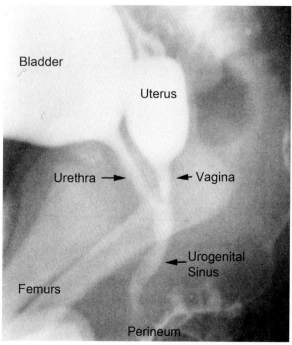

Figure 40-2. *Retrograde urethrogram of the internal
genitalia of a virilized female infant with congenital adrenal hyperplasia as a result of 21-hydroxylase deficiency. With early exposure to androgens, the urethra
and vagina do not extend to the perineum to form separate openings. An internal connection between the urethra and vagina forms a urogenital sinus, which results
in only a single opening on the perineum.*

(B) 46,XY, male internal genitalia, female external genitalia
(C) 46,XX, female internal genitalia, male external genitalia
(D) 46,XY, female internal genitalia, male external genitalia

17. At what age do females need to be exposed to excess androgens to cause labial fusion and development of a urogenital sinus (see Figure 40-2)?

(A) before 4 weeks gestation
(B) before 12 weeks gestation
(C) between 12 and 24 weeks gestation
(D) after 24 weeks gestation

18. What is the lower limit of normal of penile
length in a male term newborn?

(A) 2.0 cm
(B) 2.5 cm
(C) 3.0 cm
(D) 3.5 cm

19. In females, the genital tubercle becomes which of the following?

(A) clitoris
(B) labia minora
(C) labia majora
(D) vaginal opening

Answers

1. **(C)** Congenital adrenal hyperplasia. Congenital adrenal hyperplasia (CAH) is the most common diagnosis in virilized 46,XX infants. The ambiguous genitalia in female infants is caused by excess androgen exposure in utero and can range from mild virilization with posterior fusion to complete virilization. Maternal androgen exposure and true hermaphroditism can both cause excess virilization in girls, but they are not as common as CAH. 5α-reductase deficiency causes genital ambiguity in males.

2. **(C)** 21-Hydroxylase deficiency. 21-Hydroxylase deficiency caused by mutations in the 21-hydroxylase gene accounts for the majority of CAH. A deficiency of 21-hydroxylase impairs the conversion of 17-hydroxyprogesterone to 11-deoxycortisol, resulting in decreased cortisol production, and impairs the conversion of progesterone to deoxycorticosterone, resulting in defects in aldosterone production. Males with 21-hydroxylase deficiency do not present with genital ambiguity. However, males with 3-β-hydroxysteroid dehydrogenase deficiency, 17-α-hydroxylase deficiency and StAR deficiency are undervirilized.

3. **(A)** Possibility of a salt-wasting crisis. Children with CAH as a result of 21-hydroxylase deficiency can produce inadequate aldosterone leading to a salt-wasting crisis. Infants with a salt-wasting crisis present with failure to thrive, lethargy, vomiting, hypotension, hypovolemia, hyponatremia, and hyperkalemia. If CAH is not diagnosed and treated promptly, it can be fatal. Newborn screening programs have allowed the early detection of CAH as a result of 21-hydroxylase deficiency, especially in boys who do not present with ambiguous genitalia, and mildly virilized girls. Stress doses of hydrocortisone should be given to all infants in whom a diagnosis of CAH is considered. This will provide both glucocorticoid and mineralocorticoid coverage. Once infants with salt-wasting CAH are put on maintenance hydrocortisone, a mineralocorticoid must be added. Approximately two-thirds of infants with CAH will be salt wasters.

4. **(B)** 25%. Congenital adrenal hyperplasia as a result of 21-hydroxylase deficiency is transmitted as an autosomal recessive trait. Thus, assuming that she has more children with the same father, there is a 25% chance that they will inherit both mutant alleles and be affected with CAH. It is possible to diagnose children prenatally. In subsequent pregnancies, this mother can be started on dexamethasone early in the pregnancy (by 5 to 6 weeks) to attempt to lessen the degree of genital ambiguity in affected female offspring by lowering the excess androgen production. Screening for CAH is done either by chorionic villus sampling or amniocentesis. Dexamethasone is only continued in women carrying affected female fetuses. The excess androgen production in affected males in utero currently has no known detrimental effect.

5. **(A)** 17-Hydroxyprogesterone. The most common enzyme deficiency causing CAH is deficiency of 21-hydroxylase, which converts 17-hydroxyprogesterone to 11-deoxycortisol. Thus a deficiency of 21-hydroxylase will lead to a build-up of the precursor, 17-hydroxyprogesterone.

6. **(B)** Panhypopituitarism. This describes a baby with micropenis. The presence of other midline defects suggests panhypopituitarism. Pituitary gonadotropins are necessary for phallic enlargement after the external genitalia are formed. This baby must be screened for other pituitary hormone deficiencies. CAH is a less likely cause of genital ambiguity when other nongenital anomalies are present. Patients with true hermaphroditism have the presence of both female and male internal genitalia with dysgenetic or mixed gonads.

7. **(A)** Karyotype, pelvic ultrasound, measurement of adrenal steroids. Determination of the karyotype can help classify the infant as an undervirilized male, a virilized female or a mixed sex chromo-

some pattern. Ultrasound of the pelvis can help determine the presence of the gonads, uterus, and vagina. Measurement of adrenal steroids is necessary because CAH is a common cause of ambiguous genitalia, and patients can have life-threatening adrenal insufficiency if not diagnosed and treated. Biopsy of the gonads is not indicated in the initial evaluation. Abdominal radiograph will not help much in the initial diagnosis.

8. **(C)** Turner syndrome. Girls with Turner syndrome are usually born with normal female external and internal female genitalia, but have streak ovaries as a result of accelerated ovarian atresia. Boys with Smith-Lemli-Opitz syndrome (a disorder of cholesterol biosynthesis caused by a deficiency of 7-dehydrocholesterol reductase) often present with hypospadias, a bifid scrotum, and cryptorchidism among other phenotypic abnormalities. Patients with Prader-Willi syndrome can present with micropenis in boys and hypoplasia of the labia majora in girls. They often have hypogonadism. Patients with trisomy 18 can have cryptorchidism and hypoplasia of the labia majora.

9. **(B)** Initiate testis formation. SRY is a transcription factor expressed in gonads with a Y chromosome, which is thought to initiate the molecular events of testis formation. Mutations within SRY have been associated with 46,XY sex reversal because of testicular failure.

10. **(B)** Converts testosterone into dihydrotestosterone. The enzymatic conversion of testosterone to dihydrotestosterone is critical for virilization of external male genitalia.

11. **(D)** All of the above. Expression of SRY is thought to be the initiating factor in testis formation, thus deletion of SRY will cause sex reversal in 46,XY infants. 5α-Reductase is the enzyme that converts testosterone into the more biologically active dihydrotestosterone, and a deficiency results in undervirilization of male infants. Abnormality in the androgen receptor will cause undervirilization of males because of androgen insensitivity.

12. **(A)** Fallopian tubes, uterus, and upper vagina. The Müllerian ducts form the fallopian tubes,

uterus and upper third of the vagina. In males, Müllerian-inhibiting hormone is secreted from the testicular Sertoli cells beginning at approximately the seventh week of gestation, and causes regression of the Müllerian ducts.

13. **(D)** Epididymis, vas deferens, seminal vesicles. The Wolffian ducts differentiate into the epididymis, vas deferens, seminal vesicles and ejaculatory ducts in 46,XY males.

14. **(B)** Produce testosterone that stabilizes the Wolffian ducts. Differentiation of the Wolffian ducts is dependent on local testosterone production from the Leydig cells of the testes.

15. **(D)** Dihydrotestosterone. While development of the Wolffian ducts and internal genitalia is dependent on local production of testosterone, development of the external genitalia in males is dependent on dihydrotestosterone.

16. **(B)** 46,XY, male internal genitalia, female external genitalia. 5α-Reductase deficiency is an autosomal recessive disorder in which 46,XY infants have bilateral testes and normal male internal genitalia (a result of normal testosterone production and production of Müllerian-inhibiting hormone that causes female internal genitalia to regress), but with undervirilized external genitalia because of defective conversion of testosterone to dihydrotestosterone. They typically present with microphallus, perineal hypospadias, and a blind vaginal pouch. At puberty, 46,XY patients will undergo progressive virilization with phallic enlargement and muscular development because of testosterone production.

17. **(B)** Before 12 weeks' gestation. The separation of the vagina and urethra is complete in females by 12 weeks. Exposure to excess androgens prior to this time can interfere with this process. Exposure to excess androgens once the vagina and urethra are separate causes clitoromegaly, and rugation of the labial folds only. Formation of a urogenital sinus is common in virilized females with CAH.

18. **(B)** 2.5 cm. A phallus smaller that 2.5 cm in a term newborn would be considered a micrope-

nis. This measurement should be adjusted for gestational age. Micropenis can be caused by decreased testosterone exposure in the second and third trimester, which can be caused by LH deficiency or partial androgen insensitivity. Growth hormone deficiency can also cause micropenis. These infants should be screened for the possibility of panhypopituitarism.

19. **(A)** Clitoris. In females the genital tubercle forms the clitoris, while in males it forms the phallus.

SUGGESTED READING

Warne GL, Zajac JD: Disorders of sexual differentiation. *Endocrinol Metab Clin North Am* 27:945, 1998.

Witchell SF, Lee PA: Ambiguous genitalia. In: Sperling MA (ed): *Pediatric Endocrinology*, 2nd ed. Philadelphia: WB Saunders, 2002, p 111.

MacGillivray MH, Mazur T: Management of infants born with ambiguous genitalia. In: Radovick S, MacGillivray MH (eds): *Pediatric Endocrinology, A Practical Clinical Guide*. Totowa, New Jersey: Humana Press, 2003, p 429.

CASE 41: A 13-YEAR-OLD GIRL WITH RAPID WEIGHT GAIN

A 13-year-old girl comes into your clinic with the complaint of rapid weight gain over the last 2 years. She claims that she does not eat more than others in the family, and she has gym class three times weekly. Her typical day consists of going to school, doing homework, and then watching television or playing video games for several hours daily. There are other family members who are overweight. On physical examination, she is overweight, but in no apparent distress.

SELECT THE ONE BEST ANSWER

1. Which formula would you use to calculate BMI?

(A) kg/m
(B) kg/m^2
(C) kg^2/m
(D) kg/cm^2

2. Which BMI defines an overweight child?

(A) between 55th and 65th percentile
(B) between 65th and 75th percentile
(C) between 75th and 85th percentile
(D) between 85th and 95th percentile

3. BMI is not a good estimate of adiposity in which of the following situations?

(A) body builder
(B) endogenous obesity
(C) short stature
(D) exogenous obesity

4. Which of the following is not an adequate method of measuring the degree of obesity?

(A) DEXA
(B) weight greater than the 90th percentile of normal
(C) skinfold thickness
(D) bioelectrical impedance analysis

5. You calculate the patient's BMI as greater than the 95th percentile for age. On further questioning, she has always been "chubby," except when she was an infant when she had feeding difficulty and hypotonia. What would be the likely diagnosis?

(A) Cushing's syndrome
(B) exogenous obesity
(C) Prader-Willi syndrome
(D) Laurence-Moon-Bardet-Biedl syndrome

6. Which of the following features would you not expect to find in the child described in question 5?

(A) tall stature
(B) developmental delay
(C) hyperphagia
(D) relatively small hands and feet

7. Her mother is convinced that her daughter has hypothyroidism as a cause of her obesity. Which of the following would rule against this diagnosis?

(A) normal growth velocity
(B) delayed bone maturation
(C) fatigue
(D) family history

8. On physical examination, your patient is short and has purple striae on the abdomen. Which of the following would you be most concerned about?

(A) hypothyroidism
(B) genetic obesity syndrome
(C) exogenous obesity
(D) Cushing syndrome

9. On physical examination, the patient's BMI is greater than the 95th percentile and you notice that she has darkening and thickening of the skin on the posterior neck and in the axilla. Which of the following would you be most concerned about?

   (A) Addison's disease
   (B) hyperinsulinism
   (C) prolactinoma
   (D) Cushing syndrome

10. Your patient reports that she has had several vaginal yeast infections recently. Which of the following tests is most important in your work-up?

   (A) complete blood count
   (B) cortisol
   (C) immunoglobulin levels
   (D) fasting blood sugar

11. Which of the following is not a feature of the metabolic syndrome?

   (A) hypertension
   (B) insulin resistance
   (C) dyslipidemia
   (D) type 1 diabetes mellitus

12. On physical examination, your patient is of normal stature, but you notice hirsutism and moderate inflammatory acne. What part of the history will be important to narrow your differential diagnosis?

   (A) nutrition history
   (B) menstrual history
   (C) developmental history
   (D) school performance

13. Which of the following is the best test to diagnose the condition in question 12?

   (A) fasting insulin level
   (B) hemoglobin A1c
   (C) free testosterone
   (D) follicle-stimulating hormone

14. Excess body fat in which area of the body has been associated more strongly with health risks than fat stored elsewhere?

   (A) chest
   (B) abdomen
   (C) buttocks
   (D) thighs

15. How likely is a 13-year-old child with a BMI in the 90th percentile to be overweight as an adult?

   (A) <20%
   (B) 40%
   (C) 60%
   (D) >70%

16. Which of the following is not a comorbid condition associated with exogenous childhood obesity?

   (A) short stature
   (B) sleep apnea
   (C) type 2 diabetes mellitus
   (D) slipped capital femoral epiphysis

17. Which of the following is true regarding the prevalence of obesity in children?

   (A) It has been stable over the last 10 years.
   (B) It has been stable over the last 5 years.
   (C) It has been increasing over the last 10 years.
   (D) It has been decreasing over the last 5 years.

18. Which of the following statements regarding obesity is true?

   (A) Genes have a more important role than environment in the obesity epidemic.
   (B) Severe obesity can result from human gene mutations.
   (C) Obese children can easily lose weight if they eat properly.
   (D) Obesity occurs when energy intake is balanced by energy expenditure.

Answers

1. **(B)** kg/m^2. Body mass index provides a satisfactory index of adiposity.

2. **(D)** Between 85th and 95th percentile. Cutoff criteria for overweight and obese children are based on the 2000 CDC BMI for age growth charts. If a child's BMI falls between the 85th and 95th percentile they are considered to be overweight. If their BMI is >95th percentile, they are defined as being obese. Obesity implies excess

body fat. Body fat mass reflects the long-term balance between energy expenditure and energy intake.

3. **(A)** Body builder. The major limitation to BMI is that it does not differentiate between weight that is fat and weight that is muscle. Thus, very muscular people may be improperly classified as being overweight or obese.

4. **(B)** Weight greater than the 90th percentile of normal. Tall children who are proportional will have weights greater than the 90th percentile of normal and not be obese. However, if a child's weight is on the height curve, they are likely obese! DEXA scans can demonstrate the distribution and extent of adiposity, but the disadvantage is that sophisticated equipment is necessary. Skinfold thickness is measured with the use of specific calipers. Age- and sex-specific percentiles for triceps and subscapular skinfolds are available, and skinfold thickness >85th percentile for age and sex suggests obesity. The disadvantages of using skinfold thickness to classify obesity are that there is significant interobserver error and the measurement becomes less reliable as body fatness increases. Bioelectrical impedance estimates adiposity by measuring resistance to a low-frequency electrical current. The advantages of this method are that it is portable, noninvasive, and reliable in many populations. Disadvantages are that it can be variable, and measurements are compromised with altered hydration and extreme obesity.

5. **(C)** Prader-Willi syndrome. A history of feeding difficulty and hypotonia as an infant is found in Prader-Willi syndrome, which is the most common genetic syndrome associated with obesity. Impaired paternal imprinting in the chromosomal region 15q11–13 is found in Prader-Willi syndrome. Laurence-Moon-Bardet-Biedl syndrome, an autosomal recessive disorder characterized by retinal degeneration, mental retardation, obesity, polydactyly, renal dysplasia, and short stature, is a rare cause of pediatric obesity.

6. **(A)** Tall stature. One of the characteristic features of Prader-Willi syndrome is short stature for the genetic background. Patients present

with hyperphagia, relatively small hands and feet, developmental delay, and a characteristic behavioral disorder.

7. **(A)** Normal growth velocity. Children with a hormonal cause of obesity are typically short with a poor growth velocity. Long-standing hypothyroidism would cause short stature, delayed bone age, and fatigue. With hypothyroidism secondary to autoimmune thyroiditis, there is often a family history of thyroid dysfunction.

8. **(D)** Cushing syndrome. Short stature associated with obesity should raise the concern of an endocrinologic cause of obesity such as Cushing syndrome or hypothyroidism. Cushing syndrome describes any form of glucocorticoid excess. In children, the first signs of Cushing syndrome are typically growth attenuation and weight gain, and the attenuation of growth often occurs before the excessive weight gain.

9. **(B)** Hyperinsulinism. Acanthosis nigricans, or hyperpigmented, thick, velvety areas of skin most commonly on the posterior neck, groin, and axilla, is often seen in obese patients and is a marker of insulin resistance. Although hyperpigmentation is seen in Addison's disease, it is most prominent in areas of the skin exposed to the sun, and in flexors surfaces such as knees, elbows, and knuckles. In addition, Addison's disease presents with anorexia and weight loss, not gain.

10. **(D)** Fasting blood sugar. Obese children are at risk of developing type 2 diabetes mellitus, which usually has an insidious onset. History of frequent vaginal yeast infections should raise the concern of hyperglycemia.

11. **(D)** Type 1 diabetes mellitus. The metabolic syndrome combines atherogenic risk factors with underlying insulin resistance. Key features include hyperinsulinemia, abnormal glucose metabolism (impaired glucose tolerance or type 2 diabetes), hypertension, dyslipidemia, obesity (especially visceral) hyperuricemia, microalbuminuria, and hypercoagulability. With the marked increase in obesity in children, this syndrome will become much more common in children, and will eventually lead to increased mortality overall.

12. **(B)** Menstrual history. Obesity in a girl is a feature of polycystic ovary syndrome (PCOS) and is often the presenting complaint. Other features include menstrual irregularity, hirsutism, acne and insulin resistance.

13. **(C)** Free testosterone. PCOS is the most common cause of hyperandrogenism and typically presents after the onset of puberty. The best way to screen for PCOS is by measuring androgens, including total testosterone, free testosterone, and DHEA sulfate. Measurement of free testosterone is the most sensitive test for the detection of androgen excess.

14. **(B)** Abdomen. Many studies have shown that excess abdominal fat increases the risk of complications independent of and additive to that caused by the degree of obesity.

15. **(D)** >70%. Overweight children (age 10 to 16 years) with at least one overweight parent have a >70% likelihood of being overweight as an adult. The persistence of obesity into adulthood is among the most serious consequence of pediatric obesity as there is a tight association between length of time spent at an abnormal body weight as an adult and atherosclerosis, cardiovascular disease, type 2 diabetes mellitus, and dyslipidemia.

16. **(A)** Short stature. Most children with exogenous obesity are tall for age and may appear older than their chronological age. Obese children are more likely to have high fasting insulin levels, and in the past few years, there has been a significant increase in type 2 diabetes, which tends to correlate with the increase in prevalence of obesity in children. Few organ systems are unaffected by excessive adiposity in childhood.

17. **(C)** It has been increasing over the past 10 years. The prevalence of childhood obesity has been increasing rapidly over the past 20 years and shows no evidence of slowing.

18. **(B)** Severe obesity can result from human gene mutations. Many factors can result in an imbalance between energy intake and energy expenditure, leading to the promotion of excess fat deposition. Although genes play an important role in the regulation of body weight, behavioral and environmental factors are likely primarily responsible for the dramatic increase in obesity in the past two decades. A number of human gene mutations have been described that result in severe obesity, including mutations in leptin and melanocortin 4 receptor.

SUGGESTED READING

Goran MI: Metabolic precursors and effects of obesity in children: A decade of progress, 1990–1999. *Am J Clin Nutr* 73:158, 2001.

Maffeis C, Tato L: Long-term effects of childhood obesity on morbidity and mortality. *Horm Res* 55(suppl 1):42, 2001.

Ebbeling CB, Pawlak DB, Ludwig DS: Childhood obesity: Public-health crisis, common sense cure. *Lancet* 360:473, 2002.

O'Rahilly S: Insights into obesity and insulin resistance from the study of extreme human phenotypes. *Eur J Endocrinol* 147:435, 2002.

CASE 42: A 16-YEAR-OLD MALE WITH FATIGUE, ANOREXIA, INTERMITTENT VOMITING, AND WEIGHT LOSS

A 16-year-old patient presented to the emergency department with the complaints of fatigue, anorexia, intermittent vomiting, and weight loss. He had no diarrhea or fever, but did complain of right upper quadrant abdominal pain. He was previously healthy and was taking no medications. An abdominal CT scan was performed which revealed hepatosplenomegaly, and a presumptive diagnosis of mononucleosis was made. He was treated with prednisone for 4 days with marked improvement of his symptoms. His symptoms eventually returned, and following further tests, he was diagnosed with delayed emptying of the gallbladder. He underwent a cholecystectomy 4 months after his initial presentation. He tolerated the surgery well, but on postoperative day 1 he became very sleepy and began to have mental status changes. He now presents back to the emergency department and you find him to be hypotensive with a blood glucose of 50 mg/dL. Further history revealed that he has lost 35 pounds over the last 4 months. On physical examination, he appears dehydrated, and you notice marked hyperpigmentation on the neck, elbows, knuckles, and lower abdomen. In addition, he appears tan even though he has not recently been in the sun.

SELECT THE ONE BEST ANSWER

1. Which of the following would be the most appropriate initial management of this patient?

   (A) intravenous fluids and stress dose glucocorticoids
   (B) intravenous fluids
   (C) emergency exploratory laparotomy
   (D) consult to the pediatric oncology team

2. Which of the following laboratory results would you expect to find in this patient?

   (A) serum sodium 127, potassium 3.5 mEq/L; urine potassium 15 mEq/day
   (B) serum sodium 127, potassium 7.5 mEq/L; urine potassium 100 mEq/day
   (C) serum sodium 147, potassium 7.5 mEq/L; urine potassium 5 mEq/day
   (D) serum sodium 127, potassium 7.5 mEq/L; urine potassium 5 mEq/day

3. What would you expect this patient's ACTH and cortisol level to be prior to treatment?

   (A) low ACTH, low cortisol
   (B) low ACTH, high cortisol
   (C) high ACTH, low cortisol
   (D) high ACTH, high cortisol

4. All of the following signs and symptoms except which one should have clued you in to a diagnosis of primary adrenal insufficiency?

   (A) hyperpigmentation
   (B) anorexia
   (C) weight loss
   (D) hepatosplenomegaly

5. Which of the following is not a clinical manifestation of Addison's disease?

   (A) unexplained hypoglycemia
   (B) vitiligo
   (C) neutropenia
   (D) nausea

6. Which of the following statements regarding adrenal insufficiency is true?

   (A) Adrenal crisis is rare in patients with secondary adrenal insufficiency.
   (B) Hyperpigmentation is common in secondary adrenal insufficiency.
   (C) Hyperkalemia is commonly seen at presentation in secondary adrenal insufficiency.
   (D) The major cause of adrenal crisis is glucocorticoid deficiency.

7. Which of the following would be the preferable treatment for a child in adrenal crisis?

   (A) intravenous methylprednisolone
   (B) intravenous hydrocortisone
   (C) intravenous dexamethasone
   (D) any of the above

8. On physical examination, the patient has candidiasis in the mouth and noticeable vitiligo on the face and trunk. Which of the following tests should you check to help with your diagnosis?

   (A) magnesium
   (B) complete blood count
   (C) calcium
   (D) urinalysis

9. Your patient also describes neurologic symptoms. What would be at the top of the differential?

   (A) adrenoleukodystrophy
   (B) infectious adrenalitis
   (C) drug induced adrenal failure
   (D) autoimmune adrenalitis

10. Which of the following has not been associated with adrenal hemorrhage in children?

    (A) *Pseudomonas aeruginosa* sepsis
    (B) *Escherichia coli* sepsis
    (C) meningococcemia
    (D) neonatal asphyxia

11. Addison's disease is most commonly caused by which of the following?

    (A) infectious adrenalitis
    (B) autoimmune adrenalitis
    (C) adrenal hemorrhage
    (D) metastatic cancer

12. Which of the following statements regarding serum cortisol concentrations is true?

(A) Serum cortisol concentrations are highest in the early evening.

(B) Serum cortisol concentrations are highest in the early afternoon.

(C) Serum cortisol concentrations are highest in the early morning.

(D) Serum cortisol concentrations do not vary during the day.

13. You diagnose your patient with Addison's disease. Which of the following is true regarding outpatient treatment?

(A) He should be discharged on Florinef, but only needs glucocorticoid during times of stress.

(B) He should be discharged on glucocorticoid and Florinef.

(C) He should be discharged on glucocorticoid, but only needs Florinef during times of stress.

(D) He only needs glucocorticoid at discharge.

14. Your patient is doing well at home on his medications and his skin pigmentation has faded. His mother calls because he has developed a low-grade fever with gastroenteritis. Which of the following would be the most appropriate management?

(A) He should double his Florinef.

(B) He should come directly to your clinic.

(C) He should double his hydrocortisone.

(D) He should make no changes in his medications.

15. One year after discharge, the patient notes that his skin pigmentation is beginning to darken again. What would be your major concern?

(A) poor compliance with the glucocorticoid

(B) poor compliance with the Florinef

(C) development of ACTH resistance

(D) development of insulin resistance

16. Which of the following is not a cause of secondary adrenal insufficiency?

(A) panhypopituitarism

(B) autoimmune adrenalitis

(C) isolated ACTH deficiency

(D) megestrol acetate

17. Which of the following statements regarding secondary adrenal insufficiency is not true?

(A) Hyponatremia can occur.

(B) Hyperkalemia can occur.

(C) Skin hyperpigmentation does not occur.

(D) Weakness and fatigue are common symptoms.

18. Which of the following is the most common cause of tertiary adrenal insufficiency?

(A) cranial radiation

(B) hypothalamic tumors

(C) head trauma

(D) chronic administration of high doses of glucocorticoids

Answers

1. (**A**) Intravenous fluids and stress dose glucocorticoids. This adolescent has many clinical manifestations of Addison's disease and is likely in adrenal crisis. Thus, it is imperative to treat him with intravenous fluids and stress doses of glucocorticoids prior to any other management. Normal saline should be used in the intravenous fluids to replace sodium loss. An emergency exploratory laparotomy without pretreatment with stress dose glucocorticoids could lead to a catastrophic outcome.

2. (**D**) Serum sodium 127, potassium 7.5 mEq/L; urine potassium 5 mEq/day. Hyponatremia is a common feature of primary adrenal insufficiency secondary to mineralocorticoid deficiency and inappropriate vasopressin secretion caused by glucocorticoid deficiency. Mild hyponatremia can also occur in secondary or tertiary adrenal insufficiency because of inappropriate vasopressin secretion. Hyperkalemia is only seen in primary adrenal insufficiency.

3. (**C**) High ACTH, low cortisol. In adrenal insufficiency of any cause, serum cortisol will be low. The ACTH level will help distinguish between primary adrenal insufficiency (in which ACTH levels will be high) and secondary or tertiary adrenal insufficiency (in which ACTH levels will be low).

4. (**D**) Hepatosplenomegaly. The onset of adrenal insufficiency is often insidious. The presenting signs and symptoms are dependent on how quickly adrenal function is diminished and whether mineralo-

corticoid production is affected along with gluco-corticoid production. Adrenal insufficiency is often first detected when a stress precipitates an adrenal crisis. Hyperpigmentation in areas exposed to sunlight, areas such as the palmar creases, axilla, areola, and areas exposed to friction such as the elbows, knees belt line and knuckles, is the most characteristic finding of Addison's disease and is present in the majority of patients. Anorexia and weight loss are also seen in primary adrenal insufficiency along with other gastrointestinal symptoms such as vomiting, abdominal pain, diarrhea, and constipation. Dehydration caused by vomiting and diarrhea can often precipitate an adrenal crisis. Although splenomegaly can be seen in primary adrenal insufficiency, hepatomegaly is not a common finding.

5. **(C)** Neutropenia. Unexplained hypoglycemia is found in Addison's disease, but tends to be more common in younger patients. In adults, it can be precipitated by fever or infection. Although hyperpigmentation is the major manifestation of Addison's disease, vitiligo can be seen in patients with autoimmune causes of adrenal insufficiency, because of autoimmune destruction of dermal melanocytes. Patients can have eosinophilia. Neutropenia is not a typical clinical manifestation of Addison's disease. Other clinical manifestations include generalized weakness, fatigue, postural dizziness, diffuse myalgia, behavioral changes, and splenomegaly.

6. **(A)** Adrenal crisis is rare in patients with secondary adrenal insufficiency. The major cause of adrenal crisis is mineralocorticoid deficiency and not glucocorticoid deficiency. Secondary adrenal insufficiency is because of ACTH deficiency, which affects only the glucocorticoid production. Patients with secondary or tertiary adrenal insufficiency typically have normal aldosterone production, which is under the control of the renin-angiotensin system, thus they have normal serum potassium and rarely present in adrenal crisis. The hyperpigmentation is found only in primary adrenal insufficiency and occurs because of chronic ACTH hypersecretion.

7. **(B)** Intravenous hydrocortisone. In a patient in adrenal crisis, it is important to replace both the deficient glucocorticoid as well as the deficient mineralocorticoid. Of the above, only hydrocortisone has significant mineralocorticoid activity if given at stress doses intravenously. Unfortunately, there is currently no intravenous form of mineralocorticoid available. Fludrocortisone (Florinef) is a potent oral synthetic mineralocorticoid that can be used once the child is stable and ready to discontinue intravenous saline.

8. **(C)** Calcium. The presence of vitiligo with primary adrenal insufficiency suggests an autoimmune etiology. Autoimmune polyglandular syndrome type 1 is a rare autosomal recessive disorder in which primary adrenal insufficiency is associated with chronic mucocutaneous candidiasis and hypoparathyroidism. The candidiasis and hypoparathyroidism typically appear first in early to mid-childhood, and adrenal insufficiency usually develops in mid to late adolescence. Thus, it would be important to screen this patient for hypocalcemia. Other common associated manifestations include primary hypogonadism and malabsorption syndromes. Patients rarely develop diabetes mellitus and autoimmune thyroiditis. In contrast, in autoimmune polyglandular syndrome type 2, adrenal insufficiency is typically the initial manifestation. Hypoparathyroidism does not occur in this disorder, and diabetes mellitus and autoimmune thyroiditis are common.

9. **(A)** Adrenoleukodystrophy. The presence of X-linked adrenoleukodystrophy needs to be ruled out in any young male with primary adrenal insufficiency. Not all patients have neurologic symptoms when the adrenal insufficiency is diagnosed. Very long-chain fatty acid concentrations are increased in affected males. If a patient is diagnosed with adrenoleukodystrophy, all male siblings should be screened.

10. **(B)** *E. coli* sepsis. Adrenal hemorrhage in children has been associated with pseudomonas aeruginosa sepsis, meningococcemia (Waterhouse-Friderichsen syndrome), and in neonates following a difficult labor or asphyxia. Patients may have a sudden fall in hemoglobin with hyponatremia and hyperkalemia.

11. **(B)** Autoimmune adrenalitis. Autoimmune adrenalitis accounts for greater than 70% of cases of

Addison's disease. The most common detectable antibody is against 21-hydroxylase. Autoimmune destruction of other endocrine glands is often seen. In the past, infectious adrenalitis caused by tuberculosis was the most common cause of Addison's disease, but now is seen in less than 20% of new cases. Adrenal insufficiency occurs at a low incidence in metastatic cancer, as a significant proportion of the adrenal gland must be destroyed for adrenal insufficiency to become evident.

12. **(C)** Serum cortisol concentrations are highest in the early morning. There is a diurnal rhythm of serum cortisol, and concentrations are typically highest in the early morning between 4 AM and 8 AM In patients with normal adrenal function, cortisol levels typically increase markedly with stress.

13. **(B)** He should be discharged on glucocorticoid and Florinef. Patients with Addison's disease are deficient in both glucocorticoid and mineralocorticoid, and thus need replacement of both on a daily basis. The importance of diligence taking the medications needs to be stressed to avoid adrenal crisis. Patients with secondary or tertiary adrenal insufficiency typically only need treatment with hydrocortisone, as ACTH is not an important regulator of aldosterone release.

14. **(C)** He should double his hydrocortisone. The major risk to the patient with primary adrenal insufficiency is the lack of an appropriate adrenal response to stress. Thus, patients who are ill or undergoing any type of procedure should be treated with additional glucocorticoid. The dose of mineralocorticoid is typically not adjusted during illness. If patients are unable to keep down the medications and fluids, they need to come to the emergency department for intravenous therapy to avert an adrenal crisis. It is important that patients with adrenal insufficiency wear a Medic Alert tag.

15. **(A)** Poor compliance with the glucocorticoid. Darkening of the skin pigmentation in a patient with primary adrenal insufficiency would suggest that treatment with glucocorticoids is not adequate and ACTH levels are elevated. Either the child has outgrown the glucocorticoid dose and

will need an adjustment, or more commonly in an adolescent, they have not been as compliant as desired.

16. **(B)** Autoimmune adrenalitis. Secondary adrenal insufficiency is caused by any process that affects the pituitary gland and interferes with ACTH secretion. Autoimmune adrenalitis is a disorder of the adrenal gland and causes primary adrenal insufficiency. Isolated ACTH deficiency is rare. Megestrol acetate is a progestin with some glucocorticoid activity that is used in children with cancer or cystic fibrosis to increase appetite. It is associated with secondary adrenal insufficiency in some patients.

17. **(B)** Hyperkalemia can occur. Hyponatremia can be seen in secondary adrenal insufficiency because glucocorticoid action is required for appropriate renal free water clearance. However, hyperkalemia does not occur because the renin-angiotensin-aldosterone system remains intact. Hyperpigmentation of the skin is typically only seen in primary adrenal insufficiency.

18. **(D)** Chronic administration of high doses of glucocorticoids. With the widespread use of supraphysiologic doses of glucocorticoids, suppression of the hypothalamic-pituitary-adrenal axis is a frequent cause of adrenal insufficiency in children. Tertiary adrenal insufficiency can be seen with prolonged use of high-dose glucocorticoids (greater than 7 days), and the timing of recovery of hypothalamic-pituitary-adrenal function can be variable. Glucocorticoids should never be discontinued abruptly in patients who have been on a prolonged course, but rather should be weaned slowly.

SUGGESTED READING

Miller WL: The adrenal cortex. In: Sperling MA (ed): *Pediatric Endocrinology*, 2nd ed. Philadelphia: WB Saunders, 2002, p 385.

Bethin KE, Muglia LJ: Adrenal insufficiency. In: Radovick S, MacGillivray MH (eds): *Pediatric Endocrinology, A Practical Clinical Guide*. New Jersey: Humana Press, 2003, p 203.

Brenner K, Frohna JG: Index of suspicion. Case 3. Diagnosis: Acute adrenal insufficiency. *Pediatr Rev* 22:245, 2001.

6

Gastroenterology

CASE 43: A 1-MONTH-OLD WITH JAUNDICE

A 1-month-old boy is brought to your office for a routine check-up. The baby was a product of a full-term gestation and his birth weight was 4.1 kg. His mother had routine prenatal care and no complications during the pregnancy. The child is exclusively breast-fed and was first noted to be jaundiced at 3 days of age. His bilirubin peaked on day of life 6 and then began to decrease. Mom reports he has "always been yellow." She denies irritability, fever, vomiting, or diarrhea. She reports that the child eats well and has yellow seedy stools each time he feeds.

On physical examination, the child's weight is 5 kg. He is in no apparent distress. He has jaundiced skin and icteric sclera. His cardiac and respiratory systems are unremarkable. His abdomen is non-distended with normal bowel sounds. His liver is palpable 2 cm below the right costal margin and his spleen tip is palpable. The remainder of his examination is unremarkable.

SELECT THE ONE BEST ANSWER

1. The first laboratory test indicated in the evaluation of this patient is:

   (A) conjugated bilirubin
   (B) blood culture
   (C) hepatic function test
   (D) because of earlier bilirubin testing no further testing is necessary

2. Below are results for this child's laboratory evaluation.

Hemoglobin	12.5 g/dL
Platelets	256,000
Albumin	3.8 g/dL
ALT	70 IU/L
AST	65 IU/L
GGT	458 IU/L
Alkaline phosphatase	606 IU/L
Conjugated bilirubin	4 mg/dL
Total bilirubin	7 mg/dL
Prothrombin time (PT)	13 seconds, INR 1.0

Which entity is least likely in the differential diagnosis?

   (A) biliary atresia
   (B) Alagille syndrome
   (C) choledochal cyst
   (D) congenital acquired hepatitis B

3. The additional immediate evaluation for this child should include:

   (A) ultrasound, $\alpha 1$ antitrypsin level, urine reducing substance, urine culture
   (B) hepatitis B surface antigen, hepatitis C antibody, TORCH titers
   (C) serum amino acid, urine organic acids
   (D) all of the above

4. If this patient had an ultrasound that demonstrates a choledochal cyst, the next step in management is to:

   (A) call interventional radiology for drainage of the cyst and a cholangiogram to define the entire cyst

(B) call a surgeon because intraoperative drainage and a cholangiogram are more successful than percutaneous drainage

(C) consult a surgeon because complete resection of cyst is necessary

(D) treat conservatively with ursodiol

5. If this child had a history of vomiting and no red reflex on ophthalmologic examination, the first thing you would do is:

(A) check amino acids levels
(B) check ammonia level
(C) have mother stop breast feeding the child
(D) consult ophthalmology

6. If the child from question 5 has a fever and looks ill, then this child is at significant risk for:

(A) liver failure
(B) *E. coli* sepsis
(C) group B streptococcal sepsis
(D) all of the above

7. If the child has laboratory results as outlined in question 2 and a serum $\alpha 1$ antitrypsin level of 40 (normal, 93 to 224 mg/dL), then this child's possible diagnoses include:

(A) $\alpha 1$ antitrypsin deficiency
(B) $\alpha 1$ antitrypsin deficiency and biliary atresia
(C) $\alpha 1$ antitrypsin deficiency and neonatal hepatitis
(D) laboratory error; $\alpha 1$ antitrypsin levels are measured only in liver tissue

8. If this child had a systolic ejection murmur with a fixed split second heart sound, what additional test would you order?

(A) chest radiograph
(B) echocardiogram
(C) ophthalmology examination
(D) all of the above

9. If this child's weight was 4.3 kg at presentation, what further evaluation is indicated?

(A) sweat test
(B) thyroid function
(C) serum glucose level
(D) all of the above

10. If this child had been treated with amoxicillin suspension for the past week for otitis media, what additional evaluation is indicated?

(A) serum glucose, lactic acid, uric acid, magnesium, and phosphate levels
(B) serum fructoaldolase level
(C) PT, ammonia level
(D) A and C

11. The patient from question 2 had an additional workup, which appears below.

Urine culture: no growth in 48 hours
Urine reducing substances: negative
$\alpha 1$ Antitrypsin level: 198
Ultrasound: normal liver echogenicity, no biliary dilatation and no masses

This patient's diagnosis is:

(A) neonatal hepatitis
(B) biliary atresia
(C) congenitally acquired hepatitis B
(D) there is not enough information to make a diagnosis

12. Which test is best used to distinguish biliary atresia from neonatal hepatitis?

(A) hepatobiliary scintigraphy
(B) liver biopsy
(C) ERCP
(D) abdominal CT

13. It is vital to a patient's long-term prognosis for the diagnosis of biliary atresia to be made prior to:

(A) 1 month of age
(B) 3 months of age
(C) 2 months of age
(D) repair can be done anytime

14. If this patient is diagnosed with biliary atresia, the next step is:

(A) liver transplantation
(B) Kasai procedure
(C) Roux-en-Y procedure
(D) dependent on the age the diagnosis is made

15. If this patient is diagnosed with neonatal hepatitis, the next step is:

(A) liver transplantation

(B) medical support for cholestasis

(C) reassuring the parents there is less than a 10% chance of need for a liver transplant

(D) both B and C

16. Standard medical treatment for cholestasis includes:

(A) ursodiol treatment

(B) vitamin A, D, E, and K supplementation, nutritional support, ursodiol treatment, and treatment for pruritus

(C) vitamin K supplementation and nutritional support

(D) A and C

17. If the patient in the vignette were 4 days old instead of 4 weeks old, his differential diagnosis would include:

(A) biliary atresia

(B) viral infection

(C) bacterial sepsis

(D) all of the above

18. If the patient in question 17 had laboratory results as outlined in question 2 and a palpable spleen and no palpable liver, further evaluation would include:

(A) bacterial cultures, viral cultures, abdominal MRI

(B) bacterial cultures, viral cultures, liver biopsy

(C) bacterial cultures, viral cultures, bone marrow biopsy

(D) viral cultures, abdominal MRI, liver biopsy

Answers

1. **(A)** The most important thing to determine is whether this child has conjugated or unconjugated hyperbilirubinemia. All other diagnostic and therapeutic steps are based on this distinction.

2. **(D)** Although the term "LFTs" (liver function tests) is commonly used, its meaning is often unclear. There are three distinct groups of "liver labs." Serum transaminase (ALT and AST) elevation indicates hepatocellular damage and death (many causes). GGT and alkaline phosphatase are enzymes found in high concentration in the biliary system and elevations indicate biliary tree disease. Bilirubin, prothrombin time, albumin and ammonia are true "LFTs" and are indicators of liver function. The laboratory values indicate cholestatic liver disease secondary to biliary disease with normal liver function.

Congenital hepatitis B causes a carrier state in most infants and they have normal "liver labs." In a small percentage of infants, it can cause fulminant hepatic failure. Neither of those scenarios is consistent with the laboratory values.

3. **(A)** The differential diagnosis of cholestatic liver disease in an otherwise healthy 1-month-old is as follows:

Cholestatic disorders
Biliary atresia
Idiopathic neonatal hepatitis
Choledochal cyst
Alagille syndrome
Persistent familial intrahepatic cholestasis (PFIC)
Metabolic disorders
$\alpha 1$ Antitrypsin deficiency
Galactosemia
Disorders of bile acid synthesis
Other
Urinary tract infection

4. **(C)** Because there is an increased risk of cholangiocarcinoma in cyst remnants, choledochal cysts require complete surgical removal.

5. **(C)** Vomiting and cataracts in a cholestatic 1-month-old is galactosemia until proven otherwise. The treatment is elimination of exposure to galactose (in the lactose of breast milk and cow milk formula).

6. **(B)** In patients with galactosemia, continued exposure to galactose causes inhibition of leukocyte bactericidal activity. This puts them at increased risk for *E. coli* sepsis.

7. **(A)** The diagnosis of $\alpha 1$ antitrypsin deficiency is confirmed by a low serum level of $\alpha 1$ antitrypsin. Although it is not impossible, it would be incredibly rare for a patient to have two rare diseases.

8. **(D)** The murmur described is consistent with pulmonic stenosis. In infants with pulmonic stenosis and cholestatic liver disease, your index of suspicion for Alagille syndrome must be high. Other features include characteristic facies (difficult to distinguish in an infant), pulmonic stenosis (echocardiogram), butterfly vertebrae (chest x-ray), and posterior embryotoxon (ophthalmologic exam).

9. **(D)** Clearly, this child has failure to thrive and cholestasis. The differential diagnosis includes cystic fibrosis and hypopituitarism. All of the tests listed would be indicated.

10. **(D)** Most pediatric drug suspensions contain sucrose and can induce symptoms in patients with hereditary fructose intolerance. Fructoaldolase levels are measured in liver tissue. The metabolic consequences of the disease are secondary to accumulation of fructose-1-phosphate. See Figure 43-1. In addition to the metabolic consequences, the child may develop hepatic failure. Therefore each child should have a prothrombin time test and an NH_3 level measured.

11. **(D)** It is impossible to distinguish between biliary atresia and neonatal hepatitis based on these laboratory results.

12. **(B)** Hepatobiliary scintigraphy can (under the right conditions) distinguish between biliary atresia and neonatal hepatitis. In neonatal hepatitis, dye will be excreted from the liver into the gut, while in biliary atresia it will not. The test, however, has significant limitations. It is most reliable when the patient has been pretreated with phenobarbital for 5 days to induce biliary flow. Even with pretreatment, the liver often will not excrete bile in the presence of significant cholestasis. If the serum bilirubin level is >10 mg/dL, failure to excrete is almost universal and this test is unreliable and unhelpful. Because of the issues of patient size, ERCP is very difficult to perform in a 1-month-old. Very few gastroenterologists are skilled enough to do a successful ERCP in this age. Liver biopsy will best be able to distinguish between these two diseases and provide an accurate and expeditious diagnosis. Percutaneous liver biopsy can safely be performed by many gastroenterologists and radiologists.

13. **(C)** See below.

14. **(B)** The procedure to correct biliary atresia is known as a Kasai procedure. In the Kasai procedure, an intrahepatic bile duct is connected directly to a loop of bowel to provide bile drainage and delay hepatic damage. The likelihood of success of the Kasai decreases dramatically when performed after 8 weeks of age. Because of this, making a definitive diagnosis and instituting therapy quickly is vital. Without a successful Kasai procedure, the patient will be committed to early liver transplantation. Because of the difficulty in obtaining ideally size matched organs in a very young patient, long-term prognosis is greatly decreased.

15. **(D)** Neonatal hepatitis will resolve in the majority of patients. Ten percent of patients will develop end-stage liver disease and require liver transplantation. Any pediatric patient with cholestasis requires medical support for their cholestasis.

16. **(B)** Patients with cholestasis have a decreased ability to absorb fats (nutritional support) and fat-soluble vitamins (A, D, E, and K). Ursodiol has been shown to protect the liver during cholestatic injury. Pruritus can also develop in cholestatic patients and can be treated with antihistamines, rifampin, or naltrexone.

17. **(D)** In newborns, the differential diagnosis includes infectious etiologies. There are two types of biliary atresia. The most common is detailed

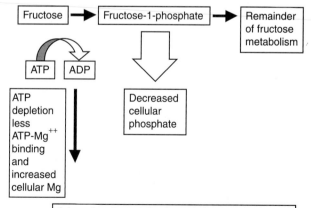

Figure 43-1.

in previous discussions, but there is also a neonatal form that is more likely associated with other congenital anomalies and can present in the first week of life.

18. **(A)** The laboratory data reveal a child with liver failure and disseminated intravascular coagulopathy (DIC). Bacterial infections can cause DIC and should be evaluated. Viral infections can cause hepatosplenomegaly and liver failure. Neonatal hemochromatosis is a disease where infants are born with cirrhosis (small liver and splenomegaly) and liver failure. The diagnosis is made by demonstration of iron deposits in the pancreas on MRI. Liver biopsy in this child would be extremely dangerous and should be avoided if possible.

SUGGESTED READING

McKiernan PJ: Neonatal cholestasis. *Semin Neonatol* 7(2): 153–165, 2002.
Bezzerra JA, Balistreri W: Cholestatic syndromes in infancy and childhood. *Semin Gastrointest Dis* 12(2):54–65, 2001.

CASE 44: AN 11-YEAR OLD WITH CRAMPING ABDOMINAL PAIN

An 11-year-old girl is brought to your office with a complaint of periumbilical abdominal pain for 5 weeks. The pain is increased when the patient eats and relieved by stooling. The pain has awakened her from sleep several times. Ranitidine did not improve her symptoms. She denies melena or weight loss but she has seen blood in her stool.

On physical examination she is a tired-appearing young lady whose weight is 34 kg (25%) and her height is 134 cm (10% to 25%). She has nonicteric sclera and a moist oropharynx. Her abdomen is nondistended with positive bowel sounds. There is no hepatosplenomegaly or masses. There is diffuse suprapubic tenderness. Rectal examination demonstrated normal sphincter tone and heme-positive stool.

SELECT THE ONE BEST ANSWER

1. Possible diagnoses for this child include:

   (A) inflammatory bowel disease
   (B) infectious colitis
   (C) irritable bowel syndrome
   (D) all of the above

2. Stool studies are ordered and should include:

   (A) bacterial cultures
   (B) assay for *Clostridium difficile* toxin
   (C) ova and parasite examination
   (D) A and C

3. Likely stool pathogens include:

   (A) *Campylobacter jejuni*
   (B) *Yersinia enterocolitica*
   (C) *E. coli* O157:H7
   (D) all of the above

4. If the child's CBC demonstrated a platelet count of 50,000, the next laboratory study(ies) you should check is/are:

   (A) hemoglobin
   (B) hepatic function panel
   (C) creatinine
   (D) all of the above

5. If the stool cultures were negative, the patient's weight was 23 kg (<5th percentile), and the height was 123 cm (<5th percentile), your next step would be to check:

   (A) CBC, sedimentation rate, and C-reactive protein
   (B) CBC, prothrombin time, bleeding time
   (C) CBC, differential, and platelet count
   (D) viral stool cultures

6. Below are the laboratory values for the patient in question 5.

Hemoglobin	8.5 g/dL
Platelets	550,000/mm^3
MCV	75 fL
Sedimentation rate	58 mm/sec
Albumin	2.8 g/dL
GGTP	300 IU/L
Alkaline phosphatase	550 IU/L

   The first radiology study you should order is:

   (A) abdominal radiograph
   (B) barium enema
   (C) upper GI with small bowel follow-through
   (D) upper GI

7. The findings you might expect on the study ordered in question 6 include:

   (A) bowel wall thickening in the ileum
   (B) strictures in the jejunum
   (C) fistulas
   (D) all of the above

8. What additional symptoms might your patient have suffered?

   (A) early satiety
   (B) right upper quadrant pain
   (C) perianal abscess
   (D) A and C

9. What nutritional therapies can be employed to treat this child?

   (A) high-residue diet
   (B) high-protein diet
   (C) diet of elemental formula
   (D) none of the above

10. The child in the original vignette undergoes a colonoscopy that demonstrates pancolitis with erythema, edema, and granularity. The patient's diagnosis is:

    (A) ulcerative colitis
    (B) Crohn's disease
    (C) either
    (D) neither

11. The patient with pancolitis has a perinuclear antineutrophil cytoplasmic antibody (pANCA). Her diagnosis is:

    (A) ulcerative colitis
    (B) Crohn's disease
    (C) both
    (D) neither

12. First-line treatment of this moderately severe case of inflammatory bowel disease includes:

    (A) aminosalicylate
    (B) steroids
    (C) A and B
    (D) no medications are needed because 20% to 30% of patients will have spontaneous remission

13. The patient in question 11 begins treatment and returns with severe abdominal pain, fever, and continued colitis. Evaluation should begin with:

    (A) abdominal radiograph
    (B) abdominal CT
    (C) repeat colonoscopy
    (D) barium enema

14. The risk of the patient from question 11 developing colon cancer in her life is:

    (A) higher than in the general population and screening should begin after 10 years of active disease
    (B) so high prophylactic colectomy is recommended after 10 years of active disease
    (C) the same as the general population. Medications to treat the disease have improved in the last decade so that there is no longer any increased risk.
    (D) only high in those patients who have liver disease in addition to bowel disease

15. Based on the laboratory values in question 6, the liver disease of the patient in question 11 most likely is:

    (A) autoimmune hepatitis
    (B) sclerosing cholangitis
    (C) gallstones
    (D) cholangiocarcinoma

16. If the child in the original vignette had a physical examination where there was no abdominal tenderness and a fissure noted on the rectal examination, your next step would be:

    (A) screening studies including a urinalysis, CBC, erythrocyte sedimentation rate
    (B) reassurance and treatment for the fissure
    (C) colonoscopy to ensure there is no additional pathology
    (D) stool cultures

17. The laboratory studies for the patient in question 16 are listed below.

Hemoglobin	13.5 g/dL
Platelets	240,000/mm^3
MCV	86 fL

Sedimentation rate	9 mm/sec
Albumin	3.9 g/dL
GGTP	30 IU/L
Alkaline phosphatase	250 IU/L

Other symptoms that may occur in this patient are:

(A) epigastric pain and nausea
(B) constipation
(C) right lower quadrant pain
(D) all of the above

18. Initial treatment for this disorder includes:

(A) dietary change and reassurance
(B) medications
(C) further radiology or endoscopic testing
(D) all of the above

Answers

1. **(D)** This vignette describes symptoms that may reflect any of the listed diagnoses. Although heme-positive stools are less likely in irritable bowel syndrome compared with patients with inflammatory bowel syndrome, up to 35% of patients with irritable bowel syndrome report rectal bleeding. In this scenario, the red flags include pain in the middle of the night, blood in the stool, and the findings on physical examination.

2. **(A)** Without a history of antibiotic exposure, *C. difficile* is an unlikely pathogen. Giardia does not usually present with blood in the stool.

3. **(D)** Any of the pathogens listed can cause acute gastroenteritis with bloody stool.

4. **(C)** The most dangerous complication of an acute gastroenteritis with bloody stool is hemolytic-uremic syndrome associated with *E. coli* O157:H7. The laboratory findings of hemolytic-uremic syndrome may present before the culture for *E. coli* is positive. Those findings include renal insufficiency, hemolysis, thrombocytopenia and, in severe cases, cerebral edema.

5. **(A)** The height and weight given are far below the 5% for age. With the symptoms described

you must be concerned the patient has Crohn's disease. Looking for signs of inflammation, anemia, and protein-losing enteropathy are the appropriate next steps.

6. **(C)** A patient with iron deficiency anemia (low hemoglobin and low MCV), protein-losing enteropathy (low albumin), and increased inflammatory marker levels is likely to have Crohn's disease. The appropriate radiologic test would be an upper GI with small bowel follow-through. The radiologic finding in a patient with Crohn's disease is evidence of small bowel disease, particularly in the terminal ileum.

7. **(D)** See above.

8. **(D)** In Crohn's disease there is likely to be upper GI involvement (early satiety) and perianal disease (perianal abscess). Although there are some patients who have liver disease (right upper quadrant pain), that is more likely to occur in a patient with ulcerative colitis.

9. **(C)** Elemental formula is known to cause remission in patients with Crohn's disease. The difficulty in this treatment is that the formulas have poor palatability and require a nasogastric tube for infusion. Other recommendations include a low-residue diet in patients with colitis.

10. **(C)** Crohn's colitis and ulcerative colitis can look exactly the same on colonoscopy. Granulomas must be present on histology to make the diagnosis of Crohn's. Serology can also assist in making the distinction.

11. **(A)** pANCA antibodies are specific for ulcerative colitis.

12. **(C)** In a moderately severe case of inflammatory bowel disease (pancolitis), both steroids and aminosalicylates should be initiated.

13. **(A)** The most dangerous complication for a patient with ulcerative colitis is toxic megacolon. Risk factors for megacolon include drugs that interfere with intestinal motility, narcotics, antidiarrheal agents, and recent instrumentation. The megacolon can be seen on abdominal radio-

graph. Treatment with bowel rest and antibiotics should be initiated when the diagnosis is suspected. Patients who do not respond to this conservative treatment may require colectomy.

14. **(A)** The risk for developing colon cancer depends on the extent of the colitis (pancolitis >left-sided colitis >proctitis) and the length of time it has been clinically apparent. The risk increases after 10 years. Patients with Crohn's colitis are equally at risk for developing colon cancer.

15. **(B)** The patient in question 11 has ulcerative colitis. The most commonly associated liver disease is sclerosing cholangitis. The disease affects the biliary system. Therefore you would expect increased GGTP and alkaline phosphatase concentrations. Autoimmune hepatitis affects the hepatocytes, thereby causing an increased ALT and AST level. Gallstones are not associated with ulcerative colitis. Cholangiocarcinoma is a complication of long-standing sclerosing cholangitis, not an initial presentation of liver disease in an 11-year-old.

16. **(A)** Although the patient has a normal abdominal examination, the presence of perianal disease and pain severe enough to be awakened is enough to order screening laboratory tests looking for inflammatory markers.

17. **(D)** The laboratory values in the table are all normal. It is unlikely for a patient with Crohn's colitis or ulcerative colitis to have a normal hemoglobin, MCV, albumin, and sedimentation rate. Your conclusion is that this patient had irritable bowel syndrome, a variant of recurrent abdominal pain. Ten percent to 15% of 4- to 16-year-old children have recurrent abdominal pain. The symptoms can include nonacid dyspepsia (epigastric pain and nausea), constipation, diarrhea, and migrating abdominal pain.

18. **(A)** Conservative therapy with dietary changes, particularly increasing dietary fiber and limiting lactose, is the first-line approach. In addition, reassurance about the benign nature of recurrent abdominal pain is crucial. Recognizing that the patient is in pain is important. You want to avoid overtesting, thereby contributing to the patient's worry about the condition. Surgery is never necessary for recurrent abdominal pain or irritable bowel syndrome.

SUGGESTED READING

Kohli R, Li BU: Differential diagnosis of recurrent abdominal pain: New considerations. *Pediatr Ann* 33: 113–122, 2004.

Hyams JS: Crohn's disease in children. *Pediatr Clin North Am* 43:255–277, 1996.

Kirschner BS: Ulcerative colitis. *Pediatr Clin North Am* 43:235–254, 1996.

CASE 45: A 4-YEAR-OLD BOY WITH RECTAL BLEEDING

A 4-year-old boy is brought to your clinic by his mother with a complaint of having two large, maroon-colored stools on the morning of the visit. The mother is unsure whether the stools were accompanied by abdominal pain. She does report that the child seems less active than usual.

On examination, this is a quiet child with a heart rate of 165 and a respiratory rate of 40. He has nonicteric sclera and dry mucous membranes. His abdomen is nondistended with decreased bowel sounds and nontender without palpable masses. The remainder of the examination is unremarkable.

SELECT THE ONE BEST ANSWER

1. Your first step is:

   (A) reassure the parent because this is likely a fissure
   (B) transfer to an emergency room for stabilization and evaluation
   (C) admit to the hospital, collect stool cultures, and monitor closely
   (D) send home to collect stool cultures before further workup

2. The initial management should include:

   (A) gastric lavage
   (B) fluid resuscitation
   (C) abdominal ultrasound
   (D) all of the above

3. The most likely diagnosis in this child is:

   (A) juvenile polyp
   (B) Meckel's diverticulum

(C) inflammatory bowel disease

(D) intussusception

4. The diagnostic procedure required is:

(A) barium enema

(B) abdominal ultrasound

(C) technetium-99m pertechnetate (Meckel's scan)

(D) colonoscopy

5. Had the mother described cramping abdominal pain prior to these "currant jelly" stools, the likely diagnosis would be:

(A) Meckel's diverticulum

(B) juvenile polyp

(C) intussusception

(D) infectious colitis

6. The treatment of choice for the patient in question 5 is:

(A) barium enema

(B) antibiotics to treat infectious colitis

(C) colonoscopy and removal of polyp

(D) exploratory laparotomy

7. The mother asks what the chance is that the problem in question 5 will recur. Your answer is:

(A) 10%

(B) 2% to 5%

(C) 20%

(D) It depends on the treatment rendered.

8. Had the child passed bright red blood per rectum, had a heart rate of 98 and a respiratory rate of 24, and had a normal physical examination, your first step would be to:

(A) reassure the parent because this is likely a fissure

(B) transfer the child to an emergency room for stabilization and evaluation

(C) admit the child to the hospital, collect stool cultures, and monitor closely

(D) send the child home to collect stool cultures before further workup

9. In the patient from question 8, what is the possibility that this condition is a precursor to cancer?

(A) 50%

(B) less 10%

(C) no chance

(D) there is not enough known about this entity to make a prediction

10. Had the child in question 8 had dark, pigmented lips, his diagnosis would be:

(A) Peutz-Jeghers syndrome

(B) Gardner syndrome

(C) Turcot syndrome

(D) multiple juvenile polyps

11. If the child from the original vignette was 15 years old and had a family history of colon cancer in multiple family members in their 30s, the likely diagnosis would be:

(A) Peutz-Jeghers syndrome

(B) Gardner syndrome

(C) Turcot syndrome

(D) multiple juvenile polyps

12. If the child from the original vignette had come in with a complaint of vomiting a large amount of bright red blood, your first step would be to:

(A) refer the child to an emergency room for stabilization and treatment

(B) send the child home to start H_2 blocker therapy

(C) admit the child to the hospital for IV H_2 blocker therapy and a GI consult

(D) refer the child to a gastroenterologist

13. The management of the patient in question 12 should include:

(A) fluid resuscitation

(B) gastric lavage

(C) PT, hepatic function panel

(D) all of the above

14. The most likely diagnosis of the patient in question 12 is:

(A) peptic ulcer/gastritis

(B) swallowed blood from epistaxis

(C) gastroesophageal reflux

(D) *Helicobacter pylori* infection

15. Had the vomiting of blood occurred after multiple episodes of vomiting, then the most likely diagnosis would be:

    (A) viral gastritis
    (B) malrotation
    (C) Mallory-Weiss lesion
    (D) arteriovenous malformation rupture

16. If the patient in question 12 was a 15-year-old from a lower socioeconomic background, then the most likely diagnosis would be:

    (A) peptic ulcer/gastritis
    (B) herpetic esophagitis
    (C) gastroesophageal reflux
    (D) *H. pylori* infection

17. In regard to *H. pylori* infection, the most sensitive test for diagnosis and treatment is:

    (A) serum antibodies and therapy with a proton pump inhibitor, clarithromycin, and amoxicillin or metronidazole
    (B) stool antigen and therapy with a proton pump inhibitor, amoxicillin, and clarithromycin or metronidazole
    (C) endoscopy and therapy with a proton pump inhibitor, clarithromycin, and amoxicillin or metronidazole
    (D) there is no "gold standard" and any of the above are acceptable

18. If on physical examination the patient from question 12 had a small, firm liver and spleen with ascites, the treatment would be:

    (A) correction of coagulopathy and the low platelet count
    (B) somatostatin infusion
    (C) endoscopic banding
    (D) all of the above

19. If the patient in question 12 had normal vital signs and a normal physical examination, the most likely diagnosis would be:

    (A) peptic ulcer/gastritis
    (B) esophageal foreign body
    (C) swallowed epistaxis
    (D) *H. pylori* infection

Answers

1. **(B)** Patients with evidence of hemodynamic compromise (HR 165 in a 4-year-old) must be stabilized prior to any workup.

2. **(B)** Fluid resuscitation should be the first step. Gastric lavage is not necessary. The description of the bleeding is from the lower GI tract. Although a vigorous upper GI bleed could cause passage of red blood per rectum, it is likely that the patient would be more unstable than the vignette describes. It is unlikely that abdominal ultrasound would reveal the source of this bleeding.

3. **(B)** The description of the bleeding could correspond to any of the entities listed. It is the remainder of the history and physical examination that reveals the answer. Meckel's diverticulum causes significant bleeding in this age group. It is not always associated with abdominal pain. A juvenile polyp does not cause significant blood loss and is not associated with hemodynamic instability. Intussusception is usually associated with cramping abdominal pain prior to bloody stool. A small percent of children with intussusception will present with extreme lethargy, pallor, and heme-positive stools. Infectious colitis causing this amount of bleeding would be associated with cramping abdominal pain and diarrhea.

4. **(C)**

5. **(C)** See explanation for answer 3.

6. **(A)**

7. **(D)** If the intussusception is reduced surgically, the rate of recurrence is 2% to 5%. If the intussusception is reduced with a barium enema, the chance of recurrence is 10%.

8. **(D)** Painless bright blood per rectum in this age group is likely because of a juvenile polyp. Most present between the ages of 2 to 10 years.

9. **(C)** There is no chance of malignancy from solitary juvenile polyps. The risk is much higher in patients who have three or more polyps.

10. **(A)** There are several syndromes associated with multiple polyps throughout the colon. Familial adenomatous polyposis coli is an autosomal dominant condition characterized by large numbers of adenomatous (premalignant) lesions throughout the colon. All are caused by mutations in the tumor suppressor gene adenomatous polyposis coli (APC). These patients are at risk for colon cancer in the third decade of life. Definitive treatment is prophylactic colectomy. Mutations in the APC gene are responsible for Gardner syndrome (multiple colorectal polyps, osteomas, lipomas, fibromas epidermoid cysts, and dermoid tumors). APC mutations are responsible for some cases of Turcot syndrome (primary brain tumor and multiple colonic polyps). Peutz-Jeghers syndrome is a rare autosomal dominant syndrome characterized by mucosal pigmentation of the lips and gums and hamartomas throughout the GI tract. Symptoms include GI bleeding and cramping, abdominal pain, and obstruction because of intussusception. Cancer develops in 50% of patients. Colorectal, breast, and gynecologic tumors are seen most frequently.

11. **(B)** See above.

12. **(A)** Same explanation as for question 1.

13. **(D)** Of course, the first step is to fluid-resuscitate the child. In this child there is an upper GI bleed with hemodynamic instability. This is very unusual for a 4-year-old. The nasogastric lavage will allow you to determine whether there is continued bleeding. There is a possibility that this could be a variceal bleed, so it is important to check liver numbers and function.

14. **(A)** Peptic acid disease is the most common cause of upper GI bleeding in a 4-year-old. It would be unlikely for a 4-year-old to have an *H. pylori* infection causing a GI bleed. Gastroesophageal reflux would have long-standing symptoms. Swallowed epistaxis would not cause hemodynamic changes in an otherwise healthy individual.

15. **(C)** Mallory-Weiss tears occur after several episodes of vomiting. The tear usually occurs in the gastroesophageal junction. In children the bleeding is usually self-limited.

16. **(D)** In developing countries, *H. pylori* infections occur later in childhood. The rate of infection in lower socioeconomic groups is much higher. Gastroesophageal reflux would be expected to have more symptoms. Herpetic esophagitis is very rare in immunocompetent hosts.

17. **(C)** There are several tests to diagnose *H. pylori*. Endoscopic mucosal biopsy is the most sensitive test. The *H. pylori* bacteria produce the enzyme urease. Christensen's urea medium (CLOtest) will have a color change if *H. pylori* is present in a biopsy. Detection of serum IgG antibodies is sensitive and specific if done correctly. The sensitivity varies among commercial laboratories. Stool antigen tests are available but have lower sensitivity. Treatment consists of a proton pump inhibitor, clarithromycin, and a second antibiotic (amoxicillin or metronidazole).

18. **(D)** A small, firm liver with a large spleen is characteristic of cirrhosis with portal hypertension. The bleeding can come from esophageal varices or gastropathy. The patient's coagulopathy (from liver disease) and thrombocytopenia (from hypersplenism) must be corrected in order to stop the bleeding. Somatostatin infusions will decrease the pressure in the splanchnic vascular bed and decrease portal pressure. The final treatment is an endoscopic procedure to determine the source of the bleeding and treat the varices. The most common treatments are banding and sclerotherapy. A variceal bleed can be a life threatening event and more than one treatment modality may be used to treat it.

19. **(C)** In children without GI symptoms and no obvious GI disease, the blood they vomit is unlikely to be from the GI tract.

SUGGESTED READING

Fox VL: Gastrointestinal bleeding in infancy and childhood. *Gastroenterol Clin North Am* 29(1):37–66, 2000.

Heikenen JB, Pohl JF, Werlin SL, et al: Octreotide in pediatric patients. *J Pediatr Gastroenterol Nutr* 35(5): 600–609, 2002.

Hyer W, Beveridge I, Domizio P, et al: Clinic management and genetics of gastrointestinal polyps in children. *J Pediatr Gastroenterol Nutr* 31(5):467–479, 2000.

CASE 46: A 6-WEEK-OLD WITH VOMITING

A 6-week-old boy comes to your office with several days of vomiting and irritability. He vomits "everything he eats." The vomiting does not have any blood in it and is not associated with diarrhea or fever. The vomitus is described as being light in color but not green. The baby is the product of a full-term gestation with no complications. His birth weight was 3.2 kg.

On physical examination this is a well-nourished child: the weight is 4.4 kg, the HR is 180, and the RR is 38. His anterior fontanel is slightly sunken and there are dry mucous membranes. The abdomen is nondistended with normal bowel sounds. The remainder of the examination is unremarkable.

Laboratory studies:
Na 135 mEq/mL
Cl 99 mEq/mL
K 4 mEq/mL
HCO_3 30 mEq/mL

SELECT THE ONE BEST ANSWER

1. This child's diagnosis most likely is:

   (A) gastroesophageal reflux
   (B) malrotation
   (C) pyloric stenosis
   (D) viral gastroenteritis

2. The diagnostic test to confirm this diagnosis is:

   (A) pH probe
   (B) upper GI series
   (C) ultrasound of the abdomen
   (D) the diagnosis should be made on clinical grounds and no further testing is necessary

3. If the laboratory investigation and physical examination were normal, the most likely diagnosis is:

   (A) gastroesophageal reflux
   (B) malrotation
   (C) pyloric stenosis
   (D) viral gastroenteritis

4. The diagnostic test to confirm the condition in question 3 is:

   (A) pH probe
   (B) upper GI series
   (C) ultrasound of the abdomen

   (D) this is a diagnosis made on clinical grounds and no further testing is necessary

5. The first-line treatment for gastroesophageal reflux includes:

   (A) surgery
   (B) thickened feeds
   (C) antacid medication
   (D) B and C

6. If the child in the opening vignette had bilious vomiting, the most likely diagnosis is:

   (A) duodenal atresia
   (B) malrotation
   (C) pyloric stenosis
   (D) Hirschsprung's disease

7. The least helpful diagnostic test you could use to confirm the condition in question 6 is:

   (A) abdominal radiograph
   (B) barium enema
   (C) upper GI
   (D) ultrasound

8. The true statement about Ladd's bands is:

   (A) Ladd's bands obstruct the duodenum
   (B) Ladd's bands originate from the duodenum
   (C) Ladd's bands are peritoneal bands associated with an annular pancreas
   (D) all of the above

9. If the child in question 6 was 6 hours old and had Down syndrome, then the likely diagnosis is:

   (A) gastroesophageal reflux
   (B) malrotation
   (C) duodenal atresia
   (D) Hirschsprung's disease

10. The diagnostic test you would order in this instance is:

    (A) abdominal radiograph
    (B) upper GI
    (C) barium enema
    (D) pH probe

11. When you go back and review this child's prenatal ultrasound, you would likely see:

(A) oligohydramnios

(B) the renal agenesis associated with this syndrome

(C) polyhydramnios

(D) there would be no consistent intrauterine finding

12. If the 6-hour-old infant with vomiting had a normal radiograph and a normal upper GI series but had a serum glucose of 20 mg/dL, your first step would be:

(A) start ranitidine (Zantac) for the reflux

(B) start IV fluids with antibiotics

(C) encourage more PO feeds for hypoglycemia

(D) give IV glucose

13. If the patient in the original vignette was a 2-year-old with vomiting and minimal abdominal pain whose vital signs and laboratory studies were those outlined in the vignette, the diagnosis is likely:

(A) viral gastroenteritis

(B) malrotation

(C) gastroesophageal reflux

(D) cyclic vomiting

14. Despite giving the patient in question 13 a 20-mL/kg fluid bolus, correcting the abnormal laboratory studies, and improving the vital signs, the child continues to vomit. Your next step is:

(A) prochlorperazine suppository

(B) IV H₂ blocker

(C) IV ondansetron

(D) upper GI series to rule out malrotation

15. The 2-year-old in question 13 has intermittent, severe cramping abdominal pain without diarrhea and between episodes has no symptoms. To make the diagnosis you need a:

(A) blood culture

(B) upper GI series

(C) barium enema

(D) renal ultrasound

16. The 2-year-old vomits several times in the morning with no abdominal pain and has a normal physical examination. The remainder of the day he has no GI symptoms but is irritable. The likely diagnosis is:

(A) gastroesophageal reflux

(B) hydronephrosis

(C) intermittent volvulus

(D) brain tumor

17. The child in question 16 has one episode of "coffee ground" emesis. What is your concern?

(A) She needs more aggressive antacid therapy.

(B) She needs endoscopy to rule out malignancy.

(C) She needs an upper GI series because she likely has a malrotation.

(D) A and C

18. The child in question 16 is noted to have weight loss despite her normal appetite. Your first concern is which of the following?

(A) She needs more aggressive antacid therapy.

(B) She needs a renal ultrasound.

(C) She needs an upper GI series.

(D) She needs a CT scan of the brain.

Answers

1. **(C)** Pyloric stenosis is a thickening of the pylorus muscle. A patient usually becomes symptomatic after 3 weeks of age. It is characterized by nonbilious vomiting and hypochloremic alkalosis.

2. **(C)** The diagnosis of pyloric stenosis may be confirmed by palpation of the thickened pylorus on physical exam. The pylorus will be a firm, mobile, olive-shaped mass. However, this is very difficult to palpate and the diagnosis is usually confirmed on ultrasound. Although changes will be seen on an upper GI series, it has increased risk compared with ultrasound and is therefore not considered the best diagnostic test.

3. **(A)** Gastroesophageal reflux is the most common diagnosis for a healthy child with nonbilious vomiting. In a patient with severe viral gastroenteritis you would not expect normal vital signs, no fever, and no diarrhea.

4. **(D)** Gastroesophageal reflux is a clinical diagnosis. Although pH probes and endoscopy can be used to document changes consistent with reflux, neither is needed to confirm the diagnosis.

5. **(D)** The first-line treatments for reflux are conservative changes. These include limiting the volume the baby consumes per feed, positioning the baby upright after feeds, and thickening the child's formula with 1 tablespoon of rice cereal per ounce. Infants who fail these measures should then initiate antacid therapy.

6. **(B)** Bilious vomiting is indicative of distal obstruction. The most common cause of obstruction in this age group is a malrotation.

7. **(A)** In a malrotation, the duodenal jejunal loop is on the right side of the abdomen. The cecum is on the left side instead of the right. The malrotation occurs around the superior mesenteric vessel, and the superior mesenteric vein lies to the left of the artery instead of to the right. A barium enema can be used to locate the cecum, and an upper GI series can be used to visualize the duodenum. An ultrasound can be used to locate the superior mesenteric vessel. The least helpful test is a radiograph.

8. **(A)** Ladd's bands are peritoneal bands that come from the malrotated cecum to the right upper quadrant and can cause duodenal obstruction.

9. **(C)** Duodenal atresia is apparent in the first 24 hours of life. Thirty percent of children with duodenal atresia have Down syndrome.

10. **(A)** Abdominal radiograph will demonstrate the "double bubble" sign. There is gas in the stomach and the proximal duodenum but no gas in the distal bowel.

11. **(C)** The amniotic fluid produced cannot travel through a gut with an atresia. Therefore there is an excess (polyhydramnios) of fluid. Fifty percent of children with esophageal and duodenal atresia will have polyhydramnios.

12. **(D)** Although the likely cause of hypoglycemia and vomiting is sepsis and further evaluation is indicated, it is imperative that the hypoglycemia be corrected immediately.

13. **(A)**

14. **(C)** Ondansetron is a serotonin 5-HT$_3$ receptor antagonist with excellent antiemetic effects. When given in the emergency room, ondansetron decreases vomiting and the need for hospital admission.

15. **(C)** The signs described are likely those of an intussusception but could be from a malrotation with intermittent volvulus. A barium enema could be used to diagnose either condition.

16. **(A)** Although morning vomiting is concerning because of its association with CNS pathology, in a patient with a normal physical examination and no other symptoms, the diagnosis is likely GE reflux.

17. **(A)** GI bleeding in this patient is likely secondary to peptic acid disease. GI malignancy in this age group is rare. Malrotation would be associated with abdominal pain.

18. **(D)** Morning vomiting is concerning. In a patient who is eating a normal diet and losing weight, you must be concerned about a brain tumor.

SUGGESTED READING

Maclennan AC: Investigations in vomiting children. *Semin Pediatr Surg* 12(4):220–228, 2003.

Reeves JJ, Shannon MW, Fleisher GR: Ondansetron decreases vomiting associated with acute gastroenteritis: A randomized controlled study. *Pediatrics* 109(4):e62, 2002.

Colleti RB, DiLorenzo C: Overview of pediatric gastroesophageal reflux disease and proton pump inhibitor therapy. *J Pediatr Gastroenterol Nutr* 37(Suppl 1):7–11, 2003.

CASE 47: AN 8-YEAR-OLD WITH JAUNDICE

An 8-year-old girl presents to your office with a 3-day history of decreased appetite and abdominal pain. She denies fever or diarrhea but has nausea and intermittent vomiting.

Physical examination reveals a jaundiced girl with a height and weight at the 50th percentile for age. The abdomen is soft and nondistended with positive bowel sounds, but the patient has diffuse right upper quadrant pain and an enlarged liver without splenomegaly.

SELECT THE ONE BEST ANSWER

1. Your initial evaluation includes:

   (A) hepatitis A antibody
   (B) Monospot

(C) hepatitis B surface antigen

(D) all of the above

2. If the patient in the vignette had not been jaundiced, your initial evaluation would include:

(A) hepatitis A antibody

(B) Monospot

(C) hepatitis B surface antigen

(D) all of the above

3. If the hepatitis A serology is negative, the next step in your evaluation of this 8-year-old jaundiced child is:

(A) hepatic function panel, PT, GGTP

(B) α1 antitrypsin level, ceruloplasmin, anti-smooth muscle antibody, ANA, anti-liver kidney microsomal antibody

(C) hepatitis B antigen, hepatitis C antibody

(D) All of the above

4. In Wilson's disease:

(A) ceruloplasmin is increased and the urine copper is increased

(B) ceruloplasmin is decreased and the urinary copper is increased

(C) ceruloplasmin is increased and the urinary copper is decreased

(D) ceruloplasmin is decreased and the urinary copper is decreased

5. Suppose the level ceruloplasmin is consistent with Wilson's disease. Left untreated, the other organ system(s) most likely to be affected includes:

(A) neuropsychiatric

(B) cardiac

(C) respiratory

(D) all of the above

6. In Wilson's disease:

(A) the disease is autosomal dominant and all family members should be screened for asymptomatic disease

(B) the disease is autosomal recessive and all family members should be screened for asymptomatic disease

(C) the disease is autosomal dominant; only symptomatic patients need to be treated so no screening is necessary

(D) the disease is autosomal recessive; only symptomatic patients need to be treated so no screening is necessary

7. If the patient's ANA titer is 1:640 and the anti-smooth muscle antibody is 1:320, the patient's diagnosis is:

(A) type I autoimmune hepatitis

(B) type II autoimmune hepatitis

(C) type III autoimmune hepatitis

(D) there is not enough information to make the diagnosis

8. The treatment for autoimmune hepatitis would include:

(A) steroids

(B) cyclosporine

(C) azathioprine

(D) A and C

9. If the symptoms of the patient in the initial vignette were because of hepatitis B, the infection would be:

(A) acute hepatitis B

(B) chronic hepatitis B

(C) you need a hepatitis B surface antigen to be able to distinguish between acute and chronic infection

(D) you need a quantitative hepatitis B DNA level to distinguish between acute and chronic infection

10. Had the patient in the vignette presented with a small firm liver, splenomegaly, and ascites, the disease that created these symptoms could have been any of the following, except:

(A) hepatitis B

(B) Wilson's disease

(C) type I autoimmune hepatitis

(D) hepatitis A

11. While you are awaiting the lab results from question 3, the patient's mother calls to say she is "difficult to wake up." Your next step is:

(A) repeat her liver numbers

(B) see her in your office before repeating the labs

(C) increase her fluid intake because her lethargy is likely secondary to dehydration

(D) refer her to an emergency room for evaluation

12. Fulminant hepatic failure is defined as:

    (A) a patient with liver disease who develops encephalopathy and coagulopathy
    (B) a patient with liver disease who develops encephalopathy
    (C) a patient without preexisting liver disease who develops encephalopathy and coagulopathy within 8 weeks of the onset of liver disease
    (D) a patient without preexisting liver disease who develops encephalopathy within 8 weeks of the onset of liver disease

13. The problems that arise in children with fulminant failure include:

    (A) hypoglycemia
    (B) coagulopathy
    (C) renal failure
    (D) all of the above

14. If the child in the opening vignette had been ill for several days with viral URI symptoms, which additional laboratory study would you send?

    (A) adenovirus culture
    (B) acetaminophen level
    (C) enterovirus culture
    (D) all of the above

15. If the acetaminophen level was elevated, the likelihood of successfully treating the patient's toxicity is:

    (A) less likely than an asymptomatic patient
    (B) more likely than an asymptomatic patient
    (C) equivalent to an asymptomatic patient
    (D) there are no data to predict the chance of successful treatment

16. Suppose that the child was 2 years old and had right upper quadrant pain and an enlarged liver. Suppose further that she was anicteric and the hepatitis A serology was negative. In this instance, the next step would be:

    (A) ultrasound and an α-fetoprotein level
    (B) hepatitis B and C serology
    (C) α1 antitrypsin level, ceruloplasmin, ANA, anti-smooth muscle antibody, anti-liver kidney microsomal antibody determinations
    (D) all of the above

17. The likely diagnosis for that patient is:

    (A) hepatocellular carcinoma
    (B) hepatoblastoma
    (C) rhabdosarcoma
    (D) angiosarcoma

18. Had the child in the original vignette had a sudden onset of right upper quadrant pain, fever and jaundice, the likely diagnosis would be:

    (A) cholecystitis
    (B) choledochal cyst
    (C) viral hepatitis
    (D) liver hematoma

Answers

1. **(A)** A child with RUQ pain and jaundice must be assumed to have some form of hepatitis. Hepatitis A causes 50% of acute hepatitis in the United States. Transmission is via person to person or by water- and foodborne outbreaks. In utero maternal-child transmission has not been recognized. The incubation period is about 4 weeks. Most children have vague symptoms: low-grade fever, nausea, vomiting, and hepatomegaly. The vast majority of young children are anicteric. The disease is self-limited in the great majority of cases.

2. **(A)** See above explanation. Acute EBV infections frequently cause hepatomegaly but almost always there are other associated symptoms (fever, lymphadenopathy, sore throat, fatigue, and splenomegaly). Patients with hepatitis B infections are jaundiced.

3. **(D)** Table 47-1 lists the differential diagnosis and the appropriate tests required.

4. **(B)** The pathophysiology of Wilson's disease is an inability to mobilize copper from lysosomes within the hepatocytes. When the liver has reached its storage capacity, the copper will escape and begin to damage other organ systems. There is an increase in urinary copper. There are neuropsychologic symptoms, renal disease, and hemolysis. Copper is needed but not available for production of ceruloplasmin. Therefore the level is low.

Table 47-1. DIFFERENTIAL DIAGNOSIS OF JAUNDICE IN THE OLDER CHILD

Disease	Test
α1 Antitrypsin	α1 Antitrypsin level, protease inhibitor type
Wilson's disease	Ceruloplasmin, urine copper, dry weight of copper in liver
Type I autoimmune hepatitis	ANA, anti-smooth muscle antibody
Type II	Anti-liver kidney microsomal antibody
Hepatitis B	Hepatitis B surface antigen
Hepatitis C	Hepatitis C antibody

5. **(A)** See above explanation.

6. **(B)** Wilson's disease is an autosomal recessive disease. Patients are more effectively treated before symptoms occur; therefore all family members should be screened for asymptomatic disease.

7. **(A)** Type I autoimmune hepatitis is associated with a positive ANA and anti-smooth muscle antibody. Type II autoimmune hepatitis is associated with anti-liver and kidney microsomal antibodies. There is no type III.

8. **(D)** The treatment for autoimmune hepatitis is steroids and azathioprine. Once the liver numbers have returned to the normal range, the initial high dose of steroids can be weaned.

9. **(B)** Hepatitis B is transmitted through percutaneous route, IV drugs, sexual contact, or in utero maternal-child transmission. There are reports of household contact spread, but since hepatitis B vaccine is part of routine pediatric care it is un-

likely she would be infected from a household contact. An 8-year-old is likely to have acquired the infection from mother at birth. This child would have a chronic infection. See Table 47–2 for the markers, which distinguish acute from chronic infection.

10. **(D)** The description here is of cirrhosis with evidence of portal hypertension, secondary to chronic liver disease. Hepatitis A does not have a chronic form. The other listed diseases do.

11. **(D)** A child who is jaundiced and then is "difficult to wake up" must be assumed to have encephalopathy. This should be evaluated in an emergency room where laboratory evaluations and treatment are immediately available.

12. **(D)**

13. **(D)** Patients with fulminant hepatic failure have decreased liver mass. They are at risk for hypoglycemia secondary to decreased glycogen storage and gluconeogenesis. Patients develop hepatorenal syndrome. The mechanism is unknown but the disease is characterized by decreased excretion of sodium (as opposed to acute tubular necrosis where sodium excretion is increased). Coagulopathy develops because the liver produces factors I (fibrinogen), II, V, VII, IX, and X. In addition in FHF there is frequently disseminated intravascular coagulopathy (DIC) contributing to the difficult to control coagulopathy.

14. **(B)** In a patient who has been ill acetaminophen toxicity must be included in the differential diagnosis. Parents frequently give acetaminophen and can inadvertently overdose a child. In a teenage child, you must be concerned about intentional overdose.

Table 47-2. SERUM MARKERS IN HEPATITIS B INFECTIONS

	HBsAg	HBsAb	HBc IgM	HBc IgG	HBeAg	HBeAb	HB DNA
Early acute	+	−	+	−	+	−	+
Late acute	+	−	+	−	−	+	+
Chronic	+	−	−	+	+	−	+

15. **(A)** The treatment for acetaminophen toxicity is N-acetyl-cysteine. The treatment is most effective if given within the first 10 hours after ingestion. Jaundice and increased liver numbers occur 3 days after the ingestion. Although the N-acetyl-cysteine may be less effective at that time, it is still given.

16. **(A)** The description of a 2-year-old with a large liver not because of a viral illness, e.g., hepatitis, is characteristic of hepatic malignancy. The initial evaluations would include an ultrasound and a serum α-fetoprotein level. Wilson's disease does not present before age 4 to 5 years. Autoimmune hepatitis rarely presents at 2 years old. The presentation for $\alpha 1$ antitrypsin deficiency or hepatitis B or C in this age group would be an asymptomatic elevation in the ALT and AST.

17. **(B)** The most common hepatic malignancy in this age group is hepatoblastoma. Hepatocellular carcinoma presents in older children and is usually associated with hepatitis B or C. Rhabdosarcomas and angiosarcomas are incredibly rare tumors.

18. **(B)** The description is the classic presentation for a choledochal cyst in this age group. Choledochal cysts can present as neonatal cholestasis. Gallstones are incredibly rare in children.

SUGGESTED READING

Whitington PF, Soriano HE, Alonso EM: Fulminant hepatic failure. In: Suchy F (ed): *Liver Disease in Children*, 2nd ed. Philadelphia: Lippincott, Williams & Wilkins, 2001, p 63.

Schwarz K, Balistreri W: Viral hepatitis. *J Pediatr Gastroenterol Nutr* 35(Suppl 1):S29–S32, 2002.

Bezerra JA, Balistreri W: Cholestatic syndromes in infancy and childhood. *Semin Gastrointest Dis* 12(2):54–65, 2001.

CASE 48: A 6-YEAR-OLD WITH FECAL INCONTINENCE

A 6-year-old boy presents with a complaint of fecal incontinence. His mother reports he stools every other day in the toilet but in between he has 4 to 6 "accidents." The mother denies abdominal distention, decreased appetite, or nausea.

Physical examination shows his height and weight to be at the 50th percentile. The abdomen is soft, with normal bowel sounds and no palpable liver or spleen. Examination of the head, ears, eyes, nose, and throat is normal. Similarly, the cardiac and respiratory examinations are normal.

SELECT THE ONE BEST ANSWER

1. Your most important next step is:

   (A) barium enema
   (B) rectal exam
   (C) lumbar spine MRI
   (D) start behavioral program for bowel training

2. If this was a low-segment Hirschsprung's disease, you would expect:

   (A) increased rectal tone compared with functional constipation
   (B) decreased rectal tone compared with functional constipation
   (C) the same rectal tone compared with functional constipation
   (D) normal rectal tone

3. If the child has a sacral dimple, then associated clinical feature(s) may include:

   (A) urinary incontinence
   (B) loss of lower extremity reflexes
   (C) anterior placed anus
   (D) A and B

4. The most appropriate next step in the management for the patient in question 3 is:

   (A) abdominal radiograph
   (B) rectal exam
   (C) lumbosacral spine MRI
   (D) start behavioral program for bowel training

5. The child in the opening vignette has a large amount of hard stool and decreased tone on his rectal exam. The next diagnostic test is:

   (A) abdominal radiograph
   (B) rectal exam
   (C) lumbar spine MRI
   (D) no diagnostic test

6. The treatment for the child in question 5 includes:

   (A) enema
   (B) osmotic laxatives

(C) behavioral intervention

(D) all of the above

7. The length of time this child will need to be treated is:

(A) 1 weeks

(B) 1 month

(C) 2 months

(D) >6 months

8. The chance of successful treatment at a year out from diagnosis is:

(A) 30% to 50%

(B) 50% to 75%

(C) 75% to 90%

(D) >90%

9. If the child in the vignette had rectal prolapse with his constipation, the next step would be:

(A) sweat test

(B) rectal biopsy

(C) treat the constipation

(D) do a detailed calorie count

10. Had the weight and height of the child in the vignette been less than the 5th percentile for age and there was rectal prolapse, your next step would be:

(A) sweat test

(B) rectal biopsy

(C) treat the constipation

(D) do a detailed calorie count

11. Had the child in the vignette been treated for urinary incontinence by a urologist and his constipation began after his treatment,

(A) the constipation and urinary incontinence are secondary to spinal tumor

(B) urinary incontinence is usually treated with anticholinergics and the constipation is secondary to the drug

(C) the constipation was previously undiagnosed and the urinary incontinence is secondary to the constipation

(D) B or C

12. Had the child in the vignette had painless bright red blood per rectum, the likely diagnosis would be:

(A) juvenile polyp

(B) fissure

(C) hemorrhoid

(D) Meckel's diverticulum

13. If this child was 6 weeks old, breast-fed and stooled once every 5 days, the treatment would be:

(A) reassurance

(B) mineral oil

(C) Maltsupex

(D) rectal stimulation

14. If the child in question 13 was well-disposed but a poor feeder with constipation, your first step is:

(A) a barium enema

(B) a rectal biopsy

(C) TSH and T_4 determinations

(D) a sweat test

15. Regarding Hirschsprung's disease, which statement is true?

(A) Male-to-female ratio is 4:1.

(B) Female-to-male ratio is 4:1.

(C) There is an even gender distribution.

(D) Male-to-female ratio is 8:1.

16. In an infant with Hirschsprung's disease, the findings on physical examination include:

(A) empty rectum

(B) rectal impaction

(C) abdominal distention

(D) A and C

17. The findings on barium enema would be:

(A) a transition zone between the dilated aganglionic section and the normal colon

(B) a transition zone between the contracted aganglionic section and the dilated colon

(C) a transition zone between the rectum and the dilated colon

(D) there are no consistent findings on barium enema and rectal biopsy is the diagnostic test of choice

18. The true statement about children with Hirschsprung's disease is:

(A) >90% do not pass their meconium in the first 24 hours of life

(B) 75% do not pass their meconium in the first 24 hours of life

(C) 50% do not pass their meconium in the first 24 hours of life

(D) 25% do not pass their meconium in the first 24 hours of life

Answers

1. **(B)** A rectal examination is the part of the physical examination that gives you the most information in this case. A patient with the functional constipation and encopresis described in this vignette is going to have loose rectal tone and stool within the vault.

2. **(A)** Children with Hirschsprung's disease have aganglionosis in certain sections of the colon. A 6-year-old presenting with Hirschsprung's disease would have to have an ultrashort segment of Hirschsprung's involvement. The rectal tone is increased in Hirschsprung's disease. The vault is likely to be empty.

3. **(D)** Spina bifida, meningomyelocele, sacral agenesis, and spinal cord tumors can be associated with fecal incontinence. Other neurologic symptoms and signs such as urinary incontinence and loss of reflexes can be associated.

4. **(C)** Evaluation of the spine by an MRI is the most appropriate diagnostic test.

5. **(D)** Functional constipation is a clinical diagnosis. The vignette and the rectal examination findings are consistent with functional constipation.

6. **(D)** The aim of therapy is to alleviate the impaction, prevent recurrence, and retrain the child to appreciate normal bowel signals.

7. **(D)** Once a child has developed encopresis and is successfully treated by the plan outlined above, the laxatives must be weaned slowly. This will frequently take >6 months. Parents should be warned about the length of time it takes to treat.

8. **(A)** The chance of successfully weaning children off all laxatives and having normal bowel habits is 30% to 50% at 1 year and only 78% at 5 years.

9. **(C)** Rectal prolapse is most frequently associated with constipation. In developing countries, it is associated with malnutrition. There is also an association with cystic fibrosis. In a child who has constipation and no other problems, it is unnecessary to look for cystic fibrosis simply because of rectal prolapse.

10. **(A)** In a child who has other symptoms possibly attributed to CF the sweat test is necessary. In this instance, the small stature "tips the scale" to doing the sweat test.

11. **(D)** Because constipation and urinary symptoms are frequently seen together, it is important to treat both ailments. It is important to remember to also look closely for constipation when a child presents with urinary incontinence. The treatment with anticholinergic drugs can lead to constipation. Drugs associated with constipation include analgesics, antacids, anticholinergic, bismuth, iron, cholestyramine, and anti-psychotics.

12. **(A)** Painless bright red blood is likely to be a polyp in this age group. Although hemorrhoids are associated with constipation in adults, they are very unusual in children. Fissures lead to painful bleeding. A Meckel's diverticulum can cause a significant bleed and can be associated with cramping abdominal pain.

13. **(A)** It is not the frequency of stool that defines constipation even in breast-fed babies. As long as the stool is of normal consistency and easily passed, several days between stools is acceptable.

14. **(C)** A "well-disposed" 6-week-old is concerning. Poor feeding secondary to abdominal pain or reflux is usually associated with an irritable baby. Here you must be concerned with hypothyroidism. The signs can be subtle.

15. **(A)**

16. **(D)** The physical findings consistent with Hirschsprung's include increased rectal tone, lack of stool

in the vault, and abdominal distention. The treatment involves resection of the poorly inner-vated colon. The most dangerous complication is enterocolitis and toxic megacolon. With this di-agnosis, the baby will present with explosive di-arrhea, fever, and shock.

17. **(B)** The aganglionotic area is contracted, hence the increased tone on rectal examination. The proximal colon will be dilated. The barium enema is diag-nostic in over 75% of patients with Hirschsprung's.

18. **(A)**

SUGGESTED READING

Loening-Baucke V: Encopresis. *Curr Opin Pediatr* 14(5): 570–575, 2002.
DiLorenzo C, Benniga MA: Pathophysiology of pediatric fecal incontinence. *Gastroenterology* 126(1 Suppl 1): S33–S40, 2004.

CASE 49: A 15-MONTH-OLD WITH DIARRHEA

A 15-month-old boy presents with a complaint of di-arrhea. He is having three to five large "explosive" stools per day. They are not malodorous, there is no blood or mucous, and they are not bulky or oily. Mom frequently sees food particles such as corn, carrots, and raisins in the stool.

On physical examination his vitals signs are HR 102, RR 28, BP 88/50. He is in no apparent distress. His breath sounds are equal and clear. His abdomen is nondistended with positive bowel sounds. There are no masses and no hepatosplenomegaly. There are no perianal lesions and the stool is heme-negative. His growth curve is in Figure 49-1.

SELECT THE ONE BEST ANSWER

1. The first studies you would order include:

    (A) stool for fat, reducing substances, and pH
    (B) a stool culture and assay for fecal leukocytes
    (C) stool examination for ova and parasites
    (D) all of the above

2. The likely diagnosis for this child is:

    (A) nonspecific diarrhea of childhood (toddler's diarrhea)
    (B) carbohydrate malabsorption

    (C) postinfectious malabsorption
    (D) you cannot distinguish among these entities

3. Chronic diarrhea of childhood can be secondary to:

    (A) excess intake of fruit juice
    (B) excess intake of carbohydrate
    (C) too little fat in the child's diet
    (D) all of the above

4. The treatment for chronic nonspecific diarrhea includes:

    (A) reassurance and limiting dietary excess
    (B) reassurance, limiting dietary excess, and clear liquids when number of stools is >5 per day
    (C) reassurance, limiting dietary excess, and Lo-motil when the number of stools is >5 per day
    (D) B or C

5. If the growth curve for the child in the vignette was the curve in Figure 49-2, your concern would be:

    (A) celiac disease
    (B) early Crohn's disease
    (C) sucrose-isomaltase deficiency
    (D) there is not enough information to make the diagnosis

6. The laboratory studies that would allow you to make the diagnosis include:

    (A) hydrogen breath test
    (B) CBC, sedimentation rate, and serum albumin
    (C) tissue transglutaminase IgA
    (D) A and C

7. Treatment for this disease includes:

    (A) gluten-free diet
    (B) sucrose-free diet
    (C) steroids
    (D) without laboratory results from question 6, you cannot make recommendations.

8. Had the child in the vignette had a rectal pro-lapse with the diarrhea, the test from question 1 that would be abnormal is:

    (A) stool examination for ova and parasites
    (B) stool evaluation for reducing substances
    (C) stool evaluation for fat content
    (D) stool culture

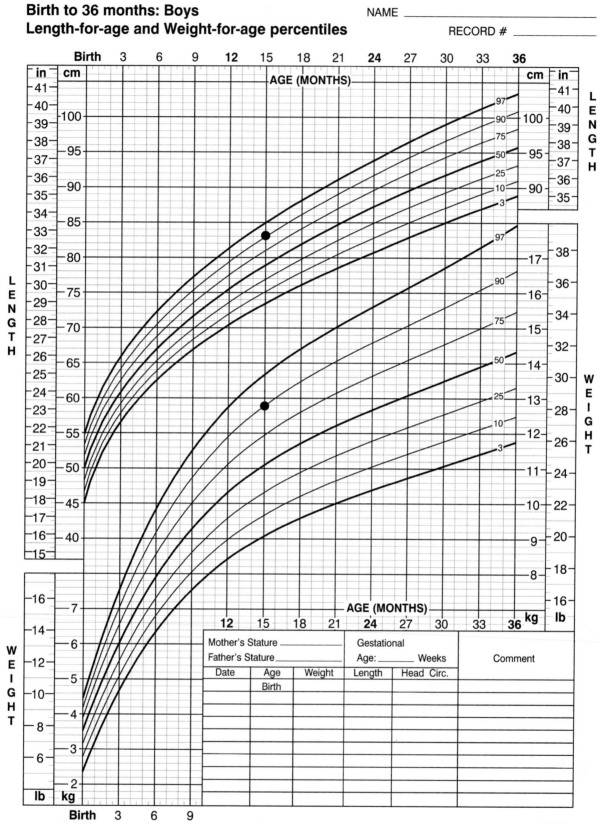

Birth to 36 months: Boys
Length-for-age and Weight-for-age percentiles

NAME _____

RECORD # _____

Figure 49-1.

Published May 30, 2000 (modified 4/20/01).
SOURCE: Developed by the National Center for Health Statistics in collaboration with
the National Center for Chronic Disease Prevention and Health Promotion (2000).
http://www.cdc.gov/growthcharts

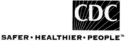

SAFER · HEALTHIER · PEOPLE™

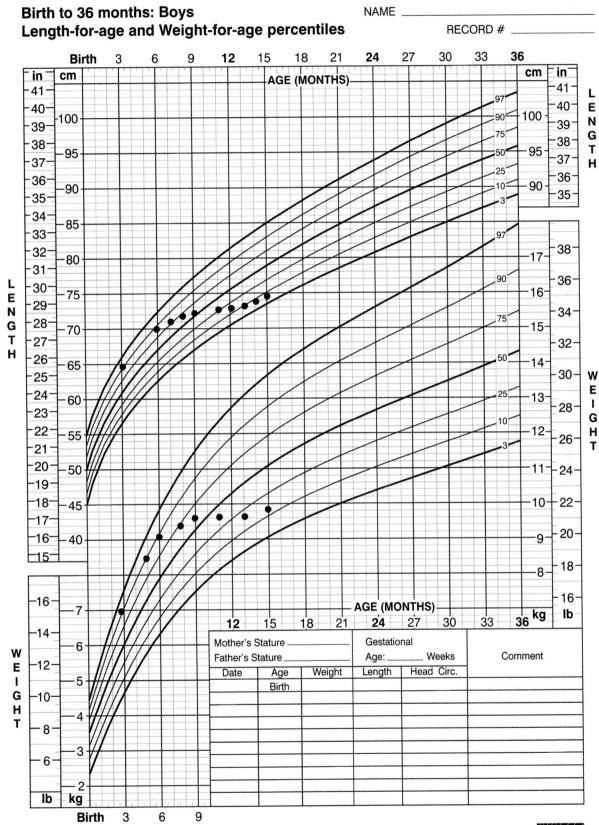

Birth to 36 months: Boys
Length-for-age and Weight-for-age percentiles

NAME _____

RECORD # _____

Published May 30, 2000 (modified 4/20/01).
SOURCE: Developed by the National Center for Health Statistics in collaboration with
the National Center for Chronic Disease Prevention and Health Promotion (2000).
http://www.cdc.gov/growthcharts

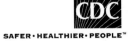

SAFER·HEALTHIER·PEOPLE™

Figure 49-2.

9. The most appropriate next test for the child in question 8 is:

   (A) abdominal radiograph
   (B) barium enema
   (C) sweat test
   (D) endoscopy

10. Later in life, the child in question 8 may suffer from:

    (A) constipation
    (B) distal intestinal obstruction syndrome (a meconium ileus equivalent)
    (C) focal biliary cirrhosis
    (D) all of the above

11. If the mom in the vignette described the stools as covered with mucous and the stools were heme-positive, the patient's history would include:

    (A) exposure to well water
    (B) exposure to antibiotics
    (C) exposure to other ill children
    (D) family history of inflammatory bowel disease

12. If the patient was 5 years old and had a history of duodenal atresia repair, the additional tests you would order include:

    (A) upper GI series with small bowel follow-through
    (B) hydrogen breath test
    (C) endoscopy with biopsy
    (D) upper endoscopy with biopsy

13. If the child had stools that "burned," the likely malabsorption would be

    (A) carbohydrate
    (B) fats
    (C) proteins
    (D) vitamins and minerals

14. The antibiotic that most often leads to *Clostridium difficile* infection in pediatric patients is:

    (A) amoxicillin
    (B) clindamycin
    (C) erythromycin
    (D) all of the above cause an equal incidence of *C. difficile*

15. If the child in the vignette was a 6-week-old with five loose watery stools with blood, the likely diagnosis is:

    (A) infectious colitis
    (B) protein intolerance
    (C) lactose intolerance
    (D) congenital chloride diarrhea

16. If the child was feeding on cow milk formula, the treatment would be:

    (A) soy formula
    (B) hydrolyzed formula
    (C) await stool culture results before making recommendations
    (D) await stool electrolytes before making recommendations

17. The stool culture yields *C. difficile*. The treatment in neonates:

    (A) would be the same as older children
    (B) would be extended compared with older children
    (C) would be shortened compared with older children
    (D) no treatment is necessary

18. If the child in question 15 was breast-fed, then the treatment would be:

    (A) soy formula
    (B) hydrolyzed formula
    (C) await stool cultures
    (D) restrict the cow milk in mom's diet

Answers

1. **(D)** The initial evaluation for a child with chronic diarrhea should concentrate on the history and physical examination. The screening laboratory tests are examinations of the stool looking for malabsorption. In addition, an intestinal infection should be ruled out.

2. **(A)** A 15-month-old child who has normal growth and diarrhea without accompanying GI symptoms likely has nonspecific diarrhea of childhood. Parents will frequently see food in the stool. The symptoms of carbohydrate malabsorption are de-

tailed below. There was no history of gastroenteritis prior to the onset of this diarrhea.

3. **(D)** Nonspecific diarrhea of childhood can be because of any of the dietary problems listed. Children can have increased diarrhea if they are put on a clear liquid diet frequently.

4. **(A)** Reassurance and restricting the dietary excesses is the treatment.

5. **(A)** This is a classic growth curve for celiac disease. It would be incredibly unusual for Crohn's disease to begin at 6 months of age.

6. **(C)** The evaluation of a child suspected to have celiac disease initially should be serologic. Detection of anti-gliadin antibodies is a sensitive test but not specific to celiac disease and these antibodies can be present in other GI diseases. Detection of anti-endomysial antibodies is much more specific. Tissue transglutaminase is a specific anti-endomysial antibody. Caution should be used in interpretation because 2% to 5% of celiac patients are IgA deficient.

7. **(A)** The treatment for celiac disease is a gluten-free diet.

8. **(C)** A patient with diarrhea, growth failure, and rectal prolapse has CF until proven otherwise. The fat content in the stool will be abnormal secondary to pancreatic insufficiency that commonly occurs in CF patients.

9. **(C)** A sweat test should be done to ensure the clinical findings are from CF.

10. **(D)** Later in life, children with CF can suffer from multiple GI symptoms. Constipation and GERD are common associated symptoms. DIOS presents with partial or complete bowel obstruction. It responds to medical therapy with Gastrografin enemas. It can recur. In chronic cases, it is important to ensure there is adequate pancreatic enzyme replacement. Two percent to 3% of CF patients will develop biliary cirrhosis.

11. **(B)** The stool description is consistent with *C. difficile* infection. Therefore it would be likely that the child had previous antibiotic exposure.

12. **(B)** Patients with previous bowel surgery are predisposed to have bacterial overgrowth. This can be diagnosed with a breath hydrogen test. The patient ingests sugar. Bacteria will convert sugar into hydrogen. In small bowel bacterial overgrowth, the peak of expired hydrogen will be early because the bacteria are in the small bowel, not the colon. In carbohydrate malabsorption there will be a later peak when the unabsorbed sugar reaches the colon.

13. **(A)** Carbohydrate malabsorption leads to delivery of unabsorbed carbohydrate to the colon. The bacteria in the colon convert it to acid. Reducing substances will be positive.

14. **(A)** Although in adults clindamycin is the antibiotic most associated with *C. difficile*, in pediatrics many more patients take amoxicillin; therefore it is the antibiotic most frequently associated with *C. difficile*. This situation may change as epidemic community-acquired MRSA necessitates increasing use of clindamycin.

15. **(B)** The most common cause of diarrhea in this age group is protein intolerance. Children with congenital chloride-losing diarrhea present earlier and are very ill. Lactose intolerance is rare in this age group.

16. **(B)** The protein intolerance is to cow's protein. Up to 50% of those children will be allergic to soy formula.

17. **(D)** Up to 70% of infants will be carriers of *C. difficile* and no treatment is necessary. The toxin receptor is absent from the intestinal cells of a neonate.

18. **(D)** The symptoms are because of exposure to cow's protein. The treatment is to restrict the exposure to cow milk, which crosses into the mother's breast milk.

SUGGESTED READING

Pietzak MM, Thomas DW: Childhood malabsorption. *Pediatr Rev* 24:195–206, 2003.

Book L: Diagnosing celiac disease in 2002: Who, why, and how. *Pediatrics* 109:952–954, 2002.

Leung AK, Robson WL: Evaluating the child with chronic diarrhea. *Am Fam Physician* 53:635–643, 1996.

General

7

CASE 50: A 12-YEAR-OLD WITH EAR DISCHARGE

A 12-year-old child comes to your office during the summer because of "smelly stuff" coming out of his left ear for 2 days. This has never happened before. For the last day he has had worsening ear pain, which does not respond to acetaminophen. It hurts his jaw to chew food. He has had no fever and no upper respiratory tract symptoms.

SELECT THE ONE BEST ANSWER

1. Which of the following are possible diagnoses from this history?

   (A) foreign body
   (B) otitis externa or otitis media with perforation
   (C) chronic suppurative otitis media
   (D) A and B
   (E) all are in the differential diagnosis

2. On examination, you note thick, yellow-white foul smelling discharge in the ear canal with underlying erythema. After flushing with water you see that the tympanic membrane is intact and appears slightly erythematous. His examination also reveals tenderness when you gently tug on the pinna of the left ear and some small (<1 cm), tender, mobile anterior cervical and preauricular lymph nodes on the left.

   Of the following, which is the least likely pathogen that contributes to this problem?

   (A) candida
   (B) *Staphylococcus aureus*
   (C) *Pseudomonas aeruginosa*
   (D) group A streptococci
   (E) C and D are both unlikely

3. Which of the following is not a risk factor for otitis externa?

   (A) otitis media
   (B) swimming
   (C) Q-tip use
   (D) foreign body
   (E) all are risk factors

4. Which of the following is the best treatment for otitis externa?

   (A) oral amoxicillin
   (B) oral amoxicillin-clavulanic acid
   (C) ceftriaxone IM
   (D) ciprofloxacin/hydrocortisone otic drops
   (E) oral ibuprofen and water lavage of the external auditory canal

5. Which of the following is a possible cause of bloody otorrhea?

   (A) acute otitis media
   (B) Langerhans cell histiocytosis
   (C) chronic otitis externa
   (D) bullous myringitis
   (E) all of the above

6. What is the most important test to perform on clear fluid associated with otorrhea?

   (A) bacterial culture
   (B) glucose level
   (C) pH
   (D) KOH prep
   (E) none of the above need to be done

7. Which of the following is a potential source of clear otorrhea?

   (A) bullous myringitis
   (B) acute otitis media
   (C) fungal otitis externa
   (D) perforated tympanic membrane
   (E) A and D

8. A 3-year-old boy is brought to the emergency room by his mother because of ear pain that started the day before and is progressing in intensity. He has had minimal relief from acetaminophen given at home. He has not been ill in the last 2 weeks but was at a birthday party 3 days earlier, where his mother is "sure he caught something from one of the other kids." On examination he has normal vital signs, profuse white, slightly foul-smelling discharge from the right ear, clear nares, normal oropharynx, and no lymphadenopathy.

   What is the best course of action?

   (A) placement of an ear wick
   (B) ciprofloxacin/hydrocortisone otic drops
   (C) water lavage
   (D) topical lidocaine
   (E) oral amoxicillin

9. On further otoscopy, you find what you believe to be a small disk-shaped battery, presumably from a toy. You attempt a gentle removal, but it is unsuccessful. You should next:

   (A) observe for 24 hours
   (B) send him to the emergency room for ENT consultation
   (C) apply topical lidocaine into the ear
   (D) start preventive ciprofloxacin/hydrocortisone drops
   (E) start oral amoxicillin

10. A 6-year-old is brought to your office for her routine check-up. Her mother says that she "failed" her hearing screen performed at the school and was instructed to get further hearing testing. She reminds you that her daughter has had multiple ear infections in the last year. On examination you note no conjunctival injection, clear nares, normal oropharynx, no lymphadenopathy, but clear effusion behind a mobile tympanic membrane on the left.

    What is the most appropriate next step?

    (A) reevaluate her effusion in 3 months
    (B) try automated auditory brainstem response
    (C) otoacoustic emissions
    (D) audiometry
    (E) tympanometry

11. What is the most common type of hearing loss in children?

    (A) sensorineural
    (B) conductive
    (C) combined
    (D) none of the above
    (E) A and B are about equal

12. What is the most common cause of that type of hearing loss in a U.S. population?

    (A) cholesteatoma
    (B) middle ear effusion
    (C) impacted cerumen
    (D) foreign body
    (E) perforated tympanic membrane

13. What is the most common infectious cause of sensorineural hearing loss in a U.S. population?

    (A) rubella
    (B) syphilis
    (C) cytomegalovirus
    (D) toxoplasmosis
    (E) herpesvirus

Match the following syndromes with the type of hearing loss associated with it.

14. Down

15. Treacher-Collins

16. Pierre-Robin

17. Hunter-Hurler

18. Alport

19. Crouzon

   (A) conductive
   (B) sensorineural

20. Which of the following does not indicate the need for hearing screening, or rescreening if newborn hearing screening was performed?

   (A) recognition of developmental delay
   (B) meningitis
   (C) exposure to CMV
   (D) otitis media with effusion for 4 months
   (E) skull fracture

Answers

1. **(D)** Chronic suppurative otitis starts more insidiously, is often asymptomatic, and should have a longer history of otic discharge. Both otitis media with a perforated tympanic membrane and otitis externa can cause purulent discharge and cannot be differentiated always by history. Likewise, a foreign body lodged in the external auditory canal can cause foul-smelling discharge and pain.

2. **(D)** This scenario depicts otitis externa, which presents with the main complaint of ear pain, especially with movement of the pinna or tragus, and thick white discharge from the external auditory canal. *P. aeruginosa* is the most common isolate when the onset of symptoms follows swimming (80%), but *S. aureus*, *Streptococcus pyogenes*, gram-negatives such as *Proteus* or *Klebsiella*, and fungi such as *Candida* or *Aspergillus* are also possibilities. The last presents with a more insidious ear discharge that is white and fluffy, sometimes with small black spores visible.

3. **(A)** Anything that causes trauma to the external canal (Q-tips, foreign body) or changes the microbial environment (swimming, and thus the nickname "swimmer's ear" for otitis externa) predisposes to bacterial invasion of the external canal.

4. **(D)** Topical therapy is best in uncomplicated cases with an antibiotic with activity against *Pseudomonas*. Topical steroids are not a recom-

mended treatment. A fungal infection would require cleansing and topical antifungal solutions.

5. **(E)** Both otitis media and otitis externa can present with bloody otic discharge. Likewise, rupture of a bulla when bullous myringitis is present may produce bloody discharge. Langerhans cell histiocytosis is a spectrum of disorders, the most systemic of which is Letterer-Siwe disease, most often associated with chronic otitis externa.

6. **(B)** The most important condition to rule out in the presence of clear otorrhea is a leakage of CSF. Measurement of glucose (CSF is 45 to 70 mg/100 mL), protein (<200 mg/mL), and β_2-transferrin levels may be of assistance since very low concentrations of these should be present in inflammatory fluid. In addition, a CT of the area is warranted to rule out congenital or malignant causes.

7. **(E)**

8. **(C)** Because the main diagnostic possibilities include acute otitis media with tympanic membrane perforation, otitis externa, and the presence of a foreign body, and because the discharge is prohibiting you from making a diagnosis, attempting gentle water lavage is the best next step. The foul-smelling discharge should alert you to the probability of a foreign body, which should be removed in as timely a manner as possible to prevent secondary infection and traumatic puncture of the tympanic membrane. Sometimes small foreign bodies can even be removed simply by gentle warm water lavage.

9. **(B)** Of the foreign bodies that 3-year-olds place in their ear, batteries are the most urgent. They leak an ototoxic fluid that can be very damaging to the ear canal. They must be removed as promptly as possible. Both topical lidocaine and topical antibiotics are often used for treatment. Lidocaine can numb the ear canal for removal of the foreign body, and antibiotics may be useful for infection of the canal associated with the foreign body. Neither should be prescribed until the procedure for battery removal is imminent.

10. **(B)** Conventional audiometry is most appropriate for evaluation of hearing in children older

than 4 to 5 years. Although this child may have otitis media with effusion, the larger problem is that even 3 months ago she failed a screening hearing test, suggesting that there may be a more chronic problem involved. ABR (automated brainstem response) and OAE (otoacoustic emission) tests are less dependent on patient cooperation and are therefore more useful in infants. Tympanometry may support your finding of middle ear effusion, but will not assess hearing.

11. **(B)**

12. **(B)** A middle ear effusion is the most common cause of conductive hearing loss. In addition to those listed above, other potential causes include congenital anomalies of the external auditory canal, tympanosclerosis, trauma, and masses in the inner ear (histiocytosis, rhabdomyosarcoma).

13. **(C)** The incidence of congenital CMV in the United States ranges from 0.2% to 2.0% of newborns. Of those, 10% have clinical manifestations at birth. Seventy-five percent of symptomatic infants and 5% to 15% of asymptomatic infants have sensorineural hearing loss that often may be progressive and present at 4 to 5 years old.

14. **(B)** Down syndrome is one of the most common and well-studied trisomies. The incidence is 1/700 births and increases in women older than 35 years old. Major associated anomalies include congenital heart disease, GI disorders, thyroid disease, leukemia, and mental retardation. Associated minor anomalies are numerous and include delayed puberty, short stature, hearing loss, rapid aging, and sterility in males.

15. **(A)** Treacher-Collins, or mandibulofacial dysostosis, is an autosomal dominant syndrome characterized by hypoplasia of the facial bones. The clinical findings vary, but often include: microtia, hearing loss, cleft palate, colobomas, and facial deformities.

16. **(A)** Pierre-Robin syndrome is an autosomal recessive disorder characterized by severe mandibular hypoplasia, leading to cleft palate, hearing loss, congenital heart disease, and other oral deformities.

17. **(B)** Hunter-Hurler syndrome is an autosomal recessive lysosomal disorder characterized by dwarfism, hunchback, coarse facies, mental retardation, hearing loss, and cardiac abnormalities. Affected children may appear normal until 1 year of age.

18. **(B)** Alport syndrome is an X-linked dominant or recessive disease that causes hearing loss, hematuria, and renal failure.

19. **(A)** In general, syndromes that involve craniofacial abnormalities are more likely to display conductive hearing loss. Both Crouzon (1/25,000 births) and Apert (1/100,000 births) syndromes have craniosynostosis as their most prominent clinical feature, associated with multiple other facial dysmorphisms. Crouzon syndrome is an autosomal dominant disorder with variable clinical presentation.

20. **(C)** Congenital CMV is associated with sensorineural hearing loss although acquired CMV infection is not.

SUGGESTED READING

Behrman RE, Kliegman RM, Jenson HB, et al: *Nelson Textbook of Pediatrics*. Philadelphia, PA, WB Saunders, 2004, pp 1813, 1938–1963.

Gürtler N: Etiology of syndromic and nonsyndromic sensorineural hearing loss. *Otolaryngol Clin North Am* 35(4):891–908.

Hone SW: Medical evaluation of pediatric hearing loss. Laboratory, radiographic, and genetic testing. *Otolaryngol Clin North Am* 35(4):751–764.

Sander R: Otitis externa: A practical guide to treatment and prevention. *Am Fam Physician* 63(5):927–942, 2001.

CASE 51: A 2-YEAR-OLD WITH EYE REDNESS

A 30-month-old is brought to you by his mother, who has noticed redness of his left eye for the last few weeks. She reports very little discharge and no surrounding swelling or redness. He attends daycare 5 days a week and has had several colds in the last 3 months, most recently 3 weeks prior. He currently has no associated upper respiratory symptoms. His mother does not think that he is bothered by it.

On examination you find a friendly, interactive toddler. He points to animals on the wallpaper, smiles at his mother, and plays interactively with his toys. You note unilateral moderate conjunctival injection but no discharge. There are no other findings, including on your funduscopic examination, during which he is quite fussy.

SELECT THE ONE BEST ANSWER

1. What is your BEST next action?

   (A) Begin antibiotic eye drops.
   (B) Begin steroid eye drops.
   (C) Ask them to return for a follow-up visit.
   (D) Begin anti-allergy eye drops.
   (E) Begin an oral antihistamine.

2. The mother misses the 1-month follow-up appointment and comes in 3 months later, because she now has the sense that the left eye is "growing" faster than the other. She says that the redness is still present and he also has some tears that leak out of that eye. On examination you note the same unilateral moderate conjunctival injection, but now also tearing and an enlarged globe. You cannot perform a funduscopic examination because of lack of cooperation from the child.
   What is your working diagnosis?

   (A) corneal abrasion
   (B) viral conjunctivitis
   (C) allergic conjunctivitis
   (D) bacterial conjunctivitis
   (E) glaucoma

3. Which test that can be conducted in the office of a general pediatrician is most indicated during the evaluation of the suspected condition for the patient in this case?

   (A) Snellen chart testing
   (B) funduscopic examination
   (C) corneal diameter
   (D) pupillary reaction to light
   (E) B and C

4. Which of the following is the best treatment for a 2-year-old with glaucoma?

   (A) β-blocker
   (B) α-agonist
   (C) trabeculotomy
   (D) A and B
   (E) none of the above

5. All of the following are associated with glaucoma in childhood except:

   (A) congenital rubella
   (B) congenital syphilis
   (C) Sturge-Weber syndrome
   (D) Marfan syndrome
   (E) neurofibromatosis

6. A 12-year-old who wears contact lenses comes to see you because of several days of right eye redness, pain, and now light sensitivity and blurry vision. She has no other symptoms, does not wear glasses, and recalls no trauma to the eye.
   What is the most likely diagnosis?

   (A) glaucoma
   (B) viral conjunctivitis
   (C) allergic conjunctivitis
   (D) bacterial conjunctivitis
   (E) corneal abrasion

7. What is the best way to diagnose the condition suspected in question 6?

   (A) slit lamp examination
   (B) funduscopic examination
   (C) visual acuity testing
   (D) corneal diameter
   (E) pupillary reaction to light

8. In addition to discontinuing contact lens use, which additional treatment(s) would be best to treat the condition in question 6?

   (A) topical antibiotics
   (B) oral antibiotics
   (C) eye patch
   (D) topical steroids
   (E) B and D

9. You see a 3-day-old healthy full-term infant in the hospital for her newborn examination and on your funduscopic examination you note the absence of a red reflex on one side. Instead you see a white discoloration. If you suspect congenital cataracts, which of the following tests would be part of your workup?

   (A) TSH and free T_4
   (B) Rubella titers
   (C) Galactose-1-phosphate

(D) G₆PD

(D) G_6PD

(E) B and C

10. Approximately what percent of unilateral congenital cataracts is hereditary?

    (A) 5%
    (B) 25%
    (C) 50%
    (D) 75%
    (E) 90%

11. Approximately what percent of bilateral congenital cataracts is hereditary?

    (A) 5%
    (B) 25%
    (C) 50%
    (D) 75%
    (E) 90%

12. You see a 6-month-old girl in your office for a health prevention visit and on your funduscopic examination notice a unilateral white discoloration in place of her red reflex.

    What is the most common cause of this finding?

    (A) retinoblastoma
    (B) infantile cataract
    (C) retinopathy of prematurity
    (D) incontinentia pigmenti
    (E) retinal detachment

13. After referral to an ophthalmologist, you are told that she has a cataract. Which of the following are associated with infantile cataracts?

    (A) trisomy of chromosome 13
    (B) trisomy of chromosome 18
    (C) deficiency of galactose-1-uridyltransferase
    (D) chromosome 5 short arm deletion
    (E) all of the above

14. You see a 2-week-old in your office for a newborn checkup and on eye examination find that he has a very small amount of iris tissue. You diagnose aniridia. His mother and father say that no one else in the family has anything similar. What other test does this infant most need?

    (A) echocardiogram
    (B) renal ultrasound

(C) spinal ultrasound

(D) EEG

(E) CBC with differential

15. What is the mode of inheritance for most children with this disease?

    (A) sporadic
    (B) autosomal dominant
    (C) autosomal recessive
    (D) X-linked
    (E) not known

16. Which of the following is NOT associated with a coloboma?

    (A) trisomy 13
    (B) trisomy 18
    (C) VATER association
    (D) CHARGE syndrome
    (E) sebaceous nevus

17. The mother of a 4-year-old brings her daughter in after she was hit in the eye with a small toy. She has been very irritable since it happened and says that her eye hurts.

    On examination you note frank red blood filling the lower third of the anterior chamber. You cannot perform a funduscopic examination because she is uncooperative.

    What is her most likely diagnosis?

    (A) intraorbital tumor
    (B) hyphema
    (C) keratitis
    (D) coagulopathy
    (E) foreign body

18. Which of the following is NOT a recommended treatment for this disorder?

    (A) bed rest
    (B) oral steroids
    (C) head elevation
    (D) surgical drainage
    (E) topical steroids

19. What is the MOST common complication of this disorder?

    (A) glaucoma
    (B) blood loss

(C) rebleeding

(D) loss of vision

(E) corneal abrasion

Answers

1. (C) Because the diagnosis at this point is unclear, and possibilities include viral, bacterial, allergic, and ophthalmologic origin, the best action is none, with a follow-up visit if it does not resolve spontaneously.

2. (E) Infantile glaucoma (2 months to 3 years of age) is diagnosed mainly by signs and symptoms. The triad of tearing, photophobia, and blepharospasm is typical, but only occurs in 30% of children with glaucoma. Findings on examination may include increased corneal diameter (>12 mm), cloudy cornea, conjunctival injection, and ocular enlargement.

3. (E) Funduscopic examination needs to be performed both to look for orbital nerve cupping (secondary to the increase in pressure) and to rule out intraorbital pathology. A 2-year-old is too young to cooperate with a Snellen chart. The pupillary reaction to light should be maintained in glaucoma. An ophthalmologist will have better luck at performing a successful funduscopic examination in a child this age and will also be able to measure intraocular pressure, the gold standard for diagnosis.

4. (C) Surgical management is the mainstay of congenital and pediatric glaucoma. Side effects from medical therapies and the difficulty of instilling drops into children's eyes each day keep these medications from being as useful as they are in adults.

5. (B)

6. (E) These are the classic symptoms of a corneal abrasion—an acute onset with no other symptoms except photophobia and loss of visual acuity.

7. (A) After installation of fluorescein dye, inspection of the cornea with a blue-filtered light is necessary. Slit lamp examination is considered the ideal, but use of a Wood's lamp or the blue light on an ophthalmoscope is an acceptable alternative.

8. (A) Prophylactic antibiotics should be applied until the epithelium is completely healed—usually 7 to 10 days. Although use of an eye patch has been a mainstay of treatment, several studies in the last few years have suggested no benefit from the use of the patch. Steroids are not necessary in this situation. Contact lenses should not be used during the healing process.

9. (E) The most common cause of leukocoria in infants is a congenital cataract. The workup includes: rubella titers for congenital infection, galactose-1-phosphate for galactosemia, glucose for hypoglycemia, VDRL for syphilis, urine protein for Alport's syndrome, urine amino acids for Lowe's syndrome, homocysteine for homocystinuria, copper level for Wilson's disease and karyotype for the trisomies. Thyroid abnormalities are unrelated.

10. (A)

11. (C)

12. (B) Cataracts are the most common cause of leukokoria in children, and all the other answers are the differential diagnosis. About 55% of infants with congenital cataracts have a positive family history.

13. (E) Trisomy 13 (Patau's syndrome), trisomy 18 (Edward's syndrome), deficiency of galactose-1-uridyltransferase (galactosemia) and cri-du-chat syndrome (deletion of short arm of chromosome 5) are all associated with cataracts in infancy and children with these genetic diseases require regular ophthalmologic evaluation. The cataracts associated with galactosemia can be prevented by appropriate diet.

14. (B) Of patients with sporadic aniridia (see next question), one-fifth will develop Wilms' tumor. Thus, these patients require renal ultrasounds as screening tools every 3 to 6 months until they are 5 years old. Also, aniridia leads to glaucoma in 75% of patients.

15. **(B)** Two-thirds of cases are autosomal dominant, and one-third is sporadic. The gene for aniridia has been isolated to 11p13. Aniridia is bilateral in 98%.

16. **(C)** CHARGE syndrome (coloboma, heart disease, atresia choanae, retarded growth and development, genital anomalies, and ear anomalies), the trisomies, and nevus sebaceous are all associated with colobomas. VATER association (vertebral defects, anal atresia, tracheoesophageal fistula, radial dysplasia, renal anomaly) is not.

17. **(B)** Blood in the anterior chamber almost always represents a hyphema in children. Tumors and coagulopathies can present similarly but are rare.

18. **(D)** Treatment for hyphema is supportive with bed rest and head elevation to 30 to 45 degrees to promote resorption. Steroids, both topical and oral, have been used as have topical mydriatics. Surgical drainage is not a recommended treatment.

19. **(C)** Rebleeding most often occurs 3 to 5 days after the initial bleed and can lead to other complications. The treatments discussed above are aimed at preventing rebleeding.

SUGGESTED READING
American Academy of Ophthalmology web site. Available at: www.aao.org. Last accessed 5/25/06.
Beck AD: Diagnosis and management of pediatric glaucoma. *Ophthalmol Clin North Am* 14(3):501–512, 2001.
Fallaha N: Pediatric cataracts. *Ophthalmol Clin North Am* 14(3):479–492, 2001.
Michael JG: Management of corneal abrasion in children: a randomized clinical trial. *Ann Emerg Med* 40(1):67–72, 2002.

CASE 52: A 5-YEAR-OLD BOY WITH A PAINLESS LIMP

A 5-year-old boy has come to your office today because his mother has noticed him limping for 3 to 4 days on his right leg. He does not recall any trauma to the area and has not been ill in the last month. He has had no fevers, and denies any pain in the back, hip, knee, or ankle.

On examination he is afebrile. His weight is 18 kg (50%) and the height is 39.5 inches (<5%). Upon walking across the examination room, you note an obvious limp on the right. Examination of the leg reveals no swelling, erythema, or warmth. You note that he is holding the leg in external rotation, and has discomfort and decreased range of motion on internal rotation and abduction. His knee and ankle examination are normal.

SELECT THE ONE BEST ANSWER

1. What is the most likely diagnosis?
   (A) transient synovitis
   (B) SCFE (slipped capital femoral epiphysis)
   (C) Legg-Calvé-Perthes disease
   (D) septic arthritis
   (E) growing pains

2. What is the cause of this disorder?
   (A) rapid growth
   (B) dislocation of femoral head
   (C) bacterial invasion of the femoral head capsule
   (D) poor blood supply to the femoral head
   (E) immature bone development

3. What is the best test to order first?
   (A) CBC with differential
   (B) ultrasound
   (C) radiograph
   (D) CT scan
   (E) MRI

4. If a radiograph of the hips is normal, what is the best course of action at this time for this 5-year-old boy?
   (A) brace
   (B) serial casting
   (C) surgical correction
   (D) observation
   (E) physical therapy

5. A 6-year-old boy is brought in for a painful limp of 2 days' duration on the left side. He recalls no trauma to the affected leg and has only been getting mild relief with nonsteroidal anti-inflammatory compounds. His recent medical history includes a "viral illness" several weeks ago and an increased temperature of 100°F (37.7°C) each day. On examination you note that he holds the left hip in a flexed, externally rotated position,

and he has pain on internal rotation. There is no erythema or warmth over the area.

What is the most likely diagnosis?

(A) transient synovitis or septic arthritis
(B) SCFE (slipped capital femoral epiphysis)
(C) Legg-Calvé-Perthes disease
(D) growing pains
(E) none of the above

6. Which of the following tests would be most helpful to make a diagnosis for the patient in question 5?

(A) radiographs
(B) CBC
(C) ESR
(D) synovial fluid aspirate with Gram stain and culture of the fluid obtained
(E) MRI

7. A 14-year-old boy is in your office for a sports physical examination for football and on questioning admits that he has had a limp for about 1 month that he insists is a result of a "pulled muscle" that occurred during a workout session. He complains of intermittent pain in his right knee and thigh. He has been afebrile and has been able to play sports, although there is pain with activity.

On examination his BMI is 31 kg/m² (>95%). His musculoskeletal examination is significant for his right leg that is held in external rotation. He has pain in the right hip on internal rotation. He is able to weight bear, but walks with a limp on the right. What is the most likely diagnosis?

(A) inguinal hernia
(B) SCFE (slipped capital femoral epiphysis)
(C) Legg-Calvé-Perthes disease
(D) septic arthritis
(E) growing pains

8. Which of the following is true of the disorder described in question 7?

(A) It has equal incidence in males and females.
(B) It is more common in overweight or obese adolescents.
(C) It is more common in rapidly growing adolescents.

(D) It is almost always bilateral.
(E) B and C

9. What is the most appropriate way to treat the disorder described in question 7?

(A) rest and ice compresses
(B) NSAIDs
(C) surgical pinning
(D) serial casting
(E) observation

10. In a sports physical examination performed on a 14-year-old soccer-playing male, you are told about pain below the knee that worsens without other symptoms when he is playing soccer. On physical examination he has a hard prominence over the tibial tubercle that is tender on palpation. The rest of his examination is normal. What is your diagnosis?

(A) osteosarcoma
(B) Osgood-Schlatter disease
(C) septic arthritis
(D) patellofemoral stress syndrome
(E) stress fracture

11. What other physical examination findings might there be in question 7?

(A) kinee effusion
(B) tight quadriceps and/or hamstring muscle(s)
(C) diminished deep tendon reflexes
(D) B and C
(E) none of the above

12. What is the best treatment for the patient's problem in question 10?

(A) brace
(B) surgical correction
(C) rest and NSAID
(D) corticosteroid injection
(E) no treatment is indicated

13. During a sports physical examination of a 10-year-old girl, you note mild lateral asymmetry of her thoracic spine on standing, and moderate to severe asymmetry of her posterior chest on forward bending. She is Tanner 2 breast, Tanner 1 pubic hair. What is the next appropriate action?

(A) observation and re-examination next year
(B) surgical consultation for back brace placement
(C) physical therapy
(D) AP radiographs
(E) PA radiographs

14. Which of the following is associated with congenital scoliosis?

   (A) horseshoe kidney
   (B) hip dysplasia
   (C) spinal dysraphism
   (D) congenital heart disease
   (E) all of the above

15. At what age should girls begin to have scoliosis screening examinations?

   (A) 2 years
   (B) 5 years
   (C) 7 years
   (D) 12 years
   (E) 15 years

16. Greater than what Cobb angle is a patient likely to develop pulmonary problems because of their scoliosis?

   (A) 10 degrees
   (B) 20 degrees
   (C) 40 degrees
   (D) 60 degrees
   (E) 80 degrees

17. Which of the following is true of kyphosis in adolescents?

   (A) It is usually postural.
   (B) Therapy is exercise to strengthen abdominal muscles.
   (C) Kyphosis corrects with hyperextension.
   (D) Patients have normal radiographs.
   (E) All of the above.

18. What distinguishes postural kyphosis from Scheuermann's kyphosis in adolescents?

   (A) etiology
   (B) examination
   (C) radiographic findings
   (D) treatment
   (E) all of the above

Answers

1. **(C)** This is the classic presentation of Legg-Calvé-Perthes disease, a disorder of the femoral head that causes a "painless limp" in prepubertal, immature children, 2 to 12 years old (mean, 7 years old). There is a predilection for boys (4 to 5:1). It is sometimes associated with delayed bone age, disproportionate growth, and short stature, as in this boy's case.

2. **(D)** A poor blood supply to the femoral head causes avascular necrosis, the cause of which is unknown.

3. **(C)** AP and lateral (frog) views are the gold standard for diagnosis. Often the radiographs are normal, although several groups have developed diagnostic criteria that depend on the degree of growth cessation of the capital femoral epiphysis, presence of any subchondral fracture, and degree of resorption and reossification.

4. **(D)** Observation is the rule in children younger than 6 years old (possibly younger than 5 years old for girls), unless there is significant deformity of the capital femoral epiphysis on the radiographs. If pain is present, temporary physical therapy and bedrest may be in order.

5. **(A)** Transient synovitis and septic arthritis can be difficult to differentiate without further testing. Both usually present with a unilateral, painful limp and often with fever. Transient synovitis is the most common cause of nontraumatic hip pain in children. It is an inflammatory process that often follows viral illness, although no specific virus has been implicated. The painful limp can be acute or gradual and is usually unilateral.

6. **(D)** Although hematologic abnormalities (increased leukocyte count and band count) are similar in both, the ESR is more often elevated with septic arthritis, but it is nonspecific. The serum CRP, on the other hand, is more reliably complete in a patient with a septic joint. Radiographs may show effusion in either illness and MRI is not indicated although ultrasonography may be helpful. A positive culture from a joint aspirate remains the gold standard for diagnosing septic arthritis.

7. **(B)** This is the classic presentation of SCFE (slipped capital femoral epiphysis), i.e., a painful limp in an obese pubertal male. The patient may complain of pain in the hip, thigh, or knee but on examination holds the leg in external rotation.

8. **(E)** SCFE is more common in obese or rapidly growing pubertal males. It is bilateral 20% to 50% of the time, but even when bilateral, each side usually presents at different times.

9. **(C)** Because further slippage of the capital femoral epiphysis will occur without treatment, surgical correction is necessary. The most popular technique is pinning through the femoral head and neck to stabilize the area.

10. **(B)** Osgood-Schlatter disease is a common cause of knee pain in athletic adolescents, males more than females. It manifests as pain and sometimes swelling over the tibial tubercle that is made worse by activities that involve pressure with bending of the knee: squatting, jumping, and kneeling.

11. **(B)**

12. **(C)** NSAIDs, ice, and rest as needed are the preferred and common treatments of Osgood-Schlatter disease. Steroid injections are not advised, and overall treatment is almost always nonsurgical. Braces offer minimal support.

13. **(E)** When noting more than a mildly abnormal Adams test (forward bending to assess for posterior chest asymmetry—the screening tool for scoliosis) in a premenarchal girl, radiographic evaluation is an appropriate first step to assess the degree of severity of the scoliosis. The risk for progression of scoliosis is much greater in premenarchal girls and should be pursued more aggressively. Posterior to anterior radiographs of the thorax should be ordered to determine the Cobb angle of deviation (the angle made by the intersection of two lines drawn parallel to the uppermost and lowermost vertebrae involved in the curve). Incidentally, PA radiographs subject the breast tissue to less radiation than anterior to posterior films.

14. **(E)** Twenty percent of patients with congenital scoliosis have genitourinary defects and 15% have congenital heart disease. Other skeletal malformations are also common.

15. **(C)** Screening exams should start at 6 to 7 years old when girls are premenarchal as the risk of progression is highest at this time.

16. **(D)** An angle of ≥60 degrees is severe scoliosis and often leads to cardiopulmonary sequelae. When the angle is ≥25 degrees, observation is recommended. Between 25 degrees and 45 degrees, close follow-up, physical therapy, and occasionally a brace are sufficient treatment. When ≥45 degrees, surgical treatment is often required.

17. **(E)**

18. **(E)** Scheuermann's kyphosis is a separate clinical entity than postural kyphosis, which has a clearly understood cause and can be corrected by the patient during the examination. On radiographs of the back, Scheuermann's kyphosis has typical findings of wedging of ≥3 thoracic vertebrae and loss of the anterior height of the affected vertebrae. Patients with this disorder, when mild, require no treatment. But unlike postural kyphosis, many require brace and exercise programs.

SUGGESTED READING

Behrman RE, Kliegman RM, Jenson HB, et al: *Nelson Textbook of Pediatrics*. Philadelphia: WB Saunders, 2004, pp 2075–2089.

DeLee JC, Drez D Jr: *DeLee & Drez's Orthopaedic Sports Medicine Principles and Practice*. Philadelphia: WB Saunders, 2003, pp 1831–1835.

Kim MK: The limping child. *Clin Ped Emerg Med* 3(2): 129–137, 2002.

Sassmannshausen G: Back pain in the young athlete. *Clin Sports Med* 21(1):121–132, 2002.

CASE 53: A 4-YEAR-OLD WITH EAR PAIN

A 4-year-old boy comes to your office because of ear pain. It began the night before and woke him from sleep several times. Appropriate doses of analgesics for the pain did not help much. His mother reports temperatures as high as 102°F (38.8°C). He had a cold approximately 1 week ago that has been improving the last several days.

On examination he is afebrile. His nares have scant, clear rhinorrhea; the oropharynx is normal. His right tympanic membrane and ear canal appear normal. His left ear canal is normal, but the tympanic membrane is bulging outward and is light yellow in color with erythema around the rim. His lungs are clear to auscultation bilaterally.

SELECT THE ONE BEST ANSWER

1. Which of the following is the least likely pathogen involved in his ear pain?

   (A) *Haemophilus influenzae*
   (B) *Streptococcus pneumoniae*
   (C) influenza virus
   (D) *Moraxella catarrhalis*
   (E) chlamydia

2. Which of the following is/are risk factors for this problem?

   (A) craniofacial abnormality
   (B) exposure to smoking
   (C) formula use
   (D) gastroesophageal reflux
   (E) all of the above

3. Besides direct observation of the tympanic membrane, which of the following methods is/are helpful to diagnose otitis media?

   (A) tympanogram
   (B) radiographs of the skull
   (C) audiology/hearing test
   (D) pneumatic otoscopy
   (E) A and D

4. Which of the following tympanograms would you expect with this patient?

   (A) completely flat, high on the *y* axis (high volume)
   (B) rounded or somewhat flattened peak
   (C) sharp peak at 0 daPa
   (D) completely flat, low on the *y* axis
   (E) none of the above

5. All of the following are complications of otitis media except:

   (A) mastoiditis
   (B) pneumonia
   (C) brain abscess
   (D) meningitis
   (E) Facial palsy

6. If you choose to put him on an antibiotic, which is your FIRST choice?

   (A) azithromycin
   (B) amoxicillin-clavulanic acid
   (C) ciprofloxacin ear drops
   (D) ceftriaxone
   (E) amoxicillin

7. If he returned 3 days later because of no change in his symptoms and his examination was exactly the same, what would your next step be?

   (A) tympanocentesis
   (B) tympanogram
   (C) change antibiotic
   (D) add oral steroids
   (E) add topical ear drops

8. In which of the following scenarios would you choose observation over antibiotic treatment?

   (A) a 4-year-old with purulent effusion, limited tympanic membrane mobility, minimal pain, no fever, or other generalized symptoms
   (B) a 6-week-old with same findings as above
   (C) a 3-year-old with purulent effusion, limited tympanic membrane mobility, and severe otalgia
   (D) all of the above
   (E) none of the above

9. If you had begun a patient with unilateral acute otitis media on antibiotic therapy and he returned 1 week later, still on medication, with a new otitis media on the other side, which is your next course of action?

   (A) tympanocentesis
   (B) tympanogram
   (C) change antibiotic
   (D) add oral steroids
   (E) add topical ear drops

10. His mother calls you very worried 2 days later because he has a very high fever, 103°F (39.4°C) axillary, and it appears that his "ear is bulging outward." What is his likely diagnosis?

    (A) otitis media with perforation
    (B) subdural abscess
    (C) acute mastoiditis

(D) meningitis

(E) foreign body

11. Of the following choices, what is the next best action for the case in question 10?

(A) admission for additional evaluation and IV antibiotics

(B) change to a stronger oral antibiotic

(C) tympanostomy tubes

(D) biopsy of mastoid

(E) course of oral steroids

12. Which of the following is NOT an indication for tympanocentesis?

(A) otitis media in an immune-compromised patient

(B) acute otitis media and temperature of 102.6°F (39.2°C) in a 3-week-old

(C) mastoiditis

(D) a 2-month history of clear effusion with some conductive hearing loss

(E) failure of second-line treatment of acute otitis media

13. You see a 2-year-old child in your office for a check-up and note on examination a clear effusion with air-fluid levels behind his left tympanic membrane (TM), which is mobile on pneumatic otoscopy. He has no ear pain, fever, or other symptoms. What is your diagnosis?

(A) otitis media

(B) recurrent otitis media

(C) resistant otitis media

(D) otitis media with effusion

(E) chronic serous otitis

14. You see the 2-year-old from question 13 back in your office 3 months later with the same physical findings and still no symptoms. His parents note that he seems to say "what" a lot when they are talking to him. What is your next action?

(A) no testing

(B) audiology referral for hearing test

(C) antibiotics

(D) speech therapy

(E) tympanostomy tubes

15. You see an 8-year-old for ear pain that she has had for 4 days straight. She had a cold last week, but most of the congestion and cough has resolved. She has had no fevers, no drainage from the ear, and analgesics help the pain minimally. On examination her tympanic membrane appears retracted, and your in-office tympanogram shows a flattened peak between 200 and 0 daPa. What is her diagnosis?

(A) otitis externa

(B) otitis media

(C) otitis media with effusion

(D) eustachian tube dysfunction

(E) cholesteatoma

16. A 3-year-old girl with bilateral tympanostomy tube placement 6 months ago comes to you with purulent discharge from her left ear for 1 day. She has had a temperature of 102°F (38.8°C) in the last day and is eating less than her usual amount. She has no other symptoms. What is the best management of this patient?

(A) amoxicillin

(B) Augmentin

(C) topical fluoroquinolone drops

(D) topical steroid and fluoroquinolone drops

(E) oral steroids

17. What is the least likely pathogen involved in chronic suppurative otitis?

(A) *Pseudomonas aeruginosa*

(B) *Staphylococcus aureus*

(C) *Escherichia coli*

(D) *Proteus mirabilis*

(E) *S. pneumoniae*

18. All of the following are possible treatments and managements for chronic suppurative otitis media except:

(A) surgical intervention since most of these patients have a CSF leak

(B) topical antibiotics

(C) close observation

(D) oral antibiotics

(E) hearing evaluation

Answers

1. **(E)** Tympanocentesis studies have revealed the etiology of otitis media to be *S. pneumoniae* in 20% to

35% of cases, *H. influenzae* in 20% to 30%, *M. catarrhalis* in 20%, no isolate in 20% to 30%, and a virus in 17% to 44%. *Chlamydia* species are not believed to be common causes of acute otitis media, although in several studies *Chlamydia* species have been identified by tympanocentesis culture in children with otitis media with effusion.

2. **(E)** Smoking, reflux, and craniofacial abnormalities, especially cleft lip, put children at increased risk for acute otitis media (children with cleft lip have recurrent otitis). Multiple studies have shown that infants fed formula have a higher rate of otitis media than breast-fed infants. It is likely both in part to reflect a protective effect of the breast milk and the practice of "propping" bottles up.

3. **(E)** Radiographs have no role in diagnosing otitis media and a hearing test may indeed be abnormal, but will not help the practitioner distinguish between acute otitis media, otitis media with effusion, or other forms of conductive hearing loss.

4. **(B)** Tympanograms estimate air pressure and volume of the middle ear space. The normal pressure, or compliance, of a healthy tympanic membrane fluctuates from –200 to +200 daPa when a tone, sound energy, is applied to it. A graph is produced with air pressure on the *x* axis and volume on the *y* axis. A tympanogram of a normal middle ear space should have a high peak at atmospheric pressure (0 on the graph). The pressure should range from –200 to +200 daPa. With middle ear effusion of any cause, there is some mobility of the TM, but it is dampened, producing a rounded curve instead of a sharp peak and often more negative middle ear pressures.

   With eustachian tube dysfunction (most commonly secondary to a cold or sinusitis), there is negative pressure in the middle ear space compared with the nasopharynx, and so middle ear pressures are in the more extreme negative range, –400 to –200 daPa. With a perforated tympanic membrane, the ear canal and the middle ear are at the same pressure, so that applying a force to the ear canal produces a flat tracing, often with high volume (higher on the *y* curve).

5. **(B)** Mastoiditis, brain abscess, and meningitis are all possible complications of acute otitis media (AOM), either through direct extension or hematogenous spread. Facial nerve palsy occurs because of its proximity to the middle ear on its anatomical course.

6. **(E)** Despite growing resistance of the major otitis pathogens to penicillin and amoxicillin, amoxicillin is still the first choice for treatment. Low-dose amoxicillin (45 mg/kg/d) is no longer used and so-called high dose (90 mg/kg/d) should be instituted. Amoxicillin-clavulanic acid (Augmentin) should be reserved for resistant or recurrent OM that has been clinically refractory to high-dose amoxicillin previously. Cephalosporins, either ceftriaxone IM for 3 days, or an oral second or third generation, should be reserved for penicillin-allergic patients, as should azithromycin. Ear drops play no role in the management of acute otitis media, unless there is a perforation in the tympanic membrane, in which case recent studies have shown similar benefit with antibiotic- and steroid-containing drops versus oral amoxicillin.

7. **(C)** After beginning antibiotic therapy for acute otitis media, resolution of symptoms should begin within 24 and 48 hours. In this case, it is appropriate to try a different antibiotic, since one-fourth of *S. pneumoniae* have penicillin resistance, while one-fourth to one-third of *H. influenzae* are resistant (β-lactamase positive). All *Moraxella* species are resistant because of β-lactamase production. Tympanocentesis may be helpful in guiding a change in therapy but is not the first step. A tympanogram will not give any extra knowledge. Steroids have no role in otitis media.

8. **(A)** The most recent guidelines for management of acute otitis media recommend observation for children with uncomplicated otitis—no high fever or severe pain. Otitis in a 6-week-old always requires treatment, follow-up, and sometimes further workup.

9. **(C)** In this case it also is appropriate to try a different antibiotic, for the same reasons as in answer 7.

10. **(C)** This is the clinical picture of acute mastoiditis, which is a complication of otitis media. Offending organisms are usually *S. pneumoniae*, *S.*

pyogenes, S. aureus, Pseudomonas species, and *H. influenzae.* Sixty percent of mastoiditis occurs in children younger than 2 years old. Clinical findings include fever, point tenderness and fluctuance over the mastoid, prominence of the pinna, and usually otitis media. Incidentally, all cases of uncomplicated AOM by virtue of anatomy will show some inflammation of the mastoid air cells. Beyond that, when the infection spreads to the overlying periosteum but *not* the underlying bone, the diagnosis is acute mastoiditis. Spread to the underlying bone constitutes acute mastoid osteitis, a more urgent surgical case.

11. **(A)** All cases of suspected mastoiditis should first be confirmed by CT of the temporal bone to distinguish between acute mastoiditis and mastoid osteitis. For acute mastoiditis, myringotomy and parenteral antibiotics are the next step.

12. **(D)** Otitis media in young infants who have systemic symptoms should warrant tympanocentesis as part of the sepsis workup. Two months of clear effusion is otitis media with effusion and is not deserving of tympanocentesis in this time frame.

13. **(D)** Because of the lack of purulent fluid, outward bulging of the TM, and the presence of a freely mobile TM, all other answers are excluded.

14. **(B)** An otitis media with effusion is considered "persistent" when it has been present for 4 months or more. At 3 to 4 months after diagnosis, if no resolution or improvement is seen, a hearing test is the next appropriate step, especially if clinical hearing loss is still evident and not resolving. A conductive hearing loss would likely be found.

15. **(D)** Eustachian tube dysfunction is common in the weeks following an upper respiratory infection. The only finding on examination is a retracted TM, and symptomatically the child may complain of frequent popping, pain, or pressure. Various OTC remedies have been employed against this, including pseudoephedrine and nasal saline sprays.

16. **(A)** Recent studies have proven that topical eardrops that are a combination of antibiotics and steroids are equivalent if not superior in eradicating otitis media with tympanostomy tubes. However, use of quinolones in this fashion encourages antimicrobial resistance and should be therefore avoided.

17. **(A)** *P. aeruginosa* in the absence of a perforated eardrum and otorrhea is a rare cause of otitis media.

18. **(C)** Surgery may be required if there is an anatomical defect that is acting as a continued bacterial medium, i.e., cholesteatoma. Observation is not an acceptable treatment plan, as hearing loss often ensues with chronic OM and worsens with time.

SUGGESTED READING

Behrman RE, Kliegman RM, Jenson HB, et al: *Nelson Textbook of Pediatrics.* Philadelphia: WB Saunders, 2004, pp 1938–1963.
Hendley JO: Otitis media. *N Engl J Med* 347:1169–1174, 2002.

CASE 54: A 14-YEAR-OLD BOY WITH A SORE THROAT AND ENLARGED SPLEEN

A 14-year-old boy comes into your office complaining of sore throat of 1 week's duration. It is getting worse by the day, and this morning he felt as if he could not swallow his breakfast, both because of the pain on swallowing and because it felt as if something was "blocking it down there." He has been feeling hot and cold but has not measured his temperature. He is feeling fatigued, but the rest of his review of systems is negative. He has had multiple episodes of "tonsillitis" this year.

On examination, he is cooperative, but appears quite tired. His temperature is 101.5°F (38.6°C) orally; the other vital signs are normal. His conjunctivae are clear, tympanic membranes are normal, and oropharynx is quite erythematous, with enlarged erythematous tonsils covered by diffuse white exudates bilaterally. No petechiae are seen. His lymphatic exam reveals anterior and posterior cervical lymphadenopathy, all 1 to 2.5 cm in diameter, mobile, and moderately tender. His lungs are clear. The cardiovascular examination is normal, and the abdominal examination reveals a palpable spleen tip 4 cm under the rib cage. There is no rash.

SELECT THE ONE BEST ANSWER

1. What is his most likely diagnosis?

   (A) streptococcal pharyngitis
   (B) viral upper respiratory tract infection
   (C) adenoviral pharyngotonsillitis
   (D) mononucleosis
   (E) peritonsillar abscess

2. What kind of microorganism most likely caused this infection?

   (A) gram-positive coccus
   (B) enterovirus
   (C) herpesvirus
   (D) echovirus
   (E) Coxsackie virus

3. Which of the following is NOT associated with this patient's disease?

   (A) Guillain-Barré syndrome
   (B) maculopapular dermatitis
   (C) pharyngoconjunctival fever
   (D) transient thrombocytopenic purpura
   (E) bilateral orchitis

4. During what time of year is this illness most common?

   (A) spring
   (B) summer
   (C) fall
   (D) winter
   (E) no seasonal association

5. What is the incubation period of this illness?

   (A) 1 to 4 days
   (B) 4 to 7 days
   (C) 7 to 14 days
   (D) 14 to 28 days
   (E) 30 to 50 days

6. What is the best specimen to diagnose this disease?

   (A) sputum
   (B) oropharyngeal secretions
   (C) blood
   (D) urine
   (E) stool

7. If this is infectious mononucleosis caused by EBV, what is the most timely test(s) to support the diagnosis?

   (A) EBV titers
   (B) complete blood count
   (C) throat culture
   (D) Monospot test to detect heterophil antibody
   (E) nasal swab

8. If you found that this patient had mononucleosis, what is your treatment?

   (A) no treatment
   (B) oral steroids
   (C) amoxicillin
   (D) ceftriaxone
   (E) azithromycin

9. Under which age does the Monospot test to detect heterophil antibody lose its sensitivity?

   (A) 1 year
   (B) 2 years
   (C) 4 years
   (D) 8 years
   (E) 10 years

10. Another child who was thought to have mononucleosis had the following test results:

    IgG to viral capsid antigen (VCA) +
    IgM to VCA –
    Early antigen (EA) –
    Antibody against EBNA (EBV nuclear antigen) +

    What can be deduced from these results?

    (A) no present or past EBV infection
    (B) definite past infection
    (C) acutely infected
    (D) either past infection or recent infection
    (E) none of the above

11. How long does infection with EBV last?

    (A) 1 month
    (B) 6 months
    (C) 1 year
    (D) 2 years
    (E) lifelong

12. The most reasonable indication for treating mononucleosis with steroids is:

(A) severe splenomegaly
(B) severe pain from sore throat
(C) severe airway obstruction
(D) hemolytic anemia
(E) myocarditis

13. A patient with mononucleosis and splenomegaly should be advised to avoid contact sports for at least how long?

    (A) 1 to 2 weeks
    (B) 3 weeks to 6 months
    (C) 1 year
    (D) life
    (E) none of the above—no recommendation to avoid contact sports.

14. The 14-year-old boy from the vignette calls you 10 days after you saw him in your office and diagnosed him with mononucleosis. He now has a fever of 103.2°F (39.5°C), cannot swallow, and feels that he cannot open his mouth easily. You see him hours later in the office and you note that his voice is quite muffled. On examination his temperature is 100.6°F (38.1°C) (he took acetaminophen 2 hours prior). The BP is 110/65. He cannot open his mouth wide, but on minimal opening you note white exudates covering both tonsils, marked tonsillar enlargement, right greater than left, and a visible bulge at the superior aspect of the right tonsil.
    What is his diagnosis?

    (A) secondary strep pharyngitis
    (B) peritonsillar abscess
    (C) retropharyngeal abscess
    (D) *Mycoplasma pneumoniae* cellulitis
    (E) *Corynebacterium diphtheriae*

15. Which of the following should be part of his overall management?

    (A) IV clindamycin
    (B) surgical incision and drainage
    (C) IV ampicillin
    (D) tonsillectomy
    (E) A, B, and D

16. Which of the following is NOT a relative indication for tonsillectomy?

(A) more than 8 episodes of viral pharyngitis in 1 year
(B) more than 6 episodes of group A streptococcal pharyngitis in 1 year
(C) acute airway obstruction concurrent with peritonsillar abscess
(D) peritonsillar abscess following recurrent tonsillitis
(E) obstructive sleep apnea

17. A patient's mother is worried about the complications of tonsillectomy. Which of the following is not a known complication?

    (A) velopharyngeal insufficiency
    (B) hemorrhage
    (C) sinusitis
    (D) eustachian tube injury
    (E) dehydration

18. Adenoidectomy is potentially beneficial in all of the following except:

    (A) chronic recurrent sinusitis
    (B) hyponasal speech
    (C) hypernasal speech
    (D) submucous cleft palate
    (E) excessive snoring

Answers

1. **(D)** The most likely diagnosis for this boy is mononucleosis because of his age, presenting symptoms, and examination. Mononucleosis can present with a wide range of severity, but the majority of cases include fever that averages 6 days' duration, exudative pharyngitis, lymphadenopathy that is most often anterior and posterior cervical but can be generalized, fatigue, and hepatosplenomegaly in 50% of patients.

2. **(C)** Seventy-nine percent of infectious mononucleosis syndromes are caused by EBV, one in the family of Herpesviruses. The other 21% are caused by CMV. Sore throat with exudative tonsillitis is more common with EBV than CMV mononucleosis, while fever is a predominant feature of CMV mononucleosis. With CMV, the heterophil agglutinin test (Monospot test) is negative.

3. (C) Pharyngoconjunctival fever is associated with adenovirus.

4. (E)

5. (E)

6. (C) Despite the location of the physical findings of mononucleosis, often centered in the oropharynx, blood is the most useful specimen because serologic testing will produce a more timely diagnosis. Viral culture is possible by pharyngeal swab, but is performed in only a few laboratories and may be positive for many years after acute infection.

7. (D) The EBV heterophil antibody, which is largely IgM, rises in the second week of illness, disappears by 6 months, and identifies approximately 90% of cases in children. Even though a single EBV serology determination might give you helpful information, often repeat testing for convalescent serology is necessary, and thus, this serologic approach may not be timely. A CBC with an absolute lymphocytosis in the second week of illness is supportive of the diagnosis. Throat cultures for viral isolation do not necessarily indicate acute infection in any disease where viral persistence is common.

8. (A) Since mononucleosis has a viral etiology (EBV), no antibacterial therapy is warranted. A high percent of patients with mononucleosis who are exposed to ampicillin or amoxicillin develop a nonallergic morbilliform rash. Penicillin is an acceptable alternative if antibacterial therapy is indicated. Ten percent to 30% of patients with mononucleosis are concomitantly group A strep positive; the treatment of the latter can complicate the diagnosis of the former. Steroids should only be considered in severe cases of mononucleosis.

9. (C) Children younger than 4 years of age may have EBV infectious mononucleosis but lack heterophil antibodies. The reason is not known. If infectious mononucleosis is suspected in these young children, EBV serology should be performed.

10. (D) The VCA (viral capsid antigen) IgM and IgG occur in high titers early after infection begins. The IgM response lasts for 3 to 5 months and IgG can be detected indefinitely. The EA likewise is positive in the first 2 weeks of infection and peaks at about 3 months. It is important to note that if tested too early, the EA and the IgM VCA may not yet be positive. EBNA antibodies are not present until several weeks to months after onset of infection. So, while a positive EBNA result excludes acute infection, it cannot differentiate between recent or past infection.

11. (E) EBV, like other herpesviruses, establishes lifelong, latent infection. As opposed to the other herpesviruses, reinfection with EBV is usually asymptomatic.

12. (C) There are few objective data that document the effectiveness of corticosteroids in infectious mononucleosis. Many clinicians use them in the management of impending or actual airway obstructions. They should otherwise be avoided as unnecessary therapy that may even increase the rate of occurrence of certain complications like encephalitis. Severe pain may be treated adequately with other medications.

13. (B) Splenic enlargement is common in mononucleosis, but splenic rupture is rare (0.1% to 0.2%). Rupture most commonly occurs within the first 3 weeks following diagnosis. Athletes are sometimes counseled to wait up to 6 months before resuming contact sports. At the time of activity resumption, neither the spleen nor the liver should be palpable.

14. (B) Although peritonsillar abscesses are most often complications of group A streptococcal pharyngitis, EBV infectious mononucleosis and group A streptococci are commonly simultaneously present. This patient has fever, trismus, and an obvious bulge, the triad of which makes the diagnosis.

15. (E) In addition to standard treatment of peritonsillar abscess, parenteral antibiotics, and surgical drainage, this patient is a candidate for tonsillectomy because of his history of recurrent tonsillitis. This would be performed after the acute episode resolves. Ampicillin is an unwise choice because of the known increase in the incidence of rash when patients with mononucleosis are given ampicillin or derivatives. This rash does not represent ampicillin allergy. It presents as a maculopapular pruritic confluent rash mainly over the trunk and includes the palms and soles.

16. **(A)** Viral pharyngitis is never an indication for tonsillectomy. Repeated bacterial infection of the tonsils may be, although the number of infections per year that warrant tonsillectomy is controversial. Some recommend it when there are >3 episodes per year, others wait for >6 per year, and yet others await >3 episodes a year for 3 consecutive years. Other reasons for performing tonsillectomy are obstructive sleep apnea or, rarely, acute airway obstruction.

17. **(C)** In addition to those listed above, complications of tonsillectomy include risks of anesthesia, infection, and atlantoaxial subluxation. Velopharyngeal insufficiency may occur because tonsillectomy increases the space in the nasopharynx leading to inability of the nasopharyngeal sphincter to close properly, causing hypernasal speech and regurgitation. The incidence of these complications is increased in children with craniofacial abnormalities or orofacial problems, such as Down, Treacher-Collins, and Pierre-Robin syndromes.

18. **(C)** Hyponasal speech is an indication for adenoidectomy, not hypernasal. Children with cleft palate and submucous cleft palate should have preventive adenoidectomy performed. Excessive snoring is a likely sign of chronic adenoid hypertrophy. A patient with excessive snoring should undergo further evaluation to determine whether adenoidectomy may be beneficial.

SUGGESTED READING

Behrman RE, Kliegman RM, Jenson HB, et al: *Nelson Textbook of Pediatrics.* Philadelphia: WB Saunders, 2004, pp 1266–1268.

Discolo CM: Infectious indications for tonsillectomy. *Pediatr Clin North Am* 50(2):445–458, 2003.

Gross, CW, Harrison, SE: Tonsils and adenoids. *Pediatr Rev* 21(3):75–78, 2000.

Pickering LK et al: *Red Book 2003 Report of the Committee on Infectious Diseases.* Elk Grove Village, IL: American Academy of Pediatrics, 2003, pp 190–192, 271–273.

CASE 55: A 5-YEAR-OLD WITH NOSEBLEEDS

A 5-year-old is brought for evaluation during winter by his mother because of recurrent nosebleeds. They happen between one and three times a week, last 10 minutes, and are difficult to stop. This has been going on for about 6 weeks.

SELECT THE ONE BEST ANSWER

1. All of the following would prompt you to explore the etiology of this boy's nosebleeds except:

    (A) duration of ≥10 minutes
    (B) family history of bleeding disorder
    (C) age younger than 2 years
    (D) low hematocrit on screening
    (E) gum bleeding

2. The differential diagnosis for recurrent epistaxis in an adolescent includes which of the following malignancies?

    (A) squamous cell carcinoma
    (B) adenocarcinoma
    (C) nasopharyngeal angiofibroma
    (D) malignant melanoma
    (E) nasal lymphoma

3. An 8-year-old girl with a history of seasonal allergic rhinitis comes in during the fall because she is "always congested." Her regular OTC allergy medicine is not working. She feels the congestion is getting worse each week and is worse on the left side.

    On examination you note allergic shiners, an allergic salute sign, mild conjunctival injection bilaterally, and a 0.75 cm soft gray bulge in the left nare, adjacent to the septum. There is some clear rhinorrhea, no foul smell, and no bleeding. What is her most likely diagnosis?

    (A) foreign body
    (B) nasal polyp
    (C) sinusitis
    (D) juvenile nasopharyngeal angiofibroma
    (E) hematoma

4. Which chronic diseases is the problem in question 3 associated with?

    (A) chronic sinusitis
    (B) asthma
    (C) cystic fibrosis

(D) aspirin sensitivity

(E) all of the above

5. What are possible treatments used for nasal polyps?

(A) intranasal steroids

(B) antihistamines and decongestants

(C) surgical removal

(D) oral steroids

(E) A, C, and D

6. A 6-year-old boy comes to your office in August with a "runny nose." His mother states that it has been going on for approximately 3 weeks and is not improving. He has been afebrile but has a nonproductive cough each night.

What findings would lead you to diagnose him with allergic rhinitis?

(A) cobblestoning of the posterior pharynx

(B) dark circles under both eyes

(C) pale, blue turbinates

(D) a horizontal indentation across the bridge of the nose

(E) all of the above

7. Which of the following is *not* a comorbid disorder of allergic rhinitis?

(A) speech impairment

(B) eczema

(C) failure to thrive

(D) otitis externa

(E) pharyngitis

8. Which of the following is *false* regarding allergic rhinitis?

(A) Prevalence peaks in adolescents.

(B) Its incidence is increasing.

(C) Higher socioeconomic status is a risk factor.

(D) Serum IgE >100 IU/mL in childhood is a risk factor.

(E) Early introduction to solid foods in infancy is a risk factor.

9. You see a new patient in your office who is 1 week old. He is there for his preventive 1-week visit. His medical history is significant for a cleft lip and palate, and no other known conditions.

All of the following are true regarding cleft lip and palate except:

(A) cleft lip is more common in males

(B) cleft lip alone is more common than cleft palate alone

(C) cleft lip and palate are inherited in an autosomal dominant pattern

(D) sensorineural hearing loss is common with cleft palate

(E) all of the above are true

10. Which of the following statements is *false*?

(A) The most immediate problem facing a child with an uncomplicated cleft lip is feeding difficulties.

(B) Surgical closure of a cleft lip is usually performed in the first 3 months of life.

(C) Surgical closure of a cleft palate is usually performed by age 1 year.

(D) Children with uncomplicated cleft lip do not require subspecialist involvement with the exception of the surgical repair.

(E) Often children with cleft palate require prophylactic tympanostomy tubes.

11. Which of the following syndromes are associated with cleft lip and/or palate?

(A) histiocytosis

(B) TAR syndrome

(C) CATCH 22 syndrome

(D) Waardenburg syndrome

(E) all of the above

12. You see a 1-month-old child in your office for a preventive visit. You note on examination that the infant is at the 80th percentile for height and weight and is developing well. She is breast-fed and her mother reports that it is going "well." You note on examination that she has a very short lingual frenulum. What will you recommend to her mother be done?

(A) nothing

(B) surgical correction

(C) cease breast-feeding

(D) early speech therapy

(E) oral motor physical therapy

13. The mother from question 12 asks you about when her 1-month-old might start to develop teeth. What can you tell her?

(A) most often by 2 months
(B) most often by 3 months
(C) most often by 4 months
(D) most often between 4 and 5 months
(E) most often between 6 and 12 months

14. At a child's 2-year routine visit, the mother asks how she can help prevent dental cavities in her child. You recommend:

    (A) using fluoride-containing toothpaste
    (B) flossing regularly and a low-sugar diet
    (C) discontinuing sleeping with the bottle
    (D) B and C
    (E) all of the above

15. Which of the following is the main etiology of dental caries?

    (A) *S. pyogenes*
    (B) *S. viridans*
    (C) *S. mutans*
    (D) *S. pneumoniae*
    (E) *Enterococcus* species

16. Which of the following are associated with delayed dentition?

    (A) Down syndrome
    (B) hypothyroidism
    (C) hypopituitarism
    (D) rickets
    (E) all of the above

17. Which of the following is *true* regarding fluoride use in children?

    (A) It is recommended starting at 1 month of age.
    (B) There is no risk to fluoride use.
    (C) The dosage is dependent on where the patient lives.
    (D) Patients with gastroesophageal reflux do not require extra fluoride.
    (E) Fluoride does *not* slow the decay process.

18. A mother calls you frantically on the phone because her 7-year-old has "knocked an adult tooth out" by getting hit in the face with a baseball. He initially cried hysterically but is now calm. She has the tooth in her hand and is wondering what to do next. Which of the following is the *best* action for her to take?

    (A) Vigorously scrub the tooth and reinsert it at home.
    (B) Gently rinse the tooth and reinsert it as soon as possible.
    (C) Immediately transport the tooth in water and the patient to the dentist.
    (D) Immediately transport the tooth in milk and the patient to the dentist.
    (E) Wait at least 24 hours before having the tooth reinserted; keep it on ice in the meantime.

Answers

1. **(A)** The duration of epistaxis that should prompt further workup is 30 minutes. Most nosebleeds can be stopped sooner, if proper technique is used—blowing the nose first, tilting the head forward, followed by firm and constant pressure just below the bridge of the nose for a minimum of 5 minutes. Children younger than 2 years old should be evaluated further because epistaxis in this age group is rare, and because most epistaxis in children is secondary to self-inflicted trauma (vigorous nose rubbing or picking).

2. **(C)** Nasopharyngeal angiofibromas occur in children and 30- to 40-year-old adults but have a peak incidence in adolescent males. They present with nasal obstruction and recurrent epistaxis. A CT of the relevant structures can define the extent of the tumor. Surgical excision is universally performed.

3. **(B)** Nasal polyps are benign pedunculated tumors of the nasal mucosa that are associated with multiple chronic diseases. Presentation includes nasal obstruction, hyponasal speech, rhinorrhea, and mouth breathing.

4. **(E)** Approximately 30% of children with cystic fibrosis develop nasal polyps. In any child younger than 12 years old in whom nasal polyps are diagnosed, regardless of other risk factors, sweat testing for CF should be performed. All the other diseases listed are associated with nasal polyps, including the Samter triad of aspirin sensitivity, nasal polyps, and asthma.

5. **(E)** Besides surgical removal, steroids are the most successful treatment for nasal polyps. Intra-

nasal steroids should be tried first, and systemic steroids are an alternative depending on the severity of disease. Neither antihistamines nor decongestants will shrink a polyp, although they may provide symptomatic relief from associated illnesses, such as allergic rhinitis.

6. **(E)** The "allergic salute" (rubbing the nose upward) causes a long-term crease across the bridge, which is indicative of chronic allergic rhinitis. "Allergic shiners" are dark circles under the eyes, caused by repeated lid edema. Postnasal drip eventually leads to a cobblestoned appearance in the posterior pharynx.

7. **(D)** Otitis media with effusion is associated with allergic rhinitis, not otitis externa.

8. **(A)** The prevalence of allergic rhinitis peaks in late childhood. The incidence of allergic rhinitis is increasing, especially in affluent societies. Risk factors include high socioeconomic status, high IgE in childhood, family history of atopy, heavy indoor allergen concentrations, mothers who smoke near their children in the first year of life, and early introduction of solids in infancy. This last risk factor has led to the more recent recommendation by the American Academy of Pediatrics that solid food not be started until infants are 6 months old.

9. **(D)** Cleft lip with or without associated cleft palate is present in 1 in 750 Caucasian births; cleft palate alone is present in 1 in 2500 Caucasian births. It is more common in males, and can be inherited dominantly in Van der Woude syndrome. It has the highest incidence ethnically in Asians, and lowest in African Americans. Conductive hearing loss is commonly associated with cleft palate but not sensorineural hearing loss.

10. **(D)** From birth, a team of services should be alerted and develop a management plan for the child with the family. These would likely include, but are not limited to, a pediatrician, an otolaryngologist, a pediatric dentist, a speech therapist, a geneticist, and a social worker, and/or psychologist.

11. **(C)** CATCH 22 syndrome includes *c*ardiac, *ab*normal facies, *t*hymic hypoplasia, *c*left palate,

and *h*ypocalcemia. TAR syndrome is *t*hrombocytopenia and *a*bsent *r*adii. Waardenburg syndrome, or partial albinism, includes acrocephaly, facial dysmorphism (not cleft lip or palate), ocular problems, deafness, and abnormal dentition.

12. **(A)** Ankyloglossia, or "tongue tie," is an abnormally short lingual frenulum. In the majority of children, the frenulum grows with them and does not cause any difficulties. In some, feeding trouble ensues in early infancy because of restricted extension of the tongue. These children should see a general pediatric surgeon early on and be counseled regarding surgical correction, especially if they are failing to gain weight appropriately. In others, speech difficulties arise later on. The majority of such speech-delayed children still do not require surgery but will benefit from speech therapy.

13. **(E)** Most often children start eruption of their primary teeth at 6 months and continue until 22 months. Primary eruption can be as early as 4 months but more often occurs after 6 months.

14. **(E)** Dental caries are one of the most common chronic diseases of childhood. Caused by bacterial overgrowth and stagnation in the oral cavity, caries can be prevented by several means, including all of the given choices. Fluoride-containing toothpaste is generally recommended starting at 2 years of age, at a time when children can begin to spit out the paste after use (the danger being an overdose of fluoride if too much is used at an early age and the child swallows it all). Sucrose is the most likely carbohydrate involved in caries formation and is contained in sweetened drinks that children often start drinking at a young age today.

15. **(C)**

16. **(E)**

17. **(C)** Fluoridation of water has been one of the most successful public health steps to prevent dental infections in children. Recommendations were made in the 1950s and 1960s to add fluoride to public drinking water, and, since then, the rate of caries has dropped 50% to 70%. Additional supplementation is usually not needed, as

the majority of public drinking water today contains adequate fluoride levels (>0.3 ppm), but in some cases supplements are required, starting at 6 months of age. The amount needed varies by how much is in the water. Careful prescribing is in order as fluoride overdose can lead to severe staining of permanent teeth. Patients with some diseases where tooth enamel can be destroyed, such as severe gastroesophageal reflux and bulimia, require fluoride supplements even if drinking fluoridated water.

18. **(B)** If the child was calm and cooperative, the best thing for the parent to do is to gently rinse the tooth and reinsert it at home, then go to the dentist's office. Avulsed teeth should never be scrubbed or scratched. If the child were not calm enough to gently reinsert the tooth, the parent should bring the tooth to the dentist as soon as possible to reinsert. The tooth should be transported in an isotonic solution—saline, lactated Ringer's, or milk. Teeth left out more than 1 hour have a poor prognosis for reinsertion. Primary teeth should not be reimplanted.

SUGGESTED READING

Behrman RE, Kliegman RM, Jenson HB, et al: *Nelson Textbook of Pediatrics*. Philadelphia, WB Saunders, 2004, pp 1111–1113, 1260–1261, 1362.

Kirschner RE: Cleft lip and palate. *Otolaryngol Clin North Am* 33(6):1191–1215, 2000.

Lack G: Pediatric allergic rhinitis and comorbid disorders. *J Allergy Clin Immunol* 108:S9–S15, 2001.

Martof A: Consultation with the specialist: Dental care. *Pediatr Rev* 22(1):13–15, 2001.

CASE 56: 4-YEAR-OLD GIRL WITH "PINK EYE"

A 4-year-old girl comes in with eye swelling of 3 days' duration. She is a new patient and has brought her old records with her. Her mother confirms that she has had no immunizations, based on parental refusal. The girl is rubbing at her eye a lot, and it is red and puffy. Her mother says that she thinks her daughter "has pink eye" and saw a doctor at another office several weeks ago for it. At that time she was congested and had a cough, and was sent home with no medication.

On examination you note that she is afebrile and slightly fussy. She has 2 cm of erythema and edema surrounding the right eye and it is very tender. She is

able to follow your finger in all directions and has no proptosis. Her nose, throat, and lung examinations are normal.

SELECT THE ONE BEST ANSWER

1. What is her most likely diagnosis?

   (A) Pott's puffy tumor
   (B) acute bacterial sinusitis
   (C) preseptal cellulitis
   (D) orbital cellulitis
   (E) type I hypersensitivity reaction

2. In this case, what is the most helpful information to make the diagnosis?

   (A) physical examination and history
   (B) CBC with differential leukocyte count
   (C) blood culture
   (D) culture of eye discharge
   (E) CT of orbits

3. How would you treat this child?

   (A) oral cephalexin
   (B) oral dicloxacillin
   (C) oral prednisone
   (D) IV ceftriaxone and clindamycin
   (E) IV ceftriaxone alone

4. A 6-year-old boy is brought to your office by his mother because he has had some increasing swelling around his eye for the last several days that seems worse today. This morning he was having difficulty "looking around" with that eye and is complaining that it hurts.

   On examination he is afebrile, has right-sided lid edema and erythema, proptosis, and lateral gaze is decreased.

   What is his diagnosis?

   (A) Pott's puffy tumor
   (B) acute bacterial sinusitis
   (C) preseptal cellulitis
   (D) orbital cellulitis
   (E) type I hypersensitivity reaction

5. What is the most common associated finding of this disease?

   (A) paranasal sinusitis
   (B) frontal sinusitis

(C)   conjunctivitis

(D)   bacteremia with hematogenous spread

(E)   trauma to orbit

6.   Which organism is the *least* likely to cause this disease in young children?

(A)   group A streptococci

(B)   *S. pneumoniae*

(C)   *H. influenzae*

(D)   *S. aureus*

(E)   *M. pneumoniae*

7.   Which of the following tests is the "gold standard" in diagnosing orbital cellulitis?

(A)   testing of visual acuity and extraocular movements

(B)   ultrasound

(C)   radiographs of the sinus and orbits

(D)   CT of orbit

(E)   MRI of orbit

8.   For how long should he receive antibiotics for his disease?

(A)   7 days

(B)   10 days

(C)   14 days

(D)   21 days

(E)   30 days

9.   Preseptal cellulitis occurs in an older age group than orbital cellulitis.

(A)   true

(B)   false

10.   Sinusitis more commonly is an associated finding of orbital cellulitis than preseptal cellulitis.

(A)   true

(B)   false

11.   A 12-year-old boy is seen in your office with redness in both eyes of 3 days' duration. They do not itch. He also has had nasal congestion and a cough for 5 days.

   On examination he is afebrile, has audible congestion and scant clear rhinorrhea. His turbinates are red and swollen. His eyes are bilaterally mildly injected and watery, with no discharge currently. There is no surrounding erythema or edema, and his funduscopic examination is normal bilaterally. His lungs are clear bilaterally. What is the most likely diagnosis?

(A)   bacterial conjunctivitis

(B)   viral conjunctivitis

(C)   allergic conjunctivitis

(D)   herpes simplex conjunctivitis

(E)   dacryocystitis

12.   The child from question 11 returns several days later with the same eye complaints but has developed a sore throat. He has been intermittently febrile (101.2°F [38.4°C] orally), and his eye examination has only changed in that the conjunctival erythema has become more intense. His posterior pharynx is slightly red, there is no exudates or petechiae, and the oral cavity is normal. He has a few tender cervical and preauricular lymph nodes, all less than 2 centimeters.

   What is the most likely pathogen of this disease?

(A)   EBV

(B)   Coxsackie virus

(C)   herpes simplex virus

(D)   adenovirus

(E)   influenza virus

13.   You see a 13-year-old boy in your office because of redness in one eye that is persisting for 3 days. It does not itch, but he is concerned because this morning there was thick, yellow discharge from the eye. Upon waking, his eyelids were stuck together. He had a "cold" last week, but that has resolved.

   On examination he is afebrile, and his left eye is severely injected, with dried and crusted yellowish discharge. His extraocular movements are intact. There is no preseptal erythema or edema. The rest of his examination is normal. What is his diagnosis?

(A)   bacterial conjunctivitis

(B)   viral conjunctivitis

(C)   allergic conjunctivitis

(D)   herpes simplex virus conjunctivitis

(E)   dacryocystitis

14.   What will you give the boy from question 13 to treat this condition?

(A) steroid and antibiotic eye drops
(B) oral amoxicillin
(C) oral doxycycline
(D) antibiotic eye drops
(E) warm compress only

15. You see a 6-month-old in the office because of "stuff coming out of his eye." His father describes a yellowish watery discharge that makes his left eye stuck closed in the morning. This has been going on for 3 days.

On examination, the baby smiles while you examine him. You note unilateral watery discharge and some scant yellow discharge. The conjunctiva is white. The infant fixes and follows on your hand 180 degrees. What is his diagnosis?

(A) dacryocystitis
(B) nasolacrimal duct obstruction
(C) viral conjunctivitis
(D) *Chlamydia trachomatis*
(E) *Neisseria gonorrhoeae*

16. You see a 5-year-old boy in your office because of a "lump" in his eye. It has been there for several weeks, is not red, does not hurt, but he does play with it frequently, which bothers his parents.

On examination he is afebrile and cooperative. You note a firm, nontender nodule in the lower left lid. There is no overlying erythema. His extraocular movements and gross visual acuity are intact. Which gland does this involve?

(A) gland of Zeis
(B) lacrimal gland
(C) gland of Moll
(D) meibomian gland
(E) none of the above

17. You get a call at night from a mother worried about her 8-year-old daughter, who has a "red lump" in her eye. It developed 2 days ago, and looks worse to her mother today. She describes a red, tender lump about 0.5 cm across that is just at the edge of the lower eyelid.

From her description, what is the *most* likely diagnosis?

(A) internal hordeolum
(B) external hordeolum

(C) chalazion
(D) dacryocystitis
(E) blepharitis

18. Which of the following is *not* associated with childhood ptosis?

(A) botulism
(B) myasthenia gravis
(C) trisomy 13
(D) amblyopia
(E) muscular dystrophy

Answers

1. **(C)** This is most likely preseptal cellulitis based on the physical findings. Preseptal (or periorbital) is differentiated from orbital cellulitis anatomically, symptomatically, and by physical findings (see below for further discussion).

2. **(A)** In cases where orbital cellulitis is not suspected, history and physical examination should lead to the correct diagnosis. A CBC may be somewhat helpful if a leukocytosis or "left shift" is present, but these changes are nonspecific. A culture of any eye discharge takes too long to be helpful in immediate decision making. A CT is not indicated for preseptal cellulitis unless orbital involvement cannot be excluded.

3. **(D)** Because of the lack of vaccination receipt in this child, *H. influenzae* type b should probably still be considered even though it is unlikely. Once a major pathogen causing preseptal cellulitis, it is now quite rare because of the vaccination program against it in the United States. The patient is also 4 years old, on the tail end of what was the *H. influenzae* type b age-specific curve. *H. influenzae* type b causes a rapidly progressive preseptal cellulitis and therefore it is appropriate to presumptively treat with parenteral antibiotics that cover it as well as the other common causes, *S. aureus*, *S. pneumoniae* and *S. pyogenes*. Patients with preseptal cellulitis should be hospitalized and initial therapy should be parenteral. Clindamycin is now an agent of choice in the many areas where methicillin-resistant *S. aureus* (MRSA) isolates are prevalent.

4. **(D)** Orbital cellulitis is differentiated from preseptal cellulitis based on anatomy (anterior vs. posterior to the orbital septum), symptomatically (pain on eye motion, decreased vision), and by physical findings (proptosis, decreased extraocular movement).

5. **(A)** Paranasal sinusitis is the most common associated finding with orbital cellulitis in children. Direct extension of infection or venous spread can also occur from the lid, conjunctiva, globe, lacrimal gland, or nasolacrimal sac. Frontal sinusitis also can cause contiguous spread of infection, though less frequently than paranasal sinusitis. In addition, because of the age at which sinuses anatomically develop, paranasal sinusitis occurs in a younger group (frontal sinuses begin to develop at approximately 7 years old).

6. **(C)** Although all of the above are implicated, the incidence of *H. influenzae* has decreased dramatically since widespread vaccination began in 1985. It is still found in older children with frontal sinusitis extending into orbital cellulitis.

7. **(D)** Although physical examination can often lead to the differentiation between orbital and preseptal cellulitis, a CT of the orbits makes the definitive diagnosis. It is superior to MRI in its ability to distinguish the orbital soft tissues and surrounding bone. Some experts believe that known orbital abscesses can be followed with ultrasound to limit radiation exposure, but this modality is not useful as an initial evaluation.

8. **(D)** He should receive parenteral antibiotics for 7 to 10 days, depending on the rapidity of improvement. Oral antibiotics may then be used to complete a 21-day course.

9. **(B)** Preseptal cellulitis occurs most often in children younger than 5 years old, whereas orbital cellulitis occurs in older children and, less commonly, adults.

10. **(A)** While orbital cellulitis is commonly an associated finding of sinusitis, preseptal cellulitis is commonly an associated finding of trauma, upper respiratory tract infections, or dacryocystitis.

11. **(B)** Viral conjunctivitis is common during an upper respiratory tract infection. It is more commonly bilateral, watery, and mild to moderate conjunctival injection.

12. **(D)** This is pharyngoconjunctival fever, caused by adenovirus. The diagnostic triad is fever, conjunctivitis, and pharyngitis.

13. **(A)** As opposed to viral conjunctivitis, bacterial conjunctivitis is more often unilateral, severe injection and thick and sometimes copious yellow discharge. It often follows a viral upper respiratory tract infection.

14. **(D)** Topical antibiotic drops are the best way to treat bacterial conjunctivitis. The fluoroquinolones are heavily promoted for the therapy of conjunctivitis but select for resistance frequently. Sulfacetamide drops are almost always effective and still constitute inexpensive, front-line therapy.

15. **(B)** This is typical nasolacrimal duct (NLD) obstruction that can occur in the newborn period and can be relapsing. It most often resolves by 9 to 12 months of age. Symptoms include watering and yellow discharge. In the newborn period the conjunctivae are sometimes mildly erythematous, making the differentiation between NLD obstruction and chlamydia or gonococcal infection difficult. In most cases, treatment for NLD obstruction is not pursued unless it persists past 9 to 12 months, at which time conjunctant is therapeutic probing of the NLD can be performed by an ophthalmologist.

16. **(D)** This is a chalazion, a granulomatous inflammation in the meibomian gland. These can be chronic, and on examination inflammatory signs are absent. Treatment most often is not warranted, although surgical excision may be needed in instances of large growth obstructing vision.

17. **(B)** This is most likely an external hordeolum, or stye. Internal hordeolums are on the inner lid and appear to be bulging from underneath. Dacryocystitis, or infection of the lacrimal gland, is located inferiorly and medially to the medial tear duct. Blepharitis is inflammation of the lid margins and typically has erythema and crusting or scaling.

18. (**C**) Amblyopia may occur as a result of ptosis, either from the lid covering the visual axis or astigmatism secondary to the weight of the lid on the globe.

SUGGESTED READING

Behrman RE, Kliegman RM, Jenson HB, et al: *Nelson Textbook of Pediatrics.* Philadelphia, WB Saunders, 2004, pp 1911–1914, 1934–1935.

Greenberg MF: The red eye in childhood. *Pediatr Clin North Am* 50(1):105–124, 2003.

Mawn LA: Preseptal and orbital cellulitis. *Ophthalmol Clin North Am* 13(4):633–641, 2000.

CASE 57: A 9-MONTH-OLD IN A CAR ACCIDENT

You see a 9-month-old infant in the emergency room with his mother, who was rear-ended in a car accident 1 hour prior. At the time of the accident, he was in his infant carrier car seat, in the backseat, facing forward. Since that time he has been acting his usual self, smiling and laughing, playful, and hungry.

On examination he weighs 22 pounds, is alert, and interactive. His neurological examination is normal, as is the rest of his examination.

SELECT THE ONE BEST ANSWER

1. What can you tell his mother about his car seat?

   (A) It should be forward-facing in the front seat.
   (B) It should be rear-facing in the front seat.
   (C) It should be forward-facing in the backseat.
   (D) It should be rear-facing in the backseat.
   (E) He should be in a booster seat.

2. She is wondering if the airbags in her four-door car are a danger to him while he is restrained in his car seat. What will you tell her?

   (A) Airbags in the front seat should be disabled.
   (B) Airbags in the backseat should be disabled or she should place her infant in the center of the backseat to avoid side airbags.
   (C) She should place her infant in the front to avoid backseat airbags.
   (D) She should place her infant next to the side airbag for protection.
   (E) None of the above are true.

3. Approximately what percentage of caregivers has installed their infant car seat correctly?

   (A) 10%
   (B) 30%
   (C) 50%
   (D) 70%
   (E) 90%

4. Which of the following is the safest choice in car seats for a 13-month-old 23-pound infant?

   (A) rear-facing convertible car seat
   (B) rear-facing infant car seat
   (C) front-facing convertible car seat
   (D) belt-positioning booster seat
   (E) shield booster seat

5. At what age is it acceptable for children to ride in the front seat with a passenger belt?

   (A) 2 years
   (B) 5 years
   (C) 8 years
   (D) 10 years
   (E) 13 years

6. In the event of an accidental ingestion, what is the best *first* recommended action that parents take?

   (A) Go the emergency room.
   (B) Administer syrup of ipecac.
   (C) Administer activated charcoal.
   (D) Call the poison control center.
   (E) Parent should perform the Heimlich maneuver.

7. At what age does the American Academy of Pediatrics generally recommend starting the regular use of sunscreen?

   (A) 1 week
   (B) 1 month
   (C) 2 months
   (D) 6 months
   (E) 1 year

8. A parent calls you from their vacation on the east coast. This morning, their 7-year-old son found a tick on his leg that is still embedded. They are wondering how to get the tick off.

   (A) Put rubbing alcohol on it.
   (B) Smother it with a cloth.
   (C) Try to burn it off with a match.

(D) Pull it out with tweezers.

(E) Break the body off at the skin level.

9. At what temperature should household hot water heaters be set at or below to prevent accidental burns?

(A) 90 degrees

(B) 100 degrees

(C) 110 degrees

(D) 120 degrees

(E) 130 degrees

10. What is the leading cause of death for all childhood age groups (1 to 21 years old) in the United States?

(A) suicide

(B) unintentional injuries

(C) malignancies

(D) homicide

(E) heart disease

11. What is the leading cause of death for children younger than 1 year of age?

(A) congenital anomalies

(B) SIDS

(C) unintentional injury

(D) malignancies

(E) sepsis

12. Who is the most likely person to be involved in a motor vehicle accident?

(A) 17-year-old male

(B) 17-year-old female

(C) 25-year-old male

(D) 25-year-old female

13. By what percent do helmets reduce the risk of bicycle-related traumatic brain injuries?

(A) 10%

(B) 25%

(C) 50%

(D) 75%

(E) 95%

14. Which of the following would you *not* include in counseling a family on fire safety and prevention?

(A) Replace their fire detector batteries every 6 months.

(B) Place portable heaters 1 foot or more from bedding.

(C) Store matches and other fire-starting materials out of reach.

(D) Smoke is more dangerous than the fire.

(E) Discontinue smoking.

15. Of these common myths regarding water safety and drowning, which is true?

(A) Children don't need life vests after they have learned to swim.

(B) Fences that surround pools won't prevent a child from drowning.

(C) Drowning children make lots of noise like splashing and will be heard easily.

(D) Continuous supervision at pools is not necessary when life vests are used.

(E) Children can drown in several inches of water.

16. Which of the following will you counsel parents on regarding safety with lawnmowers?

(A) Children should be at least 10 years old to use sit-down riding mowers.

(B) Use eye protection during mowing.

(C) Children must be at least 7 years old to use push-type mowers.

(D) Children older than 10 years can ride as passengers on sit-down mowers.

(E) A, B, and C.

17. You get a call from a mother who is taking her child to the northern Midwest during late summer and is worried about her 1-year-old and 3-year-old getting West Nile virus.

Which of the following statements would you use to counsel her on this disease?

(A) Approximately 20% of those infected develop *mild* disease.

(B) The incubation period is 3 to 14 days.

(C) One in 150 who are infected develop severe neurological disease.

(D) Encephalitis and meningitis are the most common complications of disease.

(E) All of the above.

18. Which of the following statements regarding the prevention of West Nile Virus is(are) true?

(A) DEET (N,N-diethyl-3-methylbenzamide) should not be used for infants under 2 months of age.

(B) The maximum acceptable concentration of DEET for children is 30%.

(C) DEET should be applied before clothing is put on.

(D) A and B.

(E) A, B, and C.

Answers

1. **(D)** The American Academy of Pediatrics (AAP) and the National Highway Traffic Safety Administration (NHTSA) recommend that infants remain in their rear-facing car seat in the backseat until they are both 1 year of age and over 20 to 22 pounds, and then for as long as possible. This is so that the deceleration forces are distributed over the infant's entire trunk during a crash, and it is also to protect their incompletely ossified vertebrae and corresponding weak connecting ligaments from injury. For infants who reach 20 pounds well before 1 year of age it is acceptable to change from an infant carrier seat (which typically only can fit infants <20 to 22 pounds) to a "convertible" type car seat, which has the ability to face forward or backward, as the age of the child dictates.

2. **(B)** In vehicles that have a front passenger airbag, infants must be in the backseat, since riding in the front seat puts them in a direct path of the front airbag and can lead to fatality. When children start riding in the front seat (see question 5 below), or for cars in which there is no backseat, several rules should be put into effect. Older children should be seated as far back as possible from the airbag. If a child is in a car seat of any type, the passenger airbag should be disabled. If an infant is rear facing in the front seat (in a two-seater car, for example), the passenger air bag should be disabled. For the back seat, some cars come with side airbags. Since they are difficult to disable, it is best to center infant car seats in the back to avoid the side airbags.

3. **(B)** A study conducted for the NHTSA in the mid-1990s found that approximately 72% of child restraints were being used incorrectly. A recently completed NHTSA-sponsored study updates that research. Interestingly, all rear-facing seats (infant and convertible) had the highest rate of misuse, approximately 84% for both. The NHTSA passed new regulations that require all passenger vehicles made after 2002 to be equipped with the LATCH system (Lower Anchors and Tethers for Children), which significantly reduces the complexity of installing a car seat.

4. **(A)** In general, as stated above, infants should be 20 pounds and 1 year of age to face forward. Convertible car seats are made to face forward or backward and vary in their weight limits. It is safest to keep infants facing backward for as long as possible, up to the rear-facing maximum weight limit indicated on the convertible car seat. Almost every convertible car seat on the market today has a rear-facing weight limit of 30 pounds. Booster seats are made for toddlers, and almost all have a minimum weight limit of 30 to 40 pounds. Information about any age, length, or weight parameters for a specific car seat should be affixed to the car seat.

5. **(E)** The NHTSA suggests all children 12 years and under should ride in the back seat. Please check the law in your local jurisdiction.

6. **(D)** Parents should be advised at preventive visits to always have the poison control center number nearby and to call there in case of accidental ingestions. The number is 800–222–1222. In 2003, the AAP reversed their position on the use of syrup of ipecac in the home. Because multiple studies did not show a difference in outcome in children on whom ipecac was used, and because activated charcoal is considered to be far superior, most physicians prefer to treat ingestions in an emergency room setting with charcoal.

7. **(D)** In 1999 the AAP changed its policy from recommending never using sunscreen in infants under 6 months to generally not using it for that age group unless adequate clothing and/or shade are not available. During those instances, applying small amounts to areas like the face and hands is acceptable. Sunscreen should always be SPF 15 or greater, and be reapplied after water exposure.

8. **(D)** Ticks must be removed as completely as possible. Grasping the part of the tick that is sticking out of the skin as close to the surface as possible and slowly pulling directly out most likely will aid in getting both the body and the head, which is buried underneath the skin. Old methods considered useful, including smothering with petroleum jelly or other substances, burning the tick off, or using rubbing alcohol have not been proven to be as effective.

9. **(D)** At 160°F (71.1°C), a full-thickness scald burn can occur in less than 1 second. At 120°F (48.8°C), many minutes of exposure are required for the same injury.

10. **(B)** For the past 5 years, unintentional injuries (includes motor vehicle accidents, poisoning, drowning, falls, fire/burns, firearm injuries, etc.) have ranked as the number one cause of mortality for all age groups of children older than 1 year of age.

11. **(A)** For children younger than 1 year of age, congenital anomalies are the number one cause of death.

12. **(A)** Male teen drivers are the most likely group to be involved in a motor vehicle accident (MVA). In addition, teens are five to ten times more likely to be involved in a fatal MVA while driving at night versus driving during the day.

13. **(D)**

14. **(B)** Portable heaters should always be placed ≥3 feet from any material that could be flammable (bedding, curtains, etc.). Children younger than 5 years and the elderly are at highest risk of injury from residential fires. Smoke detectors decrease the risk of fatality in a house fire by approximately 60% to 70%, but among smoke detectors that failed to alarm in a fire, 59% had been disconnected because of false or battery-related alarms. Smoke inhalation kills more people than direct fire-related injuries do.

15. **(E)** Infants and children can drown in as little as 2 to 3 inches of water in a bucket or bathtub. Children often do NOT splash or make noise when they are drowning. Reports from survivors have suggested that they either are too young to maneuver out of the water, or if older, simply cannot think of what to do at that moment, and quietly slip underneath the water. Full 5-foot surround fences are the only proven way to prevent pool drownings as children too easily climb over chain-link and picket fences. Children should wear properly fitting life vests or use personal flotation devices for a minimum of 2 years after they learn to swim, at which time constant supervision is still necessary.

16. **(B)** The AAP recommends that children younger than 12 years of age not use push-type mowers, that children younger than 16 years not use sit-down mowers, and that no children ride on sit-down mowers as passengers. Sturdy shoes and eye protection should always be worn during mowing.

17. **(E)**

18. **(D)** DEET-containing products are the most successful insect repellents. They should never be applied under clothing, and cannot be combined with other insect repellants. The concentration of DEET ranges from 5% to 30%, at which point the maximum efficacy is obtained. The percent directly correlates with the number of hours of protection given (10% gives about 2 hours of protection; 24% give about 5 hours).

SUGGESTED READING

American Academy of Pediatrics Web site. Available at: www.aap.org. Last accessed 5/26/06.
McKay MP, Curtis L: Children in cars: keeping them safe at every age. *Contemp Pediatr* 65–81, 2003.
Johnston B, Rivara F: Injury control: new challenges. *Peds Rev* 24:111–117, 2003.
National Highway Traffic Safety Administration Web site. Available at: www.nhtsa.gov. Last accessed 5/26/06.

CASE 58: AN 8-YEAR-OLD WITH CONGESTION

An 8-year-old boy comes to your office with his mother because of congestion for 5 days. In addition he has sneezing, rhinorrhea, and a mild cough. He has no fever and his symptoms are worse at night. He has no previous medical conditions.

On examination he has mild bilateral conjunctival injection, clear rhinorrhea, red swollen turbinates, and a mildly erythematous pharynx.

SELECT THE ONE BEST ANSWER

1. What is his most likely diagnosis at this time?

    (A) allergic rhinitis
    (B) rhinovirus
    (C) influenza
    (D) sinusitis
    (E) Coxsackie virus

2. How many typical upper respiratory tract infections per year does a healthy child have?

    (A) 2 to 3
    (B) 3 to 4
    (C) 4 to 5
    (D) 5 to 6
    (E) more than 6

3. He returns 14 days later with continued congestion. He no longer has a "runny" nose or sneezing, although his cough is still present and worse at night. His mother is concerned because he has never had a "cold" for this long before. On examination he is afebrile, has mild bilateral preseptal edema, thick purulent nasal discharge, swollen turbinates, and a mildly erythematous pharynx.
   What is his most likely diagnosis at this time?

    (A) allergic rhinitis
    (B) rhinovirus
    (C) influenza
    (D) sinusitis
    (E) immotile cilia syndrome

4. Which of the following is *not* implicated in causing acute bacterial sinusitis?

    (A) *Streptococcus pneumoniae*
    (B) *Moraxella catarrhalis*
    (C) *Haemophilus influenzae*
    (D) adenovirus
    (E) Coxsackie virus

5. At what time would you diagnose his condition as "chronic"?

    (A) 4 weeks
    (B) 6 weeks

   (C) 8 weeks
   (D) 12 weeks
   (E) 16 weeks

6. By what age could this child develop frontal sinusitis?

    (A) 1 year
    (B) 2 years
    (C) 3 years
    (D) 4 years
    (E) 5 years

7. A 9-year-old girl comes in to see you with fever. She had a "runny" nose several days ago, which has now changed to thick yellow discharge. Three days ago she developed a fever of 103°F (39.4°C), which has remained until today. She also has a mild headache and a nighttime cough, but no other symptoms. What is her diagnosis?

    (A) allergic rhinitis
    (B) rhinovirus
    (C) influenza
    (D) sinusitis
    (E) immotile cilia syndrome

8. What should your next course of action be with the patient in question 7?

    (A) plain films of the sinuses
    (B) intranasal steroid spray
    (C) antibiotics
    (D) CT of sinuses
    (E) prescription nondrowsy antihistamine

9. If you chose to use antibiotics, which would be your first choice?

    (A) amoxicillin at 45 mg/kg/d
    (B) amoxicillin at 90 mg/kg/d
    (C) amoxicillin (600 mg/5 mL)–clavulanate (42.9 mg/5 mL) at 90 mg/kg/day of amoxicillin
    (D) azithromycin
    (E) trimethoprim-sulfamethoxazole

10. For what duration will you treat her?

    (A) 7 days
    (B) 10 to 14 days
    (C) 3 weeks

(D) 1 month

(E) 2 months

11. After beginning antibiotics, by how many days do most show clinical improvement (decrease in symptoms and increase in well-being)?

(A) 1 day

(B) 3 days

(C) 7 days

(D) 10 days

(E) 14 days

12. Which of the following might prompt you to change your medical therapy?

(A) daycare attendance

(B) recent treatment with amoxicillin

(C) frontal or sphenoidal sinusitis

(D) B and C

(E) all of the above

13. She returns 10 days later still on your original prescription with eye pain. On examination she has left-sided preseptal edema, erythema, proptosis, and a fever of 103°F (39.4°C). What is your next step?

(A) change to a different oral antibiotic

(B) start intravenous antibiotics

(C) ophthalmology referral

(D) sinus aspiration

(E) oral prednisone

14. You see a 12-year-old boy who has had a month and a half of congestion and cough, day and night. He does not have fever but has a mild sore throat every day. On examination you confirm nasal congestion. His pharynx is mildly erythematous. He has normal-appearing tonsils, no lymphadenopathy, and no wheezing. What is his most likely diagnosis?

(A) allergic rhinitis

(B) rhinovirus

(C) influenza

(D) sinusitis

(E) immotile cilia syndrome

15. Which of the following can predispose an individual to develop sinusitis?

(A) viral upper respiratory tract syndrome

(B) dental infections

(C) allergic rhinitis

(D) cystic fibrosis

(E) all of the above

16. What should your next course of action be with the above patient?

(A) radiographs of the sinuses

(B) intranasal steroid spray

(C) oral antibiotics

(D) CT of sinuses

(E) prescription antihistamine not associated with drowsiness

17. How long should this patient receive antibiotics if clinical improvement is apparent?

(A) 7 days

(B) 10 to 14 days

(C) 21 days

(D) 30 days

(E) 45 days

18. Under which conditions would a maxillary sinus aspiration not be indicated?

(A) failure to respond to multiple courses of antibiotics

(B) severe facial pain

(C) orbital or intracranial complications

(D) symptoms for 30 days

(E) evaluation of an immunocompromised patient

Answers

1. **(B)** The vignette above is a typical story for the common cold, most often a result of rhinovirus.

2. **(E)** Most healthy children have between six and eight upper respiratory tract infections per year.

3. **(D)** The definition of acute bacterial sinusitis is persistent symptoms lasting >10 and <30 days. Nasal discharge of *any* quality, cough that is present daytime and nighttime (though usually worse at night), foul breath, and facial pain and/or headache are the most common presenting symptoms. On examination, preseptal swelling, facial pain or tenderness over the sinuses, and findings of an upper respiratory tract infection are often

present. Immotile cilia syndrome, or primary ciliary dyskinesia, is an inherited disease affecting the respiratory cilia. The majority of patients with this disease have chronic respiratory illnesses (including URIs, chronic sinusitis, chronic otitis media) throughout their childhood.

4. **(E)**

5. **(D)** Subacute sinusitis is defined as persistent symptoms from 4 to 12 weeks. Chronic sinusitis lasts longer than 12 weeks.

6. **(E)** The frontal sinuses develop from the anterior ethmoid cells and move into their position by 5 to 6 years old. The maxillary and ethmoid sinuses form in utero and are present at birth.

7. **(D)** This is another, less common, presentation of acute bacterial sinusitis: high fever (>102°F [38.8°C]) and purulent nasal discharge for at least 3 to 4 consecutive days. Viral upper respiratory tract infections can also present with fever and thick nasal discharge, although the timing is different. With a viral URI, the quality of the nasal discharge may change several times throughout the course of the illness, from clear to thick and back to clear. Fever is usually present at the outset and resolves after several days, and other constitutional symptoms are usually present.

8. **(C)** When children meet the criteria for acute bacterial sinusitis, whether in the case above or the case from question 3, antibiotic therapy is warranted. See the next question and answer for a discussion on antibiotic choices. Although amoxicillin is still considered the first choice, penicillin resistance to *S. pneumoniae* should be considered. The rates of resistance vary by location. Routine radiographic examination of uncomplicated acute bacterial sinusitis is not helpful. CT scans of patients with suspected sinusitis may be helpful but changes consistent with mild sinusitis are often found during uncomplicated upper respiratory tract infections (i.e., mucosal changes within the sinuses that are indistinguishable from acute bacterial sinusitis). Recent studies investigating the use of intranasal steroids in patients with acute bacterial sinusitis are promising but not conclusive.

9. **(B)** Despite penicillin resistance of *S. pneumoniae* (approximately one half of sinus aspirates are intermediately resistant to penicillin and one half are highly resistant), amoxicillin is still the first choice for uncomplicated acute bacterial sinusitis, although at the higher dose of 90 mg/kg per day. Both azithromycin and trimethoprim-sulfamethoxazole have less efficacy against the primary agents of sinusitis and should not be used.

10. **(B)** Most patients should be treated for 10 to 14 days. Some require longer courses if symptoms persist. Treatment beyond a few weeks is not recommended or supported by clinical studies.

11. **(B)** Most patients who are treated with an appropriate antibiotic respond promptly, within 48 to 72 hours.

12. **(D)** Recent amoxicillin therapy and the presence of frontal or sphenoid sinusitis are situations in which an alternative to amoxicillin may be appropriate. Symptomatology for more than 30 days is another indicator. Reasons include the higher likelihood of a resistant organism and the need for higher drug levels than oral amoxicillin can provide. Clinically important frontal or sphenoid sinusitis may require parenteral therapy.

13. **(B)** This is likely to be an orbital process, either cellulitis or abscess, which are two complications of acute bacterial sinusitis. They require parenteral antibiotics and in-patient observation. Other complications of sinusitis include subperiosteal intraorbital abscess, sinus-associated osteomyelitis (frontal bone osteomyelitis is also known as Pott's puffy tumor), epidural abscess, meningitis, and brain abscess.

14. **(D)** This is consistent with chronic sinusitis, with protracted respiratory symptoms (congestion and cough are most common). At this point it is important to consider other possibilities with your examination such as cystic fibrosis (poor growth, clubbing, barrel chest, nasal polyps, respiratory findings), allergic rhinitis (dark circles under eyes, horizontal crease across nose, Morgan-Dennie lines characterized by skin folds under the lower eyelid), adenoidal hypertrophy, or immunodeficiency.

15. (E) All of the other illnesses or situations listed predispose patients to sinusitis, acute and bacterial. Immune disorders, immotile cilia syndrome, facial trauma, choanal atresia, and foreign bodies are also implicated.

16. (C) Because the microbial nature of chronic sinusitis is somewhat different from that of acute bacterial sinusitis, the treatment also is different, although antibiotics remain the first step in therapy. Aspiration studies reveal that anaerobes and enterics play a greater role in chronic sinusitis. Aerobic isolates are predominantly *H. influenzae*, *S. aureus*, and *M. catarrhalis*. Therapy should be directed against these. One reasonable choice is amoxicillin-clavulanate except in areas where MRSA are prevalent. If oral antibiotic therapy is not successful, surgical drainage and parenteral antibiotics are often required.

17. (C) Treatment for chronic sinusitis should continue for at least 21 days.

18. (D) Maxillary sinus aspiration can be performed by an otolaryngologist on an outpatient basis, but this should be reserved for the other situations listed above. Sinus symptoms for 30 days are still considered subacute and an initial trial of oral antibiotics is appropriate.

SUGGESTED READING

Brook I: Microbiology and antimicrobial management of sinusitis. *Otolaryngol Clin North Am* 37(2):253–266, 2004.
Nash D, Wald E: Sinusitis. *Pediatr Rev* 22(4):111–116, 2001.

CASE 59: AN 8-YEAR-OLD GIRL WITH SORE THROAT

An 8-year-old girl comes to your office during winter complaining of worsening throat pain for 2 days, tactile temperatures at home, and abdominal pain. She has not vomited, has no diarrhea, and she has noticed no rashes. She is barely able to eat food this morning because of the pain. No one else is ill at home, but several of her friends at school have the "same thing."

On examination you note a temperature of 101.5°F (38.6°C), clear nares, white conjunctivae, oropharynx with palatal petechiae, a swollen and erythematous uvula, enlarged erythematous tonsils, and no tonsillar exudates. She has tender anterior cervical lymphadenopathy, left greater than right, all <1 cm in diameter. Her lungs are clear bilaterally; she has mild periumbilical tenderness, no hepatosplenomegaly, and no rash.

SELECT THE ONE BEST ANSWER

1. What is the most likely diagnosis?

    (A) viral pharyngitis
    (B) mononucleosis
    (C) group A streptococcal pharyngitis
    (D) Coxsackie virus
    (E) group B streptococcal pharyngitis

2. What is the most appropriate next step?

    (A) in-office Monospot test
    (B) CBC and EBV titers
    (C) rapid latex test for group A streptococcus
    (D) reassurance
    (E) start antibiotics

3. Which of these is *not* a complication of this illness?

    (A) retropharyngeal abscess
    (B) splenic rupture
    (C) glomerulonephritis
    (D) peritonsillar abscess
    (E) rheumatic fever

4. If this patient's rapid strep test was positive, what is your *first* choice of medication?

    (A) cephalexin
    (B) penicillin
    (C) azithromycin
    (D) ceftriaxone
    (E) prednisone

5. If she came back after taking the prescribed antibiotic for 10 days, still had a sore throat, and similar findings on examination, what would you do next?

    (A) reculture for group A streptococcus
    (B) Monospot test
    (C) diagnosis as a group A streptococcus carrier
    (D) A and B
    (E) admission for IV antibiotics

6. If her repeat throat culture grew group A strepto-coccus, what medication would you start her on?

(A) Tylenol or ibuprofen
(B) penicillin
(C) azithromycin
(D) ceftriaxone
(E) prednisone

7. Her mother wants to know if her 6-year-old brother, who is at home, should also be tested for group A streptococcus. He has no symptoms and is otherwise healthy. Which is the next appropriate step for you to take for her brother?

(A) rapid strep test
(B) throat culture for strep
(C) no tests
(D) prophylactic oral antibiotics
(E) prophylactic IM ceftriaxone

8. One week later her 2-year-old brother developed a fever of 101°F (38.3°C) axillary, serous rhinitis, and mild cough. On examination he was found to have a temperature of 100.5°F (38°C) rectally, a normal respiratory rate, nasal congestion, and yel-lowish discharge in both nares. The oropharynx was moist and normal appearing, and the lungs were clear. What tests, if any, would you do?

(A) rapid strep test
(B) Monospot
(C) rapid flu test
(D) CBC with differential leukocyte count
(E) no tests

9. A 6-month-old male infant presents to your of-fice with a diaper rash for 8 days. His parents have tried OTC diaper creams but none seem to be helping. He is eating normally, has regular soft bowel movements, and has had no other symptoms except irritability for 2 days when he has a bowel movement and when they are clean-ing him afterward. On examination you note bright erythema perianally extending about 3 cm outward but no other finding. His genitals ap-pear normal, and the rest of his examination is normal. What is the likely etiology of this rash?

(A) *Candida albicans*
(B) group A streptococci
(C) group B streptococci

(D) seborrheic dermatitis
(E) pinworm infestation

10. What is the most worrisome complication of the disease from question 9?

(A) rheumatic fever
(B) abscess
(C) impetigo
(D) glomerulonephritis
(E) severe diarrhea

11. What lab test can you do to confirm your suspi-cion raised in question 9?

(A) KOH prep
(B) skin culture
(C) throat culture
(D) UA
(E) stool studies

12. What do you recommend to the parents for treatment in question 9?

(A) watchful waiting
(B) continue OTC diaper creams only
(C) topical antibiotics
(D) topical steroids
(E) penicillin orally

13. A 15-year-old girl whom you saw in your office last week and diagnosed with group A strepto-coccus pharyngitis has returned. She stopped taking her antibiotics after 3 days because her sore throat resolved. It has now returned, and she feels more pain than before. She reports a fever of 104°F (40°C) last night and this morn-ing is having difficulty opening her mouth to eat and severe pain on swallowing water. On ex-amination she is generally ill appearing. Her temperature is 102°F (38.8°C) and she has very tender anterior and posterior cervical lymph nodes bilaterally. She cannot open her mouth for you to examine her oropharynx. Her ab-dominal examination is normal. What is your diagnosis?

(A) group A streptococcal pharyngitis
(B) EBV mononucleosis
(C) retropharyngeal abscess
(D) peritonsillar abscess
(E) gonococcal pharyngitis

14. What is the study to best diagnose the problem from question 13?

(A) radiograph of lateral neck
(B) CT
(C) MRI
(D) throat culture
(E) fine-needle aspiration

15. All are useful treatment measures for the diagnosis in question 13 except:

(A) parenteral antibiotics
(B) oral steroids
(C) surgical drainage
(D) PCA pump
(E) all are appropriate treatment measures

16. A 21-month-old girl is brought in by her mother because of fever (101°F to 103°F [38.3°C to 39.4°C]) and anorexia for 2 days. She has not urinated in 12 hours. She has no other symptoms, specifically, no cough, rhinorrhea, rash, vomiting, or diarrhea.

On examination she appears quite ill, has an axillary temperature of 102.5°F (39.1°C), HR of 140, capillary refill of 3 seconds, is holding her head hyperextended, and resists examination of her oral cavity. She has tender bilateral cervical lymphadenopathy and has mild stridor. The rest of her examination is normal. What is the most likely diagnosis?

(A) group A streptococci pharyngitis
(B) EBV mononucleosis
(C) retropharyngeal abscess
(D) peritonsillar abscess
(E) gonococcal pharyngitis

17. What is the most pressing complication in this child from question 16?

(A) febrile seizure
(B) airway occlusion
(C) dehydration
(D) sepsis
(E) aspiration pneumonia

18. On arrival in the emergency room, the child from question 16 is examined by an otolaryngologist who notes a right-sided anterior bulge in the posterior oropharynx.

Which of the following is the first step of your management?

(A) airway securing and monitoring
(B) placement of IV and NPO order
(C) surgery consult
(D) radiographs
(E) all of the above

Answers

1. **(C)** Although bacteria are the etiology in only 5% to 10% of cases of pharyngitis, this presentation is most likely group A β-hemolytic streptococcal pharyngitis. It is most common among school-age children and causes rapid-onset pharyngitis with associated symptoms of fever, headache, neck tenderness, abdominal pain, and emesis. Viral pharyngitis is more common in conjunction with other upper respiratory tract symptoms (congestion, rhinorrhea, cough, ear pain). Coxsackie virus is an enterovirus that can cause typical symptoms of the common cold, ulcerative pharyngitis, and hand-foot-mouth disease. EBV mononucleosis can cause exudative pharyngitis, and often splenomegaly is found on examination. Group B streptococcus does not cause pharyngitis; it is a major cause of perinatal infections and urinary tract infections in pregnant women.

2. **(C)** If you are suspicious of streptococcal pharyngitis, a rapid latex test should be performed in your office. Several rapid tests are available, and all require vigorous swabbing of the palate and tonsils, and/or the posterior pharynx. Sensitivities and specificities are similar and are approximately 80% to 90% and 95%, respectively. Because of the high specificity, a positive latex test does *not* require a confirmatory throat culture. Conversely, a negative rapid test should prompt a throat culture to screen for group A streptococci. Starting antibiotics without documenting streptococcus by latex or throat culture is not appropriate.

3. **(B)** All of these are possible complications of group A streptococcal pharyngitis except splenic rupture, which is associated with trauma to the enlarged and friable spleen of EBV mononucleosis. A retropharyngeal abscess presents as high fever, drooling, trismus (inability to open jaw), painful pharyngitis, and, sometimes, a toxic appearance. Rheumatic fever in children younger than 3 years old is uncommon. With improved testing and treatment, rheumatic fever in the United States today is uncommon (0.3% in non-epidemics, 3% in epidemics), although it may still occur in association with group A streptococci outbreaks. All the complications listed above are preventable by timely testing and antibiotic treatment.

4. **(B)** Penicillin is still the antibiotic of choice for group A streptococcal pharyngitis. Oral (penicillin V) or intramuscular benzathine penicillin G are acceptable. Other β-lactams such as amoxicillin (Augmentin) are also acceptable. Azithromycin (Zithromax) or erythromycin have activity against group A streptococci (although rare resistance is reported) but should be reserved for penicillin-allergic patients. First-generation oral cephalosporins (cephalexin, cefadroxil) can be used against group A streptococci but are expensive and have wider antimicrobial spectra. They should be also reserved for allergic, nonanaphylactic patients. IV or IM cephalosporins are not indicated. Steroids have no role in treating group A streptococci pharyngitis.

5. **(D)** Reculturing this patient for group A streptococci is an appropriate next step. Posttreatment throat cultures should be reserved only for those patients who are still symptomatic, or those patients who are at very high risk for rheumatic fever. Those who are asymptomatic at the end of treatment but still culture positive should not receive additional antimicrobial treatment since carriage of group A streptococci in the pharynx can continue for several weeks after active infection. One might also consider the possibility of concomitant EBV pharyngitis and group A streptococci since approximately 10% of patients with mononucleosis concomitantly are group A streptococci + group A streptococci carriers (10% to 50% of the population at various times) may be asymptomatic. This patient may be a carrier and have prolonged viral pharyngitis. The repeat group A streptococci test will help clarify this. Treating with a "stringer" antibiotic is unnecessary even if the patient is still positive for group A streptococci.

6. **(B)** For persistent group A streptococci, the same antibiotic is recommended (penicillin). A persistently positive test for group A streptococci after a second course of penicillin suggests that the patient is a group A streptococci carrier. In this case, the problem is not one of resistance, but one of continued infection, since no penicillin-resistant group A streptococci has ever been reported in the United States.

7. **(C)** Any testing on children exposed to group A streptococci is unwarranted since carriage during an outbreak can be as high as 25% to 40%. Only symptomatic children should be examined and a rapid group A streptococci test and culture considered.

8. **(E)** In toddlers <3 years old, group A streptococcal infection may present with serous rhinitis, fever, irritability, and anorexia, instead of the pharyngitis typically seen in older children. However, because the risk of rheumatic fever in this age group is extremely low in developed countries, culturing for group A streptococci is *not* recommended in this age group unless the patient is at high risk for rheumatic fever, or the illness occurs during a rheumatic fever outbreak. In this case, "E" (no test) therefore is the correct answer. Testing for mononucleosis or influenza is not indicated based on the symptoms. The Monospot test is insensitive in a 2-year-old child.

9. **(B)** This is the classic presentation of perianal group A streptococci dermatitis. It occurs more often in males between the ages of 6 months and 10 years. Presenting symptoms and findings are itching, pain on defecation, blood-streaked stool, and a well-circumscribed erythematous rash from the anus extending outward. Recurrence rates are 40% to 50%. The differential diagnosis includes A, D, and E, psoriasis, and sexual abuse.

10. **(D)** Glomerulonephritis is the most serious complication associated with group A strep skin infections (and pharyngeal infections), whereas rheumatic fever is *not* associated with the skin infections caused by group A streptococci.

11. **(B)**

12. (E) Group A streptococci dermatitis, especially perianal disease, requires oral antibiotics for treatment. Topical antibiotics will be ineffective.

13. (D) This is a classic story for peritonsillar abscess, most likely caused by group A streptococci. She is experiencing trismus, the inability to open the jaw secondary to peritonsillar and lymphatic edema. If she were to open her mouth, you would find an asymmetric tonsillar bulge, perhaps with uvular and/or palatal displacement. Generally, retropharyngeal abscesses are less common in children older than 5 years old, as the retropharyngeal nodes that fill the potential retropharyngeal space involute before that time; thus the pathophysiology of this disease differs in adolescents and adults, in whom it is rare. Gonococcal pharyngitis should be considered among sexually active persons and can present with fever, sore throat, and greenish pharyngeal/tonsillar exudates.

14. (B) A CT of the neck with IV contrast will most clearly and rapidly assess for a ring-enhancing abscess or possibly a phlegmon. Fine-needle aspiration is one approach to surgical treatment but is seldom performed for diagnosis.

15. (B) IV antibiotics and incision and drainage are the mainstays of treatment of peritonsillar abscess. Pain control is usually needed and can be supplied in oral (liquid) or IV form. Oral steroids may be useful in severe mononucleosis but not for peritonsillar abscesses.

16. (C) Retropharyngeal abscesses are a disease of younger children, as stated earlier, whereby infection of the lymph nodes that are located in the retropharyngeal space is associated with fever, sore throat, trismus, drooling, stridor, and change in voice (cri du canard—cry of the duck [a duck-quacking sound]).

17. (B) Airway occlusion in this case is a most urgent concern as it appears that the patient has a pharyngeal process. The difficulty in examining a child like this further complicates the situation, but the combination of fever, ill appearance, hyperextension of the neck, and stridor should prompt the physician to immediately be prepared for airway management. The other complications listed are all concerns with this patient, but relatively less urgent. Aspiration pneumonia is a known and dangerous complication of retropharyngeal abscess.

18. (A) All of these are components of the initial management of this problem. Securing the airway is obviously the most urgent. Radiographic investigation most often begins with lateral neck films (with neck in full extension during deep inspiration), which are evaluated for the width of the retropharyngeal space. The width of the prevertebral soft tissue should be no more than 7 mm at C2 and 20 mm at C6. If more urgent evaluation is required, or if proper positioning of the neck is not possible, a CT of the neck with contrast is an alternative option.

SUGGESTED READING

Behrman RE, Kliegman RM, Jenson HB, et al: *Nelson Textbook of Pediatrics*. Philadelphia: WB Saunders, 2004, pp 1264–1266.

Long SS, et al: *Principles and Practice of Pediatric Infectious Diseases*. Philadelphia: Elsevier, 2003, pp 179–188.

Pickering LK, et al: *Red Book 2003 Report of the Committee on Infectious Diseases*. Elk Grove Village, IL: American Academy of Pediatrics, 2003, pp 271–273, 573–584.

CASE 60: A 7-MONTH-OLD WITH CROSSED EYES

A mother brings her 7-month-old full-term twins in to see you for a routine check-up. During the visit she mentions that she is concerned because they both seem to have "crossed eyes" a lot of the time, especially when they are tired or at nighttime.

On examination of the first child you note that her eyes appear asymmetric. Her left eye appears to deviate inward. She has an asymmetric corneal light reflex, with the left corneal reflex displaced temporally.

SELECT THE ONE BEST ANSWER

1. All of the following cranial nerves are involved in alignment of the eyes except:

   (A) II
   (B) III
   (C) IV
   (D) VI
   (E) all of the above are involved in alignment of the eye

2. Which type of strabismus does she have?

   (A) esotropia
   (B) esophoria
   (C) exotropia
   (D) exophoria
   (E) pseudostrabismus

3. What is the most appropriate next step for this patient?

   (A) observation with re-examination in 3 months
   (B) ophthalmology referral
   (C) Snellen visual acuity test
   (D) cover test
   (E) eye patch

4. If you send her to the ophthalmologist, and he or she confirms your diagnosis, what is the *most* likely treatment of this disorder?

   (A) surgical correction
   (B) eyeglasses
   (C) eye patch
   (D) observation
   (E) prism glasses

5. What percentage of children with strabismus who go untreated develop amblyopia?

   (A) 10% to 30%
   (B) 20% to 40%
   (C) 30% to 50%
   (D) 50% to 80%
   (E) 90% to 95%

6. You examine her twin sister and note that her eyes also appear asymmetric. Her right eye appears deviated inward throughout the examination. Her corneal light reflex is normal.

   Which type of strabismus does she have?

   (A) esotropia
   (B) esophoria
   (C) exotropia
   (D) exophoria
   (E) pseudostrabismus

7. What is the next recommended action for the patient in question 6?

   (A) reassurance
   (B) ophthalmology referral
   (C) glasses prescription
   (D) eye patch
   (E) surgical correction

8. A father brings his 3-year-old son to your office one day because of a "lazy eye" that they have been noticing for a few months. His father does not recall any trauma to the eye, and tells you that both he and the patient's mother wear glasses. His son rides a tricycle, helps dress himself, can copy a circle, and uses three-word sentences. The "lazy eye" doesn't seem to bother him. On examination you note a left esotropia, an asymmetric corneal light reflex, and an abnormal cover test.

   What will the treatment be for his *most* likely diagnosis?

   (A) eye patch
   (B) prism glasses
   (C) prescription eye glasses
   (D) surgical correction
   (E) observation

9. Which of the following children does *not* require a referral to a pediatric ophthalmologist?

   (A) 6-month-old with fetal alcohol syndrome
   (B) 2-week-old with nystagmus
   (C) 5-year-old with Down syndrome
   (D) 4-month-old with strabismus
   (E) former 26-week preemie now 9 months old

10. You see a 3-day-old for a well-baby visit in your office and her mother asks you what she is able to see. What can you tell her mother that her vision would be, approximately, if she were able to read off a Snellen chart?

    (A) 400/20
    (B) 200/20
    (C) 20/20
    (D) 20/200
    (E) 20/400

11. Which of the following children needs to be evaluated further for their vision?

    (A) a 6-week-old who cannot smile
    (B) a 1-month-old who does not fixate and follow across midline parents' faces
    (C) a 5-month-old with intermittently "crossed eyes"

(D) a 15-month-old who cannot put a peg into a round hole

(E) a 2-year-old with mild hyperopia

Questions 12 through 15. *Match* the following ages with the *most* appropriate vision tests and screening tools:

12. 6 months   (A) Allen cards

13. 2.5 years   (B) HOTV or tumbling Es

14. 4 years   (C) Fix and follow

15. 7 years   (D) Snellen charts

16. An 8-year-old girl is in your office for a routine check-up. On your questioning, she tells you that she has some difficulty seeing the blackboard in class. Her mother states that she does seem to be holding her books closer to her face lately. Sometimes she squints when they are in the car. What will you most likely find on your funduscopic examination?

(A) +1.00 to + 2.00
(B) + 4.00 to +5.00
(C) −1.00 to −2.00
(D) −4.00 to −5.00

17. Which of the following statements regarding myopia is *false*?

(A) Most infants' eyes are slightly myopic.
(B) It requires a concave lens to correct.
(C) It is often hereditary.
(D) Most myopia is physiologic.
(E) Myopia is more common in preterm compared with full-term infants.

18. At what age should children begin to have routine screening visual acuity examinations?

(A) 6 months
(B) 1 year
(C) 2 years
(D) 3 years
(E) 4 years

Answers

1. (A) CN III (oculomotor) is responsible for levator muscle constriction, pupillary constriction, and lens accommodation. CN IV (trochlear) innervates the superior oblique muscle and CN VI (abducens) innervates the lateral rectus muscle. CN II (optic) is not involved in aligning the eyes, only in the transmission of visual signals.

2. (A) This is esotropia because her eye deviated medially (eso-) and is constant (-tropia) as opposed to periodic or latent (-phoria). The corneal light reflex test is performed by the examiner shining a light onto both corneas simultaneously and watching for where on the cornea the reflection occurs. In eyes that are aligned, the reflection appears symmetric. If one eye is deviated, the normal eye will be centered and the reflex in the deviated eye will appear off-center. Infantile, or congenital, esotropia is the most common esodeviation in children.

3. (B) Referrals to ophthalmology for strabismus are not generally made before 6 months of age, since intermittent asymmetry of pursuit can be present in healthy infants and resolves by 3 to 6 months. Observation is not acceptable, since delay to treatment increases the likelihood of amblyopia. The Snellen charts are visual acuity tests for vision screening for older children. The cover test is best used to detect visual axis deviations. Each eye is covered in turn while the uncovered eye is examined for tropias. It is an appropriate test to perform when trying to confirm the presence of strabismus as suspected by abnormal corneal light reflex, but requires patient cooperation to perform and would likely be difficult in an infant this age.

4. (A) It is widely agreed that surgical correction, namely medial rectus recession, is the treatment most likely to be corrective. The timing of the surgery is controversial, some arguing for as early as 3 to 4 months, some as late as 1 year.

5. (C) The amblyopia that commonly accompanies strabismus requires separate treatment.

6. (E) This is pseudostrabismus, when one or both eyes appear deviated medially because of prominent epicanthal folds or an especially broad nasal bridge. The corneal light reflex is normal because the eyes are actually aligned and can be confirmed by a cover test in older children.

7. **(A)** Pseudostrabismus is treated by reassuring the parents that their child will grow out of the "appearance" of an eye problem as she grows.

8. **(C)** He most likely has an accommodative esotropia, which most commonly presents between 2 and 3 years old as a new-onset esotropia. Family histories of amblyopia are common. The great majority of these children have an associated hyperopia, and their esotropia is because of overaccommodation in response to the hyperopia. Treatment of the hyperopia is indicated first (with prescription eyeglasses). This often is all that is needed. If that fails, surgical correction is a possibility.

9. **(D)** Strabismus can be found in healthy infants until age 3 to 6 months, at which time the inability to symmetrically follow a target resolves. Ophthalmology referrals are needed for children with genetic syndromes, in utero drug or alcohol exposure, infants with retinopathy of prematurity (at 26 weeks premature, an infant would most likely have this), children who have evidence of ocular pathology on examination, and children with strong family histories of vision difficulties.

10. **(E)** When measured by visual evoked potential, newborns have visual acuity of approximately 20/400.

11. **(D)** Peg-in-hole games are visually related behaviors that should suggest to the practitioner possible vision impairment if this milestone is not achieved on time. By 8 to 9 months, a child should poke at the holes with pegs and by 12 to 14 months should be able to put pegs into the appropriate holes. For the incorrect answers: infants should smile at 2 to 3 months, fix and follow by 2 to 3 months (by 2 months it is a red flag, by 3 months an absolute referral), strabismus is referred to ophthalmology after 6 months, and all children are mildly hyperopic until approximately 10 years old.

12. **(C)**

13. **(A)**

14. **(B)**

15. **(D)** The most advanced test of visual acuity possible should be used for a child's developmental age. The Allen cards are a series of familiar object cards that the child is asked to identify at increasing distances. The appropriate vision screening tools for ages 3 to 5 years are the matching-type tests, namely the HOTV test (chart on wall with letters H, O, T, V and child holds matching cards) and the tumbling Es (chart on wall with the letter E in various rotations and child holds matching cards).

16. **(D)** This patient by history has myopia, nearsightedness, which is causing her to strain to see far objects—squinting in the car or pulling objects closer to her face to see them more clearly. The presence of clinical symptoms for some time suggests a higher diopter on examination, −5 to 6 as opposed to −1 to 2.

17. **(A)** Almost all infants are born with slight hyperopia that increases throughout childhood, peaks at approximately 6 years old, and then decreases again. Most myopia is physiologic, as opposed to pathologic.

18. **(D)** The AAP and the American Academy of Ophthalmology recommend routine visual acuity testing at 3 years and again at 5 to 6 years. Screening for eye disease should be performed regularly, at least in the first 3 months of age and again at 12 months.

SUGGESTED READING

Behrman RE, Kliegman RM, Jenson HB, et al: *Nelson Textbook of Pediatrics*. Philadelphia: WB Saunders, 2004, pp 1898, 1904–1907.

Committee on Practice and Ambulatory Medicine, American Academy of Ophthalmology: Eye examination in infants, children, and young adults by pediatricians. *Pediatrics* 111(4):902–907, 2003.

Curnyn KM: The eye examination in the pediatrician's office. *Pediatr Clin North Am* 50(1):25–40, 2003.

Guthrie ME: Congenital esotropia. *Ophthalmol Clin North Am* 14(3):419–424, 2001.

CASE 61: 4-YEAR-OLD WITH A NECK MASS

A 4-year-old comes to your office with his father because of a "lump in the neck" that his parents noted 4 days earlier. The boy does not seem bothered by it, and although he is not currently ill, he did have a "cold" about 1 week ago. He has not had a fever, is eating and drinking well, has no specific tooth pain, and no pain on swallowing.

On examination he is afebrile. His oropharynx is normal, nares clear, conjunctivae white. He has a tender, 4-cm submandibular lymph node on the left side that has overlying erythema. His abdominal and skin examinations are normal.

SELECT THE ONE BEST ANSWER

1. What is his most likely diagnosis?

    (A) cat-scratch disease
    (B) nontuberculous *Mycobacterium* infection
    (C) acute lymphadenitis
    (D) mumps
    (E) tuberculosis

2. What is the *least* likely pathogen causing his illness?

    (A) nontuberculous mycobacteria
    (B) *Streptococcus pyogenes* (group A streptococci)
    (C) *Staphylococcus aureus*
    (D) EBV
    (E) anaerobic bacteria

3. What antibiotic will you prescribe for him?

    (A) IM ceftriaxone
    (B) PO azithromycin
    (C) PO amoxicillin
    (D) PO cephalexin
    (E) PO amoxicillin-clavulanate

4. Which of the following are also known to cause cervical lymphadenopathy?

    (A) non-Hodgkin lymphoma
    (B) Kawasaki disease
    (C) systemic lupus erythematosus
    (D) A and B
    (E) all of the above

5. You are called by the parents of a 2-week-old newborn male, who report poor feeding for 1 day and some neck swelling on the right side. On examination you note a well-hydrated, fussy but consolable infant with a temperature of 101.2°F (38.4°C) rectally and a right-sided 2- × 4-cm spongy neck mass with overlying erythema. The rest of the examination is normal.

    What are the possible etiologies of the neck mass in this child?

    (A) *S. pyogenes* (group A streptococci)
    (B) *Streptococcus agalactiae*
    (C) group B streptococci
    (D) *S. aureus*
    (E) all of the above

6. You see a 3-year-old girl who is brought to your office because of a lump in her neck that her parents noticed about 6 weeks prior. At that time, the girl said that it has already been there for "a long time." They are concerned that it is still present and not diminishing in size. In all other regards, the parents report that she is in good health and has received all of her vaccinations. They live in a suburb and have no pets. They have not traveled in more than a year.

    On examination she is afebrile and very cooperative. She has multiple firm, mobile left-sided cervical and submandibular nodes, the largest of which is 4.5 cm. There is no erythema, warmth, or drainage present. Her oral cavity, ears, conjunctivae, and scalp are normal. Her abdominal and skin examinations are normal.

    Laboratory data include:

    CBC: WBC 8.1 (48% lymphocytes, 33% neutrophils, 15% monocytes, 4% eosinophils)
    ESR: 21
    PPD: 11 mm

    What is the next test that should be ordered?

    (A) blood culture
    (B) chest radiograph
    (C) lymph node biopsy
    (D) CT of neck
    (E) MRI of neck

7. Which of the following is the most reliable way to ascertain the etiology of infection in the patient in question 6?

    (A) gastric lavage specimen
    (B) sputum specimen
    (C) urine specimen
    (D) blood culture
    (E) surgically excised tissue

8. What is the least likely way that nontuberculous mycobacteria are transmitted?

   (A) inhalation
   (B) ingestion
   (C) person-to-person
   (D) direct contact with organism
   (E) animal contact

9. Which of the following is the least likely clinical manifestation of the organism from a nontuberculous mycobacteria infection?

   (A) skin ulcer
   (B) disseminated infection
   (C) bone infections
   (D) lymphadenitis
   (E) soft tissue infection

10. The lymph node biopsy that you ordered recovered *Mycobacterium intracellulare*, and the blood culture is negative. Which of the following is most likely to lead to a cure from question 6?

    (A) ciprofloxacin
    (B) doxycycline
    (C) azithromycin and ethambutol
    (D) azithromycin, ethambutol, and rifampin
    (E) surgical excision

11. You see a 4-year-old girl who comes in for a "lump" in her neck that she has had for about 3 weeks. Her parents do not recall any trauma to the area, toothaches, or illnesses in the last month. They are worried that she has "throat cancer" because her grandmother has just been diagnosed with this. She has two cats at home and has not traveled in the past 6 months.

    On examination you find a happy, cooperative child who is afebrile. She has a visible asymmetry of the neck. She has several left-sided tender cervical lymph nodes with overlying erythema and warmth. What is the most likely etiology of her disease?

    (A) *Yersinia pestis*
    (B) *Francisella tularensis*
    (C) *Bartonella henselae*
    (D) *Chlamydia trachomatis*
    (E) *Corynebacterium diphtheriae*

12. Which of the following are other possible clinical manifestations of the organism from question 11?

    (A) hepatitis
    (B) aseptic meningitis
    (C) Parinaud oculoglandular syndrome
    (D) pharyngitis
    (E) all of the above

13. In which seasons is this disease most common from question 11?

    (A) winter/spring
    (B) summer/fall
    (C) summer/winter
    (D) spring/fall
    (E) no seasonal variance

14. What is the best treatment for this patient from question 11?

    (A) reassurance
    (B) oral antibiotics
    (C) get rid of cats in home
    (D) fine-needle aspiration
    (E) incision and drainage

15. You see a 5-year-old girl for a check-up and her parents tell you that they are concerned about a small lump on her neck. It has been there for some time but was small and nontender, and they were waiting for their check up to ask you about it. But 7 days ago she developed an upper respiratory tract infection with sneezing, coughing, and mild fevers, and now the lump is larger than it was 2 weeks ago and somewhat tender.

    On examination you find a happy, cooperative, afebrile young girl. She has mild conjunctival injection bilaterally without discharge, red swollen turbinates and rhinorrhea, and a wet cough. Her lungs are clear. Her neck has a small 0.5-cm bulge in the midline, just above the suprasternal notch. It is tender to the touch and feels slightly boggy. There is no erythema.

    What is her diagnosis?

    (A) thyroid mass
    (B) furuncle
    (C) lymphadenitis
    (D) thyroglossal duct cyst
    (E) branchial cleft cyst

16. Another 5-year-old girl is seen for a neck mass that also has been there for some time. She

comes in because it is now tender, enlarging, and yesterday some "pus" started coming out of it. She has had no fever, had a "cold" 2 weeks ago, and is generally in good health.

On examination she is afebrile. She has a 4-cm tender, smooth, fluctuant mass along the anterior border of the sternocleidomastoid muscle on the left side. There is a small dimple in the middle with yellow crusting around it. You are able to express some serosanguineous fluid with mild pressure. The rest of her head and neck exams are normal.

What is her diagnosis?

(A) thyroiditis
(B) furuncle
(C) lymphadenitis
(D) thyroglossal duct cyst
(E) branchial cleft cyst

17. What is the best way to evaluate this lesion from question 16?

(A) radiograph of neck
(B) ultrasound of neck
(C) CT of neck
(D) MRI of neck

18. In regard to question 16, are these more often unilateral or bilateral?

(A) unilateral
(B) bilateral

Answers

1. **(C)** This is most likely to be acute unilateral pyogenic lymphadenitis, often seen in children 1 to 4 years old following an upper respiratory tract infection. In >50% of cases, it is the submandibular nodes that are affected. The tempo of the illness and the overlying illness are the most important clues. Cat-scratch disease is a possibility but less likely.

2. **(D)** EBV usually causes either bilateral or generalized lymphadenopathy and more constitutional symptoms. Group A streptococci and *S. aureus* cause >80% of these cases. Infections caused by nontuberculous mycobacteria more often have an insidious onset, although they can uncom-

monly cause a picture similar to acute pyogenic lymphadenitis.

3. **(D)** Because staphylococci and streptococci are the primary pathogens, an oral cephalosporin, cephalexin is the most appropriate choice in areas where the prevalence of MRSA in the community is low. Clindamycin would be a better choice if community-acquired MRSA is common in the patient's area.

4. **(E)**

5. **(E)** *S. aureus* is the most common cause of neonatal acute cervical lymphadenitis, but another important cause of neck mass in the newborn is a result of group B strep, in the "cellulitis-adenitis" syndrome. This most often presents at 3 to 7 weeks, 75% of patients are male, and most have the overlying cellulitis described above. *S. agalactiae* and group B streptococci are synonyms.

6. **(B)** It is essential to exclude *M. tuberculosis* as early as possible because of the abnormal PPD (a positive tuberculin skin test in an otherwise healthy 3-year-old is >10 mm). However, caution must be used in interpreting PPD results in children in whom a nontuberculous mycobacterial infection is possible, since antigens of the latter can cross-react with PPD. A chest radiograph should be the next test ordered. After that, a lymph node biopsy and a CT scan of the neck are possible avenues of investigation.

7. **(E)** Because NTM are present in the environment (soil, water), specimens from nonsterile locations such as stomach, urine, and sputum can be contaminated. A blood culture will only be positive if disseminated disease is present. Examination of the tissue obtained by surgical excision is the gold standard to diagnose this infection in the presence of an 11-mm PPD.

8. **(C)** NTM are found in soil and water, and transmission can be by inhalation, ingestion, direct contact, and animal contact by means of soil and water. Person-to-person transmission is rare.

9. **(B)** NTM can cause the other infections listed, but disseminated infection occurs only in immu-

nocompromised hosts. In children with cystic fibrosis, pneumonia is also a possible manifestation.

10. **(E)** For NTM in an otherwise healthy child, complete surgical excision almost always leads to cure. Ciprofloxacin and doxycycline may be effective against rapidly growing mycobacteria (*M. fortuitum*, *M. abscessus*). C and D are multidrug therapy, reserved for immunocompromised patients or those with disseminated disease. Ethambutol is seldom used in children.

11. **(C)** This is most likely cat-scratch disease caused by *Bartonella henselae*, although the patient is afebrile. In more than three-fourths of cases, a history of a cat or kitten exposure is given.

12. **(E)** In addition to those listed, other manifestations of *Bartonella* include encephalitis, fever of unknown origin, pneumonia, TTP, erythema nodosum, and osteolytic lesions. Parinaud oculoglandular syndrome presents as conjunctivitis and preauricular or submandibular lymphadenopathy that is ipsilateral to the primary infection.

13. **(A)**

14. **(A)** Antibiotics are used for severely ill children with cat-scratch disease. Getting rid of the cats/kittens will not help this episode, although patients should be instructed to avoid rough play with cats and kittens to avoid scratches, and if scratched, should wash the wound immediately. Fine-needle aspiration is sometimes used in especially painful enlarged lymph glands for pain relief. Incision and drainage as well as surgical excision should be avoided.

15. **(D)** Thyroglossal duct cysts appear during childhood and often enlarge rapidly in the setting of an infection. They are located midline, between the hyoid bone and the suprasternal notch, and move up when the patient sticks the tongue out or during swallowing. Thyroid tissue is a possibility, though unlikely given this history, but always must be ruled out before surgery is undertaken to correct the cyst.

16. **(E)** This is a branchial cleft cyst, located at the anterior border of the SCM muscle. When su-

perinfected, like this one, it enlarges and may drain purulent fluid.

17. **(B)** Typically, ultrasound is the preferred modality to begin the evaluation of branchial clefts in children, or fistulotomy if fistula is suspected. CT is often the second choice.

18. **(A)** 2% to 3% are bilateral.

SUGGESTED READING

Behrman RE, Kliegman RM, Jenson HB, et al: *Nelson Textbook of Pediatrics*. Philadelphia, WB Saunders, 2004, pp 1528–1529, 1973.

Chesney PJ: Nontuberculous mycobacteria. *Pediatr Rev* 23(9):300–308, 2002.

Peters TR, Edwards KM: Cervical lymphadenopathy and adenitis. *Pediatr Rev* 21(12):399–404, 2000.

Pickering LK et al: *Red Book 2003 Report of the Committee on Infectious Diseases*. Elk Grove Village, IL: American Academy of Pediatrics, 2003, pp 232–234, 661–666.

CASE 62: A 3-MONTH-OLD MALE WITH APNEA

A 3-month-old male is brought to your ER on Thanksgiving after mom noted that he "stopped breathing." He was in his usual state of health until 3 days prior to presentation when he developed nasal congestion and mild cough. The cough worsened, resulting in decreased intake, and, according to mom, progressed toward an increased effort of breathing. The night of admission mom observed a particularly harsh coughing spell, followed by a period where no breathing was noted for approximately 20 to 30 seconds. Mom denies any color changes, abnormal movements, loss of tone, emesis, or fever. After the breathing resumed, the infant was breathing abnormally fast, and mom noted increased effort to breathe. She brought him to the ER, and noted no further episodes on the way.

Past medical history and family history are unremarkable. Immunizations are up to date and he takes no known medications. The infant lives at home with his mom, dad, and 3-year-old sister, all of whom are healthy. There are no smokers in the home. He attends daycare.

On your exam, he is resting quietly, with vital signs of T 100.7°F (38.2°C) rectally, HR 144, RR 62, BP 100/70, and oxygen saturation of 90% on RA. He appears mildly dehydrated, but not toxic. The right tympanic membrane has decreased mobility with poor landmarks, and nasal congestion and discharge are noted. The lung exam reveals tachypnea with subcostal retractions and nasal flaring. He has diffuse wheezes and crackles through both lung fields. A wet cough is noted. Neurologically he has no focal deficits and is alert and responsive. The remainder of the exam is benign.

He is placed on 1 L oxygen by nasal cannula and given an albuterol nebulizer treatment with no apparent response. Chest radiograph demonstrates right middle lobe atelectasis with hyperinflation, but no focal infiltrates.

SELECT THE ONE BEST ANSWER

1. Which of the following is the most likely etiology for this patient's symptoms?

   (A) *C. trachomatis*
   (B) pertussis
   (C) RSV
   (D) reactive airway disease
   (E) none of the above

2. Which of the following would be most useful in directing the immediate course of action for this patient?

   (A) CBC with differential
   (B) rapid enzyme immunoassay
   (C) EEG
   (D) viral culture of nasopharyngeal aspirate
   (E) none of the above

3. Which of the following is proven the most useful in the patient's recovery?

   (A) nebulized albuterol
   (B) nebulized budesonide
   (C) oral prednisolone
   (D) aerosolized ribavirin
   (E) none of the above

4. Which of the following is not an important issue with regard to the infection control of RSV?

   (A) prevention of fecal-oral spread
   (B) good handwashing
   (C) institution of hospital contact isolation
   (D) parental education
   (E) patient cohorting in hospital

5. Which of the following patients is not at increased risk for RSV complications?

   (A) a 6-year-old s/p bone marrow transplant
   (B) a 7-month-old, formerly 30-week premature infant without chronic lung disease
   (C) an 8-month-old with diagnosed chronic lung disease
   (D) a full-term infant with congenital heart disease
   (E) a 9-month-old, formerly 27-week premature infant without chronic lung disease

6. Which of the following is false regarding the epidemiology of RSV?

   (A) Peak months are November through May in temperate climates.
   (B) The virus can remain viable on countertops for hours.
   (C) Peak age of onset is birth to 2 months.
   (D) Spread is via ocular or nasal direct contact with large droplets in secretions.
   (E) The virus can be shed for 3 to 8 days.

7. True or False: Prior infection with RSV confers lifelong immunity.

   (A) True
   (B) False

8. True or False: The majority of children have been infected with RSV by 4 years old.

   (A) True
   (B) False

9. In a child who presents with a staccato cough without fever, what is the most notable finding on complete blood count?

   (A) absolute lymphocytosis
   (B) neutropenia
   (C) thrombocytopenia
   (D) eosinophilia
   (E) normocytic anemia

10. True or False: Newborns of mothers with documented untreated *C. trachomatis* should be treated empirically.

   (A) True
   (B) False

11. If a newborn does acquire *C. trachomatis* during delivery, what are the chances that the infant will eventually have symptoms?

    (A) 25% to 50% for pneumonia
    (B) 50% to 75% for conjunctivitis
    (C) 5% to 20% for pneumonia
    (D) 5% to 20% for conjunctivitis
    (E) 50% to 75% for pneumonia

12. Which of the following statements is true regarding the treatment of infant chlamydial infections?

    (A) Azithromycin for 5 days is the treatment of choice.
    (B) Erythromycin should not be given to children younger than 6 weeks because of the risk of pyloric stenosis.
    (C) Topical erythromycin alone is adequate for the treatment of conjunctivitis.
    (D) Oral erythromycin should be given for both conjunctivitis and pneumonia.
    (E) None of the above

13. Which of the following is not a clinical presentation of an ALTE?

    (A) limpness
    (B) gagging
    (C) cyanosis
    (D) plethoric color changes
    (E) none of the above

14. Which of the following is a potential diagnosis to explain an ALTE?

    (A) gastroesophageal reflux
    (B) anemia
    (C) pertussis
    (D) bronchiolitis
    (E) all of the above

15. A 2-week old infant has an apneic event. The infant was born via uncomplicated vaginal delivery, and had an unremarkable postnatal course. Mom denies any complications of pregnancy or infections. All appropriate bacterial cultures are pending, and an EEG demonstrates sharp spikes in the temporal lobe. What is the most appropriate next step to help diagnose?

    (A) Send CSF for viral culture.
    (B) Send CSF for a specific PCR.
    (C) Send serum for a specific PCR.
    (D) Obtain a pH probe.
    (E) Obtain head CT.

16. What would be the appropriate therapy for HSV meningoencephalitis?

    (A) acyclovir PO for 4 weeks
    (B) acyclovir IV for 3 weeks
    (C) ganciclovir IV for 3 weeks
    (D) oseltamivir IV for 4 weeks
    (E) foscarnet IV for 3 weeks

17. What is the most important goal of hospitalization for an ALTE?

    (A) obtaining definitive diagnosis
    (B) establishing home apnea monitoring
    (C) educating family to infant CPR
    (D) involving child protective services
    (E) all of the above

Answers

1. **(C)** The patient described in the vignette most likely has an infectious etiology for his respiratory symptoms. The most likely of the infectious choices in this scenario is RSV. The most common cause of respiratory tract infection in infants and young children, RSV peaks between November and May. Hypoxia and wheezing following congestion and cough are classic symptoms of RSV infection. Chlamydia is more often found in younger patients (2 months) and they have a staccato cough with possibly a history of conjunctivitis. Pertussis, although common in infants, is less frequently seen after the 4-month immunizations and tends to present with a paroxysmal cough without wheezing. Both chlamydia and pertussis, like RSV, however, can cause apnea, although chlamydia does so rarely. Reactive airway disease is less likely with a negative family history of asthma, no prior episodes, and lack of response to bronchodilators.

2. **(B)** With clinical suspicion high for RSV, the most rapid diagnostic tool would be a rapid RSV screen by immunoassay. A positive test would prevent further unnecessary laboratory testing

and antibiotic use, as well as allow for proper infection control steps. Though a viral culture would confirm any screen, results take several days. A CBC could suggest concern for other infectious causes (e.g., lymphocytosis in pertussis or eosinophilia in *Chlamydia*) but is not specific. EEG is included in the workup of apnea, but would not be warranted until an infectious cause is ruled out.

3. **(E)** The only uncontroversial method for RSV treatment is supportive care. Careful attention should be paid to oral intake, as increased respiratory rate can prevent adequate nutritional intake, and intravenous fluids may be necessary. Supplemental oxygen may be necessary for persistent desaturation. Multiple studies have investigated the role of bronchodilators, steroids, and antivirals, with no concrete results. Though some studies have shown a correlation with ribavirin use and long-term asthma outcomes, these studies are contradictory and inconclusive. Bronchodilators and steroids have shown inconsistent benefit at best and are not cost-effective for the minimal improvement they may offer.

4. **(A)** RSV is transmitted via large-droplet secretions via nasal or ocular contact. Respiratory isolation is not necessary, though the remaining answers are all mainstays for prevention of community and nosocomial transmission.

5. **(B)** Infants between 29 and 32 weeks' gestation who do not have CLD are not at increased risk after 6 months of age.

6. **(C)** Peak age of onset is 2 to 5 months.

7. **(B)** False. Reinfection often occurs with RSV, though subsequent infections tend to be less severe.

8. **(A)** True. The majority of children in the United States will be infected by the age of 2 years, though more than 75% of hospital admissions will be in children <1 year of age.

9. **(D)** Patients with *C. trachomatis* pneumonia are notable for an eosinophilia on complete blood count. Though this is not diagnostic, it is highly suggestive of such an infection in a child who fits the classic clinical picture (staccato cough, afebrile pneumonia, 1 to 3 months of age).

10. **(B)** False. There are no studies that prove the efficacy of empiric treatment of a newborn born to a *Chlamydia*-positive mother. Treatment is based on development of symptoms (conjunctivitis, pneumonia).

11. **(C)** The risk of an infant acquiring *Chlamydia* pneumonia is 5% to 20%. The risk of conjunctivitis is greater at 25% to 50%.

12. **(D)** Oral erythromycin is currently the recommended therapy for both conjunctivitis and pneumonia caused by *C. trachomatis*. Topical therapy for conjunctivitis is ineffective. Azithromycin has not been approved for children younger than 6 months of age. Though an association between erythromycin and pyloric stenosis has been reported in infants, such an association has not been proven and thus erythromycin is still recommended for therapy even for infants younger than 6 weeks old.

13. **(E)** An ALTE (formerly known as "near-miss SIDS") is defined as any episode that is frightening to the observer. All of the above symptoms can be included in that definition. The majority of ALTE patients require admission and observation/workup.

14. **(E)** All of the above are potential etiologies for ALTE. The workup of ALTE is focused on historical and physical findings directing the investigation. A large percentage of patients will have no identifiable cause for the ALTE and will have no repeat events either in the hospital or after discharge.

15. **(B)** The patient described above has an ALTE secondary to seizure activity consistent with neonatal herpes infection. Confirmation of a herpes CNS infection could be achieved by CSF PCR. A CSF viral culture is rarely positive, although it should be attempted. CT scans do not demonstrate changes before 3 to 5 days, so an MRI would be more useful. After obtaining CSF for PCR, antivirals targeting herpes should be used pending the result.

16. **(B)** Acyclovir is the drug of choice for CNS HSV infection in neonates. The dose is 20 mg/kg/dose TID for 14 to 21 days.

17. **(C)** The most important discharge goal for ALTE is to educate parents on infant CPR. Home monitoring has not been proven to reduce the incidence of SIDS and often causes more parental stress. Most cases of ALTE will be of unknown etiology. Although child protective services may be warranted in some cases of ALTE when the clinical history is suspicious, most cases only require parental education.

SUGGESTED READING

Meissner HC, Long SS: Revised indications for the use of palivizumab and respiratory syncytial virus immune globulin intravenous for the prevention of respiratory syncytial virus infections. American Academy of Pediatrics, Committee on Infectious Diseases and Committee on Fetus and Newborn. *Pediatrics* 112:1447, 2003.

Pickering LK, ed: *Red Book: 2003 Report of the Committee on Infectious Diseases*, 26th ed. Elk Grove Village, IL: American Academy of Pediatrics, 2003.

Respiratory syncytial virus activity—United States, 1999–2000 season. *MMWR Morbid Mortal Wkly Rep* 49: 1091, 2000.

CASE 63: A 2-YEAR-OLD BOY WHO NEEDS A CHECK-UP

A 2-year-old male presents for a routine health supervision visit. He is a new patient to your clinic and arrives with few medical records. Mom reports that he has been well his whole life, although his previous doctor mentioned that he was "behind on the things he does." She does not have any concerns. He started daycare 4 months prior and is starting to attempt toilet training. Bowel movements are every other day and can be hard. His diet consists of eating most foods, with minimal vegetables, but limited "junk food," and he drinks 4 to 5 glasses of whole milk per day. Developmentally he can brush his teeth with help but does not dress/undress himself. He can build a tower of six cubes, climbs steps, but does not kick a ball. He has a 20-word vocabulary and is just starting to combine two-word phrases. Family history is negative for any chronic illness.

On physical exam, his height is 88 cm and weight is 13.2 kg. Significant findings include mild pallor of the oral mucosa, a I/VI systolic ejection murmur with good pulses, dry plaques on the antecubital fossae bilaterally, and no focal neurologic findings. Otherwise his exam is unremarkable.

SELECT THE ONE BEST ANSWER

1. What screening test should be ordered for this patient?

   (A) folate level
   (B) lipid panel
   (C) complete blood count
   (D) PPD
   (E) echocardiography

2. A CBC is obtained. The patient has a hemoglobin of 10.3, hematocrit of 30.7, and an MCV of 65. Which of the following is not on your differential?

   (A) iron deficiency anemia
   (B) thalassemia
   (C) folate deficiency
   (D) lead poisoning
   (E) anemia of chronic disease

3. Which of the following iron studies are consistent with iron deficiency anemia?

   (A) low MCV, normal RDW, normal TIBC, high FEP
   (B) low MCV, normal RDW, normal TIBC, normal FEP
   (C) low MCV, high RDW, high TIBC, high FEP
   (D) low MCV, normal RDW, low TIBC, high FEP
   (E) none of the above

4. Based on history what other tests might be warranted for this child?

   (A) Denver II developmental screening
   (B) serum lead level
   (C) environmental exposure screen
   (D) all of the above
   (E) A and B

5. Which of the following situations would not warrant a risk-based evaluation for lead poisoning?

   (A) Patient lives in a house built in 1960.
   (B) Patient has a history of pica.
   (C) Patient has a sibling with history of lead poisoning.

(D) Patient frequently visits a house built in 1960 that was renovated 4 months ago.

(E) A and D.

6. The CDC recommends universal screening for lead poising for all children between 9 and 12 months.

(A) true
(B) false

7. Which of the following is not an effect of elevated blood lead levels?

(A) colic
(B) nephropathy
(C) advanced pubertal development
(D) encephalopathy
(E) hemolytic anemia

8. The patient's lead level is 18 µg/dL. What is the next step?

(A) Begin oral chelation therapy.
(B) Repeat lead level in 1 week.
(C) Begin nutritional and environmental counseling.
(D) Stop the supplemental iron therapy.
(E) None of the above

9. At what lead level should chelation be initiated?

(A) 25 µg/dL
(B) 35 µg/dL
(C) 45 µg/dL
(D) 55 µg/dL
(E) 70 µg/dL

10. Which of the following is true regarding chelation?

(A) DMSA is initially given for 21 days.
(B) Hospitalization for therapy is not required until a level of >75 µg/dL.
(C) Parenteral agents include DMSA and calcium disodium EDTA.
(D) $CaNa_2$ EDTA is toxic when given with iron.
(E) DMSA side effects include decreased ANC and increased LFTs.

11. Which of the following is not a current potential side effect of BAL?

(A) fever
(B) anaphylaxis
(C) tachycardia
(D) hypotension
(E) salivation

12. Which of the following is a contraindication to BAL therapy?

(A) iron therapy
(B) renal insufficiency
(C) hepatic insufficiency
(D) G_6PD
(E) encephalopathy

13. Which of the following is not a potential environmental exposure for lead in the United States?

(A) old furniture
(B) food cans
(C) folk remedies
(D) nearby industry
(E) target shooting

14. According to the Second National Health and Nutrition Examination Survey (NHANES II) data, which of the following are independent risk factor for elevated blood lead levels?

(A) poverty
(B) age younger than 6 years
(C) African-American ethnicity
(D) dwelling in the city
(E) all of the above

15. Which of the following is a method of prevention for lead intoxication?

(A) frequent meals
(B) meals with high vitamin C, low calcium
(C) low-phosphate detergent for cleansing
(D) limit iron intake
(E) increase fat in meals

16. All of the following regarding lead toxicity and postexposure prevention are true except:

(A) Painting over existing lead-based paint creates only temporary protection.
(B) Soil coverage with fabric and ground cover limits ground exposure to lead.

(C) Use of glass and carbon water filters prevents water transmission.

(D) Use of HEPA vacuum for cleaning is necessary to remove lead from the home.

(E) Cleaning can temporarily increase the ingestion risk.

17. Which of the following is an indication for cholesterol screening in a child older than 2 years of age?

(A) a grandmother who died of an MI at the age of 60 years

(B) a grandfather with documented hypercholesterolemia

(C) an uncle with an MI at age 45 years

(D) a father with angina at age 45 years

(E) none of the above

18. Which of the following patients should be immediately screened for tuberculosis?

(A) an international adoptee from Thailand

(B) a sibling of an asymptomatic known HIV-infected patient

(C) the child of a mother with a positive PPD and normal chest radiograph treated with a 9-month course of isoniazid

(D) A and C

(E) B and C

19. Which of the following findings would be considered a developmental delay on the Denver II for a 2-year-old?

(A) inability to wash and dry hands

(B) inability to combine words

(C) inability to kick a ball forward

(D) having half understandable speech

(E) inability to point to four pictures

Answers

1. (C) With his nutritional history and physical symptoms, this patient is a risk for iron-deficiency anemia. A screening hemoglobin and hematocrit would be beneficial to address an immediate and treatable concern. Both a PPD and lipid screen would be appropriate at this age if history suggested risk factors. Echocardiography and folate level are not routine screening tests based on this patient's history and clinical exam.

2. (C) Folate deficiency is a macrocytic anemia, not a microcytic anemia. The remaining four disease states can all be associated with microcytic anemia.

3. (C) Iron studies can often be used to differentiate the main causes of microcytic anemia. The above iron studies are most consistent with: A, lead poisoning, B, thalassemia trait, and D, chronic disease. Iron deficiency anemia will also have a low serum iron, unlike thalassemia trait and lead poisoning.

4. (D) The given history of development is consistent with developmental delay. To assess this delay, a complete Denver II should be performed. If the patient has two or more "delays" on exam, he should be referred for evaluation for services. With developmental delay and microcytic anemia, this patient may have an elevated lead level. Both a serum lead level and an environmental exposure screen are warranted at this time.

5. (A) The AAP and CDC recommend screening questions for lead poisoning risk. Children who live in or visit homes built before 1950 or those built before 1978 with renovations in the past 6 months warrant lead screening. Also, if they have any demonstrated behavior of pica or siblings/playmates with lead poisoning, they warrant testing.

6. (B) False. The CDC recommends universal screening in all high-risk areas based on prevalence of elevated lead levels. Patients in low-to-moderate risk areas should be tested based on screening criteria noted in answer 5.

7. (C) Of the listed, the only one not seen in acute or chronic lead poisoning is advanced pubertal development. Mildly elevated blood lead levels have been associated with delayed breast and pubic hair development and decreased height in girls.

8. (C) Currently the CDC recommends retesting lead levels in 3 months if the lead level is 10 to 19 $\mu g/dL$. Nutritional and environmental counseling should be initiated in any patient with a level over 14 $\mu g/dL$. Chelation is not warranted at this lead level. Iron therapy, though controversial during IV chelation therapy for lead poisoning,

is nevertheless recommended in patients with documented iron deficiency anemia.

9. **(C)** Standard chelation should be used if the lead level is ≥45 µg/dL. According to CDC recommendations, a level of ≥45 µg/dL should be repeated and verified within 48 hours.

10. **(E)** Chelation can be given orally or parenterally. Some form of chelation is begun at a level of ≥45 µg/dL, with parenteral treatment in the hospital setting started for a level of 70 µg/dL or higher. The oral chelation agent used is DMSA (succimer), which can be given initially for 19 days. This chelation must occur in a lead-free environment. Parenteral chelation, which can be begun at levels ≥45 µg/dL, include calcium disodium EDTA and BAL simultaneously. BAL is toxic when given with iron.

11. **(D)** Side effects of BAL include fever, tachycardia, hypertension, salivation, tingling around the mouth, anaphylaxis, and hemolysis in G_6PD patients.

12. **(C)** Hepatic insufficiency is a contraindication to BAL/dimercaprol therapy. Peanut allergy is also a contraindication, since BAL/dimercaprol is dissolved in peanut oil for administration. BAL administration should be used cautiously in those with renal impairment and in the presence of G_6PD.

13. **(B)** All of the above historically have been noted to contain lead, although food cans have been lead-free since U.S. legislation in 1977 limited lead in household paint, and gasoline lead, and stopped the soldering of cans for food. The remaining items are all still possible sources of lead.

14. **(E)** All of the above are independent risk factors for elevated blood lead level.

15. **(A)** Recommendations for prevention of lead intoxication include a balanced diet with frequent meals that are high in iron, vitamin C, and calcium, all which compete with lead for GI absorption.

16. **(C)** Ion-exchange and reverse-osmosis filters, as well as distillation, are effective in removing lead from water sources. However, glass and carbon filters, the most common in homes, do not remove heavy metals, including lead.

17. **(D)** The American Heart Association recommends screening for patients over the age of 2 who have a parent or grandparent with documented premature cardiovascular disease (angina, MI, sudden cardiac death, cerebrovascular disease, coronary bypass, angioplasty or peripheral vascular disease younger than the age of 55 years), a parent with documented hypercholesterolemia, or an unknown family history.

18. **(A)** Immediate testing should be performed on 1) contacts of anyone with confirmed or suspected TB, 2) children with radiographic or clinical findings of TB, 3) children immigrating from endemic countries (e.g., Asia, Middle East, Africa, Latin America), 4) children with travel histories to endemic countries and/or significant contact with indigenous peoples.

19. **(C)** By the age of 2 years, according to the Denver II, children should be able to kick a ball forward. The remaining choices are all within normal range of abilities for a 2-year-old.

SUGGESTED READING

Campbell C, Osterhoudt KC: Prevention of childhood lead poisoning. *Curr Opin Pediatr* 12:428, 2000.

Markowitz M: Lead poisoning. *Pediatr Rev* 21: 327, 2000.

Wright RO, Tsaih S-W, Schwartz J, Wright RJ, Hu H: Association between iron deficiency and blood level in a longitudinal analysis of children followed in an urban primary care clinic. *J Pediatr* 142:9, 2003.

Wu AC, Lesperance L, Bernstein H: Screening for iron deficiency. *Pediatr Rev* 23:171, 2002.

CASE 64: A 2-YEAR-OLD WHO REFUSES TO WALK

A 2-year-old male presents to the emergency room with a 1-day history of refusing to walk. Mom reports that she had first noticed him limping slightly 3 to 4 days ago, but he was otherwise well. He was not complaining of pain, but mom noticed that when he stood, he did not bear weight on his right leg. By the day of admission she noticed that he refused to walk. She denies a history of bites or specific trauma, but she does admit that he is "always running into things." He had a cough and congestion the previous week and has "felt warm" for 1 to 2 days, but has otherwise been well. She denies any preceding sore throat or rash.

On exam the patient is fussy and uncooperative. His temperature is 101.3°F (38.5°C) rectally, HR 115, RR 22, and blood pressure normal. He has no rashes or discolorations of his skin and is well hydrated. He refuses to ambulate. On musculoskeletal exam the patient has a tender, warm and swollen right knee. There is mild erythema but no induration. He resists range of motion activities at the knee, but has full range of motion and no tenderness at the hip. Otherwise his exam is unremarkable.

SELECT THE ONE BEST ANSWER

1. All are appropriate choices for initial workup except:

   (A) bone scan
   (B) hip and knee films
   (C) CBC with differential
   (D) ESR
   (E) CRP

2. The plain films demonstrate soft-tissue swelling surrounding the knee, but no findings consistent with fracture or osteomyelitis. The hip is normal. The CBC shows a leukocyte count of 18.4×10^3 with 28% bands; the ESR is 68 mm/hr and the CRP is 94 mg/L. Which of the following is not in the differential at this point?

   (A) osteomyelitis
   (B) transient synovitis
   (C) septic arthritis
   (D) cellulitis
   (E) postinfectious arthritis

3. What would be the best test/procedure to diagnose a septic joint?

   (A) urine antigen detection test
   (B) ultrasound
   (C) CRP
   (D) joint aspiration
   (E) MRI

4. The patient's ultrasound demonstrates no effusion, and osteomyelitis is now strongly suspected. What is the most likely causative organism morphology and biochemical reaction?

   (A) gram-negative bacillus without lactose fermentation
   (B) gram-positive cocci in chains
   (C) gram-negative bacillus without sucrose fermentation
   (D) gram-negative coccobacillus
   (E) gram-positive cocci in clusters

5. Knowing the likely pathogens for osteomyelitis, in a region where MRSA isolates are common what would be an appropriate empiric therapy?

   (A) clindamycin
   (B) penicillinase-resistant penicillin
   (C) third-generation cephalosporin
   (D) combination of A and C
   (E) combination of B and C

6. Which of the following is the most specific method for confirmatory diagnosis of osteomyelitis?

   (A) MRI
   (B) conventional radiograph
   (C) bone scan
   (D) bone biopsy
   (E) CT scan

7. Which of the following is the most common pathogenesis of osteomyelitis in children?

   (A) contiguity
   (B) direct invasion
   (C) hematogenous spread
   (D) unknown
   (E) B and C are approximately equal

8. All of the following are complications of osteomyelitis except:

   (A) fracture
   (B) septic joint
   (C) subperiosteal abscess
   (D) leg shortening
   (E) all of the above are complications of osteomyelitis

9. Which of the following is the most common site of septic arthritis in children older than 1 year of age?

   (A) ankle

(B) shoulder
(C) wrist
(D) knee
(E) hip

10. Which of the following is the cornerstone of the diagnosis of septic arthritis?

(A) MRI
(B) plain films
(C) blood culture
(D) arthrocentesis and fluid analysis
(E) arthrocentesis and fluid culture

11. A 13-year-old male presents after spring break with a chief complaint of knee pain. He first noted the bilateral knee pain last summer, and it resolved until recently. He denies sports, but does note that he performs in a hip-hop dance group when on school vacations. He denies fever or any other symptoms. He is not sexually active and denies any trauma. On exam he has no trouble with ambulation, has no joint effusions, has full range of motion at the hip and knee, but complains of pain on palpation of the proximal tibia. What is the most appropriate next step in care?

(A) MRI of the knee
(B) plain films of the knee
(C) plain films of the hip
(D) arthroscopy
(E) reassurance and rest

12. What is the most common cause of septic arthritis?

(A) *H. influenzae*
(B) *S. aureus*
(C) *E. coli*
(D) *Salmonella* species
(E) *M. pneumoniae*

13. Which of the following is true regarding toddlers' fractures?

(A) They result from major injury, e.g., a fall from a great height.
(B) They are best seen on lateral radiographic view.
(C) They are seen in the distal one-third of the tibia.
(D) They are best treated with rest and NSAIDs.
(E) They are most commonly seen between 3 and 4 years old.

14. In which of the following patients are radiographs not indicated with a clinical history and exam that is consistent with Osgood-Schlatter?

(A) atypical complaints of pain
(B) erythema or warmth over the tibia
(C) pain not directly over the tubercle
(D) bilateral pain and symptoms
(E) all require imaging

15. What is the common presentation of arthritis in a child with rheumatic fever?

(A) finger/joint involvement
(B) migratory in large joints
(C) unilateral wrist
(D) bilateral ankle
(E) hip involvement

16. Which is true of the treatment of toxic synovitis?

(A) Antibiotics are the mainstay of therapy.
(B) Aggressive physical therapy should be initiated early.
(C) Joint aspiration is diagnostic.
(D) NSAIDs are the initial therapy.
(E) More than 50% will recur with or without therapy.

Answers

1. **(A)** Though a bone scan is useful in diagnosis of osteomyelitis, it is not an appropriate choice for initial investigation. Though plain films are not sensitive initially for osteomyelitis and rarely assist in the diagnosis of a septic joint, they will help to rule out more concerning diagnoses such as malignancies and detect any underlying fractures. CBC with differential, ESR, and CRP are helpful inflammatory markers for diagnosis and to follow progression of illness.

2. **(B)** The most worrisome diagnoses at this point are osteomyelitis and septic arthritis. Reactive arthritis and cellulitis must still be considered but are less likely. However, transient synovitis is most common in the hip. It can be differentiated from septic arthritis by laboratory results. Septic arthritis is more likely to have an increased leukocyte count with a left shift and an increased ESR and CRP. With

these laboratory results, transient synovitis is highly unlikely.

3. **(D)** Though ultrasound will reveal a subtle effusion, the presence of an effusion does not definitively diagnose septic arthritis. Analysis of fluid obtained from an aspiration would demonstrate a leukocytic effusion, thus differentiating it from noninflammatory causes of joint effusion. Aspirated joint fluid might reveal bacteria on Gram stain or culture.

4. **(E)** Although all the choices are known causes of osteomyelitis, the most common cause is *S. aureus*. *Salmonella* is more common in patients with sickle cell anemia, and *Pseudomonas* is seen following puncture wounds. *Kingella kingae* (D) is an emerging cause of osteomyelitis in Israel, but it is far less common than *S. aureus*.

5. **(A)** Though all the choices would provide some coverage for *S. aureus*, it is important to cover most etiologies and resistant organisms. In regions that have a high prevalence of MRSA, oxacillin, nafcillin, and related compounds would no longer be appropriate empiric choices. In this instance, clindamycin would be an appropriate first agent. Ceftriaxone might be a reasonable addition if the patient has known or suspected sickle cell anemia since *Salmonella* osteomyelitis can occur in these patients as well as *S. aureus*.

6. **(D)** Biopsy of the metaphysis of the affected bone is the most specific way to diagnose osteomyelitis. MRI and bone scan are 80% to 100% sensitive, but specificities can be lower than 50%. However, they are the preferential diagnostic imaging tools, especially in the absence of surgical aspiration, or to locate the area of inflammation. CT is not traditionally helpful. Plain films can demonstrate evidence of osteomyelitis, but only after 10 to 14 days of infection.

7. **(C)** Hematogenous spread is the most common mechanism in children. The vascularization of the metaphysis allows for bacterial seeding of the marrow cavity. Inflammation ensues and increases intraosseous pressure, which in turn hampers normal bone circulation. This can lead to necrosis and potential spread of infection to the epiphysis and joints. Direct invasion of bacteria into bone occurs in children but is most often secondary to trauma.

8. **(E)** All of these are potential complications of osteomyelitis. Septic arthritis can often result from contiguous spread of osteomyelitis. Hyperemia around the inflammation can lead to leg lengthening; proliferating cartilage can lead to leg shortening. Fractures can be a result of local destruction.

9. **(D)** Though all of the above joints may become infected, the most common site in older children (>1 year) is the knee. The hip is the most common site in infants.

10. **(E)** Though culture is key to identification of the organism to treat, blood cultures are positive in no more than 50% of patients, and joint fluid culture is positive in 35% to 80% of patients. Fluid analysis is more immediately helpful in the diagnosis of septic arthritis: WBC >100,000, depressed glucose levels, and increased lactic acid and LDH. Though synovial fluid is essential to obtain, in extremely ill patients, treatment should not be delayed as one-third of joint cultures and nearly one-half of blood cultures remain positive even after initiation of antibiotics.

11. **(E)** The most likely diagnosis for the patient is Osgood-Schlatter disease. With the patient's history of recurrence during periods of increased activity, the best treatment for the patient is rest and NSAIDs as needed. A radiograph of the knee is not unreasonable if atypical clinical features are present.

12. **(B)** The leading cause of septic arthritis in children is *S. aureus*. *H. influenzae* type b was an important cause in infants and children before the introduction of immunization. *Salmonella*, *E. coli*, and *M. pneumoniae* rarely infect joints.

13. **(C)** Toddlers' fractures are commonly seen between 9 months and 3 years, as a result of minor falls, trips, or twists. The children present with inability to weight bear and pain on dorsiflexion of the ankle. On internal oblique view, a fracture is most often noted in the distal one-third of the

tibia. A fracture that is in the midshaft would be far more suggestive of abuse. Toddlers' fractures should be casted for 5 to 6 weeks. This diagnosis should always be considered in a limping child of this age.

14. (**D**) Bilateral disease is commonly seen in Osgood-Schlatter and should not prompt further imaging. The remaining choices are all suggestive of some other pathology and warrant further radiologic investigation.

15. (**B**) The classic presentation of rheumatic fever is that of a child with migratory polyarthritis in large joints. Though smaller joints (including wrist and hand) can be involved, they are more often one of many joints in a migration. Most patients have large joints involved first.

16. (**D**) Toxic synovitis, a diagnosis of exclusion, is best treated with rest and NSAIDs. Antibiotic therapy would be appropriate for septic arthritis diagnosed by aspiration, but not for toxic synovitis.

SUGGESTED READING

Jung ST: Significance of laboratory and radiologic findings for differentiating between septic arthritis and transient synovitis of the hip. *J Pediatr Orthop* 23:368, 2003.

Kim MK, Karpas AK: The limping child. *Clin Pediatr Emerg Med* 3:129, 2002.

Miller ML, Cassidy JT: Postinfectious arthritis and related conditions. In: Behrman R, Kliegman R, Jenson H (eds), *Nelson Textbook of Pediatrics*, 17th ed. Philadelphia: WB Saunders, 2004.

CASE 65: A 2-YEAR-OLD WITH RECURRENT WHEEZING

A 2-year-old male presents to your clinic for evaluation of respiratory difficulties. His mom reports that he was in his usual state of health until yesterday when he began having shortness of breath, cough, and an occasional wheeze. Mom gave him two puffs of his brother's albuterol inhaler, which initially provided some relief. Mom denies any preceding symptoms, such as rhinorrhea, fever, or other URI symptoms. Mom also denies smokers in the home, pets, or carpets, but notes that the symptoms did start after playing next door with his 4-year-old neighbor. The patient has wheezed once before when he was 4 months old and diagnosed with RSV.

On physical exam, the patient is in moderate respiratory distress. His oxygen saturation is 92% on room air, with a respiratory rate of 44. Other vital signs are normal. His lung exam is notable for diffuse expiratory wheezing with variably decreased breath sounds at the right base, obvious retractions and nasal flaring. There is decreased air exchange and an inspiratory to expiratory ratio of 1:3.5. The rest of his exam is normal except for erythematous, dry, pruritic plaques on the flexor surface of his elbows.

SELECT THE ONE BEST ANSWER

1. What is the most likely cause of this patient's respiratory distress?

    (A) viral infection
    (B) foreign body aspiration
    (C) asthma
    (D) bacterial pneumonia
    (E) anaphylaxis

2. Your initial step in treatment in your office is:

    (A) supplemental oxygen
    (B) oral steroids
    (C) systemic steroids
    (D) inhaled bronchodilator
    (E) subcutaneous epinephrine

3. Which of the following is the most effective way to deliver inhaled albuterol?

    (A) nebulizer
    (B) metered-dose inhaler
    (C) metered-dose inhaler with a spacer device
    (D) A and B
    (E) A and C

4. After two treatments, the patient improves, and you continue to obtain a history from mom. Which topic on history would have no correlation with the prevalence of asthma?

    (A) history of breast-feeding
    (B) socioeconomic status
    (C) suburban vs. inner-city residence
    (D) gender
    (E) smoke exposure

5. Which of the following can be safely eaten by breast-feeding moms hoping to delay onset of food-associated atopic dermatitis?

(A) milk
(B) fish
(C) eggs
(D) peanuts
(E) none of the above

6. The mom reports that her son has excessive cough with viral infections. He often gets short of breath and coughs when running around almost every day. He also often coughs at night (waking up 1 to 2 times per night). You diagnose what type of asthma?

(A) mild intermittent
(B) mild persistent
(C) moderate persistent
(D) moderate intermittent
(E) severe persistent

7. You are concerned by the patient's respiratory status and obtain a chest radiograph. It demonstrates hyperinflation with peribronchial cuffing and a right upper lobe volume loss. He is afebrile. What is the next appropriate step?

(A) chest tube
(B) ceftriaxone IM
(C) azithromycin PO
(D) bronchoscopy
(E) no procedure or antibiotic

8. What is the best treatment for discharge from the outpatient facility?

(A) inhaled bronchodilator daily
(B) inhaled bronchodilator PRN
(C) inhaled bronchodilator PRN and oral leukotriene inhibitor daily
(D) inhaled steroid daily and oral leukotriene inhibitor daily
(E) inhaled bronchodilator PRN and daily inhaled steroid

9. All of the following are true regarding asthma education except:

(A) Asthma action plans are warranted and efficacious.

(B) Peak flow monitoring and/or symptom monitoring are not reliable methods of self-management.
(C) Asthma action plans must be reviewed and revised by the physician.
(D) All action plans should include contacts for urgent care.
(E) Skill sets to be taught include inhaler use, self-monitoring, and environmental control.

10. What are the long-term adverse effects of daily use of inhaled low-to-medium doses corticosteroids?

(A) suppression of the hypothalamic-pituitary axis
(B) irreversible linear growth reduction
(C) decreased bone density
(D) cataracts
(E) none of the above

11. Which of the following patients would be classified as a mild intermittent asthmatic?

(A) symptoms two to three times per week, rare night symptoms, and 90% FEV_1
(B) symptoms daily, night symptoms one to two times per week, and 75% FEV_1
(C) symptoms once per week, night symptoms less than two times per month, and 85% FEV_1
(D) symptoms daily, night symptoms nightly, and <60% FEV_1
(E) none of the above

12. Which of the following is not known to exacerbate asthma symptoms?

(A) weather changes
(B) mite exposure
(C) beta-agonist drugs
(D) aspirin
(E) smog

13. All of the following are true regarding a child's risk of having an atopic disease based on family history except:

(A) 29% chance of an atopic disease if a sibling has an atopic disease
(B) 50% chance of an atopic disease if one parent has an atopic disease
(C) 72% chance of the same atopic disease as the parents if the parents share a common atopic disease

(D) 13% chance of atopic disease if neither parent has an atopic disease

(E) none of the above

14. Which of the following statements is true regarding atopic diseases?

(A) More than 50% of atopic dermatitis cases do not present until after 2 years of age.

(B) Allergic rhinitis usually precedes asthma and atopic dermatitis.

(C) Atopic dermatitis is the most common atopic disease.

(D) Hot and humid climates are risk factors for atopic dermatitis.

(E) Allergic rhinitis prevalence is increasing most in 2- to 5-year-olds.

15. Which of the following contribute to or exacerbate asthma or allergies?

(A) maternal tobacco smoking

(B) indoor pets

(C) dust mites

(D) B and C

(E) all of the above

16. All of the following are recommended for prolonged dust mite exposure reduction except:

(A) Encase mattress and pillow in allergen-impermeable cover.

(B) Wash sheets in water >130°F (54.4°C) weekly.

(C) Reduce indoor humidity.

(D) Remove bedroom carpet.

(E) Use of chemical cidal agent such as benzyl benzoate.

17. The underlying pathology of asthma is characterized by inflammation of the airway. This inflammation is mediated by many factors, one of which is major basic protein. What is the source of major basic protein?

(A) mast cells

(B) IgE receptors

(C) neutrophils

(D) IL-2

(E) eosinophils

18. What percentage of asthmatic children will outgrow symptoms by adulthood?

(A) 10%

(B) 20%

(C) 30%

(D) 40%

(E) 50%

Answers

1. **(C)** The combination of a history of RSV, current wheezing, and a family history of asthma suggests the most likely diagnosis is asthma. Although foreign body is a consideration for this patient with his history of playing with a neighbor his age, the diffuse symptoms on physical examination do not support such a diagnosis. Viral infection and bacterial pneumonia are not likely considering his lack of associated symptoms, and anaphylaxis is not supported by the vitals signs (which would demonstrate hypotension and laryngeal edema along with bronchospasm).

2. **(D)** The first-line therapy for an acute asthma exacerbation is an inhaled bronchodilator (such as albuterol). Oral steroids are often used in conjunction with inhaled steroids to decrease the airway edema, but have a much slower onset of action. Supplemental oxygen is a good supportive measure but will not treat the underlying pathology.

3. **(E)** Studies have demonstrated that when used properly, both the nebulizer and inhaler with spacer are equally efficacious in the treatment of acute asthma.

4. **(A)** Although breast-feeding in the first year of life in combination with certain food avoidance can delay the onset of atopic disease, this is mostly with respect to food-associated atopic dermatitis. There is no change in the incidence or age of onset of asthma or incidence of allergic rhinitis. Male gender, low socioeconomic status, inner-city residence, and smoke exposure (both second-hand and maternal smoking) are all risk factors for asthma.

5. **(E)** All of the foods should be avoided by any breast-feeding mom with a strong family history of food-associated atopic dermatitis, urticaria, or

al disease. Though such avoidances will reduce the incidence of such illness at 1 year, there is no such reduction at 2 years of age.

6. **(C)** Based on the history of night symptoms greater than once a week and possible daily symptoms, this patient would be considered a moderate persistent asthmatic. For more information on classification and treatment of asthma, please see http://www.nhlbi.nih.gov/guidelines/asthma/execsumm.pdf

7. **(E)** The patient has all the symptoms of an asthma exacerbation with a chest radiograph that is consistent with atelectasis. This requires no additional treatment beyond the treatment for the asthma exacerbation. The use of antibiotics in asthma is reserved for the occurrence of comorbid infections such as sinusitis or bacterial pneumonia.

8. **(E)** Current asthma guidelines recommend a controller medication of an inhaled steroid with a rescue medicine of inhaled bronchodilator for moderate-persistent asthma. Though leukotriene inhibitors with steroids are recommended as an alternate therapy for moderate persistent asthma, bronchodilators with inhaled steroid are first-line therapeutic agents.

9. **(B)** It is the opinion of the National Asthma Education and Prevention Program (NAEPP) that asthma education include the development of an action plan. Key to this plan is the ability to self-assess and manage symptoms and medications. Peak flow measurements and symptom monitoring individually or in combination are methods toward this end, and are recommended for all moderate-to-severe asthmatics.

10. **(E)** Current studies have demonstrated that low-to-medium doses of inhaled corticosteroids have no significant adverse effects. Though some studies suggest an association of reduction in linear bone growth with long-term inhaled steroids, this effect is likely nonprogressive and reversible.

11. **(C)** Mild intermittent asthmatics have day symptoms less than two times per week with night symptoms less than two nights per month. PFTs show FEV_1 >80% and PEF variability of <20%.

Mild persistent asthmatics are different only by more frequent symptoms and PEF variability of 20% to 30% (as for patient in answer A).

12. **(C)** β-Agonist drugs are part of the treatment plan for asthma. Conversely, β-adrenergic blocking drugs are known to trigger asthma exacerbations. Weather changes, allergen exposures such as mites, aspirin, and smog can all exacerbate asthma as well.

13. **(B)** There is a 50% chance of atopic disease in a child born to parents who both have an atopic disease. The percent if one parent has an atopic disease is lower. Those odds increase to 72% if the parents have the same disease. Though 20% to 30% of the population has an atopic disease, a family history is a strong predictor of a patient's risk, though environmental influences also play a strong role. Also, when a patient has one atopic disease, he/she has a threefold increase in risk for another atopic disease.

14. **(D)** Both hot and humid and cold and dry climates are risk factors for atopic dermatitis. Atopic dermatitis presents by 2 years of age in about 90% of patients. Allergic rhinitis, the most common atopic disease, is normally preceded by asthma and/or atopic dermatitis, and is increasing in prevalence in 8- to 13-year-olds.

15. **(E)**

16. **(E)** Though cidal agents such as benzyl benzoate kill the mites and denature the antigens, the effects are not maintained for prolonged periods, nor are the effects largely significant. These methods are not recommended routinely. The other answer choices are all recommended and proven to be effective in consistently reducing the exposure to dust mites.

17. **(E)** Although all of the above are involved in the pathology of asthma, it is the eosinophil that is the source of major basic protein, which injures airway epithelium and enhances bronchial responsiveness.

18. **(E)** At least half of all asthmatic children will outgrow symptoms by adulthood, though those with

severe asthma or multiple allergies are far less likely to do so.

SUGGESTED READING

The NAEPP Expert Panel Report Guidelines for the Diagnosis and Management of Asthma—Update on Selected Topics 2002. NIH Publication No. 97–4051. Washington, DC: National Institutes of Health, 2002.

Lemanske RF Jr, Busse WW: Asthma. *J Allergy Clin Immunol* 111:s502, 2003.

Nimmagadda SR, Evans RE 3rd: Allergy: etiology and epidemiology. *Pediatr Rev* 20:110, 1999.

CASE 66: A 5-YEAR-OLD WITH HIVES AFTER 10 DAYS OF ANTIBIOTICS

The mother of a 5-year-old boy calls one summer night to ask about her son's hives that developed earlier in the evening. The rash is described as red splotches with central clearing. Mom reports that he is itching quite a bit but is breathing well and has no lip involvement. There is no joint pain or abdominal pain. He had an upper respiratory infection 10 days ago, and was started on penicillin at a local emergency room yesterday for a "throat infection." Mom does report that he has been playing outside a lot and has been "getting eaten by bugs." His diet has not changed significantly, containing no seafood or peanuts, but he has been drinking a lot of fruit punch. Otherwise he has been doing well with no vomiting, diarrhea, or change in activity or appetite.

SELECT THE ONE BEST ANSWER

1. Which of the following is the most likely cause of the patient's rash?

   (A) type I immediate allergic reaction
   (B) type I accelerated allergic reaction
   (C) type II allergic reaction
   (D) type III allergic reaction
   (E) type IV allergic reaction

2. The single most important intervention for this patient is:

   (A) discontinuation of the antibiotic
   (B) antihistamines
   (C) topical steroids
   (D) topical antipruritics
   (E) all of the above are potential therapies

3. True or False. An immediate (<24-hour) reaction to penicillin is most likely IgE-mediated, whereas a reaction occurring later than 24 hours is probably not.

   (A) true
   (B) false

4. You decide to test this patient for a penicillin allergy. Which of the following is the most appropriate method for diagnosing a penicillin allergy?

   (A) penicillin challenge in the ICU
   (B) skin testing
   (C) RAST testing
   (D) CAP-RAST testing
   (E) none of the above

5. Regarding skin testing for penicillin allergy, which of the following is not true?

   (A) Negative skin tests occur in the majority of those with a clinical history.
   (B) Positive skin tests occur in 4% of patients without a clinical history.
   (C) Patients may be tested once off prescription antihistamines for 48 hours.
   (D) The risk of severe reaction during skin testing is <1%.
   (E) Skin testing is more sensitive than RAST testing.

6. Which of the following is not a contraindication to penicillin skin testing?

   (A) presence of a diffuse rash
   (B) use of diphenhydramine the previous day
   (C) absence of positive skin controls
   (D) history of Stevens-Johnson after penicillin exposure
   (E) history of moderate allergic reaction

7. Which of the following is true regarding RAST testing?

   (A) It provides immediate results.
   (B) The presence of a rash limits its use.
   (C) It is not effected by steroid use.
   (D) It has a mild risk of allergic reaction.
   (E) It can be used with a broad selection of antigens.

8. Besides drug exposure, all of the following are well-known causes of urticarial reaction except:

   (A) artificial flavoring/coloring
   (B) vancomycin
   (C) latex
   (D) radiocontrast media
   (E) all of the above can cause urticaria

9. If the boy mentioned in the vignette was having bronchospasm, hypotension, and airway edema, what is the initial treatment of choice?

   (A) epinephrine IV (1:1000 dilution)
   (B) epinephrine SC (1:1000 dilution)
   (C) epinephrine IV (1:10000 dilution)
   (D) diphenhydramine IV
   (E) hydrocortisone IV

10. Which of the following is not a known etiology of anaphylaxis?

    (A) milk ingestion
    (B) radiographic contrast media
    (C) hymenoptera stings
    (D) siphonaptera bites
    (E) exercise

11. All of the following are true in regards to risk for anaphylaxis except:

    (A) Reactions to food occur more frequently in children than adults.
    (B) Atopic children have a higher risk of reactions to drugs than the general population.
    (C) Asthmatic children have a higher risk of reaction to food than the general population.
    (D) Males have a higher risk of reaction to hymenoptera stings than females.
    (E) A recent exposure to the offending allergen increases the risk of reaction.

12. Which of the following do not support the diagnosis of anaphylaxis?

    (A) laryngeal edema, bronchospasm, hypotension
    (B) elevated plasma histamine levels
    (C) demonstration of immediate hypersensitivity by skin test/RAST
    (D) lowered plasma tryptase levels
    (E) all of the above are supportive

13. What is the risk of recurrent anaphylaxis after an insect sting?

    (A) 20%
    (B) 40%
    (C) 60%
    (D) 80%
    (E) 100%

14. True or False. Large local reactions to insect stings are IgE mediated (allergic) in origin.

    (A) True
    (B) False

15. Which of the following is true regarding venom skin testing?

    (A) It is available only in honey bee and yellow jacket preparations.
    (B) It indicates reactivity of the patient.
    (C) Testing should be delayed for at least 2 weeks after sting.
    (D) Antihistamines can interfere with results.
    (E) A negative test excludes the presence of venom-specific IgE antibodies.

16. Which of the following is true regarding radio-contrast media reaction?

    (A) The etiology is unknown but appears to be IgE-mediated.
    (B) Allergic and asthmatic patients have an increased incidence.
    (C) Reactions are immediate in all cases.
    (D) Anaphylaxis is the most common reaction.
    (E) Approximately 80% experience vasomotor reactions.

Answers

1. **(B)** This clinical description is most consistent with accelerated hypersensitivity in the form of urticaria. The proposed mechanism of such a reaction is a delayed type I hypersensitivity reaction. Although antibiotics can also cause a type IV hypersensitivity reaction, the reaction would appear more as a morbilliform, erythematous, pruritic rash with possible associated fever.

2. **(E)** The primary therapy is to discontinue the offending agent. The remaining therapies all can

be helpful depending on the extent and severity of the reaction.

3. (**A**) True

4. (**B**) Skin testing is said to be a reliable method for documenting a true penicillin allergy but in practice is seldom performed. Benzylpenicilloyl poly-L-lysine, the major determinant, is formed as a result of the beta-lactam ring opening. This major determinant is generally responsible for the urticarial reactions, whereas the minor determinants predict anaphylaxis more consistently but are not currently available commercially. Penicillin is the only antibiotic for which skin testing is available.

5. (**C**) Patients who are to undergo skin testing must have ceased taking short-acting OTC antihistamines such as diphenhydramine for at least 48 hours prior to testing. Generally, medium-acting antihistamines should be stopped for 5 days, and longer-acting antihistamines for 6 weeks. Skin testing may also be clinically affected by long-term corticosteroids, topical steroids, and tricyclic antidepressants.

6. (**E**) Although skin testing is contraindicated in those with severe allergic reaction, a moderate reaction does not limit the use. Those with severe reactions should either be given an alternate drug choice, or if none is available, desensitization without skin testing should be considered.

7. (**C**) RAST, or radioallergosorbent test, is an in vitro option for people who cannot discontinue use of antihistamines or other medications/conditions (rash) that interfere with skin testing. It is also useful in those whom anaphylaxis is a distinct risk. Its disadvantages include the delay in results and the limited specificity to clinically significant antigens.

8. (**E**) All of the substances listed can cause urticaria. Although rapid vancomycin infusion is known to cause red man syndrome (a histamine release syndrome associated with rash and occasionally hypotension), it can have accompanying urticaria.

Latex is being seen more frequently as a cause of allergic reaction, including urticaria and anaphylaxis.

9. (**C**) The treatment of choice for severe anaphylaxis, as demonstrated by the symptoms above, is intravenous epinephrine in 1:10000 dilution, administered every 5 to 10 minutes while on a cardiac monitor. Initially subcutaneous administration of a 1:1000 dilution may be a more available option and should be used when an IV is not yet in place. Hydrocortisone and diphenhydramine are both adjunctive therapies.

10. (**D**) Siphonaptera, or flea bites, are not a known cause of anaphylaxis, though they can cause a significant local reaction. All the remaining items have been known to cause anaphylaxis, including exercise-induced anaphylaxis.

11. (**B**) Though atopic children do have a greater severity of reaction to drugs, they do not have an increased risk of reaction over the general public. Males have a higher risk of reaction to stings most likely as a function of their greater exposure as a result of outdoor activities.

12. (**D**) Plasma tryptase levels will be elevated in anaphylaxis, as it is a protease specific to mast cells. Similarly, histamine is released during mast cell activation.

13. (**C**)

14. (**B**) False. Large local reactions to insect stings are IgE-mediated and therefore not allergic in origin. However, approximately 50% of these patients will develop IgE antibodies, and 5% will develop systemic symptoms on repeat exposure.

15. (**D**) Venom skin testing is available in five preparations, including honey bee, yellow-jacket, yellow hornet, white-faced hornet, and wasp. The testing can only determine prior exposure, not reactivity. A positive test with a strong clinical history is predictive, although a negative test does not exclude the possibility in such a patient. Testing should be delayed for 6 weeks after a reaction. Antihistamines will interfere with results, as in penicillin skin testing.

16. (**B**) Despite the noted increased incidence of radiocontrast media reactions in allergic and asthmatic patients, recent studies have demonstrated

a probably non–IgE-mediated mechanism. Instead, these reactions are perceived to be mast-cell mediated. Nonetheless, approximately 5% to 8% of patients will experience some type of immediate vasomotor response, with a small portion having delayed reactions. Urticaria is the most common of the reactions.

SUGGESTED READING

Hay WW Jr, Hayward AR, Levin MJ, et al: *Current Pediatric Diagnosis Treatment.* New York: McGraw-Hill, 2001.

Lasley MV, Shapiro GG: Testing for allergy. *Pediatr Rev* 21:39, 2000.

Weiss ME, Adikinson NF: Immediate hypersensitivity reactions to penicillin and related antibiotics. *Clin Allergy* 18:515, 1988

Winberry SL, Liberman PL: Anaphylaxis. *Immunol Allergy Clin North Am* 15:477, 1995.

CASE 67: A 3-MONTH-OLD WITH POOR WEIGHT GAIN, RECURRENT INFECTION, AND DIARRHEA

A 3-month-old infant has been brought to your clinic for evaluation of diarrhea. Mom reports that he has had diarrhea "since birth," and has seen at least three doctors over the course of 3 months. Each doctor switched the patient's formula, initially from breast milk through multiple types of standard cow's milk and soy formula followed by elemental formula, all with no relief. The stools are described as non-bloody, runny, and seven times per day. Mom denies any emesis or difficulty with feeds (no cyanosis, diaphoresis, arching, or discomfort). On review of systems she does note that he has had several episodes of cough and respiratory distress requiring antibiotics, as well as recurrent thrush. Birth history is unremarkable except mom's lack of prenatal care. Birth weight was 3.6 kg, length 50 cm, HC 35.5 cm. Both mom and infant were discharged on postnatal day 2.

Physical exam is significant for a small child who weighs 4.0 kg, length 55 cm, HC 39.5 cm. He is alert and active. His oral cavity has white plaques, but no vesicles or other lesions. Cardiac exam has RRR, no murmurs with good pulses. Chest has coarse breath sounds, with intermittent crackles at left base. Abdominal exam demonstrates liver edge approximately 2 cm below costal margin, with a spleen edge 1.5 cm below costal margin. There is no lymphadenopathy. Otherwise the physical exam is unremarkable.

SELECT THE ONE BEST ANSWER

1. What is the most likely cause of the patient's symptoms?

   (A) B-cell deficiency
   (B) T-cell deficiency
   (C) phagocyte deficiency
   (D) abnormal mucociliary clearance
   (E) lactase deficiency

2. Which of the following would not be included in the initial workup of this patient?

   (A) Western blot for HIV
   (B) CBC with differential
   (C) quantitative immunoglobulins
   (D) lymphocyte subsets
   (E) stool culture

3. The results of the above tests are as follows:

   HIV ELISA: nonreactive
   Absolute lymph: 2200/mm^3
   CD3$^+$ T cells: 15%
   Immunoglobulins: Normal
   HIV DNA PCR: nonreactive

   Which of the following is the most likely diagnosis with this information?

   (A) DiGeorge syndrome
   (B) Wiskott-Aldrich syndrome
   (C) congenital HIV
   (D) SCID
   (E) chronic mucocutaneous candidiasis

4. Which of the following tests can confirm the definitive diagnosis of SCID?

   (A) JAK3 mutation
   (B) RAG1 or RAG2 mutation
   (C) IL-7Rα mutation
   (D) <2% activity in ADA control
   (E) all of the above

5. Which of the following is the best treatment for the above patient?

   (A) routine IVIG transfusions
   (B) HLA-identical stem-cell transplantation
   (C) haploidentical donor stem-cell transplantation

(D) gene therapy

(E) none of the above

6. Which of the following lymphocyte subset markers reflect B cells?

(A) CD3

(B) CD4

(C) CD14

(D) CD16

(E) CD20

7. Which of the following is the most common immunodeficiency?

(A) hyper IgM syndrome

(B) cystic fibrosis

(C) IgA deficiency

(D) common variable immunodeficiency

(E) cyclic neutropenia

8. A defect in which of the following would most account for a patient with recurrent staphylococcal infections, partial albinism, and long-term risk of hemophagocytosis?

(A) leukocyte adhesion

(B) lysosomal transport

(C) phagocyte oxidase

(D) elastase

(E) none of the above

9. A 6-year-old male comes to the ER with fever, cough, and chest pain. While in the ER he is noted to have hemoptysis and is saturating 87% on room air. Chest radiograph reveals bilateral lower lobe infiltrates. He is admitted and begun on ceftriaxone and vancomycin. With no improvement after 36 hours and an unchanged chest radiograph, bronchoscopy reveals large mucous plugs and positive culture for *Aspergillus nidulans*. Which of the following immunodeficiencies would be most likely to underlie this illness?

(A) Wiskott-Aldrich

(B) leukocyte adhesion deficiency, type I

(C) common variable immunodeficiency

(D) chronic granulomatous disease

(E) Kostmann's syndrome

10. Which of the following bacterial infections are commonly seen in chronic granulomatous disease?

(A) *S. pneumoniae*

(B) Klebsiella

(C) *S. aureus*

(D) A and C

(E) B and C

11. The genetic defect in chronic granulomatous disease results in abnormal function of what chemical reactant?

(A) leukocyte integrins

(B) myeloperoxidase

(C) NADPH-oxidase

(D) adenosine deaminase

(E) LYST protein

12. Which of the following is suggestive of chronic granulomatous disease?

(A) positive Rebuck skin window

(B) abnormal neutrophil flow cytometry

(C) abnormal nitroblue tetrazolium test

(D) abnormal giant granules in neutrophils

(E) none of the above

13. Treatment strategies for chronic granulomatous disease include all except:

(A) trimethoprim-sulfamethoxazole prophylaxis

(B) IFN-γ

(C) aggressive bacteria-specific antibiotic therapy

(D) protective isolation

(E) gene therapy

14. Which of the following is true regarding cutaneous delayed-type hypersensitivity testing?

(A) It is reliable after the age of 6 months.

(B) It employs tetanus toxoid, rubella antigen, and *Candida* antigens.

(C) It is a definitive diagnostic tool.

(D) A positive test is considered more than 5 mm in all cases.

(E) A positive test reflects abnormal cellular immunity.

15. Which of the following is not true regarding humoral deficiencies?

(A) Presentation is after 6 months of life.

(B) Sinopulmonary infections are common.

(C) *H. influenzae* is a common virulent organism.

(D) Bone marrow transplant is the mainstay of therapy.

(E) Hypogammaglobulinemia is hallmark.

16. Which of the following viruses is not inactivated during IVIG preparation?

(A) hepatitis A
(B) hepatitis B
(C) hepatitis C
(D) HIV
(E) herpes viruses

17. How often should IVIG be given for humoral immunodeficiencies?

(A) every 1 to 2 weeks
(B) every 3 to 4 weeks
(C) every 1 to 2 months
(D) every 3 to 4 months
(E) weekly

18. Which humoral immune disorder cannot receive standard IVIG?

(A) common variable immunodeficiency
(B) Bruton's gammaglobulinemia
(C) selective IgA deficiency
(D) IgG subclass deficiency
(E) none of the above

Answers

1. **(B)** The most likely etiology for this patient's symptoms is a defect in T-cell function and/or number. Isolated B-cell deficiencies do not normally present until after 6 months, when maternal protection wanes. Phagocyte deficiencies do not present with recurrent pulmonary infection or FTT. A combined deficiency could present like this, but at this age, the T-cell deficiency would be the primary etiology of symptoms until maternal antibodies disappeared. Though lactase deficiency could explain the diarrhea, it would not explain the recurrent infections. Abnormal mucociliary clearance, as seen in cystic fibrosis, could present with the diarrhea, FTT, and respiratory symptoms, but is less likely to cause thrush and lack of lymphoid tissue.

2. **(A)** Initial evaluation for this patient is to determine an underlying immune deficiency. Though

HIV should be considered, the Western blot should not be used as a screening test; a DNA PCR would be the appropriate initial laboratory evaluation in this age group. A CBC with differential, quantitative immunoglobulins and lymphocyte subsets would all reflect the cell line of deficiency. Stool culture would screen for any pathogens causing the diarrhea.

3. **(D)** Severe combined immunodeficiency best explains the symptoms and laboratory findings of this vignette. Though congenital HIV can present this way, most HIV-positive children will have a positive DNA PCR by 2 to 3 months. Though not noted, mom would be tested for HIV as well. With a negative maternal result, HIV is unlikely. Wiskott-Aldrich presents with recurrent pneumonia, thrombocytopenia, and eczema, the latter of which this patient does not have. DiGeorge syndrome normally has dysmorphisms, hypocalcemia, and only mildly lymphopenic. The laboratory results do not support chronic mucocutaneous candidiasis.

4. **(E)** SCID is a heterogenous group of disorders that stem from an abnormality in function of T cells and B cells. All of the above are distinct types of SCID, although not all fit this patient, as they differ in B-cell activity and severity. Probable diagnosis of SCID requires only that the patient have either: 1) <20% $CD3^+$ T cells, absolute lymphs <3000/mm^3, and proliferative responses to mitogens <10% of control, *or* 2) the presence of maternal lymphocytes in circulation. These patients have a 85% chance (compared with 98% with a definitive diagnosis) that they will have the diagnosis in 20 years.

5. **(B)** Though both HLA-identical and haploidentical donor stem cell transplantation are used in SCID, HLA-identical has the lowest risk of GVHD and a more favorable prognosis. Haploidentical donor stem cell transplantation does not have as high a success rate, but is used if necessary. IVIG is utilized in B-cell disorders. Although there is a promising future in gene therapy for some forms of SCID, it is currently not an approved approach to care. Without a stem-cell transplantation, most patients with SCID

will die prior to their first birthday; with transplantation prior to 3.5 months, the chance of survival increases to 97%.

6. **(E)** Lymphocytes are represented by CD3, CD4, and CD8 markers among others. Natural killer cells are represented by CD16, CD56, and CD57 markers. Monocytes are represented by CD14. B cells are represented by CD19 and CD20.

7. **(C)** IgA deficiency occurs in about 1/333 people; 1/700 U.S. whites are estimated to have IgA deficiency. The majority are asymptomatic.

8. **(B)** The described patient has Chediak-Higashi, a disorder caused by mutation in the lysosomal transport protein. Affected individuals have recurrent skin and respiratory pyogenic infections, partial oculocutaneous albinism, and neurologic disturbances (neuropathy, photophobia, seizures). Patients who survive the infections eventually enter the "accelerated phase" of lymphocytic infiltration of most organ systems, leading to death. Laboratory findings include mild decrease in neutrophil counts with giant cytoplasmic granules.

9. **(D)** Invasive and pulmonary aspergillosis are commonly seen in several immunodeficiencies, with *Aspergillus nidulans* representing a species particularly virulent in chronic granulomatous disease. Kostmann's syndrome, or congenital neutropenia, would have presented by now with recurrent infections and fever. Wiskott-Aldrich is an X-linked disorder that involves eczema, thrombocytopenia, and immunodeficiency. Common variable immunodeficiency, a B-cell disorder, would have presented after 6 months of age with encapsulated organism infections. Although LAD is also a disorder of phagocytes, it is not as commonly associated with aspergillosis.

10. **(E)** Patients with chronic granulomatous disease are susceptible to catalase-producing organisms. These organisms include, among others, *Staphylococcus*, *Burkholderia*, *Aspergillus*, *Serratia*, and *Klebsiella* species. *Pneumococcus*, however, is catalase-negative.

11. **(C)** Chronic granulomatous disease results from a genetic defect in one component of the NADPH-oxidase system in phagocytes. These defects limit the enzyme activity that allows phagocytes to produce superoxide, which forms other reactive oxidants. This leads to an inability to defend against catalase-producing organisms.

12. **(C)** The initial screening test for CGD is the nitroblue tetrazolium (NBT) test. In this study, normal neutrophils will produce superoxide that is reduced by NBT and create a dark blue coloration to cells. When the superoxide is absent or low, an abnormally low number of cells are altered to blue color. This test can then be confirmed by other more quantitative tests, such as cytochrome *c* reduction assay.

13. **(E)** Although all of the above are possible treatments for CGD, gene therapy is currently only theoretical and studies are ongoing to test their efficacy and stability.

14. **(D)** Cutaneous delayed-type hypersensitivity testing is an in vivo test for cellular immunity. A positive test (>5-mm response in all subjects) reflects intact cellular immunity. The test utilizes intradermal injections of tetanus toxoid, mumps antigen, and *Candida* antigen. All negative tests should be either repeated or followed by flow cytometry and in vitro assays of T-cell function, as age of <1 year and concurrent infection can limit reliability of results.

15. **(D)** The mainstay of therapy for humoral deficiencies is IVIG replacement therapy.

16. **(A)** The incubation of fractionated immune globulin during the manufacturing of IVIG results in the inactivation of enveloped viruses (e.g., HIV, hepatitis B, hepatitis C, herpes viruses). It does not, however, inactivate nonenveloped viruses, which include parvovirus and hepatitis A.

17. **(B)** IVIG is given every 3 to 4 weeks, based on its half-life, which is 21 to 28 days.

18. **(C)** Anaphylaxis may occur in patients with selective IgA deficiency as a result of anti-IgA antibodies attacking trace IgA in the IVIG. For this

reason, IgA-deficient patients should receive IVIG with lower IgA content.

SUGGESTED READING

Bonilla FA, Geha RS: Primary immunodeficiency diseases. *J Allergy Clin Immunol* 111(2 Suppl):S571–S578, 2003.

Buckley RH: Primary cellular immunodeficiencies. *J Allergy Clin Immunol* 109:747–757, 2002.

Schubal SJ: Treatment of antibody deficiency syndromes. *Pediatr Rev* 21:358–359, 2000.

Winkelstein JA, Marino MC, Johnston RB Jr, et al: Chronic granulomatous disease. Report on a national registry of 368 patients. *Medicine (Baltimore)* 79:155–169, 2000.

8

Adolescent Medicine

CASE 68: A 14-YEAR-OLD GIRL WHO NEEDS A SCHOOL PHYSICAL

A 14-year-old comes into the clinic for a school physical examination. She will be entering high school in the fall. She has always been healthy. Her mother reports no new problems since the last visit to her previous pediatrician 2 years earlier. She mentions that her daughter has been showing a growing interest in boys lately, but has no other behavioral concerns. Menses started a year ago and have been irregular. The patient wonders whether a pelvic examination will be needed on this visit. The past medical history is unremarkable. She is an excellent student and has a "good group of friends." She is dating but denies ever being sexually active; she confides that many of her friends smoke cigarettes and that she has tried cigarettes in the past but did not like them. She has never used alcohol, marijuana, or other drugs. Her review of systems is negative. She lives with her mother and two siblings. Her father, who had type 2 diabetes mellitus, died 3 years ago of a myocardial infarction at age 47. The family history is otherwise noncontributory.

The physical examination is normal except for mild acne. She is 5'2", weighs 136 lbs, and her BMI is 25.

SELECT THE ONE BEST ANSWER

1. How would you conduct an adolescent clinical encounter to foster adequate rapport and maximize accurate data collection?

   (A) Always interview the adolescent and parent at the same time.

   (B) Interview parent and patient separately in that order.

   (C) Interview patient and parent separately in that order.

   (D) Interview patient only.

   (E) None of the above.

2. Which of the following options would you choose for conducting a physical examination in an adolescent patient?

   (A) Always have a parent in attendance during the physical examination.

   (B) Never have a parent in attendance during the physical examination.

   (C) Always have a chaperone in the examining room when examining a teenager.

   (D) Have a parent in attendance during the physical examination only according to patients' wishes.

   (E) Tailor your decision according to patient's age, level of cognitive and emotional maturity, and personal wishes.

3. Which of the following statements regarding confidential care of adolescents is true?

   (A) Confidential care should only be provided to emancipated minors.

   (B) The law generally requires parental consent for the provision of medical care to minors.

   (C) All patients younger than age 18 need parental consent to receive mental health services, including diagnosis and treatment of substance abuse.

(D) Minors cannot obtain confidential reproductive services if they are younger than 15 years.

(E) In some states, minors cannot consent to care of STD/HIV-related issues.

4. Which of the following topics would be appropriate to explore with this 14-year-old girl in her first visit?

(A) school performance

(B) history of physical and/or sexual abuse

(C) use of alcohol, cigarettes, marijuana, and/or inhalants

(D) dating and need for birth control

(E) all of the above

5. What are the most common causes of death among boys age 15 to 19 years and in what order are they ranked?

(A) unintentional injury, homicide, suicide, malignancies, heart disease

(B) unintentional injuries, suicide, malignancies, HIV, congenital conditions

(C) unintentional injuries, suicide, homicide, malignancies, congenital conditions

(D) homicide, unintentional injury, heart disease, malignancy, suicide

(E) unintentional injury, malignancy, homicide, suicide, heart disease.

6. Regarding mortality rates in teenagers, which of the following is not true?

(A) The rates of unintentional injury in 15- to 19-year-olds are more than twice as high in males as in females.

(B) In white youth, suicide rates in 15- to 19-year-old are more than four times higher in males than in females.

(C) Homicide is the leading cause of death among African-American males, age 15 to 24 years.

(D) In African-American youth age 15 to 19 years, suicide rates are higher in females than in males.

(E) Both for males and for females, unintentional injury is responsible for close to 50% of all deaths among 15- to 19-year-olds.

7. What are the main elements you will need to assess in this patients' physical examination?

(A) height, weight, blood pressure, and heart rate

(B) sexual maturity rating

(C) thyroid examination

(D) scoliosis

(E) all of the above

8. According to the American Medical Association Guidelines for Adolescent Preventive Services (GAPS), how often should an adolescent have a comprehensive examination?

(A) once a year

(B) every 6 months during the growth spurt

(C) three times, during early, middle, and late adolescence.

(D) whenever it is requested

(E) every other year

9. Under what circumstances is a pelvic examination recommended in an adolescent girl?

(A) in all cases of primary dysmenorrhea

(B) history of sexual intercourse and routinely after age 16 years

(C) history of sexual intercourse and routinely after age 21 years

(D) before prescribing contraceptives

(E) A, C, and D

10. During her private interview the patient denies sexual activity. Her physical examination is normal. Her last menstrual period was 4 months ago. What would be the appropriate course of action in this case?

(A) No testing is needed at this time. Reassure her about the fact that a period will soon come, since she has had irregular periods all along and has only been menstruating for a year.

(B) Have your nurse run a pregnancy test in a urine sample collected earlier in the visit to determine whether the patient may be lying.

(C) Advise the patient that it is your policy to exclude pregnancy through urine testing in all patients of reproductive age whose menses are late.

(D) Ask her mother privately for permission to perform a pregnancy test.

(E) Have the patient come back for blood testing if she has not had a period in another 3 months.

11. Which of the following laboratory screening tests would be routinely recommended in this visit?

(A) hemoglobin and hematocrit
(B) cholesterol
(C) HIV testing
(D) urinalysis
(E) none of the above

12. If she has never had chickenpox or the varicella vaccine, what statement would apply?

(A) She should receive one dose of varicella vaccine at the present visit followed by a second dose within 4 to 8 weeks.
(B) She will just need one dose of varicella vaccine.
(C) There is no need to immunize her at this time since she most likely had a subclinical case of varicella during childhood. No testing is required.
(D) Varicella immunization should be given followed by a check of varicella titers 2 months after vaccination to document immunity.
(E) Varicella immunization should be given unless the patient has household members who are immunocompromised.

13. She returns 48 hours later for a reading of her PPD. PPD indicates 10 mm of redness and 8 mm of induration. At this point you would:

(A) obtain a chest radiograph and start INH
(B) obtain further social history
(C) notify local Board of Health
(D) determine whether the patient has received the BCG abroad
(E) repeat PPD in 1 month

14. Which of the following statements regarding tuberculosis testing is not true?

(A) Incarcerated teens should have annual PPD screening.
(B) HIV infected teens should be tested for tuberculosis yearly.
(C) Tuberculosis skin testing should be performed before initiation of immunosuppres-

sive therapy, including prolonged steroid administration.
(D) Previous BCG administration is a contraindication to tuberculosis skin testing.
(E) Ten percent of immunocompetent children with culture-documented tuberculosis may be initially PPD negative.

15. How would you counsel this patient regarding pregnancy and STD prevention?

(A) There is no need to address this issue at the present time since she is only 14 and not sexually active.
(B) Refer her to a gynecologist for such discussions.
(C) This discussion should better be left to her parents' discretion.
(D) Ask her if she has any questions or concerns regarding sexuality. Congratulate her in her decision to remain abstinent and explain that you will be available to her in the future for further discussion of this issue if needed.
(E) A and C.

16. Both the patient and her mother express some concerns about her facial acne. Among the following, what pathogenic factors are *not* involved in the development of acne vulgaris?

(A) retention hyperkeratosis
(B) increased sebum production
(C) overgrowth of *Propionibacterium acnes*
(D) inflammation
(E) dietary factors

17. What medication would you use in the initial management of this patient's mild comedonal acne?

(A) azelaic acid cream 20% twice a day
(B) benzoyl peroxide gel 5% once daily or topical tretinoin 0.025% once daily
(C) oral macrolide antibiotic
(D) topical antibiotics twice daily
(E) oral tetracycline antibiotic

18. How long after starting the therapy you selected in question 17 would you like to see this patient again?

(A) 2 years
(B) 1 month

(C) 6 months

(D) 3 months

(E) 2 weeks

Answers

1. **(B)** To obtain a comprehensive health history in the adolescent patient it is necessary to interview both parents and patients. It is preferable to interview the parent first and then move on to a private discussion with the teen. Private time should be allotted to interview the parent to attend to the concerns that prompted the visit and to obtain a detailed past medical history as well as a family history. During the initial interview with the parent, it is essential to discuss the privacy and confidentiality rules that will apply to the care of his/her teenager and to explain under what specific circumstances confidentiality might be breached. These rules should then be discussed privately with the patient before eliciting the medical history. This approach improves the chances of having an honest discussion of sensitive issues with parents and teens, enhances rapport, and promotes accuracy in data collection. Some younger teens or those with developmental delay may need to be interviewed together with their parents. Special provisions apply to the evaluation and treatment of reproductive and/or mental health issues in adolescents. These provisions vary from state to state, and it is essential for health providers to become familiar with the statutes that apply to the locales in which they practice.

2. **(E)** When considering this question it is important to bear in mind the adolescent's age, developmental stage, and level of cognitive and emotional maturity. The presence of a parent during the physical examination is generally reassuring for the younger teens and for those with developmental delays. Most middle or older adolescents prefer to have parents wait outside the room during the examination. Under such circumstances, the decision is best deferred to the patient. When performing a pelvic examination in an adolescent it is recommended to have a chaperone in the room.

3. **(B)** The law generally requires parental consent for the provision of medical care to minors. However, there are legal provisions that authorize minors to consent to health care, either because of the status of the minor or the type of services requested. All states have specific provisions that allow minors to consent to certain services, including pregnancy-related care, diagnosis and treatment of STDs, HIV/AIDS, examination and treatment of sexual assault, as well as diagnosis and treatment of mental health issues, including drug and alcohol problems. Although statutes concerning the provision of confidential care vary from state to state, all 50 states allow minors to give consent for care of STD/HIV issues.

4. **(E)** All of the above. One of the most important goals of the adolescent visit is to assess the functional status of teens regarding their families, peer relationships, and school/work performance. A thorough clinical history in an adolescent should include the presenting complaint and its progression, past medical history, family history, and review of systems. In addition, it is essential to obtain detailed information about family composition and dynamics, major recent life changes, and specific health concerns. The provider should also address nutrition, including diet and eating patterns, body image, school performance, relations with friends and family, vocational goals, and use of tobacco, alcohol, marijuana, inhalants and other drugs. A developmentally appropriate, detailed sexual history should be obtained. It is also important to screen for depression, suicidal ideation, and any history of physical, emotional, and/or sexual abuse. Injury risks should be assessed with special attention to seat-belt use, helmet use, drunken driving, and use of weapons.

5. **(A)** In 2000, national vital statistics reports indicated that unintentional injuries were by far the most common cause of mortality among all young people age 10 to 24 years. Most unintentional injuries are secondary to motor vehicle accidents, of which a significant number (40%) are alcohol-related. Homicide ranks second in males and females age 15 to 24 years, while suicide ranks 3rd in males 15 to 24 years of age and 5th in females 15 to 19 years of age. These data underscore the need for appropriate screening and anticipatory guidance in adolescents, particularly regarding injury prevention, exposure to vio-

lence, alcohol and other substance use, drunken driving, and mood disorders.

6. **(D)** Among African-American youth age 15 to 19 years, suicide rates are more than 6 times higher among boys than among girls.

7. **(E)** A comprehensive physical examination should include the following:

   - Height, weight, blood pressure, and heart rate
   - Growth assessment, plotting height, weight, growth velocity, and calculated body mass index in the corresponding growth charts
   - Skin examination
   - Eyes, ears, nose and throat, dental and gum exam
   - Neck examination for thyromegaly or adenopathies
   - Cardiopulmonary examination
   - Abdominal examination
   - Genital examination and assessment of sexual maturity rating
   - Breast examination
   - Musculoskeletal examination
   - Neurologic examination
   - Vision and hearing screening

8. **(C)** According to GAPS, adolescents should have a comprehensive examination once during early adolescence (age 11 to 14 years), once during middle adolescence (age 15 to 17 years), and once during late adolescence (age 18 to 21 years). These guidelines also recommend that blood pressure and body mass index be monitored yearly.

9. **(C)** A pelvic exam should be performed in adolescents with gynecologic complaints such as pelvic pain, vaginal discharge, or severe menstrual bleeding. Sexually active adolescents should also be examined to exclude STDs. On the other hand, a pelvic examination is not indicated prior to prescribing contraceptives in the asymptomatic, nonsexually active teen. According to the U.S. Preventive Services Task Force a pelvic exam is not needed until age 21 in asymptomatic women who have not become sexually active. Most cases of primary dysmenorrhea are functional and, if the clinical history is highly suggestive of that diagnosis, a pelvic exam will not be required.

10. **(C)** Despite the fact that the patient denies sexual activity, that her periods have been irregular since menarche and that she has only been menstruating for a year, it would be prudent to document that pregnancy has been excluded as a cause of secondary amenorrhea. This should be discussed with the patient and her consent should be obtained prior to performing the test.

11. **(E)** There are no universal recommendations regarding laboratory screening tests in asymptomatic adolescents. Several national organizations have published screening guidelines but vary widely in their advice. While the AAP recommends baseline anemia screening, neither the AMA, Bright Futures, nor the U.S. Preventive Services Task Force endorse that view. An anemia screen would be indicated in an adolescent girl if the clinical history reveals inadequate diet or frequent or heavy periods. Cholesterol screening is performed in all adolescents with a family history of premature cardiovascular disease or hyperlipidemia. Screening for gonorrhea, chlamydia, and syphilis is recommended at least annually for sexually active teens while HIV should be performed in adolescents at high risk for that condition. A urinalysis to screen for glycosuria would be appropriate in this girl given her family history of diabetes.

12. **(A)** She should be immunized against chickenpox. Two doses, at least 1 month apart, are given to adolescents 13 years and older. Alternatively, varicella titers could be obtained followed by immunization if the titers are negative. Serological testing is unnecessary after immunization given the high rates of seroconversion with the use of the present vaccine. Varicella vaccination is not contraindicated in household members of immunocompromised patients, including those with HIV infection. Immunized persons who develop a rash should avoid contact with immunocompromised, susceptible hosts for the duration of the rash.

13. **(B)** Tuberculin testing should be considered positive in children 4 years and older without any risk factors if the area of induration measures >15 mm. With an induration of 8 mm it will be important to determine whether this teen has been

in close contact with a known or suspected contagious case of active or previously active tuberculosis, either untreated or inadequately treated before the exposure took place. This result would be interpreted as positive in teens receiving immunosuppressive therapy or those with immunosuppressive conditions including HIV. The interpretation of a positive tuberculin skin test should generally not be influenced by a previous history of BCG administration.

14. **(D)** According to the 2003 report of the Committee on Infections Diseases of the AAP, previous BCG administration is not a contraindication to tuberculosis skin testing. Moreover, disease caused by *M. tuberculosis* should be suspected in any symptomatic patient with a positive PPD, regardless of history of BCG immunization. In the asymptomatic teen who has received BCG, the interpretation of a positive PPD should include consideration of the following factors: exposure to a person with contagious tuberculosis, family history of tuberculosis, immigration from a country with high prevalence of the disease, and a PPD reaction >15 mm. These factors strongly suggest actual infection. Prompt radiographic evaluation of all teens with a positive PPD test is recommended regardless of their BCG immunization status.

15. **(D)** During the well-adolescent visit, the primary care provider has an invaluable opportunity to discuss a number of preventive health care issues including sexual activity and its consequences. After establishing an initial rapport and adequate communication with the patient and family the physician can elicit any questions or concerns the patient may have regarding sexuality. Pregnancy and STD prevention can then be addressed, tailoring the discussion to the teen's level of cognitive and emotional development and to his/her sociocultural background. Knowing that in the United States approximately 30% of adolescent girls are already sexually active by ninth grade and that this percentage more than doubles by twelfth grade, it is essential to discuss pregnancy prevention, including abstinence, barrier, and hormonal methods early on during adolescence. Similarly, since up to 66% of common STDs such as chlamydia and gonorrhea infections oc-

cur in people age 15 to 24 years, the importance of educating the young on STD prevention cannot be overemphasized.

16. **(E)** Acne vulgaris is the most common skin disorder in the United States. The prevalence of comedones during adolescence approaches 100%. Four pathogenic factors play a major role in this condition: 1) retention hyperkeratosis, 2) increased sebum production, 3) proliferation of *P. acnes* within the pilosebaceous follicle, and 4) inflammation. Follicular hyperkeratinization with increased proliferation and decreased desquamation of the keratinocytes lining the follicular orifice lead to the formation of a hyperkeratotic plug (a combination of sebum and keratin in the follicular canal). During adrenarche, there is an increased production of sebum as sebaceous glands enlarge. *P. acnes* organisms thrive in the presence of increased sebum, hydrolyzing triglycerides into fatty acids and glycerol which in turn, together with other factors, leads to local inflammation. According to the extent of follicular hyperkeratinization, sebum production, *P. acnes* growth, and inflammation present, the initial microcomedo will evolve into a noninflammatory closed comedo, an open comedo, or an inflammatory pustule, papular, or nodular lesion. Dietary factors play no role in the development of acne.

17. **(B)** Comedolytic agents such as benzoyl peroxide and retinoids help to prevent and/or decrease keratinocyte proliferation and retention. Initial management of mild comedonal acne includes topical 5% benzoyl peroxide gel or 0.025% tretinoin topical once daily.

18. **(D)** It would be advisable to monitor acne treatment 3 months after initiating topical medication, stressing the need for consistent, long-term compliance to achieve adequate therapeutic results.

SUGGESTED READING

Joffe A, Blythe MJ: Handbook of adolescent medicine. *Adolesc Med* 14:2, 2003.

Neinstein, LS: *Adolescent Health Care. A Practical Guide*, 4th ed. Philadelphia, PA: Lippincott Williams and Wilkins, 2002.

American Medical Association. *Guidelines for Adolescent Preventive Services*. Chicago, IL: American Medical Association, 1992. Available at: http://www.ama-assn.org/ama/pub/category/1980.html. Last accessed May 2006.

Maternal and Child Health Bureau. *US Public Health Services (MCHB)—Bright Futures: Guidelines for Health Care Supervision of Infants, Children, and Adolescents.* 1994. Available at: http://www.brightfutures.org. Last accessed May 2006.

Guide to Clinical Preventive Services. Washington, DC: The United States Preventive Services Task Force (USPSTF), 1989/1996.

Elster, AB: Comparison of recommendations for adolescent clinical preventive services developed by national organizations. *Arch Pediatr Adolesc Med* 152: 193, 1998.

Immunization of adolescents. Recommendations of the Advisory Committee on Immunization Practices, the American Academy of Pediatrics, the American Academy of Family Physicians, and the American Medical Association. *MMWR Morb Mortal Wkly Rep* 45:1, 1996.

Guidelines for Adolescent Preventive Services: Clinical Evaluation and Management Handbook. American Medical Association, Chicago, IL, 1995.

Elster AB, Levenberg, P: Integrating comprehensive adolescent preventive services into routine medical care. *Pediatr Clin North Am* 44:1365, 1997.

Pickering LK, ed: *Red Book: 2003 Report of the Committee on Infectious Diseases*, 26th ed. Elk Grove Village, IL: American Academy of Pediatrics.

Krowchuk DP, Lucky AW: Managing adolescent acne. *Adolesc Med* 12:355–374, 2001.

CASE 69: A 15-YEAR-OLD BOY WITH SHORT STATURE AND PUBERTAL DELAY

A 15-year-old boy is brought in to the teen clinic for evaluation of short stature. Records provided by his previous pediatrician indicate that he had been growing along the 5th percentile for height and weight until a year ago. During the past year he has grown approximately 6 cm. He is upset about being the shortest in his class and also worried about his acne and the tender "knots" he recently found in his breasts.

His mother states that he was born after a full-term, uncomplicated pregnancy. His birth weight was 3000 g (6 lbs, 10 oz). Delivery was normal. He attained all his early developmental milestones on time. At age 18 months he was hospitalized for acute diarrhea and dehydration. His past medical history is otherwise unremarkable and the family history is noncontributory. His mother is 5'2" and his father is 5'10". He is an average student and has several good friends. The review of systems is negative.

On physical examination he is a pleasant, slender young man with no evidence of dysmorphism. He is 5'1" (5th percentile) and weighs 105 lbs (10th percentile). His BMI is 19.5. He has mild facial acne and slight bilateral gynecomastia. His genital development is at Tanner stage 3. His testicular volume is 8 mL, bilaterally. The rest of the examination shows no abnormalities.

SELECT THE ONE BEST ANSWER

1. What is the most likely diagnosis in this case?

   (A) acquired hypothyroidism
   (B) vitamin deficiency
   (C) Klinefelter syndrome
   (D) constitutional delay of puberty
   (E) GH deficiency

2. What other clinical information will you need to assess this problem?

   (A) dietary history
   (B) time at onset and tempo of pubertal changes
   (C) adult height and growth and pubertal development patterns of all first- and second-degree relatives
   (D) history of medication intake
   (E) all of the above

3. What is this adolescent's mid-parental height?

   (A) 5'6" (168 cm)
   (B) 5'7½" (171 cm)
   (C) 5'8½" (174 cm)
   (D) 5'9" (175 cm)
   (E) 5'10" (178 cm)

4. According to his mid-parental height what would be this young man's target height?

   (A) 5'5" to 5'7" (165 to 170 cm)
   (B) 5'6" to 5'9" (168 to 175 cm)
   (C) 5'4½" to 5'10" (164 to 178 cm)
   (D) 5'5" to 6'0" (165 to 183 cm)
   (E) 5'5" to 5'9½" (165 to 176 cm)

5. Which of the following elements of the physical examination will be the least valuable in the initial evaluation of this condition?

   (A) evaluation of visual acuity
   (B) sexual maturity rating

(C) sense of smell

(D) thyroid examination

(E) arm span and upper/lower segment ratios.

6. What tests, if any, would help in the initial evaluation of this patient?

(A) no tests needed at this time

(B) CBC, urinalysis, complete metabolic panel including glucose, calcium, phosphorus, kidney, and liver function tests

(C) CBC, urinalysis, thyroid function tests, bone age

(D) CBC, urinalysis, erythrocyte sedimentation rate, complete metabolic panel including glucose, calcium, phosphorus, kidney and liver function tests, LH, FSH, testosterone, TSH, prolactin, and bone age

(E) somatomedin C and karyotype

7. Concerning bone age, which of the following statements is not true?

(A) Delayed bone age occurs in adolescents with chronic illness, hypothyroidism, and hypopituitarism.

(B) In patients with constitutional delay of puberty, the bone age equals the chronologic age.

(C) A bone age study provides clues for potential future linear growth.

(D) In familiar short stature the bone age is advanced in relation to the height age.

(E) In patients with constitutional delay of puberty, the bone age equals the height age.

8. Bone maturation is controlled by:

(A) adrenal androgens

(B) estrogens

(C) thyroid hormones

(D) testosterone

(E) all of the above

9. Pubertal linear growth accounts for what percent of final height?

(A) 10% to 15%

(B) 15% to 20%

(C) 20% to 25%

(D) 25% to 30%

(E) >30%

10. During peak height velocity, the average linear growth in boys is:

(A) 6 cm/year

(B) 8 cm/year

(C) 10 cm/year

(D) 13 cm/year

(E) 15 cm/year

11. Which of the following statements is false?

(A) Peak height velocity occurs about 18 to 24 months earlier in girls than in boys.

(B) Most linear growth occurs in boys during Tanner stages 3 and 4.

(C) Testicular growth is usually the earliest sign of pubertal development.

(D) Menarche usually happens during Tanner stage 2.

(E) Most linear growth occurs in girls before Tanner stage 3.

12. The mean age of onset of puberty in boys is:

(A) 11.6 years

(B) 12.5 years

(C) 13.2 years

(D) 14.0 years

(E) 14.5 years

13. Which of the following is not a normal finding in adolescent boys?

(A) gynecomastia during SMR 3

(B) testicular size of 4.0 mL during SMR 4

(C) attainment of SMR 3 before peak height velocity

(D) asymmetric gynecomastia

(E) facial acne at age 12 years

14. Which of the following statements concerning constitutional delay of growth and puberty (CDP) is false?

(A) Constitutional delay of growth and puberty is a diagnosis of exclusion.

(B) A family history of CDP is usually present.

(C) Most delayed puberty in boys is constitutional.

(D) In CDP, bone age is delayed in relation to chronological age and typically corresponds to height age.

(E) Absence of any sign of puberty in a boy after the age of 12.5 years merits investigation.

15. The percentage of body fat seems to play an important role in the onset of pubertal changes. What percent body fat is typically needed to reach menarche?

   (A) 15%
   (B) 17%
   (C) 20%
   (D) 22%
   (E) 25%

16. All of the following are consistent with the diagnosis of constitutional delay of puberty except:

   (A) negative detailed review of systems and evidence of adequate nutrition
   (B) linear growth velocity less than 3.7 cm/year during the previous year
   (C) normal findings on physical examination, including genital anatomy, sense of smell, and upper to lower body segment ratio
   (D) normal complete blood count, electrolyte, BUN, and sedimentation rate
   (E) delayed bone age

17. All of the following psychological features are characteristic of early adolescence except:

   (A) concrete thought
   (B) inability to perceive long-term consequences of current decisions and acts
   (C) limited dating
   (D) development of a sense of omnipotence and invincibility
   (E) emergence of sexual feelings

18. Which of the following would be an abnormal finding during middle adolescence?

   (A) growth deceleration
   (B) stature reaches 95% of final height
   (C) conformity with peer values, codes, and dress
   (D) increased competence in abstract thought
   (E) wide mood swings

Answers

1. (**D**) In evaluating a child with short stature, the first step is to determine the patient's growth and developmental pattern. Several questions should be addressed:

   - Is the child truly short, i.e., more than 2 SDs below the mean height for children of the same age and sex?
   - Are there any dysmorphic features suggesting the possibility of genetic or congenital disorders?
   - Does the child have growth failure, that is, a subnormal growth velocity for age and sex? Has he always progressed along the same percentile lines in his growth chart, or is there a pattern of attenuated growth with progressive deviation from previously normal growth channels?
   - To what extent does his present height correlate with expected height for age, as estimated by his mid-parental height?
   - Considering both his mid-parental height and his degree of pubertal development, what is his potential for further linear growth?

   In this case, the growth chart indicates that he has always grown along the 5th percentile for height and weight. He has gained 6 cm during the past year indicating that, even though he has not grown to the extent expected during the growth spurt (8 to 14 cm/yr), there has been continuous, linear growth. From his sexual maturity rating (Tanner 3) we can infer that he probably has not attained peak height velocity yet but that puberty is underway. There are no dysmorphic features that would suggest chromosomal abnormalities, intrauterine infections, or exposure to toxins, smoke, or alcohol. With an otherwise normal clinical history, review of systems and physical examination, chronic illnesses (malnutrition, chronic renal failure, cardiac disease, inflammatory bowel disease, cystic fibrosis, Cushing's disease, hypothyroidism) or skeletal dysplasias would be unlikely. Given the clinical findings and pending results of laboratory and imaging studies, familiar short stature and constitutional delay of puberty (CDP) would be among the most common conditions to explain this patient's presentation. Since his mid-parental height allows us to predict a normal final height, CDP would be the most likely diagnosis in this case.

   Acquired hypothyroidism would typically present with a pattern of attenuated or stunted linear growth, increased tiredness, weight gain, cold intolerance and dry skin, none of which are present in this patient. Klinefelter syndrome, the most frequent cause of primary hypogonadism, would also be unlikely. Phenotypic abnormalities in this condition include relatively long arms and legs, decreased virilization, and small, firm testes leading to severely subnormal sperm counts and infertility. Behavioral changes may also be present. The most common genotype in Klinefelter syndrome is 47,XXY. Growth hormone (GH) deficiency and other endocrine disorders that affect linear growth are usually associated with an increased weight/height ratio. In many cases, however, it may be difficult to distinguish GH deficiency from constitutional delay of puberty solely on clinical grounds and a full endocrinology workup will be needed to confirm the diagnosis.

2. **(E)** The single most useful tool in the evaluation of a teenager with growth retardation is a thorough clinical evaluation. Data gathering should include a complete review of system, a detailed description of linear growth patterns and pubertal changes along time, diet and exercise history, previous illnesses, medication, congenital abnormalities, headaches, visual disturbances, and anosmia. Information about growth and development patterns and adult height of first- and second-degree relatives should be obtained. Accurate serial measurements of height and determination of height velocity are fundamental components of the diagnostic workup.

3. **(C)** His mid-parental height is 5'8½". The mid-parental height is calculated in boys by adding 5" (13 cm) to the maternal height and averaging it with paternal height. For girls, the mid-parental height equals the paternal height minus 5" averaged with maternal height.

4. **(D)** His target height would be between 5'5" and 6'0" (165 to 183 cm). The target height equals the mid-parental height ± 2 SD. Each SD equals 1.67" (4.25 cm).

5. **(A)** Sexual maturity rating is an essential element in the evaluation of growth and development during the adolescent years. Since most linear growth in boys takes place during Tanner stages 3 and 4, the finding of a genital SMR 3 in this case should be reassuring about the potential for further linear growth. Anosmia and hyposmia are characteristically present in patients with Kallmann syndrome, an LHRH deficiency leading to hypogonadotropic hypogonadism. This syndrome is often associated with mid-cranial and mid-facial anomalies. A thyroid examination, arm span and upper/lower segment ratios should also be documented as a part of the evaluation of abnormal growth and development. Visual fields and funduscopic examination may help exclude intracranial masses such as craniopharyngiomas, which may be responsible for pituitary and hypothalamic dysfunction.

6. **(D)** Constitutional delay of puberty is a diagnosis of exclusion. Even though the history is highly suggestive of this diagnosis, a CBC, sedimentation rate, complete metabolic panel, bone age, and a basic hormonal workup would help exclude some other conditions included in the differential diagnosis (chronic liver or kidney failure, chronic inflammatory disorders, IBD, metabolic disorders, hypothyroidism, Cushing's syndrome, etc). IGF-1 and IGFBP-3 are very helpful to screen for GH deficiency if the condition is suspected. Karyotype determinations are needed whenever clinical and/or laboratory findings point to the possibility of chromosomal anomalies.

7. **(B)** In constitutional delay of puberty, the bone age is delayed for chronological age but closely correlates with height age. In patients with familial short stature, the bone age typically corresponds to the chronological age and is usually advanced for height age. Delayed bone age occurs in adolescents with chronic illness, hypothyroidism, and hypopituitarism. Bone age is a helpful tool to determine potential linear growth.

8. **(E)** Bone maturation is controlled by thyroid hormones, estrogen, testosterone, and adrenal androgens. During puberty, an excess of these hormones leads to accelerated bone maturation while their deficiency results in delayed bone age.

9. **(C)** Pubertal linear growth accounts for 20% to 25% of final adult height, averaging 12 to 13 inches in boys and 10 to 13 inches in girls.

10. (C) During peak height velocity (PHV), the average linear growth in boys is 10 cm/year (range, 5.8 to 13.1 cm). At PHV, girls grow an average of 9 cm/year (range, 5.4 to 11 cm). The average growth spurt lasts 24 to 36 months.

11. (D) In most girls, breast changes, including the development of breast buds and widening of the areolae represent the first physical sign of puberty (B2). On average, pubertal changes are completed in 4 years with a range of 1.5 to 8 years. Peak height velocity in girls, an early pubertal phenomenon, is attained between SMR 2 and 3 at an average age of 11.6 ± 1.2 years. Menarche, on the other hand, is a relatively late pubertal event and usually occurs at SMR 3 in 20% and at SMR 4 in 56% of girls. Menarche occurs in American girls at an average age of 12.4 years with a range of 9 to 17 years of age, usually 1 year after PHV is attained and 3 years after the start of the growth spurt.

    In boys, testicular growth is usually the earliest physical sign of puberty (G2) and occurs at an average age of 11.6 ± 1 year (range 9.5 to 13.5 years). The typical sequence in adolescent males continues with adrenarche and further genital development while PHV is a relatively late event, usually happening between SMR 3 and 4. Fertility is attained at SMR 4.

12. (A) The mean age of onset of puberty in boys is 11.6 years ± 1 year.

13. (B) Pubertal gynecomastia is seen in approximately 50% of normal boys during SMR 2 and 3. It usually appears at an average age of 13 and persists for 6 to 18 months. In boys with persistent gynecomastia, etiologies such as hypogonadism, testicular tumors, hyperthyroidism, androgen resistance syndromes, and drug use should be investigated

    Asymmetric gynecomastia is a common finding. Facial acne at age 12 years would not be unusual in a normal boy who is undergoing adrenarche. Testicular size increases from an average prepubertal volume of 5.0 mL at the start of puberty to a final volume of approximately 19 mL by age 20 years.

14. (E) Constitutional delay of puberty is the most common cause of delayed puberty in boys. These boys will eventually progress spontaneously through puberty. However, since CDP is a diagnosis of exclusion, the absence of any pubertal changes after the age of 14 years should prompt investigation to rule out other causes of delayed puberty. A thorough evaluation should include a detailed personal and family history, physical examination, review of growth charts, laboratory testing, and imaging studies. Characteristically, the bone age in boys with CDP closely approximates the height age and both are delayed in relation to chronologic age. Usually a family history of pubertal delay is present in parents, older siblings, or other family members.

15. (B) A percentage of body fat of between 17% and 18% is necessary to reach menarche, and 22% is usually required to maintain regular periods.

16. (B) The criteria for presumptive diagnosis of constitutional delay of puberty include absence of history of systemic illness, evidence of adequate nutrition, normal findings on physical examination, including genital anatomy, sense of smell, and upper to lower segment ratio, normal thyroid and growth hormone levels, normal CBC, ESR, electrolytes and BUN, delayed bone age, and height less than or equal to the 3rd percentile for age with annual growth rate velocity at the 5th percentile for age (at least 3.7 cm/year). A family history of CDP is often present but is not a necessary criterion for diagnosis.

17. (D) Early adolescence marks the beginning of the process leading from significant dependence on parents to fully independent behavior. Rapid physical changes will bring up an increased preoccupation with the self and uncertainty about one's appearance and attractiveness. As the adolescent starts to detach from his/her parents, strong emotional bonds with peers develop, usually starting with friends of the same sex. Contact with teens of the opposite sex usually happens only in the context of groups of friends. Cognitive skills remain mostly concrete during early adolescence but there is an increasing shift toward abstract thinking (formal operational thought). During this stage the adolescent strives toward self-definition and the development of a value system of his/her own. This often leads to a testing of authority both at home and at school. Typically the devel-

opment of a sense of omnipotence and invincibility leading to increased risk-taking behaviors emerges during middle adolescence.

18. **(E)** During middle adolescence, the struggle for emancipation becomes more overt as the teenager devotes more and more time and energy to his/her peer group (school friends, clubs, team sports, gangs). With the growth spurt essentially behind, there is a progressive stabilization and acceptance of one's body image and a growing preoccupation with appearance, grooming, and attractiveness. For most teens there is an increased involvement with the peer group, which helps affirm evolving identity and further emancipation from the family. Dating, sexual experimentation, and intercourse usually start during this stage in many adolescents. Wide mood swings are more frequent in younger teens and should raise concerns if they are noticed in middle adolescence.

SUGGESTED READING

Joffe A, Blythe MJ: Handbook of adolescent medicine. *Adolesc Med* 14:2, 2003.

Neinstein LS: *Adolescent Health Care. A Practical Guide*, 4th ed. Philadelphia, PA: Lippincott Williams and Wilkins, 2002.

Tanner JM, Whitehouse RH: Clinical longitudinal standards for height, weight, height velocity, weight velocity, and stages of puberty. *Arch Dis Child* 51:170, 1976.

Rosenfield RL: Essentials of growth diagnosis. *Endocrinol Metab Clin North Am* 25:743, 1996.

Marshall W, Tanner JM: Variations in the pattern of pubertal changes in boys. *Arch Dis Child* 45:13, 1970.

CASE 70: A 16-YEAR-OLD GIRL WHO HAS NEVER HAD A MENSTRUAL PERIOD

A 16-year-old Caucasian girl comes for the first time to the teen clinic because she has never had a menstrual period. She is a competitive gymnast who was home-schooled for several years so she could pursue her athletic career. She was recently diagnosed with a stress fracture for which she is undergoing physical therapy and is now taking a break from gymnastics. She has a history of asthma and uses an albuterol inhaler as needed, but has never been hospitalized. Her growth and development have always been normal. On further questioning she states that her breast development started at age 12 and that now she wears a size 34B sports bra. She noticed pubic and axillary hair about 2 to 3 years ago. She has grown 1½ inches during the past 18 months. Her mother recalls that her own periods started at age 13. The family history is otherwise noncontributory. She denies trying to lose weight at this time but admits to being on a strict diet during the previous spring, around the time of a big gymnastic competition. At that time her weight went down to 105 lbs. Now, she is back on her usual diet and estimates her caloric intake at 2000 kcal/day. She considers herself to be slightly thin, although at times she wishes she could be a little thinner. She denies ever having been sexually active or using alcohol, tobacco, or other drugs. She states that she is usually stressed around the time of athletic competitions but that she has never been depressed. She is currently a tenth grader at a public school and is a straight A student. Review of systems is negative for headaches, nausea, vomiting, abdominal pain, dysuria, or vaginal discharge.

On physical examination, she is 5'5", 112 lbs, has a heart rate of 72 bpm and a blood pressure of 110/70 mm Hg. She is at Tanner stage 3 for breast and pubic hair development. The rest of her examination is unremarkable.

SELECT THE ONE BEST ANSWER

1. In adolescent girls, what is the average and standard deviation age at menarche (in years)?

   (A) 12.7 ± 1
   (B) 11.8 ± 1
   (C) 13.5 ± 1.2
   (D) 11.5 ± 1.2
   (E) 12.0 ± 1.5

2. Which of the following statements is accurate?

   (A) Menarche occurs at SMR 3 in 60% of girls.
   (B) The peak height velocity is attained in girls before they reach Tanner stages B3 and PH2.
   (C) The average girl stops growing after menarche.
   (D) Twenty percent of girls start menses a year after attaining SMR 5.
   (E) The interval between menarche and regular periods is approximately 3 years.

3. What is the definition of primary amenorrhea?

(A) no menstrual flow by age 16 years regardless of normal secondary sex characteristics

(B) no menstrual flow by age 14 years in a girl with absent secondary sex characteristics

(C) no menstrual flow a year after attaining SMR 5

(D) no menstrual flow 4 years after the onset of puberty

(E) all of the above

4. Among the following which one is the most likely cause of primary amenorrhea in this patient?

(A) hypopituitarism
(B) hypothalamic amenorrhea
(C) physiologic delay of puberty
(D) hypothyroidism
(E) hyperprolactinemia

5. In a patient with absent breast development, which of the following would be included in the differential diagnosis of primary amenorrhea?

(A) polycystic ovarian syndrome
(B) agenesis of the Müllerian structures
(C) imperforate hymen
(D) pure gonadal dysgenesis, 46,XX with streak gonads
(E) androgen insensitivity

6. Among the causes of primary amenorrhea, which of the following does not present with hypogonadotropic hypogonadism?

(A) Kallmann syndrome
(B) eating disorders
(C) competitive athletics
(D) Turner syndrome
(E) chronic disease

7. Which of the following clinical characteristics would make complete androgen insensitivity syndrome an unlikely diagnosis in this case?

(A) absent menses
(B) normal breast development
(C) pubic hair at Tanner stage 3
(D) normal linear growth
(E) none of the above

8. Which of the following would be relevant issues to document in the clinical history?

(A) onset and tempo of pubertal changes
(B) polyuria and polydipsia
(C) changes in athletic training patterns
(D) headaches
(E) all of the above

9. Which component of the physical examination will be least relevant in this case?

(A) blood pressure
(B) acne
(C) appearance of the external genitalia
(D) evaluation of the growth chart
(E) genu valgum

10. What is the single most important finding that will guide the laboratory workup of primary amenorrhea?

(A) degree of breast development
(B) height and weight
(C) signs of virilization
(D) presence or absence of a uterus, either clinically or on ultrasound
(E) upper/lower segment ratio

11. What tests are useful in the diagnosis of primary amenorrhea?

(A) pregnancy test
(B) FSH
(C) TSH
(D) bone densitometry
(E) all of the above

12. Under what circumstance would cranial MRI be the *least* helpful?

(A) galactorrhea
(B) visual field defects
(C) progressively worsening headaches
(D) abnormal sella on skull X-ray
(E) hypergonadotropic hypogonadism

13. Which of the following statements apply to the female athlete?

(A) Pubertal development and menarche are often delayed in thin female athletes.
(B) Each year of premenarchal athletic training delays age of menarche by 5 months.
(C) Intensity of exercise correlates with incidence of amenorrhea.

(D) The female athlete triad includes amenorrhea, disordered eating, and osteoporosis.
(E) All of the above.

14. Which of the following factors is *not* associated with decreased bone density in adolescent athletes?

(A) low weight
(B) low body mass index
(C) low calcium intake
(D) delayed puberty
(E) use of combined oral contraceptives

15. Which of the following symptoms would not be suggestive of an eating disorder in this young athlete?

(A) postural dizziness
(B) diarrhea
(C) amenorrhea
(D) weight loss
(E) cold intolerance

16. Which of the following statements is not true regarding the relation between amenorrhea and anorexia nervosa?

(A) Amenorrhea occurs in almost all patients with anorexia nervosa.
(B) In half of the patients with anorexia nervosa, amenorrhea develops at the same time as weight loss.
(C) In 25% of patients, amenorrhea follows substantial weight loss.
(D) Weight loss follows amenorrhea in 25% of cases.
(E) Anorexia nervosa is never a cause of primary amenorrhea.

17. All of the following are common signs of anorexia nervosa except:

(A) nail pitting
(B) edema
(C) warm, sweaty palms
(D) increased lanugo hair
(E) bradycardia

18. Which of the following psychosocial characteristics is not typically found in teens with eating disorders?

(A) depression, anxiety, and obsessional thoughts
(B) perfectionism
(C) increased sexual interest
(D) school overachievement
(E) disturbed body image

19. Assuming that this girl's primary amenorrhea is exclusively a result of hypothalamic hypogonadotropic hypogonadism associated with strenuous athletic training, which of the following would be recommended for the management of her condition?

(A) counseling regarding appropriate activity level
(B) maintenance of adequate weight
(C) increasing calcium intake to 1500 mg/day
(D) watchful waiting
(E) all of the above

Answers

1. **(A)** The average age of menarche of American adolescents is 12.7 years with a standard deviation of 1 year. According to some studies, a minimum body mass index of 17 is needed to start menarche. Young ballet dancers, long-distance runners, and gymnasts often start their pubertal development and attain menarche at an age significantly older than the average. African-American girls, as a group, experience initial pubertal changes and menarche up to a year earlier than white girls.

2. **(B)** Breast budding in most girls signals the start of puberty. As opposed to boys, most of whom attain peak height velocity at SMR 4, the adolescent girl's growth spurt is an early pubertal event. Peak height velocity in girls occurs before they reach SMR B3 and PH2. Although linear growth later decelerates, the average girl is expected to grow 2 to 3 inches in the 2 years following menarche.

The mean interval from breast development to menarche is 2.3 years. Menarche is a relatively late event in pubertal development and occurs in 66% of girls at SMR 4. Only 25% of girls attain menarche at SMR 3. An additional 10% start menses at SMR 5. Ninety-five percent to 97% of girls have reached menarche by age 16 years and 98% by age 18 years.

3. (**E**) All of the above. Primary amenorrhea is defined as the absence of spontaneous uterine bleeding by age 14 years in a girl with absence of secondary sex characteristics and by age 16 years in a girl regardless of the presence of normal secondary sex characteristics. Girls with no menstrual flow a year after attaining SMR 5 or 4 years after onset of puberty also meet criteria for the diagnosis of primary amenorrhea.

4. (**B**) The differential diagnosis of primary amenorrhea includes conditions resulting from hypothalamic, pituitary, or ovarian dysfunction and those resulting from abnormal development of the lower genital tract. Given this patient's clinical presentation the most likely diagnosis would be functional hypothalamic amenorrhea. Eating disorders, severe or prolonged illness, stress, and exercise are common contributing factors in the pathogenesis of this condition. Functional hypothalamic amenorrhea is characterized by abnormal hypothalamic secretion of GnRH, low or normal LH, absent LH surges, anovulation, and low serum concentrations of estradiol. Both weight loss below a certain level (approximately 10% below ideal body weight or a BMI <17) and exercise can lead to amenorrhea. Constitutional delay of growth and maturation, a common condition in boys, is a relatively rare cause of primary amenorrhea.

5. (**D**) Of the conditions listed above, only pure gonadal dysgenesis with streak gonads would present with absent breast development.

6. (**D**) Turner syndrome is the most common cause of primary gonadal failure in adolescent girls and is characterized by ovarian dysgenesis (accelerated stromal fibrosis and decreased or absent oocyte production), short stature, a wide variety of phenotypical abnormalities, a 45,X0 karyotype, and elevated gonadotropins. Stigmata of Turner syndrome include micrognathia, a high-arched palate, ptosis, epicanthal folds, prominent ears, hearing loss, short webbed neck with low hairline, broad chest, coarctation of the aorta, hypertension, cubitus valgus, renal abnormalities (malrotation, horseshoe kidneys, hydronephrosis), and lymphedema.

Eating disorders, competitive athletics, and chronic disease are among the hypothalamic causes of primary amenorrhea and therefore present with decreased levels of gonadotropins. Kallmann syndrome is a genetic defect leading to isolated GnRH deficiency. It is much more common in boys than in girls. Clinical features include delayed sexual maturation, anosmia or hyposmia, and midline facial defects.

7. (**C**) The complete androgen insensitivity syndrome is an X-linked recessive disorder in which 46,XY individuals appear phenotypically as women. These patients have testosterone insensitivity because of a defect in androgen receptors, and, therefore, do not develop testosterone-dependent male sexual characteristics. At puberty, breast development occurs, but pubic and axillary hair is sparse. Although they typically present with normal-looking female external genitalia, testes may be palpable in the labia majora or inguinal area. There is regression of the müllerian structures leading to absence of the fallopian tubes, uterus and upper third of the vagina. The diagnosis can be confirmed by the finding of elevated testosterone concentrations, XY karyotype, and pelvic ultrasonography results. Surgical excision of the testes is recommended given the increased risk of testicular cancer observed in this condition.

8. (**E**) The clinical history should include a detailed account of the onset and tempo of pubertal changes, including growth spurt, family history of pubertal delay, symptoms of virilization, galactorrhea, and medications. Headaches, visual field defects, polyuria, polydipsia, and fatigue should be investigated to exclude other hypothalamic-pituitary diseases. It is also essential to document recent stressors, changes in diet or exercise patterns, changes in body weight, and recent symptoms suggestive of severe or protracted illness.

9. (**E**) Adolescents with primary amenorrhea should have a complete physical examination, including current height and weight, calculated body mass index, arm span, breast development, galactorrhea, and search for signs of thyroid dysfunction. The skin should be examined for acne, hirsutism, striae, and hyperpigmentation. Growth chart reviews will be essential to assess progression of linear growth and its temporal relation with

weight changes. A careful external genital examination is needed to evaluate pubertal development, clitoral size, and appearance of the hymen. The presence of a normal vagina, cervix, uterus, and ovaries can sometimes be determined by a gentle one-finger vaginal-abdominal or recto-abdominal examination but is most accurately defined by ultrasonography. Findings consistent with Turner syndrome and other genetic disorders should be documented. Hypertension, if present, may suggest coarctation of the aorta, one of Turner syndrome's typical stigmata. High blood pressure may also be a feature of 17α-hydroxylase deficiency, a rare disorder leading to decreased cortisol synthesis with increased production of ACTH, mineralocorticoid excess, and lack of pubertal development. The presence of acne is associated with normal or increased production of adrenal and gonadal steroids.

10. **(D)** It is essential to confirm the presence or absence of a normal vagina, cervix, and uterus (either clinically or by ultrasound) as a first step in the workup of primary amenorrhea. If the uterus is absent, a karyotype and testosterone levels are obtained to distinguish between isolated, abnormal müllerian development with absent uterus, 46,XX karyotype and normal testosterone levels, and androgen insensitivity syndrome. In the latter, the karyotype will be 46,XY and the testosterone levels will be elevated. If, on the other hand, the uterus is present and there are no outlet obstructions such as imperforate hymen or vaginal atresia, an endocrine evaluation should be performed.

11. **(E)** Pregnancy should always be excluded first by testing hCG in serum or in urine. A CBC, complete metabolic panel, and erythrocyte sedimentation rate may help to exclude undiagnosed chronic illnesses leading to hypothalamic dysfunction. It is useful to obtain FSH levels which, if elevated, will indicate primary ovarian failure and will lead to the investigation of the potential causes of hypergonadotropic hypogonadism such as Turner syndrome and mosaicism, Noonan syndrome, autoimmune oophoritis, or gonadal damage secondary to chemotherapy or radiation. Elevated FSH levels in the presence of hypertension suggest either Turner syndrome with

coarctation of the aorta or 17α-hydroxylase deficiency. An elevated serum progesterone, low cortisol, low 17α-hydroxyprogesterone, and increased serum deoxycorticosterone can confirm this latter condition, a rare form of congenital adrenal hyperplasia.

Normal or low FSH levels suggest hypothalamic dysfunction such as functional hypothalamic amenorrhea, usually secondary to weight loss, excessive exercise, stress, or severe or prolonged illness. Less common causes of hypothalamic dysfunction include inflammatory or infiltrative diseases, craniopharyngiomas and other brain tumors, cranial irradiation, and brain injury. Serum prolactin and TSH are necessary to exclude hyperprolactinemia and thyroid disorders. Testosterone and DHEA-S levels are part of the laboratory workup, particularly if there is clinical evidence of hyperandrogenism.

A bone age determination will be helpful in adolescent girls with primary amenorrhea and other signs of pubertal delay to exclude constitutional delay of puberty (a condition occurring much more frequently in boys than in girls) and hypothyroidism. A bone densitometry determination would be helpful in this case, given the history of primary amenorrhea, strenuous athletic training, and stress fractures.

12. **(E)** A cranial MRI is indicated in girls with hypogonadotropic hypogonadism, particularly in the presence of headaches, visual field defects, abnormal sella on radiographs, or any other signs of hypothalamic-pituitary dysfunction. It would be the least helpful in the workup of amenorrhea secondary to hypergonadotropic hypogonadism since the elevation of gonadotropins in that case results from ovarian failure.

13. **(E)** Exercise is clearly beneficial for young women, since it leads to improved cardiovascular fitness, weight control, lower blood pressure, and improved lipid profile. In addition, it promotes socialization, a greater sense of well-being, and self-esteem. There are, however, some potential problems associated with strenuous athletic training, including delayed pubertal development and menarche, eating disorders such as anorexia nervosa, bulimia, purging, binging and fasting, and hypoestrogenic amenorrhea. Disordered eating

has been reported in 15% to 62% of young female athletes. Strenuous exercise also increases the risk of osteoporosis and stress fractures.

14. **(E)** In female athletes, bone mineral density correlates with weight, weight/height, and estrogen and testosterone levels. Low bone density is associated with low estrogen levels, delayed puberty and menarche, low calcium and protein intake, low weight, low body mass index, low androgen levels, disordered eating, and family history of osteoporosis. Use of oral contraceptives in the postmenarchal athletic female decreases the likelihood of osteoporosis. Delayed menarche associated with hypoestrogenemia can have a significant effect on bone mineralization in adolescent athletes, given the fact that 48% of skeletal mass in women is normally attained during puberty.

15. **(B)** An eating disorder should be considered in the differential diagnosis of this 16-year-old girl with a history of weight loss in the past, strenuous exercise, and amenorrhea. Postural dizziness, depressive symptoms, constipation, hair loss, cold intolerance, epigastric pain, nausea, vomiting, fatigue, cramps, and muscle weakness would be among the common presenting symptoms of anorexia nervosa.

16. **(E)** Eating disorders are among the causes of hypothalamic dysfunction leading to primary amenorrhea. Anorexia nervosa is 10 times more common in girls than in boys. The mean age of onset is 13.7 years but it can start in children as young as 10 years. Amenorrhea is present in almost 100% of the cases, coinciding with weight loss in half of them, following it in 25%, and preceding it in 25% of anorectic girls.

17. **(C)** The most common signs of anorexia nervosa are decreased weight and cachexia, decreased temperature, bradycardia, hypotension, dry, hyperkeratotic skin, edema, acrocyanosis, nail pitting, and increased lanugo hair.

18. **(C)** Young women with eating disorders typically have a constellation of psychological features, including low self-esteem, perfectionism, depression, anxiety, obsessional thoughts, social anxiety, and

overachievement. Disturbed body image, increased preoccupation with food, and decreased sexual interest are common features in this condition.

19. **(E)** In this 16-year-old with strenuous athletic training leading to primary amenorrhea, in whom other etiologies have been excluded, it would be reasonable to offer counseling about decreasing physical activity to a level adequate to maintain appropriate weight and bone mineral density while at the same time increasing calcium intake to avoid osteoporosis and stress fractures. If estrogenization is thought to be adequate, in the absence of menses, a progesterone challenge test may help bring about her periods. If the response to this test is positive, a repeat progesterone challenge may be offered every 2 to 3 months. Some authors advocate the cyclic use of estrogens and progestins to treat girls with hypothalamic amenorrhea once an acceptable height has been attained.

SUGGESTED READING

Kaplowitz PB, Oberfield SE: Reexamination of the age limit for defining when puberty is precocious in girls in the United States: Implications for evaluation and treatment. Drug and Therapeutics and Executive Committees of the Lawson Wilkins Pediatric Endocrine Society. *Pediatrics* 104:936, 1999.

Marshall W, Tanner J: Variations in the pattern of pubertal changes in girls. *Arch Dis Child* 44:291, 1969.

Emans SJ, Laufer MR, Goldstein DP (eds): *Pediatric and Adolescent Gynecology*, 5th ed. Philadelphia, PA: Lippincott Williams and Wilkins, 2005.

Neinstein LS: *Adolescent Health Care. A Practical Guide*, 4th ed. Philadelpha, PA: Lippincott Wilkins and Williams, 2002.

Herman-Giddens ME, Slora EJ, Wasserman RC, et al: Secondary sexual characteristics and menses in young girls seen in office practice: A study from the Pediatric Research in Office Settings Network. *Pediatrics* 99:505, 1997.

CASE 71: A 17-YEAR-OLD FEMALE WITH PAINFUL MENSES

A 17-year-old girl comes to the clinic complaining of painful periods. You have been her pediatrician for several years and know that she has been a healthy, well-adjusted adolescent. She started her menses at age 14 years. Her periods have been regular for the most part although she has occasionally complained about heavy but painless periods lasting up to 6 days. Over the past year, her periods have become painful to the point that she had to miss school an average of 2 days a month. She also reports associated nausea during menses. She has tried OTC pain relievers without success. She has been dating for a year but denies sexual activity. She has heard that "the pill may help with cramps" and wants to know your opinion about that. Her past medical history is noncontributory. Her mother had a history of severe menstrual cramps during adolescence. The review of systems shows that she had vomiting on two occasions during menses during the past 3 months. She also mentions increased nervousness, headaches, and backaches, all of which have developed over the past year and usually present together with her episodes of pelvic pain.

SELECT THE ONE BEST ANSWER

1. Which of the following statements concerning prevalence of dysmenorrhea is not accurate?

   (A) Dysmenorrhea affects up to 72% of 17-year-old girls.
   (B) In 10% of adolescents, dysmenorrhea may be severe enough to be incapacitating for 1 to 3 days a month.
   (C) Forty percent of adolescent patients with dysmenorrhea have associated organic pathology.
   (D) Dysmenorrhea is the greatest single cause of lost school hours among adolescent girls.
   (E) The prevalence of dysmenorrhea doubles between SMR 3 and 5.

2. All of the following elements of the clinical history are helpful in differentiating primary from secondary dysmenorrhea except:

   (A) acute vs. gradual onset
   (B) cyclic nature of symptoms
   (C) associated clinical manifestations
   (D) duration of pain
   (E) severity of pain

3. Which among the following are factors involved in the pathogenesis of primary dysmenorrhea?

   (A) elevation of myometrial resting tone
   (B) increased frequency of myometrial contractions
   (C) increased contractile myometrial pressures above the normal range (>120 mm Hg)

   (D) dysrhythmic uterine contractions
   (E) all of the above

4. Which of the following statements concerning the role of prostaglandins in primary dysmenorrhea is not true?

   (A) Prostaglandin $F_{2\alpha}$ causes myometrial contractions, vasoconstriction, and ischemia.
   (B) Prostaglandins are synthesized in the endometrial tissue.
   (C) Anovulatory cycles are associated with lower prostaglandin levels and rarely are associated with dysmenorrhea.
   (D) Prostaglandin inhibitors increase dysmenorrhea.
   (E) Patients with dysmenorrhea have higher levels of prostaglandin levels in the endometrium.

5. Which of the following items would be relevant in the clinical evaluation of dysmenorrhea?

   (A) age at menarche
   (B) menstrual pattern
   (C) response to analgesics
   (D) vaginal discharge
   (E) all of the above

6. Regarding the value of the pelvic examination in the evaluation of dysmenorrhea, all of the following statements are true except:

   (A) A pelvic examination is helpful in the diagnosis of endometriosis, polyps, uterine, and cervical abnormalities.
   (B) A pelvic ultrasound will sometimes be needed to rule out pelvic pathology in virginal patients.
   (C) A pelvic examination is not needed in virginal patients with a history suggestive of primary dysmenorrhea who respond to prostaglandin inhibitors.
   (D) A pelvic examination is needed in all patients to rule out secondary dysmenorrhea.
   (E) A pelvic examination is mandatory in cases of acute and subacute pelvic pain.

7. Which of the following conditions should be considered in the differential diagnosis of secondary dysmenorrhea?

   (A) endometriosis

(B) congenital obstruction of the outflow tract
(C) pelvic inflammatory disease
(D) ovarian cysts
(E) all of the above should be considered

8. All of the following are helpful in the treatment of primary dysmenorrhea except:

(A) ibuprofen or naproxen sodium
(B) acetaminophen
(C) aspirin
(D) mefenamic acid
(E) continuous hormonal therapy

9. When using NSAIDs in patients with primary dysmenorrhea, what are the most common pitfalls leading to failure to achieve adequate symptom relief?

(A) starting medication several hours after the pain started
(B) poor compliance because of side effects
(C) failing to offer a loading dose
(D) taking the medication at 12-hour intervals
(E) A and C

10. All of the following statements are true regarding the role of oral contraceptives in the treatment of primary dysmenorrhea in adolescents except:

(A) Combined oral contraceptives provide relief in 70% of patients with primary dysmenorrhea.
(B) Oral contraceptives are beneficial in primary dysmenorrhea as a result of inhibition of ovulation, endometrial hypoplasia, and reduction of menstrual flow.
(C) In patients with primary dysmenorrhea but no need for birth control, "the pill" can be prescribed for 3 to 6 months, discontinued, and then reinstituted if a trial of NSAIDs fails to provide relief.
(D) Patients with severe dysmenorrhea who fail to respond to continued use of oral contraceptives should be reevaluated for organic pathology.
(E) All of the above statements are true.

11. Which of the following is not a typical symptom or sign of endometriosis in adolescents?

(A) cyclic, severe dysmenorrhea
(B) vaginal discharge

(C) abnormal uterine bleeding
(D) dyspareunia
(E) pain on defecation

12. What is the most common gynecologic cause of acute pain leading to hospitalization in women of reproductive age in the United States?

(A) adnexal torsion
(B) ovarian cysts
(C) endometriosis
(D) ectopic pregnancy
(E) pelvic inflammatory disease

13. Which of the following gastrointestinal conditions should be included in the differential diagnosis of acute pelvic pain in teens?

(A) appendicitis
(B) intestinal obstruction
(C) constipation
(D) inflammatory bowel disease
(E) all of the above should be included

14. Regarding the evaluation of acute pelvic pain in adolescents, which of the following statement is not true?

(A) A normal pelvic ultrasound excludes endometriosis and PID.
(B) A psychosocial history might reveal contributing factors such as stress or history of sexual or physical abuse.
(C) The initial laboratory workup should include a CBC with differential, sedimentation rate, C-reactive protein, urinalysis and urine culture, cervical culture, pregnancy test, and a stool guaiac test.
(D) An elevated leukocyte count reflects inflammation, ischemia, or infection and may indicate ovarian torsion.
(E) Bone and joint inflammations and infections may present as acute pelvic pain.

15. Which of the following statements apply to the evaluation of chronic pelvic pain?

(A) A normal pelvic examination and normal ultrasound are predictive of a normal laparoscopy 50% of the time.
(B) The predictive value of an abnormal pelvic ultrasound is 92%.

(C) The most common laparoscopic finding in adolescents with chronic pelvic pain is endometriosis.

(D) No obvious cause of chronic pelvic pain is found on laparoscopy in 25% of patients.

(E) All of the above.

16. If her dysmenorrhea were severe enough to merit long-term use of combined oral contraceptives, which of the following conditions would you need to exclude before prescribing them?

(A) ovarian cyst
(B) endometriosis
(C) family history of breast cancer
(D) varicose veins
(E) diastolic pressure >100 mm Hg

Answers

1. **(C)** In adolescent girls, dysmenorrhea is the most common gynecologic complaint. By definition, primary dysmenorrhea refers to pain associated with menstrual flow in the absence of organic pelvic pathology. Secondary dysmenorrhea, on the other hand, indicates menstrual pain secondary to organic disease such as ovarian cysts, adhesions, endometriosis, or PID. Primary dysmenorrhea is very common in adolescents and rarely has its onset after age 20 years. It is associated with ovulatory cycles and, therefore, typically, primary dysmenorrhea develops approximately 2 years after menarche, once normal ovulation becomes established. Secondary dysmenorrhea may occur at any age. In adolescence, however, primary dysmenorrhea is by far the most common cause of painful menses.

2. **(E)** Primary dysmenorrhea usually has a gradual onset as opposed to the acute onset of most menstrual pain associated with pelvic pathology. The cyclic nature of the bleeding and cramping helps to differentiate primary from secondary dysmenorrhea, since, in the latter, there is often irregular intermenstrual bleeding. The duration of pain is an important clinical feature, lasting 1 to 2 days in primary dysmenorrhea (usually starting right before the period), while in secondary dysmenorrhea, prolonged intermenstrual pain, worsening during periods is the rule. Nausea, vomiting, fatigue, headache, irritability, diarrhea, and backache are

common in primary dysmenorrhea. In secondary dysmenorrhea there is often a history of an STD, severe abdominal pain, and dyspareunia.

3. **(E)** All the above myometrial factors play a role in the pathogenesis of dysmenorrhea.

4. **(D)** Exogenous injections of prostaglandins induce dysmenorrhea while prostaglandin inhibitors decrease menstrual pain.

5. **(E)** When evaluating an adolescent for dysmenorrhea, it is important to determine age at menarche since primary dysmenorrhea usually starts a year after menarche (most commonly between the ages of 14 and 16 years) and peaks around 17 to 18 years. After the age of 20 years new-onset dysmenorrhea is usually secondary to pelvic pathology. Other relevant questions include the date of the last menstrual period, the onset and characteristics of pain such as location, radiation, duration, severity, and degree of functional impairment. A sexual history should be elicited, asking about condom use, contraception, number of sexual partners, exposure to STDs, dyspareunia, and vaginal discharge. Response to prostaglandin inhibitors is important to distinguish primary from secondary dysmenorrhea and to select appropriate further management.

6. **(D)** A pelvic examination is helpful in the diagnosis of organic pathologies underlying secondary dysmenorrhea. It is mandatory in cases of acute and subacute pelvic pain. Adolescent girls without a history of sexual activity and with a clinical picture consistent with primary dysmenorrhea responsive to prostaglandin inhibitors will not need a pelvic examination. Occasionally, however, a pelvic ultrasound may be needed in such patients if symptoms persist.

7. **(E)** The following conditions should be considered in the differential diagnosis of secondary dysmenorrhea: endometriosis, PID and pelvic abscess ovarian cysts, neoplasias, adhesions, congenital obstruction of the outflow tract (cervical stenosis), and complications of pregnancy such as ectopic pregnancy and miscarriage.

8. **(B)** Prostaglandin synthetase inhibitors (NSAIDs) are the drugs of choice in the treatment of pri-

mary dysmenorrhea. NSAIDs are thought to be more effective if administered just before the onset of pain. Mefenamic acid, ibuprofen, and naproxen sodium are popular choices. Both mefenamic acid and naproxen sodium require a loading dose. NSAIDs are contraindicated in adolescents with peptic ulcer disease, hepatic or renal disease, or a bleeding disorder.

9. (E) For optimal effectiveness, NSAIDs should be started as soon as the symptoms develop and even on the day prior to the one when menses are anticipated in those teens with reasonably predictable periods. A loading dose is needed when using naproxen and mefenamic acid.

10. (E) Combined oral contraceptives are useful for adolescents with primary dysmenorrhea who fail to respond to a trial of NSAIDs and for those who need both relief of menstrual pain and contraception. Oral contraceptives may take 2 to 3 months to show adequate relief of dysmenorrhea and NSAIDs can be used concomitantly in the interim.

11. (B) Endometriosis is the most common cause of chronic pelvic pain lasting more than 3 months and not responding to NSAIDs or oral contraceptives. Clinical features of endometriosis include chronic pelvic pain usually worsening during menses, pain on defecation, dyspareunia, and abnormal uterine bleeding. On physical examination, tenderness over the adnexa and cul-de-sac is more common in teens than the classical finding of thickened, nodular sacrouterine ligaments often found in adult women with endometriosis.

12. (E) Adolescent girls with acute pelvic pain deserve an urgent and thorough evaluation to rule out potentially life-threatening conditions. The differential diagnosis of acute pelvic pain includes gynecologic conditions such as PID, adnexal torsion, ovarian cysts, threatened or spontaneous abortion, and endometriosis. PID is the most common cause of acute pain leading to hospitalization in women of reproductive age in the United States. Nongynecologic causes include gastrointestinal, genitourinary, musculoskeletal, and psychological disorders.

13. (E) The list of gastrointestinal conditions responsible for acute pelvic pain in teens is quite lengthy and includes, among others, appendicitis, intestinal obstruction, gastric ulcer, inflammatory bowel disease, lactose intolerance, irritable bowel syndrome, diverticular disease, constipation, and mesenteric adenitis.

14. (A) The initial evaluation of acute pelvic pain with suspected underlying organic pathology should include a thorough clinical and psychosocial history, a physical examination, and laboratory testing. Ultrasonography is a useful procedure in the evaluation of acute pelvic pain, particularly for those in whom a thorough pelvic examination is not possible. However, a normal ultrasound does not exclude endometriosis or PID.

15. (E) While the predictive value of an abnormal pelvic ultrasound is 92%, a normal ultrasound only has a predictive value of 50%. In a large study evaluating laparoscopic findings in adolescents with chronic pelvic pain, 75% of patients had intrapelvic pathology, while no obvious cause of chronic pain was found in the remaining 25%. Among those with organic pathology, endometriosis was the leading diagnosis followed by postoperative adhesions secondary to appendectomy or ovarian cystectomy.

16. (E) According to the WHO Medical Eligibility Criteria (2001), among the above conditions, only hypertension would preclude initiation of combined oral contraceptives.

SUGGESTED READING

Emans SJ, Laufer MR, Goldstein DP: *Pediatric and Adolescent Gynecology.* 5th ed. Philadelphia, PA: Lippincott Williams and Wilkins, 2005.

Neinstein LS: *Adolescent Health Care. A Practical Guide,* 4th ed. Philadelphia, PA: Lippincott Williams and Wilkins, 2002.

Johnson BE, et al: *Women's Health Care Handbook,* 2nd ed. Philadelphia, PA: Hanley & Belfus, 2000.

CASE 72: A 14-YEAR-OLD GIRL WITH PAINFUL URINATION

A 14-year-old girl is brought in by her aunt (who is the patient's guardian) for an urgent care visit with the complaint of acute onset, painful urination. This is the first time you have met this family. The present symptoms started about 2 days ago and are now severe enough to keep her from attending school. She has been healthy except for vague, recurrent stomach aches for several years. There is no previous history of UTI. A review of systems reveals that she has been tired, "achy" and had a slight fever during the previous week. She started her menses 8 months prior to this visit and states that she had skipped her periods two or three times since then. She had her latest menstrual period 3 weeks ago. The family history is positive for arthritis in an older sister and insulin-dependent diabetes on the paternal side of the family. She lives with her aunt, her older sister, two cousins, and a niece. She used to be an average student but her grades have shown a significant decline since she started high school 6 months ago. She denies cigarette smoking or alcohol use but states that she smokes marijuana with her friends on weekends. Her aunt worries about her increasing rebelliousness. After a recent confrontation she ran away from home and eventually returned 3 days later. She is a thin, small-for-age girl who looks younger than her stated age.

SELECT THE ONE BEST ANSWER

1. The differential diagnosis of dysuria in adolescent girls includes all of the following except:

    (A) UTI
    (B) chlamydial urethritis
    (C) herpes simplex type 2 vaginitis
    (D) traumatic urethritis
    (E) endometriosis

2. Among the following, which is the most common pathogen responsible for UTI in healthy, nonpregnant adolescent girls?

    (A) *E. coli*
    (B) *Gardnerella vaginalis*
    (C) *S. saprophyticus*
    (D) Group B streptococci
    (E) *Enterococcus* species

3. What conditions are included in the differential diagnosis of dysuria in adolescent males?

    (A) gonococcal urethritis
    (B) nongonococcal urethritis
    (C) prostatitis
    (D) chemical irritation from spermicides
    (E) all of the above

4. The following factors predispose adolescent girls to UTIs except:

    (A) start of sexual activity
    (B) new sexual partner
    (C) recent history of streptococcal pharyngitis
    (D) poor perineal hygiene
    (E) use of diaphragms

5. On taking a clinical history in this young girl, which of the following is the *least* helpful?

    (A) use of douches, deodorant soaps, and bubble baths
    (B) abnormal vaginal discharge and itching
    (C) sexual history, including number of partners, condom and other contraceptive use, and potential exposure to STDs
    (D) family history of hypertension
    (E) history of fever and flank pain

6. In accordance with your office guidelines, you have already discussed the extent and limits of your privacy and confidentiality policy with both the parent (or guardian) and the patient earlier in the visit. On interviewing the patient privately, she tells you tearfully that she had unprotected vaginal intercourse with her 15-year-old new boyfriend a week earlier. She has not discussed this with her aunt and would prefer to keep it confidential. She became sexually active at age 13 years and had two previous sexual partners. She is not using hormonal contraception and uses condoms inconsistently. The physical examination should include all except:

    (A) abdominal examination
    (B) costovertebral angle tenderness
    (C) inspection of the external genitalia
    (D) speculum examination
    (E) all of the above should be included

7. You perform a physical examination with a chaperone in attendance. You find her to be a well-developed, quiet, cooperative 14-year-old girl, somewhat immature for her age. She is afebrile. There are no abnormal clinical findings on the general examination. The abdomen is soft. There are no masses, guarding, rebound, or visceromegalies. There is no costovertebral tenderness. Her pubertal development is at Tanner stage 4. The

external genital examination shows normal labia and absence of inguinal lymphadenopathy. There is some scant yellowish discharge in the introitus where you also find two small clusters of vesicular lesions, some of them ulcerated and very tender to touch. A careful and gentle speculum examination shows a red and friable cervix and thick, foamy discharge in the cul-de-sac. The bimanual examination is poorly tolerated but there are no obvious masses or cervical motion tenderness.

All of the following tests will be necessary at this time except:

(A) gonorrhea and chlamydia probe
(B) herpes culture
(C) wet prep
(D) KOH
(E) HIV

8. On the wet preparation you are likely to find:

(A) white blood cells
(B) red blood cells
(C) trichomonas
(D) epithelial cells
(E) all of the above

9. The wet preparation shows large amounts of white blood cells and flagellated organisms. With the information you have so far (including history and physical examination), this patient most likely carries a diagnosis of:

(A) trichomonal vaginitis
(B) herpes simplex infection
(C) chlamydial cervicitis
(D) a UTI
(E) all of the above

10. The following laboratory tests should now be performed except:

(A) RPR
(B) blood culture
(C) HIV
(D) urine culture
(E) pregnancy test

11. Concerning chlamydia infections, which of the following statements is false?

(A) Cervical ectopy is a risk factor for infection.

(B) Most chlamydia infections are asymptomatic.
(C) Retesting is recommended 4 to 6 months after treatment of chlamydia cervicitis.
(D) Fifteen percent of all *C. trachomatis* infections occur in females age 15 to 19 years.
(E) There is a high rate of concurrent disease in adolescents with urinary tract symptomatology evaluated for UTI and *C. trachomatis*.

12. Regarding trichomonal vaginitis, which of the following statements is true?

(A) Up to 90% of women infected with *T. vaginalis* present with vaginal discharge.
(B) Partners of patients with trichomonal infection should be treated.
(C) Most recurrences of trichomonal vaginitis are a result of resistance to treatment.
(D) Trichomonal infections in males are symptomatic in most cases.
(E) All of the above are true.

13. Regarding the clinical manifestation of primary herpes infections in adolescents, which of the following statements is false?

(A) The incubation period lasts 2 to 12 days.
(B) Re-epithelization occurs 15 to 20 days after the initial outbreak.
(C) Lesions shed the virus for 3 to 5 days.
(D) Cervicitis is present in up to 90% of first episodes but is less common in recurrent disease.
(E) Constitutional symptoms may include headaches, fever, malaise, myalgia, nuchal rigidity, and photophobia.

14. The following laboratory tests are useful for the diagnosis of HSV infections except:

(A) Tzanck smear
(B) wet mount
(C) PAP smear and colposcopy
(D) viral culture
(E) serology

15. In gonorrhea, all of the following are true except:

(A) Females have a 50% chance of contracting gonorrhea from an infected male after a single sexual encounter.
(B) Males have a 25% chance of contracting gonorrhea from an infected female.

(C) The incubation period is 2 weeks.

(D) Adolescent girls ages 15 to 19 years have the highest rates of gonorrhea infection.

(E) Most gonorrhea infections in adolescent girls are asymptomatic.

16. The risk of PID increases with all of the following:

(A) barrier methods

(B) age younger than 24 years or smoking

(C) birth control pills

(D) use of an intrauterine device

(E) B and D

17. All of the following clinical signs are considered as minimal diagnostic criteria for the diagnosis of PID except:

(A) lower abdominal tenderness

(B) fever

(C) adnexal tenderness

(D) cervical motion tenderness

(E) all are required to made a diagnosis of PID

18. Assuming that her pregnancy test is negative, that there is no suspicion of PID, and that there are no known allergies, what would be the treatment of choice in this 14-year-old adolescent girl?

(A) ceftriaxone 125 mg IM single dose, doxycycline 100 mg orally twice a day for 7 days, acyclovir 400 mg orally three time a day for 5 days, metronidazole 2 g single dose orally, symptomatic treatment for pain relief

(B) ciprofloxacin 500 mg single dose orally, doxycycline 100 mg orally twice a day for 7 days, valacyclovir 1 g orally twice a day for 7 to 10 days, symptomatic treatment for pain relief

(C) ceftriaxone 125 mg IM single dose, azithromycin 1 g single dose orally, metronidazole 2 g single dose orally, valacyclovir 1 g orally twice a day for 7 to 10 days, symptomatic treatment for pain relief

(D) metronidazole 2 g single dose orally, ceftriaxone 250 mg IM single dose, azithromycin 1 g, valacyclovir after herpes genitalis is confirmed by viral culture

(E) ceftriaxone 250 mg single dose orally, erythromycin base, 500 mg four times a day, acyclovir 200 mg orally 5 times a day, metronidazole topically for 5 days, symptomatic treatment for pain relief

19. What other management recommendations would you offer at this visit?

(A) partner needs treatment for trichomonas, chlamydia, and gonorrhea

(B) test for HIV and syphilis

(C) counseling to address runaway behavior and substance use

(D) discuss contraceptive options and STD prevention

(E) all of the above

Answers

1. **(E)** Dysuria is a common symptom in adolescent girls and may be secondary to infection, trauma, and chemical irritation. The differential diagnosis includes bacterial UTI, chlamydia and gonorrhea urethritis, candida and trichomonal vulvovaginitis, bacterial vaginosis, herpes simplex infections, traumatic urethritis, vulvovaginal chemical irritation, and vulvar dermatoses. In one study of adolescents with presenting complaint of dysuria, isolated UTI was only found in 17% of the cases and combined UTI and vaginitis was responsible for another 17%. Of the remaining two-thirds, the diagnoses were candida vaginitis, bacterial vaginosis, trichomoniasis, gonorrhea, and chlamydia or herpesvirus infection. These data underscore the importance of obtaining a detailed gynecologic and sexual history in young adolescents with dysuria.

2. **(A)** *E. coli* is responsible for up to 90% of UTIs in this age group. In most series, *S. saprophyticus* is the second most common pathogen identified. In chronic or recurrent infections, *Klebsiella* species, enterococci, *Proteus* species, or *Pseudomonas aeruginosa* may be found. The incidence of group B streptococci as a causative agent for UTI increases in pregnant adolescent girls.

3. **(E)** Gonococcal and nongonococcal urethritis (NGU), prostatitis, and chemical irritation secondary to spermicides are the leading causes of dysuria in adolescent boys. The most common etiologic agents of NGU are *C. trachomatis*, *Ureaplasma urealyticum*, *Gardnerella vaginalis*, herpes simplex virus, *Staphylococcus saprophyticus*, *E. coli*, and *T. vaginalis*.

4. **(C)** Additional risk factors for UTI in girls include delayed postcoital micturition, pregnancy, and anatomical abnormalities such as vesicourethral reflux, urethral stenosis, neurogenic bladder, and nephrolithiasis.

5. **(D)** In evaluating an adolescent girl with dysuria, the following should be investigated:

   - Onset of symptoms (acute onset suggests cystitis, while a gradual onset is more typical of urethritis)
   - Concurrent diagnoses: diabetes mellitus, HIV, pregnancy, recent use of steroids
   - Review of symptoms with emphasis on fever, abdominal, flank, and joint pain
   - Recent and past sexual activity (consensual and nonconsensual)
   - Symptoms of urethritis in the male partner
   - Internal vs. external dysuria (in the latter, the pain is triggered as urine passes over the affected skin or mucosa)
   - Vaginal discharge and itching
   - Menstrual history including date of last menstrual period
   - Use of douches, deodorant soaps, and bubble bath
   - Use of diaphragms or cervical caps
   - Past history of UTI, vesicoureteral reflex, and/or other abnormalities of the urinary tract
   - History of fever and flank pain, suggesting pyelonephritis
   - Terminal dysuria or hematuria, which would strongly favor the diagnosis of UTI

   As usual, when providing health care to adolescents, a brief psychosocial history, including family composition and dynamics, school, social, and emotional functioning and risk factors, would be invaluable in the diagnosis and management of the patient.

6. **(E)** Weight, temperature, and blood pressure should be documented. A general physical examination with special attention to skin, HEENT, neck, abdomen, and extremities will be necessary. In this case, it is important to look for rashes suggestive of STDs and to perform a throat and neck examination looking for signs of infection (e.g., oral sores, exudates, and lymphadenopathies). The eyes should be inspected for iritis and conjunctivitis complicating some STDs, and a musculoskeletal examination may be helpful to assess for STD-associated arthritis. An abdominal examination should be done looking for tenderness, guarding, masses, and visceromegalies. The costovertebral angles should be evaluated for tenderness and Tanner stage should be recorded. A thorough pelvic exam will be needed to establish the diagnosis, while a rectal exam would only be indicated in selected cases.

7. **(D)** The presence of clusters of exquisitely tender vesicular and ulcerative lesions is highly suggestive of herpes infection. However, in view of the yellowish, foamy discharge found on introitus and cul-de-sac, other STDs such as gonorrhea, chlamydia, and trichomoniasis need to be ruled out. A GC/Chlamydia probe, wet prep, and herpes culture will be necessary to confirm the diagnoses. In the absence of symptoms or signs suggesting monilial vaginitis or vulvitis, a KOH prep will not be helpful. HIV testing is indicated in view of her clinical picture and sexual history.

8. **(E)** The clinical appearance of the discharge provides important clues to the diagnosis. Leukorrhea is a normal finding in adolescent girls and results of the progressive estrogenization of the vaginal mucosa, which starts a few months before menarche and continues throughout the reproductive years. There is a normal, cyclic variation in the appearance of leukorrhea throughout the month. A thick, curdy, "cottage cheese" white discharge suggests *Candida* infection while a thin, grayish, foul-smelling discharge is consistent with bacterial vaginosis. *Trichomonas* vaginitis is usually present with a frothy, malodorous yellow or white discharge.

   Microscopic examination of the wet preparation is a helpful technique, which often provides timely information in the office setting. Normal findings include sheets of epithelial cells such as those seen in leukorrhea. Epithelial cells covered with refractile bacteria attached to their surface are known as "clue cells." Clue cells are characteristic in bacterial vaginosis and typically, leukocytes are absent in this condition. On the other hand, large numbers of leukocytes are usually seen both in trichomonal infections and in mucopurulent cervicitis. The presence of flagellated organisms will confirm the diagnosis of trichomoniasis. It is important to remember, however, that the sensitivity of the wet preparation to identify trichomonas is approximately 70% and that therefore, almost one-third of patients with this diagnosis may be missed with this technique. In this case, with a clinical picture suggestive of several coexisting genital infections and a friable cervix, the wet preparation is likely to show all the elements listed.

9. **(E)** Although trichomoniasis has already been confirmed on wet prep and herpes simplex infections is very likely from a clinical standpoint, cervicitis, either because of chlamydia or gonorrhea, and concomitant UTI still need to be excluded. In several clinical series concurrent UTI and genital infections were found in up to 20% of adolescent girls presenting with genitourinary symptoms.

10. **(B)** Even though the clinical picture is highly suggestive of vulvovaginitis and cervicitis, a urine culture will help rule out concomitant UTI. HIV and syphilis testing should be done in all patients with evidence of other STDs. A pregnancy test will be needed given this patient's history of unprotected intercourse.

11. **(D)** An estimated 3 million teenagers acquire an STD every year, with an approximate rate of 1 in 4 sexually active teens between the ages of 13 and 19 years. Approximately two-thirds of all cases of STD occur in people younger than 24 years. Chlamydial infections are the most common of all bacterial STDs at all ages. Forty percent of chlamydial infections occur in females ages 15 to 19 years. In adolescent girls in this age group, the rate of chlamydial infections is 3.5 times higher than that of gonorrhea. Both chlamydia and gonorrhea have a predilection for columnar epithelium. The high prevalence of these infections in young women may be explained, at least in part, by the presence of cervical ectopy, a normal developmental finding during adolescence. It is estimated that more than 50% of females and 25% of males with chlamydial infections may be asymptomatic. Given the high rate of recurrence after treatment of chlamydia infections, retesting in 4 to 6 months is recommended. The high rate of recurrence is most likely a result of reinfection

rather than to antibiotic resistance. According to present AAP recommendations, all sexually active adolescent girls should be screened for *C. trachomatis* infection every 6 months.

12. **(B)** As many as 50% of women and most men with trichomonal infections are asymptomatic. For those adolescent girls who present with symptoms, vaginal discharge and itching are the most common complaints. The discharge is typically yellow-green and may be frothy. On physical examination vulvar and vaginal erythema are common and a "strawberry cervix," resulting from swollen papillae and punctuate hemorrhages, may be present. Trichomonads can be detected on wet mounts (with 64% and 75% sensitivity in asymptomatic and symptomatic women respectively). Cultures and DNA amplification methods increase sensitivity to 97% and 99%, respectively. Partners of patients with *Trichomonas* infections should also be treated.

13. **(C)** A first episode of primary genital herpes infection is defined as an infection in a patient with no prior history of genital herpes who is seronegative for herpes. The incubation period lasts about a week with a range of 2 to 12 days. Vesicular lesions subsequently appear, marking the end of the incubation period. The vesicles then evolve into ulcers that may coalesce and the virus may shed for at least 10 to 12 days. Re-epithelization takes place in 2 to 3 weeks and leaves no scarring. Cervicitis is common in 70% to 90% of first episodes but is less common in recurrent disease. Recurrent genital herpes infections are usually milder, have less constitutional symptoms, present with fewer lesions, and heal faster. During recurrent infections viral shedding lasts for about 4 days. Up to 15% of genital herpes infections are caused by HSV-1.

14. **(B)** The Tzanck preparation, in which scrapings from a lesion are stained with Wright's stain, may show characteristic multinucleated giant cells. The Pap smear would show the same findings with a 60% to 70% sensitivity and 95% specificity. Colposcopy may reveal characteristic ulcers with a sensitivity of about 70%. Viral cultures are the test of choice for confirmation of infection. Virus detection, however, is dependent on the stage of the

lesions: cultures are positive in 90% of vesicles and 70% of ulcers but only on 25% of crusted lesions.

15. **(C)** The incubation period of gonorrhea is 3 to 5 days. It is estimated that 75% to 90% of women and 10% to 40% of men infected with gonorrhea are asymptomatic. Screening for gonorrhea in asymptomatic girls can be accomplished by obtaining endocervical cultures. Newer, non-culture tests such as DNA probes, LCR (ligase chain reaction) and PCR (polymerase chain reaction) tests have very good sensitivity and specificity and allow screening for gonorrhea in urine samples and vaginal swabs. Routine cultures from the pharynx and rectum in adolescents are not cost-effective in asymptomatic adolescents. The currently recommended treatments are believed to be effective in gonorrhea eradication from all sites.

16. **(E)** PID comprises a variety of inflammatory disorders of the upper genital tract in women, including endometritis, salpingitis, tubo-ovarian abscess, and pelvic peritonitis. It is a common condition that affects 1 million women and leads to 200,000 hospitalizations per year. Seventy-five percent of women with PID are younger than 25 years. In one-quarter of affected women, PID leads to sequelae such as infertility, ectopic pregnancy, and chronic pelvic pain. Teenagers account for one-fifth of all cases of PID. PID is usually polymicrobial, including aerobic and anaerobic bacteria, and results from ascending infection of bacteria from the cervix. Among the sexually transmitted infections, gonorrhea, chlamydia, and genital mycoplasma are the most common pathogens responsible for PID. Smokers have twice the risk of nonsmokers and there is also increased risk for PID in IUD users. The use of barrier methods and birth control pills lowers the risk for PID.

17. **(B)** The diagnosis of PID relies heavily on clinical judgment. Because of the lack of conclusive diagnostic indicators, the condition is correctly diagnosed on clinical and laboratory grounds in 65% of cases. The differential diagnosis is extensive and includes appendicitis, gastroenteritis, irritable bowel syndrome, cholecystitis, endometriosis, hemorrhagic ovarian cyst, ovarian torsion,

nephrolithiasis, and somatization. The most frequently found clinical features are abdominal pain (100%), adnexal tenderness (90%), and cervical motion tenderness (80%). Vaginal discharge, abdominal guarding, and rebound are less common (73% and 61%, respectively). Fever is present in only 30% of cases. Minimal diagnostic criteria include abdominal pain, adnexal tenderness, and cervical motion tenderness. Fever and vaginal discharge are additional clinical criteria. An increased erythrocyte sedimentation rate and C-reactive protein and laboratory documentation of cervical infection with gonorrhea or chlamydia will provide supportive evidence. Additional tests such as pelvic ultrasound are helpful to detect pelvic abscess and ectopic pregnancy. A pregnancy test will be needed as part of the workup.

Empiric treatment is started as soon as the diagnosis of PID is suspected. Although most women with PID are treated in the outpatient setting, adolescents may need to be hospitalized for treatment, given their often unpredictable compliance. Other indications for in-patient treatment include pregnancy as well as suspected surgical emergencies such as appendicitis, ectopic pregnancy, or pelvic abscess. Severe illnesses with nausea or vomiting also preclude outpatient management. Careful follow-up will be required in all cases.

18. **(C)** Your findings so far confirm the diagnosis of trichomoniasis and are also highly suggestive of a first episode of genital herpes. Concurrent gonorrhea and/or chlamydia are also likely in this adolescent at risk who presents with mucopurulent cervicitis. All these infections will need to be treated to avoid short- and long-term complications. Although you could treat her for trichomonas and herpes on the first visit and ask her to return for treatment of gonorrhea and chlamydia once these infections are confirmed, follow-up may be unreliable in view of this patient's psychosocial history. Thus, it would be preferable to treat her for all suspected infections on the present visit. Antibiotic resistance has been a major problem in the treatment of gonorrhea. The 2002 CDC guidelines for the treatment of STDs state that resistance to quinolones (ciprofloxacin and ofloxacin) precludes their use in certain areas of the country, particularly in the western United

States. The recommended dose of ceftriaxone for the treatment of uncomplicated gonorrhea cervicitis is 125 mg IM single dose. Regimens that include ceftriaxone or doxycycline would also cover incubating syphilis. Azithromycin, doxycycline, and erythromycin will all be effective in treating chlamydia. However, azithromycin is a preferred treatment in adolescents because of its easy one-time dose schedule. There are several antiviral agents available for the treatment of first episode of genital herpes. Among them, valacyclovir is the one that requires the least frequent dosing, increasing the potential for compliance. Many experts do not prescribe antivirals for uncomplicated herpes infection. Ciprofloxacin has not been approved for use in patients younger than 18 years.

19. **(E)** This patient's sexual partner should be treated for trichomonas, chlamydia, and gonorrhea infections. HIV and RPR testing is recommended and the patient is advised to abstain from sexual activity until all her lesions are healed. Underlying her presenting concerns, this 14-year-old has a host of risk factors, including school failure, high risk for pregnancy and STDs, runaway behavior, and drug use. A brief initial discussion on this visit will need to be followed up with more extensive evaluation and interventions including individual and family counseling.

SUGGESTED READING

Emans SJ, Laufer MR, Goldstein DP, eds: *Pediatric and Adolescent Gynecology*, 5th ed. Philadelphia, PA: Lippincott Williams and Wilkins, 2005.

Pickering LK, ed: *Red Book: 2003 Report of the Committee on Infectious Diseases*, 26th ed. Elk Grove Village, IL: American Academy of Pediatrics, 2003.

Neinstein LS: *Adolescent Health Care. A Practical Guide*, 4th ed. Philadelphia, PA: Lippincott Williams and Wilkins, 2002.

Johnson BE, et al: *Women's Health Care Handbook*, 2nd ed. Philadelphia, PA: Hanley and Belfus, 2000.

Hatcher RA, et al: *Contraceptive Technology*, 17th rev. ed. New York: Ardent Media, 1998.

CASE 73: A 17-YEAR-OLD FEMALE WITH HEAVY, IRREGULAR MENSES

A 17-year-old girl presents to the teen clinic with her mother, complaining of irregular menstrual bleeding for the past 6 months. You have been her pediatrician for the past 4 years and reviewing her chart you find that she has had mild intermittent asthma and eczema in the past, but no other chronic conditions. She started her periods at age 11 years and menses have been regular every 28 days until 6 months ago. Menstrual flow has been always heavy and she reports having always used five pads a day for the duration of her periods. Lately her menses have been somewhat irregular, lasting up to 10 days. There is no history of dysmenorrhea. She lives with both parents and a younger sister. She is a good student and participates in many extracurricular activities. She started dating 18 months ago and has been sexually active for the past 7 months. She has been using condoms "most of the time." Family history is remarkable for hyperlipidemia and hypertension on maternal side of the family. Her mother had a history of heavy periods all along. The younger sister has grand mal seizures.

Physical examination is entirely normal except for mild overweight and moderate facial acne.

SELECT THE ONE BEST ANSWER

1. What other elements of the clinical history will you need to assess now?

   (A) first day of the last menstrual period
   (B) duration of bleeding
   (C) amount of bleeding
   (D) abdominal pain
   (E) all of the above

2. The following statements regarding the normal menstrual cycle in adolescents are true except for:

   (A) Normal duration is 2 to 7 days.
   (B) Average blood loss is about 100 mL.
   (C) Normal intervals are 21 to 40 days.
   (D) Menses occur approximately 14 days after the LH midcycle surge.
   (E) Ovulation occurs about 12 hours after the LH peak.

3. Which of the following definitions of abnormal vaginal bleeding patterns is incorrect?

   (A) metrorrhagia: uterine bleeding at irregular but frequent intervals
   (B) polymenorrhea: uterine bleeding at regular intervals of <28 days
   (C) menorrhagia: prolonged or excessive bleeding at regular intervals

(D) hypermenorrhea: prolonged or excessive bleeding at regular intervals

(E) menometrorrhagia: prolonged or excessive bleeding at irregular intervals

4. The overwhelming majority of cases of abnormal uterine bleeding in adolescence are a result of:

    (A) STDs
    (B) dysfunctional uterine bleeding
    (C) complications of pregnancy
    (D) coagulopathies
    (E) medications and drugs

5. Which of the following conditions would be an unlikely cause of abnormal vaginal bleeding in this patient?

    (A) spontaneous abortion
    (B) dysfunctional uterine bleeding
    (C) endometrial cancer
    (D) cervicitis
    (E) blood dyscrasias

6. Which among the following elements of the physical examination would be the least relevant for the diagnosis and immediate management of this patient's menstrual problem?

    (A) pelvic examination
    (B) heart rate
    (C) blood pressure
    (D) pallor
    (E) moderate acne

7. The laboratory evaluation of abnormal vaginal bleeding in adolescents requires all of the following except:

    (A) pregnancy test
    (B) hemoglobin and red blood cell indexes
    (C) coagulation studies
    (D) endometrial biopsy
    (E) gonorrhea and chlamydia probe

8. The physical examination reveals that the patient is hemodynamically stable with a blood pressure of 110/60 mm Hg and a heart rate of 84 bpm. The pelvic examination shows moderate bleeding. There is no clinical evidence of infection. A stat hemoglobin comes back at 10.5 g/dL and the pregnancy test is negative. All of the following treatments will be acceptable for this patient except:

    (A) hospitalization (intravenous estrogens followed by conjugated estrogens orally plus medroxyprogesterone acetate orally for 7 to 10 days)
    (B) medroxyprogesterone acetate 10 mg/day for 10 to 14 days
    (C) oral conjugated estrogens 2.5 mg four times a day for 21 days plus medroxyprogesterone 10 mg orally on days 17 through 21
    (D) any of the combined oral contraceptives 1 pill orally 4 times a day for 3 to 5 days to stop the bleeding followed by tapering to one pill a day until the pack is finished
    (E) observation, menstrual calendar, and iron therapy

9. Which among the following is not a common side effect of the monophasic combined oral contraceptive pills in adolescents?

    (A) weight gain
    (B) nausea
    (C) breast tenderness
    (D) breakthrough bleeding
    (E) headaches

10. The patient returns for follow-up 1 week later. She is now taking a combined pill containing a fixed amount of 35 micrograms of ethynyl-estradiol and 0.25 mg of norgestimate orally once a day. Her bleeding has stopped. She has not had any side effects from the medication except for some nausea during the first 2 to 3 days while she was taking "the pill" three times a day. She is also taking ferrous sulfate tablets 325 mg orally twice a day. A review of all laboratory tests obtained on the previous visit shows normal or negative results. The patient states that she is interested in long-term contraception and wants to know what methods you would recommend.

    Among the following, which contraceptive method has the lowest failure rate during typical use in adolescents?

    (A) combined oral contraceptives
    (B) male condom
    (C) progestin-only contraceptives
    (D) periodic abstinence
    (E) injectable depo-medroxyprogesterone

11. Beneficial effects of the birth control pill include the following except:

    (A) effective in the treatment of acne
    (B) improves bone mineralization
    (C) menstrual regulation
    (D) decreased risk of endometrial cancer
    (E) decreased risk of thromboembolism

12. Combined oral contraceptive pills can safely be used by an adolescent with any of the following conditions except:

    (A) post-abortion
    (B) active viral hepatitis
    (C) hypothyroidism
    (D) pelvic inflammatory disease
    (E) varicose veins

13. Which of the following antibiotic medications interferes with the contraceptive effectiveness of the pill?

    (A) amoxicillin
    (B) rifampin
    (C) cephalosporin
    (D) sulfonamides
    (E) griseofulvin

14. All of the following medications decrease the clearance of combined oral contraceptives, potentially leading to increased estrogen levels and side effects except:

    (A) selective serotonin reuptake inhibitors
    (B) ketoconazole
    (C) ritonavir
    (D) nefazodone
    (E) carbamazepine

15. The combined oral contraceptive pill decreases the clearance of all of the following medications except:

    (A) benzodiazepines
    (B) theophylline
    (C) tricyclic antidepressants
    (D) aspirin
    (E) prednisolone

16. The mother expresses some concerns about this patient's ability to take a pill every day. Of the following methods, which one has the lowest contraceptive failure rate in typical users?

    (A) contraceptive patch
    (B) progesterone intrauterine device
    (C) vaginal ring
    (D) diaphragm
    (E) medroxyprogesterone acetate IM injection

17. On discussing the benefits and disadvantages of all contraceptive options with the patient, you decide to keep her on the same combined oral contraceptive she has been on so far. She will also need to use condoms consistently to prevent STDs. All of the following statements regarding male condoms are accurate except:

    (A) when used as the only contraceptive method, the typical failure rate is 14%
    (B) condoms with spermicide have a lower typical failure rate
    (C) rates of breakage or slippage average 2%
    (D) best available method for prevention of HIV
    (E) condoms decrease the rate of cervical cancer

18. In patients on anticonvulsants, which of the following is the contraceptive of choice?

    (A) combined oral contraceptive
    (B) diaphragm with spermicide
    (C) injectable estrogen-progestin combination
    (D) depo-medroxyprogesterone
    (E) progestin-only pills

19. The patient has been on the pill for 2 weeks and now calls you to let you know that she is bleeding again. After telling you emphatically that her compliance has been perfect, she explains that she has no cramping or fever and that she is using about two to three pads a day. She has not been sexually active for the past 7 weeks and denies being on any other medication. What would you do at this time?

    (A) admit her to the hospital for evaluation
    (B) change the pill to one with a higher estrogen content
    (C) prescribe an NSAID (ibuprofen or naproxen) to decrease the flow
    (D) change her to progestin-only pills
    (E) B or D

Answers

1. **(E)** The menstrual history should always include first day of the last menstrual period, duration and amount of bleeding, interval, and regularity of menses. In this case, it will also be important to ask about ongoing abdominal or pelvic pain, history of abnormal bleeding from other sites (purpura, epistaxis, hematuria), weight changes, stress, recent use of hormonal and nonhormonal medication, and substance abuse. The date of her latest vaginal intercourse should be helpful for adequate interpretation of the pregnancy test.

2. **(B)** The normal menstrual cycle is characterized by a follicular phase, ovulation, and luteal phase. During the follicular phase, under the influence of FSH, one follicle becomes dominant by day 7. Estradiol, the main hormone promoting endometrial growth during this phase, reaches a peak shortly before the LH surge on day 14. The follicle ruptures within 12 hours of the LH surge and about 24 hours after the estradiol peak. After ovulation, estradiol levels plummet while progesterone, produced by the corpus luteum, becomes the dominant hormone as the luteal phase starts. Progesterone inhibits the growth of a new follicle and causes maturation of the proliferative endometrium. In the absence of fertilization, the corpus luteum degenerates over the following 14 days at which time progesterone levels decline steeply. Progesterone withdrawal is responsible for initiation of bleeding during the normal menstrual cycle. The normal menstrual cycle lasts 2 to 7 days, occurs at intervals of 21 to 35 days, and leads to an average blood loss of 35 to 40 mL up to a maximum of 80 mL.

3. **(B)** Metrorrhagia is defined as uterine bleeding at irregular but frequent intervals. Menorrhagia and hypermenorrhea are synonymous and describe prolonged or excessive bleeding at regular intervals, Menometrorrhagia indicate prolonged or excessive bleeding at irregular intervals. Polymenorrhea is defined as uterine bleeding at regular intervals of less than 21 days.

4. **(B)** Dysfunctional uterine bleeding is defined as heavy, prolonged unpatterned uterine bleeding unrelated to structural or organic disease. It re-

sults from anovulation and is responsible for 90% of abnormal vaginal bleeding in adolescents. In the absence of ovulation, there will not be progestins to allow for maturation and stabilization of the endometrium. Because of the effects of unopposed estrogen, the endometrium remains in a proliferative phase, becomes unstable, and bleeds erratically. Since dysfunctional uterine bleeding is a diagnosis of exclusion, a thorough history should be obtained to rule out organic causes, including complications of early pregnancy, coagulopathies, STDs, and side effects of medications and drugs among others. Regardless of the etiology, in any patient complaining of abnormal vaginal bleeding it is essential to evaluate the severity of past and ongoing bleeding and to address any potential need for hospitalization, intravenous fluids, or blood replacement.

5. **(C)** Genital cancers, although included in the differential diagnosis, would be unlikely in a 17-year-old adolescent. Most cases of abnormal vaginal bleeding in adolescence are secondary to dysfunctional uterine bleeding. However, the differential diagnosis to consider includes:

   - Pregnancy-related conditions: intrauterine or ectopic pregnancy, spontaneous abortion, and molar-trophoblastic disease
   - Infections: vaginitis, cervicitis, endometritis, salpingitis, and PID
   - Other gynecologic conditions: ovarian cysts, genital cancers, breakthrough bleeding associated to contraceptive use, ovulation bleeding, and polyps
   - Systemic diseases: renal and liver failure
   - Blood dyscrasias
   - Direct trauma and foreign body
   - Medications: anticoagulants and platelet inhibitors

6. **(E)** A pelvic examination is rarely indicated in a postpubertal, not sexually active patient within 18 months of menarche unless trauma is suspected. All other women with abnormal vaginal bleeding should have a pelvic examination, particularly when there is a pattern of increasing, protracted or very heavy bleeding. Blood pressure and heart rate, both in the upright and supine position, would be essential to assess for he-

modynamic instability and potential need for hospitalization. A complete physical examination will be needed, documenting general appearance, pallor, tachycardia, abdominal masses, guarding, rebound, or evidence of endocrinopathies. Breasts should be checked for galactorrhea. Recent weight gain or loss may play a role in dysfunctional uterine bleeding. Moderate acne, particularly in a patient with obesity and hirsutism suggests hyperandrogenism.

7. **(D)** A pregnancy test will be essential to exclude complications of pregnancy as the cause of abnormal vaginal bleeding. Hemoglobin and hematocrit determinations will help determine the magnitude of chronic bleeding. Coagulation studies may reveal coagulopathies or blood dyscrasias, particularly in patients with a pattern of excessive bleeding (hypermenorrhea) since menarche and/or family history of abnormal vaginal bleeding. Among adolescents requiring hospitalization for this problem, 20% have coagulopathies. Testing for infections will be needed in sexually active teens with abnormal bleeding since gonorrhea, chlamydia, and trichomonal infections are common causes of protracted or irregular vaginal bleeding in adolescents who previously had regular periods. Endocrine abnormalities such as hypothyroidism and polycystic ovarian syndrome frequently present with menorrhagia or irregular bleeding and thyroid function tests, FSH and LH, prolactin, and androgen studies will help confirm these diagnoses. Endometrial biopsy is not indicated in adolescents.

8. **(A)** There are numerous options for treatment of anovulatory, dysfunctional uterine bleeding. Patients with acute, very heavy, or uncontrolled bleeding should be hospitalized and treated with intravenous estrogen, 25 mg every 4 hours until bleeding abates. If bleeding is less heavy and the patient is hemodynamically stable, conjugated estrogens orally can be given in the outpatient setting until bleeding stops at which time the dose of estrogens can be reduced to 1.25 to 2.5 mg/day and oral medroxyprogesterone acetate 10 mg orally added for 7 to 10 days. On discontinuing these medications withdrawal bleeding will occur. Patients with acute, moderate bleeding can be treated with combined oral contraceptives given

up to 4 times a day with gradual tapering until bleeding subsides. At that time the patient should continue to take 1 pill a day until the pack is finished. In patients with significant anemia, taking only the pharmacologically active pills of each package for 21 days, discarding the placebo pills and starting a new package will prevent withdrawal bleeding. This method of administration may be used for 2 to 3 cycles to promote a faster resolution of the anemia. Iron therapy should be offered in all cases to correct iron deficiency and prevent further anemia. In this patient, any of the listed outpatient hormonal treatments can be used. In view of her moderate bleeding, hemodynamic stability, and moderate anemia, hospitalization does not seem necessary at this time.

9. **(A)** Weight gain is rarely a side effect of the pill. Nausea and breakthrough bleeding, on the other hand, are among the most common. Both side effects tend to abate after the first few cycles. Nausea is considered an estrogenic side effect of the pill and, if bothersome, it can be corrected by choosing a pill with a lower estrogen content. Other potential side effects of the pill include headaches, breast tenderness, hypertension, abdominal cramping or bloating, and changes in menstrual flow.

10. **(E)** Typical use failure rates reflect the percentage of women experiencing an unintended pregnancy during the first year of typical use of the method. Injectable depomedroxyprogesterone has the lowest failure rate of all hormonal contraceptive methods (0.3%) except for progestin implants. Combined oral contraceptive pills have a typical use failure rate of 2% in the general population but those rates are much higher (6% to 7%) in adolescent girls age 15 to 19 years, mostly as a result of unreliable compliance. Progestin-only pills have a somewhat higher failure rate than combined pills. For male condoms the typical failure rate is 12%, while for couples using no method the chance of pregnancy climbs up to 85%.

11. **(E)** Combined oral contraceptives have a protective effect against endometrial and ovarian cancer. They also have some other beneficial effects, including regulation of menses, decreasing the severity of dysmenorrhea, reduced iron loss, im-

proved bone mineralization, and lowered risk of ectopic pregnancy and of symptomatic pelvic inflammatory disease.

12. **(B)** Combined oral contraceptives can safely be used in all the conditions listed except active viral hepatitis in which it is absolutely contraindicated. Other absolute contraindications include:

- Pregnancy
- Breast cancer
- Migraine headaches with focal neurological signs
- Breast-feeding within 6 weeks postpartum
- Hypertension with systolic BP >160 and diastolic >100
- History of or current deep venous thrombosis or pulmonary embolism
- Vascular disease
- Major surgery with prolonged immobilization
- History or current ischemic heart disease or stroke
- Complicated valvular heart disease
- Diabetic retinopathy, neuropathy, nephropathy
- Benign hepatic adenoma

Relative contraindications to the use of combined oral contraceptives include mild hypertension, sickle cell disease, depression, and migraine without focal neurological findings.

13. **(B)** Rifampin is known to decrease the contraceptive effectiveness of the pill. According to recent WHO recommendations on oral contraceptives, griseofulvin is no longer considered to interfere with the effects of the pill.

14. **(E)** Carbamazepine as well as most anticonvulsants, including phenytoin, ethosuximide, felbamate, and topiramate, decreases the contraceptive effects of the pill. All other medications listed increase estrogen levels and may lead to potential side effects such as nausea, vomiting, headaches, and breast tenderness.

15. **(D)** Combined oral contraceptives decrease the clearance of benzodiazepines, caffeine, theophylline, tricyclic antidepressants, and prednisolone, potentially increasing their risk for toxicity. On the other hand, aspirin and morphine concentrations may decrease in users of estrogen-progestin pills.

16. **(B)** IUDs are an excellent method of long-term, reversible contraception for multiparous women in long-term mutually monogamous relationships. They are generally not recommended for nulliparous women or those with multiple sexual partners, high risk for STDs, heavy or painful menstrual periods, or abnormal Pap smears. The transdermal contraceptive patch and vaginal ring injections share all the indications and contraindications of the birth control pill but may be more convenient for teens since they do not require daily compliance on the part of the user. The "patch" needs to be replaced once a week while the vaginal ring, which delivers an estrogen-progestin combination absorbable through the vaginal mucosa, is replaced once a month. Depomedroxyprogesterone injections have the lowest contraceptive failure rate of all commonly used contraceptives and are particularly suitable for younger adolescents who need birth control and for all older teens whose compliance is unreliable. Diaphragms and cervical caps have significantly high failure rates (20% and 40%, respectively).

17. **(B)** There is little evidence that condoms with spermicide have a lower failure rate.

18. **(D)** Depomedroxyprogesterone is the contraceptive of choice in adolescent girls with seizure disorders since it increases the threshold for seizures. As opposed to progestin-only pills, which should be taken daily, injectable progestins only need to be administered every 12 weeks, which facilitates compliance. Moreover, anticonvulsants decrease the contraceptive effectiveness of combined oral contraceptives but do not affect depomedroxyprogesterone metabolism. Since according to some studies, long-term use of this method may be associated with reversible bone loss, it is recommended that young women using this method take calcium supplements to achieve a dietary intake of 1300 mg per day.

19. **(C)** Breakthrough bleeding is common in the first 3 months of therapy and usually resolves spontaneously. This should be discussed with all patients before starting them on oral contraceptives to avoid unneeded anxiety and discontinuation of treatment. Pregnancy and STDs should be considered under these circumstances, but are

unlikely in this case since she denies sexual activity for the previous 7 weeks, had a negative pregnancy test, and no evidence of sexually transmitted diseases 2 weeks earlier. Reassurance would be appropriate at this time with close follow-up if the bleeding became persistent or bothersome. In this case, an NSAID would be very effective in decreasing menstrual flow. Alternatively, she should be asked to take an extra pill a day from a different package until bleeding stops.

SUGGESTED READING

Emans SJ, Laufer MR, Goldstein DP, eds: *Pediatric and Adolescent Gynecology*, 5th ed. Philadelphia: Lippincott Williams and Wilkins, 2005.

Johnson BE, et al: *Women's Health Care Handbook*, 2nd ed. Philadelphia: Hanley and Belfus, 2000.

Neinstein LS: *Adolescent Health Care. A Practical Guide*, 4th ed. Philadelphia: Lippincott Williams and Wilkins, 2002.

Hatcher RA, et al: *Contraceptive Technology*, 17th rev. ed. New York: Ardent Media, 1998.

CASE 74: A 15-YEAR-OLD FEMALE WITH ABDOMINAL PAIN, WEIGHT GAIN, AND FATIGUE

A 15-year-old adolescent girl comes in to the clinic for a "check-up." She has been your patient for 3 years and a brief review of her chart reminds you that she only has been seen by you for yearly physical examinations. She has no history of chronic illness, allergies, or hospitalizations. Immunizations are up to date. She had been in counseling for "anger issues" for several years and 2 years ago was seen by a psychiatrist who diagnosed oppositional defiant disorder. She lives with her maternal grandmother (and guardian), who raised her since she was 2 years old, and a 17-year-old brother. Her brother has been recently released from jail. Grandma is a diabetic and is also on medication for hypertension. In the past she had often complained about her granddaughter's behavior, which she describes as rebellious, hostile, and argumentative. She does not feel that "the girl can be trusted." At times, she even suspected drug use, a notion that her granddaughter vehemently denies. The patient ran away from home for 3 days on one occasion last year. Her father lives out of state and is not involved in her life while her mother is "around sometimes," having been sporadically in rehabilitation programs for drug addiction. The patient was an average student in elementary school but her academic performance has been declining lately. She is now in eighth grade. The review of systems reveals tiredness, nausea, vomiting, and vaguely described periumbilical pain. A careful history of the pain fails to discern any patterns in onset, duration, progression, intensity, aggravating or relieving factors, or associated symptoms. Her appetite has increased lately. Neither her fatigue nor her abdominal pain has kept her from participating in sports. She became sexually active 6 months prior to this visit. She states that she is not interested at all in hormonal birth control for fear of gaining weight. Her menses have been normal since menarche at age 11. Her last period started 2 weeks before this visit and lasted 3 to 4 days. She has had some nausea and vomiting off and on for the past few weeks but denies diarrhea or constipation. During the previous week she has noticed increased urinary frequency. Her review of systems is otherwise negative.

On physical examination, she looks well but quiet, aloof, and "testy." She is a well developed at 5'5" and 140 lbs. She has gained 8 pounds since her last visit 6 months earlier. She has a large scar on her arm, the result of "a fight" about 3 years ago. Her physical examination is otherwise unremarkable except for some fullness in her lower abdomen. There is no abdominal tenderness and no guarding or rebound. There is no CVA tenderness. You ask her to empty her bladder and to return to the examination room.

SELECT THE ONE BEST ANSWER

1. What other elements of the clinical history would be important in this case?

   (A) dysuria
   (B) medications
   (C) substance use
   (D) number of sexual partners
   (E) all of the above

2. What elements of the physical examination are most important?

   (A) eye examination
   (B) cardiovascular examination
   (C) neurologic examination
   (D) pelvic examination
   (E) all of the above

3. The speculum examination shows no abnormalities. There is no uterine bleeding. The bimanual

examination reveals an enlarged uterus, the size of a grapefruit, almost palpable above the symphysis pubis. The cervix is soft. No adnexal masses are felt. There is no adnexal or cervical motion tenderness. The most likely diagnosis is:

(A) 4-week intrauterine pregnancy
(B) inaccurate dates
(C) ectopic pregnancy
(D) missed abortion
(E) threatened abortion

4. According to the uterine size, if pregnancy is confirmed, what would be the estimated gestational age?

(A) 4 weeks
(B) 6 weeks
(C) 8 weeks
(D) 12 weeks
(E) 14 weeks

5. What could explain the discrepancy between uterine size and the reported date of the last menstrual period when the uterus is larger than expected for dates?

(A) inaccurate dates
(B) twin pregnancy
(C) leiomyoma
(D) molar pregnancy
(E) all of the above

6. The following conditions could present with a uterine size smaller than expected for dates except:

(A) inaccurate dates
(B) incomplete or missed abortion
(C) ectopic pregnancy
(D) corpus luteum cyst of pregnancy
(E) hCG-secreting tumors

7. Which of the following tests would be helpful to explain discrepancies between uterine size and dates?

(A) pelvic ultrasonography
(B) maternal α-fetoprotein
(C) serial measurements of human chorionic gonadotropin
(D) measurement of fetal heart rate
(E) A and C

8. All of the following statements about hCG levels during pregnancy are true except:

(A) A sensitive urine pregnancy test can detect hCG levels as low as 10 to 25 mIU/mL.
(B) A sensitive urine pregnancy test may help diagnose pregnancy before a period is missed.
(C) Low levels of hCG early in pregnancy suggest the diagnosis of ectopic pregnancy.
(D) Between 5 and 8 weeks, hCG levels should increase by 66% in 48 hours.
(E) Between 23 and 35 days of gestation, the mean doubling time is 1.6 days.

9. All of the following would suggest the diagnosis of ectopic pregnancy except:

(A) pelvic pain
(B) amenorrhea
(C) RUQ pain
(D) irregular bleeding
(E) adnexal mass

10. All of the following laboratory tests are indicated at this time except:

(A) pregnancy test
(B) CBC, differential, and platelet count
(C) gonorrhea, chlamydia probe
(D) urinalysis
(E) amylase and lipase

11. The pregnancy test is positive. The patient receives that news without surprise and states that she is not ready for motherhood. She does not want her grandmother to know about the pregnancy. What do you do next?

(A) Discuss all her options with her.
(B) Suggest having her grandmother involved in the decision-making process.
(C) Refer to an obstetrician.
(D) Refer to a case manager.
(E) Arrange a follow-up visit in 1 week.

12. The following statements regarding abortion are correct except:

(A) Abortions after 16 weeks of gestation carry a risk for complications 15 times higher than those performed before 12 weeks.

(B) Abortions done between 9 and 12 weeks of gestation have 1/10th the complication rate of carrying the pregnancy to term.

(C) Teenagers are less likely to have a second trimester abortion than older women.

(D) Adolescents younger than 19 account for 20% of all legal abortions.

(E) Forty-one percent of teen pregnancies end in abortion.

13. During the private interview with the patient she admits to drinking "socially" on weekends, sometimes to drunkenness, and to smoking marijuana 3 times a week. All of the following statements regarding alcohol use are true except:

(A) No amount of alcohol is safe in pregnancy and total abstinence is recommended.

(B) The use of alcohol during pregnancy can lead to fetal alcohol syndrome or spontaneous abortion.

(C) By age 15, 1 in 10 boys report that they are problem drinkers.

(D) Thirty-four percent of American twelfth graders report having been drunk in the previous month.

(E) Alcohol is involved in 40% of adolescent mortality resulting from motor vehicle accidents.

14. Which among the following is not a physical consequence of acute heavy drinking?

(A) acute gastritis
(B) hyperthermia
(C) acute pancreatitis
(D) amnesia
(E) ataxia

15. Concerning marijuana use, all of the following statements are true except:

(A) Cigarette smoking is more common than marijuana use in teens.

(B) Up to 48% of high school graduates have used marijuana at least once.

(C) Marijuana can be detected in the urine for up to 30 days after single time use.

(D) The duration of action of marijuana is 3 hours if smoked.

(E) The typical potency of street marijuana is 4% to 6%.

16. All of the following symptoms and signs may be attributed to marijuana use except:

(A) conjunctival hyperemia
(B) increased appetite
(C) mood fluctuations
(D) impaired learning and cognition
(E) nausea

17. What percentage of twelfth graders report ever having used an illicit drug?

(A) 18%
(B) 30%
(C) 41%
(D) 53%
(E) 66%

18. What is the percentage of twelfth graders who report ever having used an illicit drug other than marijuana?

(A) 10%
(B) 25%
(C) 33%
(D) 40%
(E) 50%

19. Among the following, which is the most common drug of abuse (other than marijuana) used by eighth graders?

(A) smokeless tobacco
(B) amphetamines
(C) inhalants
(D) crack cocaine
(E) MDMA

20. The patient returned 2 days later with her grandmother. She stated that both she and her boyfriend had decided to seek a pregnancy termination. She had not told her family about the pregnancy yet and asks you to help her do so. Her grandmother was disheartened and upset after hearing the news, but in the end, supportive of her granddaughter's decision. The patient was seen by an obstetrician and underwent a suction curettage 2 days later, without complication. She comes to see you 2 weeks later for follow-up. All of the following should be done at this time except:

(A) ask about ongoing contraceptive methods

(B) ask about fever, pelvic pain, vaginal discharge, or continued bleeding

(C) perform a pelvic examination to confirm uterine involution and absence of tenderness

(D) check a urine pregnancy test

(E) start contraception

21. The patient wants to start depomedroxyprogesterone acetate shots. Your advice about this method will include the following except:

(A) Depomedroxyprogesterone acetate is one of the most effective hormonal contraceptions available.

(B) The most common side effects of depomedroxyprogesterone are irregular menstrual bleeding and weight gain.

(C) Depomedroxyprogesterone should not be given until a month after pregnancy termination.

(D) Osteoporosis may result from long-term use.

(E) It is a good method for adolescents who have difficulties with medication compliance.

Answers

1. **(E)** A history of medication and substance use should be elicited in all adolescents, and a detailed sexual history is essential in all sexually active teens. This includes, among others, age at first intercourse, types of sexual contact, sexual orientation, type of contraceptive use, number of sexual partners, use of alcohol or other drugs associated with sexual activity, and past history of STDs.

2. **(E)** Since the differential diagnosis of abdominal pain is quite extensive, a comprehensive physical examination will be needed. The recent onset of sexual activity and frequent urination in an adolescent girl who has been an unreliable historian in the past point to the need for a pelvic examination even if her menses are reported as normal. The pelvic examination would help to rule out pregnancy and STD as a cause of her abdominal pain. Given the history of possible marijuana use, one should look for signs of acute or chronic intoxication. For example, in acute intoxication, conjunctival hyperemia, and an abnormal neurologic examination with decreased coordination, sleepiness, slow reaction times, decreased postural stability, increased body sway, and dilated pupils are characteristic. Tachycardia may be present and orthostatic hypotension may develop at larger doses. Clinical signs suggestive of other substance use should be explored.

3. **(B)** In the absence of any clinical sign of abnormal early pregnancy, it is likely that the reported date of the last menstrual period was inaccurate. Nevertheless, a careful workup should rule out the other diagnoses.

4. **(D)** The uterine size is consistent with a 12-week pregnancy. The uterine fundus reaches the symphysis pubis at 12 weeks, the navel at 20 weeks, and the rib cage at 40 weeks.

5. **(E)** Any of the above could explain the finding of a uterus larger than expected for dates.

6. **(D)** In ectopic pregnancy, incomplete or missed abortion, and hCG-secreting tumors (a very uncommon occurrence), the uterus is smaller than expected for dates. On the other hand, in the presence of a corpus luteum cyst of pregnancy the uterus may seem to be larger than expected for gestational age.

7. **(E)** A pelvic ultrasound, including a vaginal probe, will help determine both fetal size and viability. A serial hCG measurement to assess doubling times is needed for the diagnosis of threatened abortion or ectopic pregnancy. Abdominal ultrasonography allows visualization of a gestational sac around the time hCG levels reach 4000 to 6000 mIU/mL while transvaginal ultrasonography can detect it at 1000 to 1500 mIU/mL, approximately 6 weeks from the last menstrual period. MSAFP is a marker for the detection of open neural tube defects and Down syndrome and would not be useful to explain the discrepancy between uterine size and dates.

8. **(C)** Low levels of hCG early in pregnancy can result from either intrauterine or ectopic pregnancy. Serial hCG measurements in conjunction with clinical assessments are helpful to distinguish ectopic or failed pregnancies from normal ones. Above hCG levels of 100 mIU/mL, the normal doubling time is 2.3 days in early pregnancy, 1.6 days from day 23 to 35, 2.0 days from 35 to 42, and

3.4 from 41 to 50 days. To facilitate the calculations, it is helpful to remember that in weeks 5 to 8 of pregnancy, hCG levels increase by 29% in 24 hours, 66% in 48 hours, 114% in 72 hours, 175% in 96 hours, and 255% in 120 hours. Up to 15% of normal pregnancies may show a lag in doubling and up to 13% of ectopic pregnancies may present with physiologic increases in hCG levels.

9. **(C)** Ectopic pregnancy is the leading cause of maternal death during the first trimester. This condition is more common among women age 35 to 44 years. However, 15- to 24-year-old women have the highest mortality rate compared with other age groups. Predisposing factors include the use of IUDs, use of progestin-only pills, and tubal abnormalities secondary to a history of tubal surgery, PID, or previous ectopic pregnancy. Pelvic pain, amenorrhea followed by irregular vaginal bleeding, and the presence of an adnexal mass strongly suggest the possibility of an ectopic pregnancy. Rebound tenderness is present in up to 50% of cases.

10. **(E)** A pregnancy test is most important at this time to confirm the clinical suspicion of pregnancy. A wet mount prep and cervical swabs for gonorrhea and chlamydia are obtained during the pelvic examination to exclude STDs. A urinalysis is needed to rule out UTI and/or glycosuria in this patient with abdominal pain, increased tiredness, frequent urination, and family history of diabetes. A CBC with differential leukocyte count, sedimentation rate, and CRP would be ordered if the physical examination reveals abdominal tenderness, adnexal tenderness, and cervical motion tenderness suggestive of PID. In pregnant girls, additional blood testing should include HIV, RPR, and Rh determinations. Serum amylase and lipase levels would be needed to rule out pancreatitis or cholangitis, which seem unlikely given the clinical presentation.

11. **(A)** The first step is to discuss the options available to her including:

- Continuing pregnancy and becoming a parent
- Continuing pregnancy and giving the baby up for adoption
- Pregnancy termination

The patient's feelings should be explored in the context of her present social situation, educational goals, financial status, and expectations about family support. She should be counseled about the potential effects of preexistent medical conditions, ongoing medication, smoking, alcohol, and other drugs on pregnancy outcomes. Counseling should be nonjudgmental and realistic but always supportive of the teen's choice. Although, by virtue of her pregnancy, the patient is now an emancipated minor, she should be encouraged to involve her family in the decision making process. Insurance status is an important consideration since insurers often require family involvement. Since legal requirements for parental notification vary from state to state, health providers should be familiar with the laws applying to their specific geographical area.

The decision to involve the family is best made after an individualized assessment of the patient's and family needs. Most teenagers need time to consider their options and it is helpful to arrange for a follow-up visit within a week with frequent telephone contact if needed. This is especially true for younger or emotionally immature adolescent girls. In this case, since she is already about 12 weeks pregnant, she needs to know that a decision has to be made in a matter of days rather than weeks. In the meantime, she should be referred to a case manager for further counseling. An appointment with an obstetrician should be arranged either for prenatal care or for pregnancy termination.

12. **(C)** Elective abortion is the most commonly performed surgical procedure in the United States. Of the almost 1 million teens who get pregnant every year, close to 50% carry pregnancy to term, 41% choose to have an abortion, and the rest end in miscarriages.

Teenagers are more likely to have a second trimester abortion than older women often because of failure to recognize the symptoms of pregnancy, ambivalence, fear of disclosure, and lack of awareness of services available. Morbidity and mortality from the procedure increase with gestational age and the risk doubles every 2 weeks after the eighth week. Suction curettage is the most widely used method (97% of cases) and may be performed up to a gestational age of 14 weeks. The procedure has a risk of death in 1:262,000 pregnancies when done before the eighth week and in 1:100,000 pregnancies in weeks 9 to 12. The comparable risk of death in carrying a pregnancy to term is 1:10,000. Dilatation and evacuation (D&E) is used whenever abortion is performed between 13 and 16 weeks of pregnancy (in some places up to 20 weeks). The percent of adolescents undergoing abortion in relation to the total number of abortions performed has declined significantly since the 1970s and teens now account for about 20% of all abortions reported.

13. **(C)** Alcohol is the most common substance of abuse in adolescence. In 2002, the monthly prevalence of any alcohol use in high school seniors was 48% while their annual prevalence of any use was 71%. There has been a modest decline in reported alcohol use during the past decade. Yet, almost one-third of twelfth graders report drinking five or more drinks in a row in the previous 2 weeks. MVAs are the leading cause of death among young people age 15 to 24 years. About 40% of these accidents are alcohol-related. Alcohol is also a contributing factor in a significant proportion of homicides and suicides, violence and injuries, impairment in school functioning, and deterioration in interpersonal relations. By age 15, one-fifth of adolescent boys and one-sixth of adolescent girls report that they are problem drinkers. Fewer than 5% of adolescents can be categorized as alcoholics. Adolescents who drink daily, have a family history for alcoholism, have blackouts or withdrawal symptoms, and continue to drink despite experiencing damaging consequences in their family, school, and social life fit into that category. The vast majority of teens who use alcohol but do not meet those criteria are considered problem drinkers. Problem drinkers have been drunk six or more times a year and at least twice a year have suffered negative consequences of alcohol use, including drunken driving and problems with family, friends, school, or police because of drinking. These teens are at especially high risk for MVAs and other unintentional injuries and for emotional, social, and academic difficulties. Alcohol use, particularly in early pregnancy, is responsible for fetal alcohol syndrome, a condition characterized by abnormal facies, microcephaly, thin upper lip, short palpebral fissures, hypoplastic maxilla, heart, kidney and skeletal defects, and mental retardation.

14. **(B)** Mild alcohol intoxication produces euphoria, slurred speech, and ataxia. Hypoglycemia may be present. With more severe intoxication bradycardia, hypotension, hypothermia, stupor, coma, and death may occur.

15. **(C)** Marijuana is the most common illicit drug used by adolescents, ranking a close third after alcohol and cigarette smoking. During the 1990s the prevalence of use within the past month tripled for eighth graders (from 3.2% to 10.2%) and almost doubled for twelfth graders (from 13.8% to 23.7%). In the class of 2002, 48% of twelfth graders reported ever having used marijuana. D-9-tetrahydrocannabinol (THC) is primarily responsible for the neurophysiologic, biochemical, and behavioral changes induced by marijuana. Currently most marijuana is obtained from a hybrid plant (*Cannabis sativa x indica*), and only the seedless buds of female plants (sinsemilla) are considered worth smoking. The concentration of THC has increased dramatically in the past 25 years from 2% to 10%. The dose delivered varies with the supplier. The drug may sometimes be adulterated by addition of PCP. The effects of marijuana start from seconds to minutes after inhalation and from 30 to 60 minutes after oral ingestion, peaking at 20 minutes and lasting for 3 hours. It induces feelings of well-being and relaxation and, at higher doses, it is a hallucinogen. Its serum half-life is 19 hours. It is primarily metabolized in the liver. Two-thirds of the cannabinoid metabolites are excreted in the feces and one-third in the urine. After single use it can be detected in urine for up to 5 days and for up to 1 to 2 months in chronic users.

16. **(E)** At low doses, marijuana causes euphoria, relaxation, time distortion, vision and hearing distortion or enhancement, increased appetite, tachycardia, dry mouth, and sleepiness. At higher doses, it may cause dysphoric reactions including distortions in body image, disorientation, mood fluctuation, depersonalization, paranoia, and acute panic reactions. Although delirium and hallucinations may occur with high doses of THC, they may in-

dicate that the drug has been adulterated with PCP. Conjunctival hyperemia and increased appetite are common. The major effects of marijuana use are behavioral. Long-term use may impair memory, learning ability, and perception. Performance of tasks requiring coordination is significantly affected. The same is true for tracking ability, reaction time, and visual-perceptive functioning, all important considerations when driving a car or operating complicated machinery. Attention and short-term memory are affected even in moderate doses. The existence of an "amotivational syndrome" secondary to marijuana remains controversial. Apathy, loss of energy, passivity, absence of drive, loss of effectiveness, impaired concentration and memory, and decreased interest in work and school performance and lack of concern about it, have been described as characteristic of the amotivational syndrome but it is difficult to discern whether marijuana use is the cause or a consequence of preexisting behavioral problems. Nausea is not among the symptoms of marijuana intoxication. THC has antiemetic properties. Adolescent boys with heavy marijuana use may present with gynecomastia and decreased sperm counts.

17. **(D)** In 2002, the annual prevalence of lifetime use of any illicit drug in twelfth graders was 53%. This percentage has been stable since 1997. Twenty-five percent of eighth graders reported ever having used an illicit drug. This includes use of marijuana, LSD, other hallucinogens, crack, other cocaine, heroin, amphetamines, barbiturates, and tranquilizers.

18. **(C)** In 2002, almost one-third of twelfth graders reported ever having used any illicit drug other than marijuana. The most commonly used illicit drugs in this category include hallucinogens, amphetamines, MDMA, narcotics (including OxyContin and Vicodin), and tranquilizers. Of note, 9.6% of twelfth graders reported having used Vicodin during the previous year.

19. **(C)** In 2002, a nationwide survey of the lifetime prevalence of use of various drugs by eighth graders indicated that 25% of them had ever used an illicit drug. If inhalants are included, that percentage climbs to 31%. Nineteen percent of

eighth graders reported having used marijuana. After marijuana, inhalants are the most frequent drug of abuse with a lifetime prevalence of 15% and an annual prevalence of 7.7%. Inhalants are more likely to be used by younger than older adolescents. Frequently used inhalants include model glue, gasoline, aerosols used as propellants for cleaning fluids, fabric guard, correction fluid, deodorants, and spray paint. Toluene is the most common hydrocarbon found in paints and model glues. Inhalation of toluene may result in renal and hepatic damage, neuropathy, seizures, and encephalopathy. Sudden death attributable to cardiac arrhythmias has been reported. Amphetamines rank third with a lifetime prevalence of 8.7%. Almost half of all eighth graders reported they had ever used alcohol and 1 in 5 report ever having been drunk. Thirty-one percent of teens have tried cigarettes and 11.2%, smokeless tobacco.

20. **(D)** All of the above will be necessary except for a pregnancy test, which may remain positive for up to 4 weeks after a pregnancy termination. Complications of first-trimester abortion may include excess blood loss, infection, and failed abortion. Pelvic infection should be excluded. Fever and bleeding 3 to 7 days post-abortion and uterine or adnexal tenderness suggest that diagnosis. Contraception is usually initiated at the time of the procedure. It will be important to re-examine the several psychosocial risk factors discussed on the previous visit (alcohol and marijuana use, poor school performance, anger issues) and to refer for appropriate counseling.

21. **(C)** With a typical failure rate of 0.3%, depomedroxyprogesterone is one of the most effective hormonal contraceptive available to teens. This failure rate compares very favorably with the one of combined oral contraceptives, which have a failure rate of about 2% in adult typical users and up to 6% to 7% in teens. It is an excellent method for teens who have difficulties with medication compliance, those who have significant dysmenorrhea or dysfunctional uterine bleeding, those that cannot tolerate estrogens, and particularly those with seizures undergoing anticonvulsant therapy. Irregular bleeding is a common occurrence during the first few months

of use after which most patients will develop amenorrhea for as long as they remain on the medication. Weight gain is a common complaint, particularly in those teens who are overweight when the treatment is started. Osteoporosis may result from long-term use. Depomedroxyprogesterone can be started immediately after pregnancy termination.

SUGGESTED READING

Joffe A, Blythe MJ: Handbook of adolescent medicine. *Adolesc Med* 14:2, 2003.

Neinstein, LS: *Adolescent Health Care: A Practical Guide*, 4th ed. Philadelphia: Lippincott Williams and Wilkins, 2002.

Schydlower M, ed: *Substance abuse: A guide for health professionals*, 2nd ed. Elk Grove Village, IL: American Academy of Pediatrics, 2001.

Johnson BE, et al: *Women's Health Care Handbook*, 2nd ed. Philadelphia: Hanley and Belfus, 2000.

Emans SJ: Teenage pregnancy. In: Emans SJ, Laufer MR, Goldstein DP (eds): *Pediatric and Adolescent Gynecology*, 5th ed. Philadelphia: Lippincott Williams and Wilkins, 2005.

Hatcher RA, et al: *Contraceptive Technology*, 17th rev. ed. New York: Ardent Media, 1998.

CASE 75: A 15-YEAR-OLD FEMALE WITH OBESITY, ACNE, NO MENSES IN 3 MONTHS, AND POSSIBLE DEPRESSION

A 15-year-old adolescent girl comes to the clinic with a history of deteriorating school performance. Her past medical history indicates that she was a full-term 8-lb 10-oz baby born by cesarean section after a pregnancy complicated by gestational diabetes. She attained all her developmental milestones on time. She was never hospitalized and has no chronic illnesses except for seasonal bouts of allergic rhinitis. She is always congested and has been told that her tonsils are "too big." She started her menses at age 11 years. Menses have been irregular, with no excessive cramping. Her last menstrual period was 3 months ago. She has a few friends but spends most of her free time at home watching TV. Her family history reveals that her maternal grandmother had passed away 6 months ago at age 56 years, of complications of diabetes and hypertension. Both parents are obese. While interviewing the patient alone and after being assured confidentiality, she tells you that she has never been sexually active but wants to start birth control "just to be on the safe side." She denies smoking cigarettes or us-

ing alcohol or other drugs. She has been sleepy lately and sometimes she may even fall asleep in class. She feels tired and quite irritable most of the time. She is unhappy about her appearance and frustrated about her lack of success with several of the diets she tried in the past. She admits to being a "loner" and feels hopeless at times. When asked about suicidal ideation she states that the thought has crossed her mind in the past but that she never devised a plan.

On physical examination she is 5'5" tall and weighs 215 lbs. The BMI is 40 and the BP is 128/82. She has significant comedonal acne and a small amount of facial hair on sideburns and upper lip. She has moderate acanthosis nigricans on the back of her neck. She has boggy turbinates and enlarged tonsils and breathes mostly through her mouth. The abdominal examination is normal. She has completed her pubertal development (SMR 5).

SELECT THE ONE BEST ANSWER

1. All of following statements regarding adolescent obesity are correct except:

    (A) Higher birth weight predicts increased risk of overweight in adolescence.
    (B) Genetic factors play a significant role in the development of adolescent obesity.
    (C) Dissatisfaction with body image predicts onset of depression in adolescent girls.
    (D) Obesity in adolescents is usually the result of endocrinopathies.
    (E) All of the above are correct.

2. All of the following syndromes are associated with obesity except:

    (A) Prader-Willi
    (B) pseudohypoparathyroidism
    (C) Alstrom syndrome
    (D) Kallmann syndrome
    (E) Klinefelter syndrome

3. What is the currently most commonly accepted definition of overweight/obesity in children and adolescents?

    (A) BMI greater than the 95th percentile for sex and age
    (B) BMI greater than the 85th percentile for age and sex
    (C) body weight of 20% greater than the ideal body weight for age and sex

(D) weight for height greater than the 95th percentile

(E) body weight of 30% greater than the ideal body weight

4. Which of the following conditions are associated with increased adiposity in adolescence?

(A) increased rate of valvular disease
(B) pseudotumor cerebri
(C) gallbladder disease
(D) hypertension
(E) B, C, and D

5. Regarding the epidemiology of obesity in adolescents, which one of the following statements is not accurate?

(A) The prevalence of obesity among adolescents has tripled during the past two decades.
(B) Adolescent boys and girls have the same prevalence of obesity.
(C) About 15.5% of all adolescents age 12 to 19 years are categorized as obese.
(D) The prevalence of obesity in Latino boys is 12%.
(E) The prevalence of obesity in African-American girls age 12 to 19 years is 26.6%.

6. Among the elements of the clinical history you need to explore now which would be the most relevant?

(A) detailed dietary history
(B) type, intensity, and duration of exercise
(C) television viewing time
(D) medication
(E) all of the above

7. Among the following, which clinical finding will be the least helpful to distinguish endogenous from exogenous causes of obesity?

(A) height for age
(B) linear growth rate
(C) intertrigo
(D) pigmented striae
(E) myxedema

8. In this patient, any of the following conditions could explain her menstrual delay except:

(A) thyroid dysfunction

(B) pregnancy
(C) functional adrenal hyperandrogenism
(D) polycystic ovarian syndrome (functional ovarian hyperandrogenism)
(E) androgen insensitivity

9. All of the following tests should be ordered at this time except:

(A) fasting glucose and lipid profile
(B) estradiol and progesterone
(C) FSH/LH
(D) pregnancy test
(E) DHEA-S

10. The laboratory results indicate that her LH-to-FSH ratio is 5:1. Her testosterone level is 75, while DHEA-S is 215. All other hormonal tests were within the normal range. A lipid profile showed a total cholesterol of 190 mg/dL and an LDL of 125 mg/dL. All of the following therapeutic interventions may be indicated at this time except:

(A) weight management
(B) combined oral contraceptives
(C) topical acne medication
(D) insulin sensitizers
(E) statins

11. Regarding the treatment of her moderate comedonal acne, all of the following are true except:

(A) A single daily application of 5% benzoyl peroxide will be effective in most cases of mild comedonal and inflammatory acne.
(B) 13-*cis*-Retinoic acid (isotretinoin, Accutane) may be associated with severe teratogenic effects.
(C) Oral contraceptives containing low-androgenic progestins are helpful in the management of acne in adolescent girls.
(D) Depomedroxyprogesterone acetate is effective in controlling mixed comedonal-inflammatory acne.
(E) Some oral antibiotics used for the treatment of acne may lead to photosensitivity reactions.

12. All of the following could explain this patient's increased tiredness and deteriorating school performance except:

(A) depression
(B) obstructive sleep apnea
(C) hypothyroidism
(D) pregnancy
(E) hyperandrogenism

13. Depression should be considered in the differential diagnosis of this adolescent with history of excessive tiredness, social isolation, and declining school performance. Regarding the epidemiology of depression in adolescents, all of the following are correct except:

    (A) The incidence of major depressive disorder (MDD) increases from 2% in children to 4% to 8% in adolescents.
    (B) The cumulative incidence of MDD is 15% to 20%.
    (C) In children there is no gender difference in risk.
    (D) Depression is more common in adolescent boys than in girls.
    (E) Bipolar disorder develops in 20% to 40% of children and adolescents with MDD.

14. Depression in children and adolescents is associated with increased risk of suicidal behaviors. Which of the following statements about the epidemiology of suicidal ideation and attempts during adolescence are true?

    (A) Suicide is the third leading cause of death among 15- to 24-year-olds.
    (B) The rate of completed suicides in adolescents is higher for girls than for boys.
    (C) Rates of suicidal attempts are higher for girls than for boys.
    (D) A and C.
    (E) All of the above.

15. All of the following are common symptoms suggestive of MDD in adolescents except:

    (A) irritable mood
    (B) feeling of worthlessness
    (C) psychomotor agitation or retardation
    (D) difficulty concentrating
    (E) hallucinations

16. Which among the following is a predisposing factor for depression in adolescence?

(A) family history of depression in first-degree relatives
(B) prior depressive illness
(C) chronic illness
(D) family dysfunction
(E) all of the above

17. What circumstances would indicate urgent psychiatric referral for an adolescent with depression?

    (A) history of suicidal attempt or present suicidal ideation
    (B) psychosis
    (C) coexisting substance abuse
    (D) family unable to monitor teen's safety
    (E) all of the above

Answers

1. **(D)** It has been shown that higher birth weight predicts increased risk of overweight in adolescence and that having been born to a mother with gestational diabetes is associated with increased likelihood of being overweight in adolescence. However, the effect of gestational diabetes on an offspring's obesity is controversial. Adjustment for a mother's own BMI decreases the likelihood of a causal role for abnormal maternal-fetal glucose metabolism as a cause of obesity in the offspring. Dissatisfaction with body image is a very common occurrence during adolescence, particularly among girls. It usually leads to unhealthy weight control practices and eating patterns and in some studies was found to predict the onset of depression. In most instances, obesity is a chronic multifactorial disease. Only 3% of obese adolescents have underlying endocrinopathies such as hypothyroidism, Cushing's syndrome, or hypothalamic/pituitary diseases and pseudohypoparathyroidism. An additional 2% of obese adolescents have rare genetic syndromes associated with obesity. Obesity associated with mental retardation, short stature, cryptorchidism or hypogonadism, dysmorphism, and ocular or auditory defects should suggest a genetic origin. Prader-Willi syndrome is the most frequent of the genetic disorders associated with obesity. The remaining 95% of obesity in adolescents results from a combination of genetic and environ-

mental factors not fully elucidated. Genetic factors play a significant role in the development of obesity and are known to explain 30% to 50% of its variability. Studies show that if one parent is obese, the risk of obesity for the offspring is 30%, while if both parents are obese, the risk increases to 70%. Although some of these findings may be explained by environmental factors, there is a high correlation between the BMI of identical twins, even when reared in different households. Also, a strong correlation has been shown between the BMIs of adoptees and their biological parents, while none exists between those of adoptees and their adoptive parents.

2. **(E)** Alstrom syndrome is a rare disease with autosomal recessive inheritance. Retinal degeneration, truncal obesity, diabetes mellitus, and sensorineural hearing loss are characteristic features of this condition. Further variable symptoms include chronic hepatitis, asthma, and impaired glucose tolerance test. Pseudohypoparathyroidism (PHP) is associated with biochemical hypoparathyroidism (e.g., hypocalcemia and hyperphosphatemia) because of parathyroid hormone (PTH) resistance rather than with PTH deficiency. In this condition target renal cells are unresponsive to PTH, leading to increased reabsorption of phosphate. PHP type 1 is the most common form and is associated with a combination of skeletal and developmental features known as Albright hereditary osteodystrophy. Clinical characteristics of this syndrome include short stature, obesity, round facies, short neck, brachydactyly, and mental retardation. Prader-Willi syndrome is characterized by early onset of obesity with hyperphagia, infantile hypotonia, hypogonadism, cryptorchidism, and mental retardation. Short stature, small hands and feet, strabismus, and increased incidence of diabetes mellitus are common findings in this condition. The incidence of the syndrome is 1:16,000. It results from deletions of a segment of the paternal chromosome 15. Klinefelter syndrome occurs in men who have an extra X chromosome leading to a 47,XXY karyotype. Its clinical features include small, firm testes, azoospermia, variable degrees of eunuchoidism, gynecomastia, mental abnormalities, and hypergonadotropic hypogonadism. A slim, tall body habitus is characteristic in this condition.

3. **(A)** The BMI is used to identify overweight and those at risk of overweight in children and adolescents. This index is calculated by dividing weight by squared height.

A BMI ≥95th percentile identifies children or teenagers who are overweight, while children with a BMI between the 85th and 95th percentiles for age and gender are categorized as at risk for overweight. A potential limitation to the use of the BMI results from the fact that the index is based on weight and height. Since weight is not always a measure of adiposity and may result from increased muscle or bone mass, a definitive clinical definition of obesity may require an additional measurement such as triceps skinfold thickness. Nevertheless, the vast majority of children with BMI >95th percentile for age and sex are also found to have increased percentage of body fat by other methods. BMI not only identifies children who have increased body fat, but also helps predict associated risk factors such as elevated blood pressure or increased insulin levels.

Since, prior to adulthood, adiposity varies with age and gender, BMI is age and gender specific in children and adolescents. BMI charts provide a reference that allows for longitudinal follow-up of adiposity from age 2 to 20 years. They can be used to track body size throughout childhood and adolescence.

4. **(E)** Obesity during adolescence is associated with numerous short-term and long-term health consequences, including hypertension, hyperlipidemia, type 2 diabetes mellitus, sleep apnea, gallbladder disease, pseudotumor cerebri, and orthopedic conditions such as slipped femoral capital epiphysis and tibia vara or Blount disease. Obese adolescents may suffer from low self-esteem, poor body image, social isolation, and increased incidence of depression. Long-term consequences include a higher mortality risk for cardiovascular and cerebrovascular disease during adulthood, tibia vara, gallstones, osteoarthritis, and increased risk for certain cancers (colon, rectum, prostate). Unfavorable social outcomes such as lower education levels, lower incidence of marriage, lower household income, and a higher rate of poverty as a consequence of pervasive cultural stereotypes have also been documented.

5. **(D)** National statistics from 1999 to 2000 showed that the overall prevalence of obesity among adolescents increased from 5% to 15% in the past two decades. Both adolescent girls and boys have an overall prevalence of 15.5%. However, minority adolescents have the highest prevalence of obesity with rates as high as 27.7% in Mexican boys and 26.6% in African-American girls. Several factors seem to play a role in these discouraging statistics, including increased food availability and portion sizes, sedentary lifestyles, television viewing, time spent on computer games, aggressive marketing of fast food to young people, and decreased opportunity for sports and other outdoor activities in schools and within communities.

6. **(E)** A thorough clinical history will help identify endogenous causes of obesity and determine exogenous contributing factors and existing or potential complications. A detailed dietary history should include, among others, types of food preferred, portion sizes, numbers of meals a day, and patterns of food consumption. Given the importance of physical activity in maintaining normal weight and in view of the increasingly sedentary habits of adolescents, it is essential to document a detailed exercise history. Medications such as tricyclic antidepressants, antipsychotics, depomedroxyprogesterone, and corticosteroids are associated with significant weight gain.

7. **(C)** A comprehensive physical examination in overweight adolescents should include height, weight, blood pressure, pulse, and respiratory rate. It is essential to review the growth chart since overweight patients with underlying endocrinopathies are usually short for age, while those with exogenous obesity have either normal or above normal height for age. A decline in height velocity is typically found in teens with endogenous causes of obesity. The skin examination may reveal, among others, acne, acanthosis nigricans, intertrigo, and striae. Although striae are a common finding in overweight teens, purplish striae suggest underlying hypercortisolism. Acne is present in a large percent of teenagers independent of the presence of obesity. Within a clinical scenario of obesity, irregular menses, and hirsutism in an overweight girl, significant acne could be an additional indicator of hyperandrogenism. Acanthosis nigricans is recognized as a marker of insulin resistance and, thus, a harbinger of type 2 diabetes mellitus. Intertrigo is a common finding in overweight adolescents regardless of etiology. A thorough cardiopulmonary, musculoskeletal, and neurological assessment is needed, looking for evidence of hypertension, cor pulmonale, degenerative changes of the joints, slipped capital femoral epiphysis, and pseudotumor cerebri.

8. **(E)** Obesity, thyroid dysfunction, hypothalamic amenorrhea, and functional adrenal or ovarian hyperandrogenism could explain this young woman's 3-month history of amenorrhea. Androgen insensitivity would not be in the differential diagnosis since the patient had normal menses in the past.

9. **(B)** Even though there is no history of sexual activity, it is always important to exclude pregnancy in any adolescent with secondary amenorrhea. In this patient, because of her obesity and positive family history for diabetes and hyperlipidemia, she is at higher than normal long-term risk for cardiovascular disease. A fasting glucose and lipid profile should be ordered. TSH and prolactin level would help exclude hypothyroidism and hyperprolactinemia, while total and free testosterone and DHEA-S levels will be useful to assess the cause of her clinical hyperandrogenism.

10. **(E)** Because obesity and resulting insulin resistance play a prominent role in the pathogenesis of polycystic ovarian syndrome, therapeutic interventions should first address weight management. In patients with signs of hyperandrogenism who do not desire to get pregnant, combined oral contraceptives are effective in controlling the clinical manifestations. Topical acne medication should also be recommended. Insulin sensitizers have been found useful in the treatment of patients with polycystic ovary syndrome since they correct insulin resistance, androgen excess, and clinical manifestations of hyperandrogenism.

11. **(D)** Oral contraceptives, particularly those with low androgenic effects, are effective in the treatment of acne since they decrease biologically active free testosterone and reduce ovarian androgen

production. On the other hand, depomedroxy-progesterone and long-acting progestin implants often worsen acne. Mild comedonal acne can be successfully treated with 5% benzoyl peroxide gel in a majority of cases, while moderate comedonal acne may require daily applications of tretinoin cream or gel in concentrations form 0.025% to 0.05%. Topical antibiotics are effective in the treatment of moderate inflammatory and mixed acne. They work best when combined with benzoyl peroxide. Severe acne may respond to tretinoin cream or gel but, if inflammatory, will often require oral antibiotics. If there is no response, the patient should be referred to a dermatologist. In this patient, who will also receive combined oral contraceptives to treat other manifestations of hyperandrogenism, topical 5% benzoyl peroxide with or without topical antibiotics would be helpful as initial therapy.

12. **(E)** Several elements of the history suggest the possibility of depression, including her increased tiredness, dissatisfaction with body image, deteriorating school performance, and limited social interactions. There has been a recent death in the family for which she may be appropriately grieving. She does not admit to feeling sad or depressed and specifically denies suicidal ideation. Nevertheless, depression is still a consideration in this girl and should be explored further. Obstructive sleep apnea is a likely possibility given her morbid obesity and enlarged tonsils. Additional history taking may reveal loud snoring, brief periods of apnea while asleep with continuing respiratory effort, and daytime somnolence. A polysomnogram will be needed to confirm the diagnosis. Hypothyroidism should be considered in the differential diagnosis of any adolescent with obesity, increased tiredness, and deteriorating school performance. Early pregnancy may lead to increased somnolence and weight gain.

13. **(D)** Depression is, by far, one of the most prevalent forms of psychopathology in adolescents. Its broad clinical spectrum spans from transient depressive mood, which could be a justified response to the frustrations of daily life to major depressive disorders requiring hospitalization. Despite the fact that depression is a major cause of morbidity and mortality during the second decade of life, it is estimated that two-thirds of adolescents with clinical depression go unrecognized and untreated. Moreover, depression is often associated with significant comorbidities. It has long-term effects on psychosocial functioning and, importantly, is a major risk factor for suicide. The risk of MDD increases from 2% to 8% from childhood to adolescence. While among children there is no gender difference in the risk of significant depression, during the second decade of life, the female-to-male ratio for MDD becomes 2:1, a difference that will persist throughout life. Bipolar disorder develops in 20% to 40% of children and adolescents with MDD.

14. **(D)** Suicide is the third leading cause of death among 15- to 24-year-olds in the United States after motor vehicle accidents and homicide. Twelve percent of all deaths in this age group are due to suicide. The rates of completed suicides are about five times higher in males than in females (15:100,000 and 3.3:100,000, respectively). Up to 20% of high school students report having had suicidal ideation in the previous 12 months and up to 8% of the students in the same survey had attempted suicide one or more times during that time period. It is estimated that 500,000 teens make a suicide attempt each year. The rates of suicidal attempts are higher among girls than among boys, while the rates of completion are higher in boys and in girls since boys tend to use more violent and lethal means. Rates of attempted suicide are higher in gay/lesbian and bisexual youth. Among adolescents who develop MDD, up to 7% may commit suicide in the young adult years. These data emphasize the need to screen all adolescents for emotional disorders, and specifically for depressed mood and suicidal ideation during the well-teen visit. Early diagnosis and treatment of depression, accurate evaluation of suicidal ideation, and limiting access to lethal agents—including firearms and medications—are valuable strategies in the prevention of suicide in adolescents.

15. **(E)** Even though the diagnostic criteria of MDDs are the same in adolescents as in adults, the recognition of the disorder is often more difficult in young people. In teens, irritability and acting out are more common presenting features

of depression than depressed mood. Symptoms of depression include:

- Persistent sad or irritable mood
- Loss of interest in activities once enjoyed
- Significant change in appetite or body weight
- Difficulty sleeping or oversleeping
- Psychomotor agitation or retardation
- Loss of energy
- Feelings of worthlessness or inappropriate guilt
- Difficulty concentrating
- Recurrent thoughts of death or suicide

Five or more of these symptoms must persist for ≥2 weeks before a diagnosis of major depression can be established. The symptoms must cause significant distress or impairment and represent a change from previous functioning. They must not be attributable only to substance abuse, or medication or medical condition or accounted for by bereavement. A fundamental prerequisite for the diagnosis is to exclude a history of manic, manic-depressive, or hypomanic episodes. Either depressed and/or irritable mood or loss of interest in almost all previously pleasurable activities should be present most of the day, nearly every day for ≥2 weeks, with the others occurring during the same time period. The symptoms must cause significant distress or impairment and represent a change from previous functioning. They must not be attributable only to substance abuse, medication, or medical condition or accounted for by bereavement. Other signs of depression in adolescents include:

Frequent vague, nonspecific physical complaints such as headaches, muscle aches, stomach aches or tiredness, frequent absences from school or poor performance in school, talk of or efforts to run away from home, outbursts of shouting, complaining, unexplained irritability or crying, being bored, lack of interest in playing with friends, alcohol or substance abuse, social isolation, poor communication, fear of death, extreme sensitivity to rejection or failure, increased irritability, anger, or hostility, reckless behavior, and difficulty with relationships. On the other hand, decreased need for sleep, grandiosity, and overinflated sense of self, if present, would suggest the diagnosis of bipolar disorder.

16. **(E)** All of the following are considered predisposing factors for depression in adolescence:

family history of depression in first-degree relatives, history of prior depressive episode, chronic illness, family dysfunction, peer problems, academic difficulties, learning disabilities, early losses, history of anxiety disorders or ADHD, history of abuse or neglect, stress, break-up of a romantic relationship, traumatic events (e.g., exposure to violence, natural disasters).

17. **(E)** All the above conditions would indicate urgent psychiatric evaluation and treatment. Treatment for depressive disorders in children and adolescents often involves short-term psychotherapy, medication, or a combination of both, together with targeted interventions involving the home and school environment. Optimal treatment of teens with depression calls for counseling in all cases. Certain types of short-term psychotherapy, particularly cognitive-behavioral therapy (CBT), have been helpful to relieve depression in children and adolescents. On the other hand, the use of antidepressant medication in children and adolescents remains controversial. Medication should be considered in adolescents with moderate to severe depression, severe vegetative symptoms, marked functional impairment, presence of psychotic symptoms, strong family history of depression, depressed phase of bipolar disorder, or failed psychotherapeutic intervention.

SUGGESTED READING

Joffe A, Blythe MJ: Handbook of adolescent medicine. Adolesc Med 14:2, 2003.

Neinstein LS: *Adolescent Health Care: A Practical Guide*, 4th ed. Philadelphia: Lippincott Williams and Wilkins, 2002.

Bonin L: *Depression in adolescents: epidemiology, clinical manifestations, and diagnosis*. Up-To-Date, 2004. Available at: http://www.uptodateonline.com. Last accessed May 31, 2006.

Kennebeck S, Bonin L: Epidemiology and risk factors for suicidal behavior in children and adolescents. Up-To-Date, 2004. Available at: http://www.uptodateonline.com. Last accessed May 31, 2006.

American Academy of Child and Adolescent Psychiatry: Practice parameter for the assessment and treatment of children and adolescents with suicidal behavior. *J Am Acad Child Adolesc Psychiatry* 40:24S, 2001.

American Academy of Pediatrics: Suicide and suicide attempts in adolescents. Committee on Adolescents. *Pediatrics* 105:871, 2000.

Centers for Disease Control and Prevention (CDC): *Deaths: Leading Causes for 2000*. National Vital Statistics Reports, 50(16), September 16, 2002.

General Emergency and Urgent Care

9

CASE 76: A 17-YEAR-OLD WITH KNEE PAIN

A 17-year-old female high school soccer player is brought to an urgent care clinic with a chief complaint of left knee pain. The onset of symptoms occurred during a soccer game the previous day. The athlete states as she went to kick the ball with her right foot she planted her left foot, felt her left knee buckle and heard a "pop." She then fell to the ground and had to be helped off the field. She experienced immediate swelling in the knee as well as some difficulty straightening the knee. She denied any tingling or numbness in the leg. She is using crutches as walking is painful. She denies any history of previous knee injuries and has played soccer for 7 years.

SELECT THE ONE BEST ANSWER

1. The best initial management for this athlete on the soccer field should include:

   (A) ice applied to the knee joint for approximately 20 minutes
   (B) application of a knee immobilizer after attempting to straighten the leg to full extension
   (C) ambulation on the sidelines to improve the range of motion and decrease the swelling
   (D) an immediate dose of ibuprofen 600 to 800 mg PO to prevent inflammation
   (E) immediate transport by ambulance to the nearest emergency room for evaluation

2. Based on the history alone, the most likely diagnosis is:

   (A) meniscal tear
   (B) medial collateral ligament tear
   (C) anterior cruciate ligament tear
   (D) posterior cruciate ligament tear
   (E) patellar dislocation

3. On physical examination, a moderate knee joint effusion and a 5-degree flexion contracture are noted. Valgus and varus testing performed at 30 degrees of knee flexion reveal no instability. An anterior drawer performed with the knee at 30 degrees of flexion and at 90 degrees of flexion reveals increased laxity. A posterior drawer test is negative. McMurray's test is negative. There is no pain with patellar compression, nor is patellar instability noted. Based on the above physical examination, which of the following tests performed is most helpful in confirming your suspected diagnosis?

   (A) valgus test
   (B) varus test
   (C) anterior drawer at 90 degrees of flexion
   (D) anterior drawer at 30 degrees of flexion
   (E) McMurray's test

4. Of the following physical findings, which is least likely to confirm the presence of internal derangement of the knee?

   (A) knee joint effusion
   (B) decreased range of motion
   (C) instability with a Lachman test

(D) painful clicking with a McMurray's test

(E) instability with a valgus test

5. You tell the patient that the swelling in her knee indicates inflammation is present. Which of the following statements is most accurate regarding inflammation?

(A) Inflammation is primarily an acute response to trauma, infection, and autoimmune diseases.

(B) NSAIDs work on joint inflammation by inhibiting prostaglandin synthesis in the arachidonic acid cascade at the cyclooxygenase pathway.

(C) Corticosteroids work most effectively on joint inflammation by inhibiting leukotriene production.

(D) Inflammation is characterized by erythema, edema, warmth, and pain and has a protective effect on synovium, tendons, bursae, and cartilage.

6. The patient now tells you she is in pain after you have examined her and asks what she should do. Your next step in treatment should be which of the following?

(A) apply an ace wrap

(B) knee joint aspiration

(C) corticosteroid injection

(D) knee joint aspiration followed by a corticosteroid injection

(E) knee brace

7. You are now ready to order a radiologic imaging study of the left knee. Which of the following is most helpful in confirming your diagnosis?

(A) AP and lateral plain radiograph

(B) AP, lateral, sunrise, and notch plain radiographs

(C) CT scan

(D) MRI scan

(E) no imaging study is needed

8. Which of the following treatment recommendations is likely to result in complete recovery from the above injury including eventual return to soccer?

(A) custom hinged knee brace for 3 to 6 months

(B) six to 12 weeks of physical therapy in a sports rehabilitation center

(C) arthroscopic surgery and repair

(D) arthroscopic surgery and reconstruction

(E) complete rest and crutch-assisted ambulation for 6 to 12 weeks

9. You provide the patient with a brace, refer her to physical therapy and schedule her for follow-up in 10 to 14 days. Upon her return to the office she tells you the swelling has decreased as has her pain; however, she notes severe sharp stabbing sensations of pain when she attempts to straighten her leg completely. Your physical examination reveals a 10-degree flexion contracture, a small joint effusion, and medial joint line tenderness. Attempts to straighten the knee into neutral (full extension at 0 degrees) reproduce sharp pain. Laxity is again noted with a Lachman test. McMurray testing reveals a painful "click." You are now most concerned about the following diagnosis:

(A) anterior cruciate ligament injury

(B) medial collateral ligament injury

(C) meniscal injury

(D) A and C

(E) all of the above

10. The patient now tells you she has been unable to go for an MRI because of her insurance and lack of transportation; however, she is planning to go in 10 days. She asks what you want her to do in the meantime. The most appropriate recommendation to make at this point is:

(A) continue the brace and follow-up after the MRI

(B) continue the brace and physical therapy and follow-up after the MRI

(C) resume crutch use, stop physical therapy and await the MRI

(D) referral to an orthopedic surgeon after the MRI

(E) referral to an orthopedic surgeon within 1 week, regardless of the MRI being done

11. If in the scenario described in question 1, the athlete injured while playing soccer was 12 years old, your differential diagnosis would include all of the following except:

(A) osteochondritis dissecans
(B) physeal injury
(C) meniscal tear
(D) cruciate ligament injury
(E) tibial tubercle avulsion

12. If in the scenario described in question 1, the athlete injured while playing soccer was 12 years old, the most likely diagnosis would be:

(A) osteochondritis dissecans
(B) physeal injury
(C) meniscal tear
(D) cruciate ligament injury
(E) tibial tubercle avulsion

13. Which of the following radiographic studies is least likely to reliably demonstrate the suspected diagnosis in the 12-year-old soccer player with a painful, swollen knee and inability to bear weight?

(A) plain radiographs including AP, lateral, notch, and sunrise view
(B) CT scan
(C) MRI scan
(D) bone scan
(E) All are equally sensitive and specific for diagnosis in this case as described.

14. Which of the following knee injuries occurs more commonly in skeletally immature males versus females?

(A) patellar dislocation
(B) osteochondritis dissecans
(C) patellofemoral pain
(D) anterior cruciate ligament injury
(E) meniscal injury

15. Which of the following conditions is the most common cause of knee pain in adolescent females?

(A) patellofemoral pain
(B) Osgood-Schlatter's disease
(C) plica band syndrome
(D) chronic medial collateral ligament sprain
(E) iliotibial band syndrome

16. Which of the following physical examination findings is *not* associated with an increased risk of patellofemoral pain?

(A) genu valgum
(B) pes planovalgus foot deformity
(C) Q angle of 15 degrees
(D) weak quadriceps muscles
(E) patellar hypermobility

17. Which of the following activities is least associated with increased stress on the patellofemoral joint?

(A) jumping
(B) squatting
(C) prolonged sitting
(D) stair climbing
(E) straight leg raises

18. Of the following conditions affecting the knee, which one should a primary care physician feel most uncomfortable managing without an orthopedic consultation?

(A) Osgood-Schlatter's disease
(B) patellofemoral pain
(C) patellar tendonitis
(D) osteochondritis dissecans
(E) chronic medial collateral ligament sprain

19. In a patient with knee pain which of the following is an indication for referral to an orthopedic or sports specialist for evaluation and management?

(A) knee effusion
(B) abnormal range of motion
(C) locking of the joint
(D) pain at the ends of long bones
(E) all of the above

20. If the athlete described in question 1 had recovered from her injury and came to you for clearance for return to sports, which of the following statements is true?

(A) If all swelling and pain have resolved and the athlete demonstrated walking without any limp or instability, then sports may be resumed safely with little risk of re-injury.
(B) In general, bracing is thought to help with swelling acutely via a compressive effect but has little demonstrated effectiveness in re-injury prevention immediately following a ligament sprain.

(C) An athlete must pass a functional test including running, jumping and cutting without pain or instability prior to participation.

(D) The athlete must take 8 weeks off from all sports participation because all ligament injuries take at least that long to heal.

(E) None of the above statements is true.

Answers

1. **(A)** The best initial treatment for an injured knee is ice applied to the swollen, painful area for approximately 20 minutes. It is appropriate to follow the general RICE (Rest, Ice, Compression, Elevation) principles for acute injury treatment. However, in the provided choices for an acute knee injury, one should not attempt to "force" the knee into extension as there may be mechanical limitations such as torn tissue or extreme swelling that prevent the knee from reaching full extension. The knee joint has maximal space to accommodate swelling at approximately 30 degrees of flexion. Weight bearing should be as tolerated and in this setting, keeping the athlete non–weight-bearing until a full examination is performed is appropriate. While immediate use of ibuprofen or another non-steroidal anti-inflammatory agent may be helpful for pain, it is unlikely to have any immediate effect on the post-traumatic inflammatory response. Urgent treatment is prudent in the setting of sports-related knee injuries. In the absence of gross deformity or neurovascular compromise, emergent transport is unnecessary.

2. **(C)** A non-contact deceleration injury to the knee joint resulting in a painful "pop," immediate swelling, and an inability to fully bear weight following the injury is an anterior cruciate ligament tear approximately 85% of the time in a skeletally mature patient.

3. **(D)** The maneuver most helpful to confirm your diagnosis is the anterior drawer test performed at 30 degrees of flexion, otherwise known as the Lachman test. The Lachman test is performed by using one hand to stabilize the femur while the examiner's opposite hand is placed around the leg at the level of the tibial tubercle and an attempt is made to anteriorly translate the tibia forward. The Lachman test is more clinically sensitive at diagnosing ACL (anterior cruciate ligament) tears than an anterior drawer test performed at 90 degrees of knee flexion. In that instance, it is common to find patients guarding or reflexively tightening their hamstring muscles; this results in a false negative drawer test with decreased anterior translation. The McMurray test is performed with the patient lying supine. The examiner places one hand anteriorly on the joint lines and then proceeds to cup the heel with the opposite hand and begins to flex and extend the knee while simultaneously internally and externally rotating the tibia on the femur. The test is positive, indicating a torn meniscus, if a painful click is felt.

4. **(E)** Instability with valgus stress testing indicates an injury to the medial collateral ligament (sprain versus tear); however, this ligament is extra-articular in location. An effusion almost always indicates internal derangement, especially in the setting of trauma. Decreased range of motion may be related to the knee effusion. However, the presence of a flexion contracture (or the inability to straighten the leg entirely) indicates a heightened concern for a mechanical block to the knee joint from a torn ACL/PCL, a meniscal tear or a loose body trapped in the joint. An abnormal Lachman test indicates an intra-articular ACL injury and an abnormal McMurray's test indicates a torn meniscus.

5. **(B)** Inflammation is both an acute and chronic response to trauma, infection and systemic autoimmune disease. In the acute phase, inflammation may be a healthy, self-limiting response; however, in the chronic phase it is often destructive such as in the setting of arthritis and articular cartilage destruction. Corticosteroids affect inflammation by inhibiting leukotriene production, but also by inhibiting prostaglandin synthesis at the phospholipase A2 pathway.

6. **(E)** In the setting of traumatic knee injuries there is no role for acute corticosteroid injections and no significant therapeutic role for knee joint aspiration. If a joint aspiration is performed, the hemarthrosis tends to re-accumulate quickly thus limiting the effectiveness of the therapeutic aspi-

ration. An ACE wrap is a relatively ineffective way to provide support and compression if a more supportive knee brace is available. Knee immobilizers that do not allow for range of motion are acceptable alternatives initially, but their use should be limited to a few days and active range of motion should be encouraged within the limits of pain.

7. **(D)** While plain radiographs of the knee are an appropriate initial study, a non-infused MRI of the left knee is helpful in diagnosing ligamentous injuries of the knee, as well as diagnosing other associated intra-articular injuries such as meniscal tears. Some might argue that no imaging study is needed in the case described as your diagnosis seems clinically accurate; MRIs are helpful to look for associated injuries such as collateral ligament, meniscal, and articular cartilage injuries. MRIs are generally recommended as part of the evaluation for an internal derangement of the knee.

8. **(D)** ACL injuries usually result in complete ligament tears either midsubstance or from the proximal attachment on the posterior femur. The injured ligament usually retracts and loses proper anatomic positioning, thereby preventing any reasonable chance of healing with conservative management. While bracing and physical therapy are important adjunctive treatments to decrease pain and improve strength and function, both pre- and postsurgery, the definitive treatment is an ACL reconstruction using a graft. Attempts to repair torn ACLs surgically have resulted in high failure rates and complications; therefore, in general, a surgical reconstruction is the preferred treatment of choice.

9. **(D)** Given the above information, your examination suggests ACL and meniscus injury resulting in signs of internal derangement. Bucket handle meniscal tears are most likely to result in a mechanical block in knee joint range of motion. An MCL injury should demonstrate pain to palpation over this extra-articular structure and increased laxity with valgus testing.

10. **(E)** A flexion contracture as a sign of internal derangement of the knee at 10 to 14 days postinjury is an indication for an immediate surgical

evaluation. Mechanical blocks of the joint are associated with higher complication rates such as permanent loss of normal range of motion and damage to articular cartilage from pinching and compression with knee joint movement. Therefore, while it would be helpful to expedite the MRI, if that seems unlikely to happen, it is appropriate to refer for an orthopedic consultation 10 to 21 days postinjury in the setting of a presumed mechanical block. The surgeon may recommend immediate arthroscopy to address the "locked" knee.

11. **(A)** Osteochondritis dissecans injuries are much more common in the skeletally immature athlete; however, they are more frequently associated with overuse. The etiology is multifactorial and thought to result from cumulative microtrauma to the subchondral bone leading to stress fracture and, ultimately, collapse. Treatment of this lesion depends on whether the cartilage is intact, partially attached or completely detached.

12. **(B)** It is reasonable to assume that a 12-year-old female is not yet skeletally mature. Therefore, the highest risk of injury associated with knee trauma is a physeal injury to the distal femur or proximal tibia. Physeal, or growth plate injuries are best treated with casting and crutches and merit a referral to a pediatric orthopedist as there is increased risk of growth arrest. Tibial tubercle avulsion injuries can best be diagnosed on a lateral radiograph of the knee and also merit an orthopedic evaluation. Anterior cruciate ligament injuries do occur in skeletally immature athletes. The management of ACL injuries at this age is controversial.

13. **(A)** In the setting of physeal injuries, a number of non-displaced Salter-Harris 1 to 2 fractures can be difficult to see on plain radiographs. Often a follow-up radiograph obtained 24 to 48 hours postinjury or 10 to 14 days postinjury will demonstrate the fracture line or a periosteal reaction. MRI, CT, and bone scan are all sensitive and specific for identifying physeal fractures. Clinically, pain at the end of long bones is a physeal injury until proven otherwise.

14. **(B)** Osteochondritis dissecans lesions are most common in males 9 to 18 years old. Patellofemo-

ral pain and patellar dislocations are associated with underlying patellar instability and malalignment—a clinical finding more common in females. Females tend to have valgus knee alignment that is often associated with flat feet. These cause overpronation and abnormal patellar tracking on the femur. Females often have "looser" ligaments and relatively weaker supporting muscles such as the quadriceps and hamstring muscles. ACL injuries are more common in females because of the above factors mentioned in addition to frequently having a smaller bony notch on the femur for the ligament to pass through. Hormonal influences are also thought to play a role in increasing a female's risk of ACL injury.

15. **(A)** Patellofemoral pain syndrome is the most common cause of adolescent knee pain, particularly in females. It is often referred to as anterior knee pain. There are many contributing factors (see next question). Osgood-Schlatter disease is inflammation and pain at the tibial tubercle seen in growing prepubescents. Plica syndrome is a painful band of synovial tissue that snaps on the undersurface of the patella causing pain. Iliotibial band syndrome is a tendonitis causing lateral knee pain—most common in runners.

16. **(C)** Anterior or patellofemoral pain is associated with a variety of physical findings including flat feet, knock knees (valgus knees) and increased internal hip rotation (femoral anteversion). Obesity also contributes to the presence of anterior knee pain. Functionally, weak quadriceps muscles, tight hamstrings and patellar instability contribute to the development of patellofemoral pain. The Q angle refers to the relationship of the quadriceps and patella vectors as drawn from the anterior superior iliac spine and bisecting the mid-superior pole of the patella followed by a line bisecting the mid-patella and the mid-patellar tendon. An angle >20 degrees is associated with lateral patellar tracking and increased stress on the patellofemoral joint.

17. **(E)** Patellofemoral pain has often been referred to as "theater knee" because weight-bearing activities and prolonged sitting tend to increase anterior knee pain. Sitting with the knee extended or performing exercises with a straight leg do not require stress to be placed across the patellofemoral joint, therefore usually do not hurt, and are often used as early exercises to start strengthening the leg without aggravating the patella and its surrounding structures.

18. **(D)** In general, overuse injuries are associated with genetic, biomechanical and workload problems. The factors contributing to pain and injury should be initially evaluated and treatment initiated by a primary care physician. Acute traumatic injuries or chronic, overuse injuries that don't respond appropriately to treatment may be referred for further evaluation by an orthopedic or sports specialist. Osteochondritis dissecans is the most complicated of the above conditions to manage; and the likelihood of needing surgical intervention rises in the older, more skeletally mature athlete.

19. **(E)** All of the above indicate either a physeal (growth plate) problem or other intra-articular pathology.

20. **(C)** Ligament sprains vary in the time it takes to heal depending on the location of the injury and the extent of the original injury. Ligament sprains are often graded 1 to 3: Grade 1 refers to a partial ligament tear with no joint instability. Grade 2 refers to a partial ligament tear with mild to moderate joint instability. Grade 3 refers to a complete tear with joint instability. Treatment of ligament sprains in the acute phase is aimed at decreasing inflammation and restoring strength. The definitive criteria for safe return to sports involve the athlete being able to perform sport-specific exercises such as running, jumping and cutting without pain, weakness or instability. If the athlete cannot perform sport-specific exercises properly, the risk of re-injury dramatically increases. Bracing is effective initially and provides compression and support to the joint. It also has an important role in assisting faster returns to competition by enhancing joint proprioception, thereby enhancing joint stability.

SUGGESTED READING

Bernstein J: *Musculoskeletal Medicine*. Rosemont, IL: AAOS Publications, 2003.

Sullivan, JA, Anderson SJ: *Care of the Young Athlete*. Rosemont, IL: AAOS and AAP Publications, 2000.

CASE 77: A 15-YEAR-OLD AND A 17-YEAR-OLD WHO COLLAPSE DURING A MARATHON

You are working in the emergency room on a Saturday afternoon watching the local marathon race on television. The announcer has just stated that the outside temperature is 95°F (35°C) and the humidity is 80%. You are glad to be inside in the air conditioning, yet you are sorry that you could not volunteer in the medical tent at the race. Suddenly two marathoners are brought in for urgent evaluation.

The first athlete is a 15-year-old female who is complaining of spasms in her calf muscles, mild lower abdominal pain, and thirst. She states she was competing in her first marathon, softball is her usual sport, and she didn't train much for this race. She did drink some water every 3 miles at the fluid stations then collapsed at mile 16. Her weight was 85 kg. Her vital signs were: pulse 96 bpm, BP 110/70 mm Hg, respiratory rate 28, temperature 99.9°F (37.7°C). She was wearing a tight fitting, dark-colored, long sleeve shirt over a tank top and matching shorts. Upon removal of her garments she was noted to have sunburned skin without blistering on her face, back, chest, upper and lower extremities. She appeared profusely sweaty, had tight gastrocnemius muscles with spasms.

The second athlete is a 17-year-old male cross country runner who collapsed at mile 23 complaining of dizziness, lightheadedness, headache, nausea, and had vomited twice in the field. His weight was 80 kg. His vital signs were: BP 100/60 mm Hg, pulse 110 bpm, respiratory rate 36, tympanic temperature 101°F (38.5°C). On examination he appeared confused and disoriented, and his skin was sweaty and hot to the touch. Further examination was unremarkable.

SELECT THE ONE BEST ANSWER

1. Which of the following is the most serious form of heat illness?

   (A) fever
   (B) heat syncope
   (C) heat stroke
   (D) heat exhaustion
   (E) rhabdomyolysis

2. Which diagnosis most likely explains the first athlete's symptoms?

   (A) sunburn
   (B) dehydration
   (C) heat exhaustion
   (D) heat cramps
   (E) heat stroke

3. What patient factor was most likely to predispose the first athlete to heat illness?

   (A) obesity
   (B) dehydration
   (C) clothing
   (D) sunburn
   (E) excessive exercise

4. What environmental conditions predispose an athlete to heat illness?

   (A) high ambient temperature
   (B) high winds
   (C) high humidity
   (D) A and C only
   (E) all of the above

5. What is the most important mechanism the body uses for heat dissipation?

   (A) conduction
   (B) convection
   (C) radiation
   (D) evaporation
   (E) respiration

6. Which of the following statements regarding heat dissipation is false?

   (A) Conduction occurs via indirect contact of the body with the environment.
   (B) Convection is heat transferred from a solid surface to surrounding gas molecules.
   (C) Radiation is the transfer of heat between the body and its environment via electromagnetic waves.
   (D) Evaporation is the conversion of liquid to gas.
   (E) All of the above are true.

7. Heat cramps are most likely related to the loss of which electrolyte?

   (A) Mg+
   (B) Na+
   (C) K+

(D) Cl–

(E) Ca+

8. When caring for a preadolescent athlete, all of the following statements accurately describe heat illness except:

(A) Children are at increased risk for heat illness because of a higher surface area to mass ratio.

(B) Younger athletes have slower rates of acclimatization.

(C) Children are at decreased risk for heat illness because the circulating blood volume is less.

(D) Children are less efficient at sweating.

(E) Children's motor movements are less efficient than adults' during exercise.

9. The best initial treatment of choice in the emergency room for the first athlete is?

(A) intravenous fluid replacement with normal saline

(B) salt tablets

(C) unlimited oral intake of a standard electrolyte solution

(D) unlimited oral intake of water

(E) massage and gentle calf stretching

10. Based on the initial presentation above, what is the most likely diagnosis accounting for the second athlete's symptoms?

(A) dehydration

(B) heat stroke

(C) heat exhaustion

(D) heat syncope

(E) rhabdomyolysis

11. Which of the following statements is true regarding heat exhaustion and heat stroke?

(A) Heat exhaustion and heat stroke are separate clinical conditions that do not occur in the same patient suffering from heat illness.

(B) Hemoconcentration, urinary concentration, and hypertension are common occurrences in both conditions.

(C) Both conditions can result in hyperpyrexia ≥105° F (40.5°C).

(D) Both conditions may cause an athlete to experience weakness, fatigue, dizziness, disori-

entation, myalgias, tachycardia, nausea, vomiting, or hypotension.

(E) Both conditions result in reversible tissue damage if an accurate diagnosis and prompt initiation of treatment occurs.

12. Which of the following are complications of heat stroke?

(A) permanent neurologic deficits

(B) hepatic failure

(C) uremia

(D) disseminated intravascular coagulation

(E) all of the above

13. All of a sudden you are called to the bedside of the second athlete and you observe generalized tonic-clonic seizure activity and posturing. The patient feels hot and dry to the touch. You are concerned now that the second athlete is suffering from heat stroke. Which of the following would be least likely to be found in a patient with heat stroke?

(A) a temperature of 101°F (38.5°C)

(B) an elevated creatine phosphokinase

(C) urine specific gravity of >1.030

(D) lactic acidosis

(E) blood pressure of 100/60 mm Hg

14. You instruct the nurse to obtain the patient's current temperature. What is the temperature measurement method you recommend to the nurse?

(A) rectal

(B) oral

(C) axillary

(D) tympanic

(E) the easiest and fastest method of her choice

15. Which of the following statements is true regarding measurement of core body temperature in a patient with heat illness?

(A) Rectal thermometers are used only in patients who feel "hot" to the touch.

(B) Rectal thermometers are preferred but need only to be able to measure up to 106°F (41.1°C).

(C) Oral temperatures are notoriously unreliable in exertional heat illness because of tachypnea and compliance.

(D) Tympanic membrane temperature measurement has been proven to reflect true core temperature because the tympanic membrane is adjacent to the hypothalamic temperature regulation center.
(E) All of the above

16. The nurse reports to you that the current vital signs for the second athlete are as follows: BP of 90/50 mm Hg, pulse of 120, oxygen saturation of 95% on room air, temperature of 106.7°F (41.5°C). What is the most important initial emergency room treatment for the second athlete?

(A) Prepare the patient for emergent placement of a Swan-Ganz catheter for central venous pressure monitoring.
(B) Begin rapid cooling procedures.
(C) Administer supplemental oxygen.
(D) Administer room temperature intravenous fluids using a 1/L bolus of 0.9% normal saline over 30 to 60 minutes.
(E) Administer an antipyretic medication stat.

17. In the medical tent, the most effective method to achieve rapid cooling is which of the following?

(A) whole body immersion in ice water
(B) wrapping the body in cold towels
(C) packing the body in ice
(D) spraying with water and place in front of fans
(E) ice packs in the groin and axilla

18. In the emergency room setting the preferred method of rapid cooling is?

(A) administration of cooled intravenous fluids with 0.9% normal saline
(B) iced gastric lavage
(C) ice packs in the groin and axilla
(D) rapid whole body sponging with rubbing alcohol
(E) whole body immersion in ice water

19. You have now initiated rapid cooling and the patient is more lucid, the skin is feeling cooler and clammy to the touch. At what temperature do you want to stop rapid cooling?

(A) 37°C (98.6°F)
(B) 37.3°C (99°F)
(C) 37.7°C (100°F)

(D) 38.3°C (101°F)
(E) 39.6°C (103°F)

20. After an hour, the first athlete feels much better and is ready to go home. You advise her that in the future she should try to prevent heat cramps during competition in strenuous and endurance sports lasting over 1 hour in duration. Which of the following recommendations is most effective in the prevention of heat cramps?

(A) salt tablets
(B) water only before and during intense endurance exercise
(C) water and an electrolyte drink before and during intense exercise
(D) increased warm-up time and stretching of calf muscles pre-exercise
(E) weight loss

21. If you were able to give the second athlete any advice prior to his next marathon, you would most likely want him to know all of the following principles except:

(A) The sweat rate for the average endurance athlete in a temperate climate averages 1.0 to 1.2 liters per hour and can exceed 2 liters per hour in conditions of high heat and humidity.
(B) Sweat is hypotonic and is more hypotonic in those athletes who sweat greater volumes.
(C) Athletes should voluntarily drink fluids before, during and after activities.
(D) If an athlete is participating in endurance events, he should start taking salt tablets 2 to 3 days prior to competition.
(E) Proper nutrition, adequate sleep, gradual acclimatization, avoidance of drugs/substances like alcohol, ephedra, and caffeine are important preventive measures.

Answers

1. (C) Heat stroke is the most severe form because it is associated with irreversible tissue damage.

2. (D) Heat cramps are a common mild form of heat illness that tend to occur after exercise and are associated with a large production of sweat during exercise.

3. **(B)** Dehydration and volume depletion as a result from sweating without adequate fluid replacement is the most important risk factor for heat-related illness. All of the listed factors contribute to an increased risk of heat illness.

4. **(D)** Heat and humidity are most important. Once ambient temperature equals or exceeds skin temperature, conduction, convection, and radiation cease to be effective methods of heat loss. Once ambient humidity exceeds 75% then the effectiveness of evaporation decreases. Low winds are associated with decreased heat dissipation.

5. **(D)** Evaporation (via sweating) is the dominant mode of heat dissipation or heat loss in the body.

6. **(A)** Conduction requires direct contact of the body with surrounding objects and air.

7. **(B)** Heat cramps are thought to be caused by a total body loss of sodium and are exacerbated by excessive sweating.

8. **(C)** Children are at increased risk for heat illness because circulating blood volume is less and the ability to circulate blood volume increases blood flow to the periphery resulting in a greater ability to dissipate heat.

9. **(C)** The best initial treatment for heat cramps is drinking an electrolyte solution (or administering 1 tsp of table salt dissolved in 500 mL of water). The underlying cause of heat cramps is total-body salt depletion. Cramping is often made worse by excessive intake of hypotonic fluids such as water. Gentle massage and stretching may be a helpful adjunct to treatment of the underlying problem. Intravenous fluid use is generally reserved for the more severe cases.

10. **(C)**

11. **(D)** Both conditions have similar initial signs and symptoms; however they represent a continuum of disease process. If left untreated or unrecognized, heat exhaustion can quickly become heat stroke at which time extreme hyperpyrexia (>40.5°C [105°F]—not seen in heat exhaustion), coma, seizures, and irreversible tissue damage can occur.

12. **(E)** All of the above are potential complications of heat stroke. Rhabdomyolysis, dysrhythmias, acidosis, adynamic ileus, electrolyte imbalances, and seizures are also seen.

13. **(A)** Heat stroke is associated with temperatures ≥40.5°C (105°F).

14. **(A)** In the setting of severe heat illness, it is critical to try to accurately measure core temperature. A rectal temperature is the preferred method with a probe 10 to 15 cm in length.

15. **(C)** Rectal temperature measurement is the gold standard and it is recommended that probes be accurate to at least 112°F. Tympanic membrane measurement has *not* correlated well with 10-cm rectal probe temperature measurements in research studies, despite the hypothesis described in answer D.

16. **(B)** In the setting of suspected heat stroke, it is vital that you initiate treatment before firmly establishing the diagnosis. In fever, the set point for temperature regulation is elevated and often responds to the use of antipyretics. In the setting of heat illness, the set point for temperature regulation is maintained yet hyperthermia results because more heat is gained than lost. In hyperthermia, antipyretics are likely to be ineffective and alternate methods of body cooling are necessary.

17. **(A)** Whether in the medical tent or in the emergency room it is critical to initiate treatment immediately. The most important initial treatment is the institution of rapid cooling. The treating physician must also follow the general principles of ABC, monitor the patient's vital signs, obtain appropriate laboratory tests, and start intravenous rehydration. The most effective way to achieve rapid cooling is whole body immersion in ice water. Unfortunately this method is usually not practical. The most common way to initiate rapid cooling is through the use of water sprays and fans (maximizes convection). One may also pack the athlete in ice or cold, wet towels. It is important to expose as much skin as possible. One should avoid placing ice packs over the major vessels in the groin and axilla as this may result in peripheral vasoconstriction and less efficient cooling.

Table 77-1. HEAT EXHAUSTION VERSUS HEAT STROKE

Key Factors	Heat Exhaustion	Heat Stroke
Signs and symptoms	Vague malaise, fatigue, headache, nausea, dizziness	CNS dysfunction (coma, seizures, delirium)
Core temperature	Normal or elevated < than 40.0°C	Elevated >40.5°C
Sweating	Common	Present in some cases Dry, hot skin more concerning
Treatment	Slow cooling Slow volume repletion	Rapid cooling Vigorous volume repletion if orthostatic and hypotensive <90/60 mm Hg
Antipyretics	Ineffective	Ineffective
End organ injury	Reversible injury	Often irreversible end organ damage

18. **(A)** In the emergency room setting, the preferred method for rapid cooling is administration of cooled intravenous fluids. Whole body immersion is not practical. Rubbing alcohol is generally not recommended. Ice packs in the groin and the axilla should be avoided. See Table 77-1 for summary of heat exhaustion versus heat stroke.

19. **(D)** One of the most common complications of rapid cooling is overcooling and temperatures as low as 88°F (31°C) have been reported (Boston Marathon). Therefore, the ideal temperature at which to stop rapid cooling is 101°F (38.3°C), subsequently allowing the body to further cool on its own. Shivering is a sign of overcooling and actually causes increased heat production and may cause a rebound increase in core temperature.

20. **(C)** The best prevention of heat cramps is adequate hydration before and during athletic activities. Appropriate clothing, conditioning, and, in rare cases, modest increases in dietary salt are helpful interventions. Excessive water intake often worsens heat cramps as it causes further total body sodium loss.

21. **(D)** Salt tablets are generally not recommended because the high solute load causes gastrointestinal irritation. However, adding extra table salt to food is recommended.

SUGGESTED READING

Rosen's Emergency Medicine: Concepts and Clinical Practice, 5th ed. St. Louis, MO: Mosby, 2002, pp 2002–2009.

Lugo-Amador N, Rothenhaus T, Moyer P: Heat-related illness. *Emerg Med Clin North Am* 22:315–327, 2004.

Barr SI, Costill DL, Fink WJ: Fluid replacement during prolonged exercise: effects of water, saline or no fluid. *Med Sci Sports Exerc* 27:2002–2010, 1995.

CASE 78: A 5-YEAR-OLD MALE WITH ABDOMINAL PAIN

A 5-year-old African-American male presents to a pediatric emergency department with a chief complaint of abdominal pain. His pain is periumbilical and is described as diffuse, non-radiating, waxing and waning with no relationship to meals or bowel movements. His pain began after lunch yesterday and he developed vomiting overnight. He has had three non-bilious and non-bloody episodes of emesis, two loose non-bloody stools today, and tactile elevated temperature. He states he is thirsty, but has refused to eat for the last several hours. The patient denies headache, sore throat, dysuria, frequency, or urgency. His past medical history is unremarkable.

His vital signs reveal a blood pressure of 100/60 mm Hg, pulse of 100, respiratory rate of 36 and a temperature of 100.4°F (38°C). Upon examination he is found to have dry mucous membranes, hypoactive bowel sounds with reproducible periumbilical tenderness, mild right lower quadrant tenderness and no rebound tenderness. His rectal exam is unremarkable except for a small amount of soft stool in the rectal vault.

SELECT THE ONE BEST ANSWER

1. What is the most likely diagnosis in this patient?

(A) gastroenteritis
(B) acute pancreatitis
(C) peritonitis
(D) acute appendicitis
(E) cholecystitis

2. All of the following are common non-surgical causes of acute abdominal pain in children except?

   (A) mesenteric adenitis
   (B) gastroenteritis
   (C) psoas abscess
   (D) pyelonephritis
   (E) constipation

3. All of the following are considered common extra-abdominal causes of abdominal pain in children except?

   (A) drug ingestions such as acetaminophen or salicylates
   (B) diabetic ketoacidosis
   (C) pneumonia
   (D) group A streptococcal pharyngitis
   (E) all of the above

4. Initial management steps for this patient in the emergency department should include all of the following except which?

   (A) Make the patient NPO (nothing by mouth).
   (B) Administer intravenous fluids.
   (C) Place a nasogastric tube to low intermittent wall suction.
   (D) Obtain prompt surgical consultation.
   (E) Draw appropriate laboratory studies.

5. Which of the following laboratory studies is least likely to be helpful in confirming the etiology of this patient's abdominal pain?

   (A) serum electrolytes, BUN, and creatinine
   (B) urinalysis
   (C) C-reactive protein
   (D) white blood cell count with differential
   (E) amylase and lipase

6. Which of the following statements describing acute appendicitis in a school-age child is false?

   (A) Diarrhea is rarely associated with appendicitis.

(B) The onset of abdominal pain frequently precedes the appearance of any other symptoms.
(C) Tenderness upon rectal examination is a non-specific finding for appendicitis.
(D) Anorexia and low grade fever may be associated symptoms.
(E) Pain may be either constant or colicky in nature, but almost always worsens with movement.

7. Which of the following physical examination findings is least likely to correlate with a diagnosis of acute appendicitis?

   (A) Referred tenderness from the left lower quadrant to the right lower quadrant during palpation
   (B) Bluish discoloration around the umbilicus
   (C) Tenderness at a point between the umbilicus and the anterior superior iliac spine two-thirds the distance from the umbilicus
   (D) Extension of the hip posteriorly with the patient lying prone elicits pain
   (E) Abduction of the right hip with the patient lying supine elicits pain

8. Which of the following statements is true regarding the appendix?

   (A) The appendix is funnel-shaped in infants and becomes conical shaped around 2 years of age.
   (B) The appendix may be located anterior, retrocecal, or subcecal.
   (C) The appendix may be located in any of the four abdominal quadrants (right upper, left upper, right lower, left lower).
   (D) The appendix is a diverticulum that extends from the inferior tip of the cecum with a lining interspersed with lymphoid follicles.
   (E) All of the above.

9. Which of the following statements is true regarding the management of acute appendicitis in children?

   (A) All patients should receive intravenous antibiotics.
   (B) All patients should have at least one imaging study.
   (C) All patients should have a prompt surgical consultation.

(D) All patients should receive pain medication until adequate pain control is achieved.

(E) All of the above.

10. In the 5-year-old patient described above, which of the following imaging studies is most likely to yield a definitive diagnosis and is the current preferred study of choice?

(A) abdominal radiographs
(B) ultrasonography
(C) barium enema
(D) upper GI
(E) CT

11. Which of the following statements is true regarding imaging studies in children with acute appendicitis?

(A) Computed tomography offers the advantages of better contrast sensitivity, the capability of viewing all tissue layers, reduced operator dependence and is the safest imaging modality.
(B) Ultrasonography offers the advantage of low cost, no radiation exposure and little variation among operators.
(C) Abdominal radiographs are most helpful in diagnosing other causes of abdominal pain such as constipation, bowel obstruction, free air, or renal stones.
(D) Ultrasonography offers 100% sensitivity and specificity to accurately exclude the possibility of appendicitis as a cause of acute abdominal pain in children as long as either a normal appendix is visualized or the appendix is not visualized at all.
(E) All of the above statements are true.

12. Which of the following statements is false?

(A) Appendicitis is the most common surgical abdominal emergency in children.
(B) Missed appendicitis is one of the top reasons for malpractice claims in the emergency department.
(C) In cases involving appendicitis in children, a well-documented chart will not prevent a lawsuit.
(D) All children with acute onset of abdominal pain should have an imaging study regardless of the clinical diagnosis.

(E) Males have a higher lifetime risk of suffering from appendicitis than females.

13. A delay in diagnosing acute appendicitis in children can have serious consequences. Which of the following is least likely to occur as a direct result of a delayed diagnosis?

(A) death
(B) bowel obstruction
(C) perforation
(D) peritonitis
(E) pancreatitis

14. Which of the following causes of abdominal pain in children is considered a surgical emergency besides appendicitis?

(A) intussusception
(B) peritonitis
(C) malrotation with midgut volvulus
(D) A and C only
(E) all of the above

15. You now return to the bedside of your patient and you find him lying on his side with his knees curled up. His mother tells you that he fell off his bike and landed on the handlebars the same day he started having abdominal pain. He is now complaining of worsening periumbilical pain and also mid-back pain. You find that he has hypoactive bowel sounds, guarding and right upper quadrant pain. All of the following statements are true regarding your suspected diagnosis except:

(A) A complete blood count might demonstrate a leukocytosis with a bandemia.
(B) Abnormal liver function tests as well as an elevated lipase and amylase might be present.
(C) A sentinel loop of small bowel seen best on a plain radiograph is often diagnostic.
(D) Ultrasonography is the cornerstone of diagnosis for the suspected condition.
(E) Blunt abdominal trauma is a relatively rare cause of this condition.

16. An ultrasound confirms the presence of an enlarged edematous pancreas and mild pancreatic duct dilatation. Which of the following is the least important step in appropriate management of this patient?

(A) intravenous hydration
(B) intravenous administration of antibiotics
(C) nasogastric suction
(D) serial abdominal examinations
(E) intravenous administration of meperidine

17. Which of the following is least likely to be a potential cause of acute pancreatitis in this 5-year-old?

(A) trauma
(B) cholelithiasis
(C) viral infection
(D) cystic fibrosis
(E) urolithiasis

18. You now are asked to evaluate a 2-year-old African-American female who presents with a history of sudden, sharp, crampy episodic right lower quadrant abdominal pain for 1 day and decreased oral intake. Your physical examination reveals no reproducible abdominal tenderness; however, a guaiac positive soft mucous stool on rectal examination is noted. Which of the following abdominal imaging studies would most likely aid you in confirming your suspected diagnosis?

(A) plain radiographs
(B) ultrasonography
(C) computed tomography
(D) barium enema
(E) B or D

19. Had the 2-year-old described in question 18 presented with bilious vomiting, abdominal distention, tenderness, and guarding, which of the following diagnosis would be most likely?

(A) mid-gut volvulus
(B) mesenteric adenitis
(C) peritonitis
(D) gastroenteritis
(E) Meckel's diverticulum

20. In any infant or toddler who presents with acute abdominal pain, bilious emesis, and guarding, which of the following imaging studies is the initial study of choice most likely to confirm your suspicions?

(A) magnetic resonance imaging
(B) ultrasonography

(C) computed tomography
(D) barium enema
(E) upper GI

Answers

1. **(D)** Acute appendicitis is the most likely etiology of this patient's clinical picture. While the presentation could initially be confused with gastroenteritis, the presence of hypoactive bowel sounds, anorexia, pain preceding the onset of any other symptoms, and reproducible tenderness have a higher correlation with appendicitis than any of the other diseases listed.

2. **(C)** A psoas abscess usually requires surgical drainage.

3. **(E)** All of the conditions can present with abdominal pain in children and must be included in the differential diagnosis.

4. **(C)** The placement of a nasogastric tube should be reserved for patients who appear to have the need for gastric decompression. This would include patients with suspected pancreatitis or some form of bowel obstruction such as a volvulus.

5. **(A)** Serum electrolytes, BUN, and creatinine may be helpful for assessing a patient's renal and hydration status but otherwise adds little to the diagnostic evaluation of abdominal pain. The urinalysis is useful to exclude the diagnosis of a urinary tract infection while amylase and lipase are useful in differentiating pancreatitis from other causes of abdominal pain such as appendicitis. Lastly, the combination of an increased leukocyte count with an increased blood CRP level can be suggestive of appendicitis in the setting of acute abdominal pain.

6. **(A)** In children, diarrhea can be associated with the presence of appendicitis up to 30% of the time. Many of the clinical features of acute appendicitis are non-specific; however, pain as the initial symptom and pain associated with movement—i.e., jumping up and down, riding in a bumpy car or tapping on the patient's heel—raise clinical suspicion.

7. **(B)** Bluish discoloration around the umbilicus describes Cullen's sign that, when coupled with Grey Turner's sign (bluish discoloration around the flank), is suggestive of acute hemorrhagic pancreatitis. Rovsing's sign describes referred pain from LLQ to RLQ. McBurney's point describes the classic RLQ appendiceal location for pain. Choices "D" and "E" refer to the classic psoas and obturator signs, respectively, that if present, non-specifically support the diagnosis of acute appendicitis.

8. **(E)**

9. **(C)** All suspected cases of acute appendicitis should have early surgical involvement as some children will be spared further diagnostic evaluations once the decision for surgical treatment has been made. In the absence of a perforation or peritonitis, antibiotics are not always necessary. Until the diagnosis has been made and the surgical recommendations have been made, pain should be monitored closely, but the administration of medication that could impede the evaluation and monitoring of the patient's status should be avoided.

10. **(B)** In current medical practice today, ultrasonography is the preferred diagnostic study of choice with >80% to 90% sensitivity and specificity that is comparable with abdominal computed tomography. Abdominal CT is a useful adjunct and is still often performed if the ultrasound is inconclusive. In some cases a CT is obtained as the initial study; however, it is associated with greater risks as it is an invasive procedure requiring contrast administration and high radiation exposure.

11. **(C)** Abdominal radiographs are traditionally not useful in the diagnostic evaluation of appendicitis except in the presence of a fecalith (calcified appendix). The disadvantage of CT is radiation exposure compared with ultrasound imaging that is associated with a high degree of operator dependency and variation. The presence of a normal appendix on an ultrasound effectively excludes appendicitis as a diagnosis; however, the inability to visualize the appendix renders the study inconclusive.

12. **(D)** Not all patients with acute abdominal pain need an imaging study, but a prompt surgical consultation is recommended.

13. **(E)** Pancreatitis is not a complication of acute appendicitis. Rather, it must be differentiated from appendicitis in the setting of acute abdominal pain.

14. **(E)** All of the choices have the associated risk of serious complications if the diagnosis is delayed or missed. The surgical evaluation is an important part of the work-up of acute abdominal pain and the surgical team must be ready to provide operative intervention should conservative treatment measures fail or be deemed inappropriate.

15. **(E)** All of the choices are true in the setting of suspected acute pancreatitis except that blunt abdominal trauma is actually a common cause. In fact, it is the most common cause of acute pancreatitis accounting for 13% to 33% of cases.

16. **(B)** In the setting of acute pancreatitis and the absence of peritonitis or septic shock, antibiotics have little role. Adequate pain control is an important step in treatment for this condition whereas it can interfere with a prompt diagnosis and treatment for acute appendicitis.

17. **(E)** Blunt trauma to the mid-epigastric area of the abdomen such as being struck with bicycle handlebars is the most common cause of acute pancreatitis in children. Viruses such as coxsackie B, cytomegalovirus, varicella, hepatitis A and B, influenza A and B, and Epstein-Barr virus have been implicated in addition to bacterial and parasitic causes. Gallstones can cause pancreatitis but are usually only seen in this age range in the presence of a hereditary hemolytic anemia such as hereditary spherocytosis or sickle cell disease. Cystic fibrosis can cause acute pancreatitis but the incidence is relatively low in African-Americans. Renal stones should not cause pancreatitis.

18. **(E)** Barium enemas have traditionally been the gold standard for the diagnosis (100% sensitivity and specificity) and 70% successful reduction rates of intussusception. However, current practice reflects increasing use of ultrasonography

with pneumatic reduction by an air enema. Success rates approach 90% with fewer complications than barium enemas.

19. **(A)** The presence of bilious emesis should prompt a thorough evaluation for bowel obstruction. Malrotation with intermittent volvulus is one cause in the toddler to preschool-age child.

20. **(E)** An upper GI with a contrast enema is still the gold standard for the diagnosis of volvulus. If the duodenal C-loop crosses to the left of the midline at a level greater than or equal to the pylorus, then malrotation is effectively ruled out. Conversely, a corkscrew column that ends abruptly is highly suspicious for volvulus.

SUGGESTED READING

Halter J: Common gastrointestinal problems and emergencies in neonates and children. *Clin Fam Pract* 6(3): 731, 2004.
Guzman D: Pediatric surgical emergencies. *Clin Pediatr Emerg Med* 3(1):1–2, 2002.
Reynolds S: Missed appendicitis and medical liability. *Clin Pediatr Emerg Med* 4(4):231, 2003.

CASE 79: A 3-YEAR-OLD GIRL WHO DRINKS A BOTTLE OF ACETAMINOPHEN

You are called to evaluate a 3-year-old 15-kg female brought in by ambulance. The aunt who arrived with the patient states she has been sick for 2 days with a "cold" and has had fevers up to 101°F (38°C) at home, a cough and 2 to 3 episodes of vomiting. The little girl is complaining of "stomach pain." Past medical history and family medical history are noncontributory. Medications include acetaminophen every 6 hours.

On physical examination, the blood pressure is 90/50 mm Hg, the pulse is 110, respiratory rate is 40, and tympanic temperature is 99.8°F (37.7°C). The child appears ill, somewhat diaphoretic and in mild pain. Her exam is significant for mid-epigastric tenderness without rebound or guarding. Bowel sounds are normal and a rectal exam is unremarkable. The mother arrives and brings an empty bottle to you and states "I think my baby drank her medicine." You examine the bottle and see it contains 4 oz of acetaminophen suspension 160 mg/5 mL. Mom states the bottle was newly opened yesterday and she gave only two doses.

The last dose was given 4 to 6 hours prior and she left the bottle in the room in case she needed it again during the night.

SELECT THE ONE BEST ANSWER

1. Which of the following statements regarding childhood poisonings is false?

    (A) The ingestion of a potentially poisonous substance by a young child is a common event.
    (B) Death attributable to unintentional poisoning is uncommon in children younger than 6 years of age.
    (C) Data such as signs and symptoms of toxicity, management strategies in the home, and indications for seeking emergency care are available from local and national poison control centers.
    (D) The American Academy of Pediatrics currently recommends that syrup of ipecac be kept at home for emergency use.
    (E) The storage of poisonous substances in the home should be discussed at the 6-month well-child visit.

2. All of the following statements correctly describe reasons for the decreases in the death rate attributable to unintentional poisoning in young children in the last 50 years except:

    (A) the advent of child-resistant closures for products
    (B) an increase in the OTC drug products available for parents to purchase for routine household use
    (C) improved public education and anticipatory guidance
    (D) the establishment of multiple poison control centers
    (E) all of the above are true

3. All of the following statements regarding syrup of ipecac are true except which?

    (A) The only recommended method of inducing emesis is administration of ipecac.
    (B) Syrup of ipecac is a safe emetic.
    (C) The amount of substance removed from the stomach is directly related to the duration of time from its ingestion to emesis.

(D) The induction of emesis using ipecac is an unpleasant experience.

(E) The use of home ipecac therapy has the potential to decrease the efficacy of other poison treatments such as activated charcoal or *N*-acetylcysteine.

4. Which of the following statements correctly describes the indications for administration of an emetic as treatment for a potentially toxic ingestion?

(A) anytime a young child ingests a potentially toxic substance

(B) to achieve gastric emptying prior to administration of activated charcoal or *N*-acetylcysteine resulting in increased efficacy of the treatment intervention

(C) when the child seems too lethargic to tolerate activated charcoal

(D) anytime a health care professional recommends its use

(E) none of the above

5. Which of the following statements best describes gastrointestinal decontamination in the emergency room setting?

(A) The initial management steps should always include gastric lavage or administration of an antiemetic.

(B) The use of activated charcoal alone without gastric emptying is the current recommended procedure of choice.

(C) A cathartic such as sorbitol is often used to improve the efficacy of activated charcoal.

(D) The risk of aspiration is decreased when a gastric emptying technique is performed in conjunction with the administration of activated charcoal.

(E) All of the above.

6. Which of the following should always be your initial step in the management of an overdose patient?

(A) the ABCs (airway, breathing, circulation)

(B) Administer naloxone.

(C) Obtain rapid bedside glucose measurement.

(D) Administer 20 mL/kg of 0.9% normal saline as an intravenous bolus over 30 minutes.

(E) Call the poison control center for assistance.

7. Which of the following laboratory studies is least likely to be helpful in the management of this 3-year-old patient?

(A) standard urine drug screen

(B) liver function tests

(C) prothrombin time

(D) electrolytes, BUN, creatinine, blood glucose

(E) serum acetaminophen level

8. Your laboratory tests results reveal increased AST and ALT levels about twice the normal range. The acetaminophen level is elevated. The patient is complaining of worsening abdominal pain. Which of the following statements best describes your initial management steps?

(A) activated charcoal alone

(B) activated charcoal plus gastric lavage

(C) *N*-acetylcysteine alone

(D) activated charcoal and *N*-acetylcysteine

(E) gastric lavage, activated charcoal and *N*-acetylcysteine

9. Which of the following ingested substances is least likely to adsorb activated charcoal?

(A) acetaminophen

(B) salicylates

(C) iron

(D) β-blockers

(E) TCAs

10. Acetaminophen overdose is most frequently associated with toxicity to which of the following?

(A) central nervous system

(B) liver

(C) kidneys

(D) pancreas

(E) bone

11. Which of the following statements describing acetaminophen toxicity is false?

(A) The majority of cases involve unintentional overdosing.

(B) Delays in the diagnosis and treatment of acetaminophen intoxication do not adversely affect outcome.

(C) The risk of toxicity is increased in patients taking drugs such as carbamazepine that are metabolized via the cytochrome P450 pathway.

(D) Acetaminophen toxicity includes four phases progressing from mild non-specific symptoms to onset of organ injury, peaking with maximum organ injury and ending with either recovery or irreversible injury.

(E) Conditions such as diabetes mellitus, obesity, malnutrition, and/or a family history of hepatotoxic reactions may increase the risk of acetaminophen toxicity.

12. Suppose this patient had ingested a potentially toxic amount of ibuprofen suspension. Which of the following statements is true regarding acute NSAID toxicity?

(A) The majority of ibuprofen overdoses follow a benign, rapidly reversible course.

(B) Plasma NSAID concentrations are useful and should always be obtained.

(C) As a result of high protein binding and rapid metabolism, gastric decontamination with activated charcoal is never indicated.

(D) GI toxicity is rarely associated with NSAID use or overdose.

(E) All of the above.

13. Which of the following household items is least likely to be harmful to a child if swallowed in large quantities?

(A) antidiarrheal medication

(B) ibuprofen

(C) mouthwash

(D) multivitamins

(E) bleach

14. Which of the following statements is false regarding caustic ingestions?

(A) The vast majority of all reported caustic ingestions occur in children.

(B) Caustic substances have the potential to cause tissue burns on contact with the eyes, skin, airway/lungs, and/or the GI tract.

(C) Alkalis, acids, and antiseptics are all agents capable of causing chemical injury.

(D) The transfer and storage of cleaners and caustic substances to alternative household containers has been associated with a decreased risk of ingestion in children.

(E) Button battery ingestion may cause esophageal obstruction and pressure necrosis and/or caustic injury because of leakage of alkaline material.

15. The presentation of a comatose patient with marked miosis, respiratory depression, hypotension, bradycardia, and hyporeflexia would make you most concerned about the possible overdose of which of the following?

(A) opioids

(B) organophosphates

(C) cocaine

(D) diphenhydramine

(E) pseudoephedrine

16. The presentation of a confused diaphoretic patient with miosis, abdominal cramping, fecal and urinary incontinence, profuse sweating, and drooling would cause you to be most concerned about which of the following toxic ingestions?

(A) opioids

(B) organophosphates

(C) cocaine

(D) ethanol

(E) ephedra

17. Which of the following signs and symptoms is not consistent with an anticholinergic toxic syndrome?

(A) tachycardia

(B) dry, flushed skin

(C) urinary retention

(D) miosis

(E) slightly elevated temperature

18. Which of the following pairs of toxins and antidotes does not match?

(A) opiates and naloxone

(B) benzodiazepines and flumazenil

(C) methanol and ethanol

(D) salicylates and N-acetylcysteine

(E) iron and deferoxamine

Answers

1. **(D)** The AAP no longer recommends syrup of ipecac be stored in a household for emergency use.

2. **(B)** Decreases in the death rate are attributable to safer medications and product reformulations, not the OTC availability.

3. **(C)** The amount of substance removed from the stomach is inversely related to time between ingestion and emesis. In theory, immediate administration of ipecac will result in greater, but not complete, removal of the ingested toxin from the stomach.

4. **(E)** Currently there is no recommended use in the home or in the emergency department for the administration of an emetic such as syrup of ipecac. Lethargy and vomiting are both noted contraindications because of the risk of aspiration. Induction of vomiting can actually decrease the effectiveness of activated charcoal or *N*-acetylcysteine in the presence of ongoing emesis.

5. **(B)** The current recommendation to use activated charcoal (AC) alone for GI decontamination without the use of a gastric emptying technique such as gastric lavage or syrup of ipecac has demonstrated similar or superior results. Sorbitol speeds AC clearance but does not improve efficacy. The risks of aspiration are largely avoided when AC only is used.

6. **(A)** The highest priority in the management of any acutely ill patient is the evaluation and support of airway, breathing, and circulation.

7. **(A)** Simply detecting the presence of the drug ingested is not as helpful as the actual serum measurement of the drug level. Drug screens are helpful in detecting the presence of other ingested substances.

8. **(D)** The need for gastric lavage in isolated acetaminophen overdose is rare because of the very rapid GI adsorption of acetaminophen. Activated charcoal will effectively adsorb acetaminophen and is ideally given in the first 4 hours (up to 6 to 8 hours) postingestion. *N*-acetylcysteine is an effective antidote that should be given ideally up to 8 hours postingestion.

9. **(C)** Ions, hydrocarbons, metals such as iron, and ethanol do not adsorb. Whole bowel irrigation may be considered.

10. **(B)** Hepatotoxicity is of greatest concern because hepatic metabolism accounts for up to 90% of acetaminophen elimination. It is important to note that in acute toxicity, liver injury usually presents 24 to 48 hours postingestion. Acetaminophen ingestions >150 mg/kg are associated with highest risk of hepatotoxicity.

11. **(B)** Delays in diagnosis and failure to institute treatment measures are associated with poorer outcomes. Because the early symptoms seen in stage 1 are non-specific, a heightened awareness of the potential for toxicity and the recognition of patients at risk for toxicity are vital.

12. **(A)** Unlike acetaminophen toxicity, NSAID overdoses do follow fairly benign courses. Children who ingest >300 mg/kg should have GI decontamination, evaluation and observation. High-protein binding causes urinary alkalinization, hemoperfusion and hemodialysis to be ineffective in enhancing elimination (dialysis is used in salicylate intoxication). GI side effects are the most common side effects in general that are associated with the use of NSAIDs.

13. **(E)** Bleach is non-toxic. Antidiarrheal products tend to contain salicylates. Both salicylates and ibuprofen tend to cause significant renal impairment. Many mouthwash products contain ethanol that can cause hypoglycemia. A multivitamin overdose can lead to multiple organ system impairment.

14. **(D)** The transfer of caustic substances to unlabeled or erroneously labeled containers is an associated risk factor for potential ingestion by a child.

15. **(A)** An opioid overdose results in global depression with a depressed sensorium as the hallmark.

16. **(B)** This scenario describes the cholinergic syndrome seen in organophosphate poisoning. A useful mnemonic to remember is "SLUDGE": salivation, lacrimation, urination, defecation, GI cramping, and emesis. Exposure sometimes occurs through unsuspected dermal exposure. Organophosphates are found in many pesticides and insecticides as well as drugs such as neostigmine and physostigmine.

17. **(D)** The anticholinergic effects include all the following except miosis. Dilated pupils, or mydriasis is seen. Remember mad as a hatter, red as a beet, dry as a bone, and hot as a hare. Anticholinergics are found in drugs such as atropine as well as hallucinogenic mushrooms and plants such as jimson weed.

18. **(D)** *N*-acetylcysteine is the antidote used in acetaminophen toxicity.

SUGGESTED READING

Schneider S, Wax P: Caustics. In: Mark, J (ed): *Rosen's Emergency Medicine*, 5th ed., Vol 3. St. Louis, MO: Mosby, 2002, pp 2115–2119.

Kulig K: General Approach to the Poisoned Patient. In: Mark, J (ed): *Rosen's Emergency Medicine*, 5th ed., Vol 3. St. Louis, MO: Mosby, 2002, pp 2063–2068.

Bizovi K, Parker S, Smilkstein M: Acetaminophen. In: Mark, J (ed): *Rosen's Emergency Medicine*, 5th ed., Vol 3. St. Louis, MO: Mosby, 2002, pp 2069–2075.

Seger D. Murray L. Aspirina and Nonsteroidal Agents. In: Mark, J (ed): *Rosen's Emergency Medicine*, 5th ed., Vol 3. St. Louis, MO: Mosby, 2002, pp 2076–2081.

AAP Policy Statement. Poison treatment in the home. *Pediatrics* 112(5):1182–1185, 2003.

AAP Committee on Drugs. Acetaminophen toxicity in children. *Pediatrics* 108(4):1020–1024, 2001.

Abbruzzi G. Pediatric toxicologic concerns. *Emerg Med Clin N Am* 20(1): 223–247, 2002.

10

Genetics

CASE 80: A NEWBORN WITH A HEART DEFECT AND DYSMORPHIC FEATURES

A newborn is evaluated in the regular nursery. The child was born full-term to a 39-year-old mother by a normal spontaneous vaginal delivery. A prenatal ultrasound showed the presence of a congenital heart defect most likely an atrioventricular (AV) canal defect. The family elected not to have prenatal testing. The family history is otherwise negative.

On physical examination the vital signs are within normal limits. Brachycephaly, up-slanted palpebral fissures, epicanthal folds, protruding tongue, and generalized hypotonia with otherwise normal neurologic exam are noted.

SELECT THE ONE BEST ANSWER

1. The most likely diagnosis for this child is?

   (A) trisomy 13
   (B) trisomy 18
   (C) Down syndrome
   (D) Treacher Collins syndrome
   (E) Holt-Oram syndrome

2. Which of the following is not a common feature of Down syndrome in the newborn infant?

   (A) small low-set ears with over-folded upper helix
   (B) transverse palmar (simian) crease
   (C) increased gap between toes 1 and 2
   (D) rocker bottom feet
   (E) excess nuchal skin fold

3. Which of the following investigations does not need to be considered in a newborn suspected of having Down syndrome?

   (A) echocardiogram
   (B) thyroid testing
   (C) complete blood count
   (D) renal ultrasound
   (E) none of these is necessary

4. Karyotype to determine the chromosomal basis of Down syndrome is essential for which of the following reasons?

   (A) Confirming the diagnosis as the clinical features of Down syndrome can be difficult to recognize in some newborns and can overlap with other conditions.
   (B) Karyotype is not essential in the evaluation for a child with Down syndrome.
   (C) Allows appropriate counseling regarding recurrence risks for the parents.
   (D) Helpful in assigning gender in a child with Down syndrome.
   (E) A and C.

5. Results of chromosome analysis show an unbalanced Robertsonian translocation between the long arm of chromosome 14 and 21: 46,XY, der,(14;21)(q10;q10). Part of the family counseling should include which of the following with regard to this chromosomal rearrangement?

(A) Parents should be offered chromosome analysis to see if they are carriers of a balanced Robertsonian translocation.

(B) Advise not to have any more children.

(C) Counseling that this is not really Down syndrome, as that only applies to trisomy 21.

(D) Children with unbalanced Robertsonian translocations as the cause of Down syndrome are less severely affected.

(E) None of the above.

6. All of the following are associated medical problems in children with Down syndrome except:

(A) hearing loss

(B) polycystic kidneys

(C) eye problems

(D) atlantoaxial instability

(E) sleep apnea

7. Which of the following best describes the expected intelligence and personality of a child with Down syndrome?

(A) All have severe mental retardation with IQ in the range of 30 to 40.

(B) IQ range of 35 to 65 with a mean of 54, and occasionally higher.

(C) Aggressive and violent, prefer to be alone and have little social interactions.

(D) Affectionate and docile, tend toward mimicry, enjoy music, and have a good sense of rhythm, poor coordination.

(E) B and D.

8. The most common cause of trisomy 21 is:

(A) maternal non-disjunction at meiosis I with increasing risk associated with advanced maternal age

(B) non-disjunction associated with advanced paternal age

(C) mosaicism

(D) sporadic events unrelated to maternal age

(E) environmental exposures

9. What is the overall recurrence risk for Down syndrome because of trisomy 21 (as opposed to an unbalanced translocation)?

(A) One percent in women younger than 40 years of age and age-related risk for women older than 40 years of age

(B) Age-related risk

(C) 10% in women under 35 and age-related risk in women older than 35

(D) The same as the population risk

(E) None of the above

10. Which of the following are features of trisomy 13?

(A) microophthalmia, cleft lip and palate, polydactyly, holoprosencephaly

(B) up-slanting palpebral fissures, epicanthal folds, clinodactyly

(C) hypotonia, rocker bottom feet, clenched hand, low set malformed ears

(D) obesity, hypogenitalism, almond shaped eyes, small hands and feet

(E) supravalvular aortic stenosis, hypercalcemia, short stature

11. All of the following are features of trisomy 18 except:

(A) small palpebral fissures

(B) clenched hand

(C) hypoplastic nails

(D) protruding tongue, large cheeks

(E) cardiac defect

12. Which of the following modalities can be used for screening/testing for Down syndrome?

(A) amniocentesis

(B) chorionic villus sampling

(C) maternal serum screening

(D) prenatal ultrasonography

(E) all of the above

13. A newborn is evaluated in the nursery. Pregnancy was complicated by a prenatal ultrasound that showed coarctation of the aorta. This female infant was delivered at term by normal spontaneous vaginal delivery. On physical examination the baby is noted to have lymphedema of the feet and hands, webbed neck, and shield chest. The most likely diagnosis to explain the features is?

(A) Down syndrome

(B) Klinefelter syndrome

(C) Turner syndrome

(D) Williams syndrome
(E) Marfan syndrome

14. Which of the following medical problems are not associated with Turner syndrome?

(A) coarctation of the aorta
(B) agenesis of the corpus callosum
(C) horseshoe kidney
(D) premature gonadal failure
(E) hypothyroidism

15. Standard treatment of growth failure in Turner syndrome includes:

(A) leg-lengthening procedures
(B) maximizing caloric intake
(C) estrogen replacement
(D) recombinant human growth hormone
(E) none of the above

16. Which of the following is true regarding Noonan syndrome?

(A) Noonan affects only males.
(B) Noonan syndrome is the result of a sex chromosome abnormality.
(C) The clinical features of Noonan syndrome have significant overlap with those of Turner syndrome.
(D) Noonan syndrome is not a genetic condition.
(E) None of the above are true.

17. An 8-year-old boy is noted to be tall, have gynecomastia, underdeveloped secondary sexual characteristics, and have small testes. The most likely diagnosis is:

(A) Noonan syndrome
(B) Marfan syndrome
(C) Klinefelter syndrome (47,XXY)
(D) 47,XYY
(E) mosaic trisomy 8

Answers

1. **(C)** The features described are most consistent with Down syndrome. Treacher Collins syndrome, also known as mandibulofacial dysostosis, is associated with defects of the lower eyelids, mandibular and malar hypoplasia, microtia and dysplastic ears, and hearing loss. Holt-Oram is associated with congenital heart defect, most often ASD or VSD, and upper limb abnormalities.

2. **(D)** Common newborn features of Down syndrome include those in the question and mild microcephaly, flat occiput, brachycephaly, up-slanting palpebral fissures, epicanthal folds, Brushfield spots, protruding tongue, low flat nasal bridge, clinodactyly 5th digit, transverse palmar crease and short stature. Rocker bottom feet is a common feature of trisomy 18.

3. **(D)** The medical problems listed need to be screened for in all individuals suspected of having Down syndrome independent of symptoms except a renal ultrasound. Congenital heart defects are present in 40% to 45% and not all are recognizable by physical examination. Fifteen percent to twenty percent of individuals will have hypothyroidism which can be present at birth or develop during the lifetime of the individual. Polycythemia, thrombocytopenia, and leukocytosis (with occasional myeloproliferative disorders) are common in newborns. Additional problems which should be remembered in the newborn period but do not necessarily require screening if there are no associated symptoms include intestinal abnormalities (esophageal or duodenal atresia, Hirschsprung disease), and cataracts. The incidence of renal malformations in Down syndrome is not significantly higher than the general population risk.

4. **(E)** Karyotype is helpful in confirming the clinical suspicion. The most important reason, however, is for counseling regarding recurrence risks. Trisomy 21 has low recurrence risk (either based on maternal age or 1%, whichever is higher) whereas an unbalanced translocation may be inherited from a balanced translocation carrier parent and the recurrence risk may be as high as 100% depending on the translocation.

5. **(A)** Robertsonian translocations involve acrocentric chromosomes (the acrocentric chromosomes are 13,14,15,21,22) and unbalanced rearrangements that include chromosome 21 account for 3.3% of all cases of Down syndrome. One-third of these cases are inherited from a parent with a balanced translocation and two-thirds are de novo

events in the infant. The term Down syndrome applies to individuals with the recognizable clinical phenotype described and does not imply a specific genetic mechanism. There is no clinical distinction between patients with trisomy 21 (three full copies of chromosome 21) and translocation cases.

6. **(B)** Sixty percent to eighty percent of children with Down syndrome have hearing deficits. Eye problems may include cataracts, strabismus, myopia, and so on. Fifteen percent will have atlantoaxial instability, although most are asymptomatic, one percent to two percent will require surgical correction. Other skeletal problems include patella and hip dislocation. Other medical problems in addition to those listed in question 3 include nutrition (failure to thrive in infancy and obesity in older children and adults), leukemia, seizure disorders, sleep apnea, delayed eruption of teeth, and Alzheimer disease.

7. **(E)** Intelligence is variable and cannot be readily predicted by any reliable factor. Research has shown that early intervention, environmental enrichment, and assistance to the families will result in progress that is usually not achieved by those children who have not had such educational and stimulating experiences. Intelligence deteriorates in adulthood, with clinical and pathological findings consistent with advanced Alzheimer disease. Although most children and adults have the friendly, docile personality described, 13% will have serious emotional problems including depression.

8. **(A)** Most cases of Down syndrome involve non-disjunction of maternal meiosis I, which may be related to the time from meiotic arrest between oocyte development in the fetus and ovulation. There is an increased risk for non-disjunction associated with advanced maternal age (maternal age 30: 1:1000 risk of Down syndrome; age 35: 1:365 risk; age 40: 1:100 risk; age 45: 1:50 risk). The risk is for non-disjunction of any chromosome but trisomy 21, 13, and 18 are the only trisomies that can result in live born children and the rest tend to result in miscarriage. There is no association between Down syndrome and environmental exposures in the mother. There is no proven increased risk for trisomy with advanced paternal age, but there is an increased risk of new mutation

in advanced paternal age. Mosaicism refers to the finding of two different cell lines in an individual. There are individuals with mosaic Down syndrome meaning they have some cells with trisomy 21 and some cell lines with normal chromosome number. Mosaicism may be associated with a milder phenotype.

9. **(A)** The incidence of Down syndrome is approximately 1.0 to 1.2/1000 live births. The recurrence risk in chromosomally normal parents is 1% until the age-related risk becomes higher than 1% (older than 40 years of age). Although the individual risk for Down syndrome is higher in older women, only 20% of all babies with Down syndrome are born to women older than the age of 35 as they account for only about 5% of all pregnancies. If the mother carries a balanced translocation, the recurrence risk is 10% and if the father is the carrier then the recurrence risk is 3% to 5%.

10. **(A)** See Table 80-1. The features described in answer B are most consistent with Down syndrome, those in C with trisomy 18, those in D with Prader-Willi syndrome and those in E with Williams syndrome.

11. **(D)** See Table 80-1. Protruding tongue and large cheeks are seen in Down syndrome.

12. **(E)** Amniocentesis and chorionic villus sampling (CVS) can both be used to obtain a prenatal karyotype to determine the presence of a trisomy or other chromosomal abnormality. CVS is done between 10 to 12 weeks of gestation and has a 1:100 risk of miscarriage, while amniocentesis is done at 16 weeks of gestation and has a 1:200 risk of miscarriage. Maternal serum screening results of low levels of α-fetoprotein and unconjugated estriol, and elevated levels of human chorionic gonadotropin are associated with an increased risk of Down syndrome. Ultrasound can detect major fetal anomalies as early as 16 weeks of gestation and those associated with increased risk for the presence of Down syndrome include increased nuchal thickening, congenital heart defects, duodenal atresia, and echogenic bowel.

13. **(C)** Turner syndrome has the karyotype 45,X and occurs in 1/8000 live births. Commonly associ-

Table 80-1. CLINICAL FEATURES OF COMMON AUTOSOMAL TRISOMIES

	Trisomy 21 Down Syndrome	Trisomy 18 Edward Syndrome	Trisomy 13 Patau Syndrome
Incidence	1/800	1/8000	1/5000
Head shape	Microcephaly, brachycephaly, 3 fontanels	Microcephaly	Microcephaly, cutis aplasia, sloping forehead
Eyes	Up-slanting palpebral fissures, epicanthal folds, Brushfield spots	Short palpebral fissures, corneal opacity	Microophthalmia, hypotelorism, coloboma
Ears	Small, low set	Low set, dysplastic	Low set, dysplastic
Facial dysmorphic features	Protruding tongue, low flat nasal bridge	Small oral opening, micrognathia	Cleft lip and palate (60%–80%)
Extremities	Clinodactyly of 5th finger, simian crease, short metacarpals, wide gap between 1st and 2nd toe	Overlapping clenched fingers, hypoplastic nails, rocker bottom feet	Postaxial polydactyly hands and/or feet, hypoconvex nails
Cardiac defect	40% (AV canal most common)	60%	80%
Kidney malformations		Polycystic kidney, horseshoe kidney	Polycystic kidney, duplicated ureters
Genitalia	Small penis, hypogonadism	Cryptorchidism, hypoplasia labia majora, prominent clitoris	Cryptorchidism, bicornuate uterus
Neurological findings	Hypotonia, mild to moderate mental retardation	Feeble fetal activity, weak cry, postneonatal hypertonia, severe mental defect	Hypo- or hypertonia, holoprosencephaly, seizures, apnea, severe mental defect
Dentition	Delayed eruption of teeth		

ated features include short stature, webbed neck, low posterior hairline, shield chest, lymphedema of the extremities, cubitus valgus of elbow, and short fourth metacarpal and/or metatarsal. The physical phenotype is highly variable and often normal with the exception of short stature, which is typically not present at birth with a mean length of 146 cm (5th percentile). Approximately one-third of girls with Turner syndrome are diagnosed at birth because of lymphedema, one-third are diagnosed between ages 5 and 10 because of short stature, and one-third are diagnosed secondary to delay or absence of puberty.

14. **(B)** The medical complications are highly variable with respect to severity and frequency and do not correlate with karyotype findings. Clinical manifestations include feeding problems in the newborn period, short stature, coarctation of the aorta, and/or bicuspid aortic valve (present in 17% to 45%), hypertension, mitral valve prolapse, hypothyroidism (occurring in 15% to 30%

of adults), gonadal dysgenesis (90% will require estrogen to initiate puberty and complete growth and estrogen and progesterone to maintain menses), ocular problems (strabismus), recurrent otitis media, and structural renal malformations in 40% (renal agenesis, horseshoe kidney, duplication of the collecting system, ureteropelvic and uretero vesicular obstruction). Cerebral findings include arteriovenous malformations but not agenesis of the corpus callosum or other structural brain malformations.

15. **(D)** Treatment with recombinant human growth hormone (GH) is effective in increasing height velocity. Many girls will achieve heights of 150 cm or more with early initiation of treatment. Girls should be followed closely by an endocrinologist to track growth velocity to determine the optimal time to initiate GH. Children with Turner syndrome may have excessive weight gain and careful monitoring of nutrition is essential to prevent obesity.

16. **(C)** Noonan syndrome is an autosomal dominant condition with 50% of patients having a mutation in the *PTPN11* gene on chromosome 12q24.1. Noonan syndrome is seen in boys and girls with equal frequency. It is often mistakenly referred to as male Turner syndrome because of the overlapping features. In both Noonan and Turner syndromes, patients have short stature, webbed neck, cardiac defects (coarctation of the aorta in Turner and pulmonary stenosis in Noonan), low posterior hairline, shield chest, wide spaced nipples, and edema of the hands and feet.

17. **(C)** Klinefelter is caused by a sex chromosome abnormality, 47,XXY and occurs with a frequency of 1:600 male live births. Common clinical features include tall stature which becomes evident by 5 years of age (newborns have normal growth parameters), eunuchoid habitus, slightly delayed motor and language milestones with IQ of 80 to 100, delayed sexual development, and infertility. The most frequently observed personality characteristics are shyness, non-assertiveness, immaturity, and lacking in confidence. Noonan syndrome has features that overlap with Turner syndrome and can occur in both boys and girls. Marfan is characterized by aortic root dilation, subluxed lens of the eye, and marfanoid body habitus. 47,XYY is characterized by tall stature, severe acne, normal IQ with more aggressive behavior and behavioral problems, and normal testes size and function.

SUGGESTED READING

Cohen WI, ed: Health Care Guidelines for Individuals with Down Syndrome: 1999 revision. 1999 Available at: http://www.denison.edu/collaborations/dsq/health99. Last accessed 6/5/2006.

Cassidy SB, Allanson JE, et al: *Management of Genetic Syndromes*. New York, Wiley-Liss, 2001.

CASE 81: AN INFANT WITH HYPOGLYCEMIA

A 7-month-old girl presents with lethargy, diaphoresis, pallor, and tachycardia. The mom states the child had a viral infection yesterday, had emesis one time, and did not eat very well. The girl went to bed without eating dinner, and this morning the family had a difficult time arousing her and brought her straight to the office. She has no history of other health problems in the past. The family history is significant for two healthy siblings and one sibling who died at 4 months of sudden infant death syndrome (SIDS).

On examination the vital signs show respiratory rate of 60, heart rate of 160 bpm, and blood pressure of 90/50 mm Hg. You note diaphoresis, pallor, and the child is lethargic and difficult to arouse.

SELECT THE ONE BEST ANSWER

1. Immediate investigations should include?

    (A) CT scan of brain
    (B) chest radiograph
    (C) complete blood count
    (D) blood cultures
    (E) glucose measurement by glucose oxidase reagent strip

2. The glucose oxidase reagent strip reveals a glucose of 30. The next most appropriate step in management is?

    (A) Consult an endocrinologist for advice on how to evaluate the hypoglycemia.
    (B) Intravenous dextrose 25% at a dose of 2–4 ml/kg.
    (C) Oral glucose replacement with orange juice.
    (D) Immediate intubation and mechanical ventilation.
    (E) Call for newborn screen results.

3. When starting the IV for glucose replacement, which of the following laboratory investigations are important in determining the underlying etiology of the hypoglycemia?

    (A) electrolytes, BUN, Cr, plasma glucose, liver profile, complete blood count
    (B) urine and/or serum ketones
    (C) endocrinology labs including cortisol, insulin, C-peptide, growth hormone
    (D) carnitine levels, acylcarnitine profile, urine organic acids, serum amino acids, and lactate level
    (E) all of the above

4. The initial results of laboratories are as follows: sodium 139 mEq/L, potassium 4.5 mEq/L, chloride 107 mEq/L, bicarbonate 17 mEq/L, glucose 32 mg/dL, urine ketones negative, serum ketones negative, aspartate aminotransferase (SGOT) 257 U/L, alanine aminotransferase (SGPT) 205 U/L.

The remaining labs are unremarkable. The most likely diagnosis given this information is?

(A) medium chain acyl-CoA dehydrogenase (MCAD)
(B) hyperinsulinism
(C) salicylate poisoning
(D) galactosemia
(E) physiologic ketotic hypoglycemia

5. What other additional history or physical findings in this case are consistent with MCAD?

(A) prolonged fast
(B) diaphoresis and lethargy
(C) family history of SIDS
(D) history of vomiting
(E) A and C

6. How would you counsel the family about other siblings and recurrence risks for future children?

(A) Siblings and future children are at 5% risk for MCAD.
(B) Siblings and future children are at 25% risk for MCAD.
(C) Siblings and future children are at 50% risk for MCAD.
(D) Siblings and future children are at <1% risk for MCAD.
(E) Only girls are at 50% risk; boys are not affected.

7. If this patient had hepatomegaly without splenomegaly, retarded growth, poorly developed musculature, hyperlipidemia, and hypercholesterolemia, the most likely diagnosis would be?

(A) insulin-induced hypoglycemia
(B) growth hormone deficiency
(C) fatty acid oxidation defect.
(D) glycogen storage disorder
(E) none of the above

8. Which of the following symptoms would be suspicious for galactosemia as a cause of the hypoglycemia?

(A) vomiting and jaundice
(B) *E. coli* sepsis
(C) hepatomegaly with elevated transaminases
(D) renal Fanconi syndrome
(E) all of the above

9. All of the following regarding the long-term complications of galactosemia are true except:

(A) include deficits in speech and language
(B) may be present even if appropriate treatment is initiated early
(C) include pseudotumor cerebri
(D) include liver failure
(E) include hypergonadotropic hypogonadism in females

10. Results of the laboratory screening of the child in case 1 show: sodium 139 mEq/L, potassium 4.5 mEq/L, chloride 107 mEq/L, bicarbonate 7 mEq/L, glucose 32 mg/dL, urine and serum ketones markedly positive, lactate of 7.2 mEq/L, ammonia level of 550 μmol/L, WBC of 4.2, and platelet count of 75. The most likely diagnosis would be?

(A) fatty acid oxidation defect
(B) urea cycle defect
(C) organic acidemia
(D) glycogen storage disorder
(E) none of the above

11. If an organic acidemia is suspected, what type of vitamin therapies should be considered?

(A) vitamin B_{12} (1 mg) intramuscularly
(B) multivitamin
(C) biotin (10 mg) orally or via nasogastric tube
(D) CoQ10
(E) A and C

12. Which of the following would be suspicious of a urea cycle defect?

(A) synthetic liver dysfunction with normal liver transaminases
(B) vomiting, lethargy and tachypnea
(C) respiratory alkalosis, with ammonia level of 1500 μmol/L
(D) large spleen and liver, hypercholesterolemia, and hypoglycemia
(E) no difference between organic acidemias, and urea cycle defects

13. If a urea cycle defect is suspected, appropriate treatments would include all of the following except?

(A) removal of protein source
(B) intravenous glucose

(C) carnitine supplementation

(D) hemodialysis

(E) suspicion and possible treatment for cerebral edema

14. Jaundice and liver dysfunction may be the presenting symptoms of which of the following inherited metabolic disorders?

(A) galactosemia

(B) tyrosinemia

(C) α_1-antitrypsin deficiency

(D) neonatal hemochromatosis

(E) all of the above

15. Which of the following are not true regarding phenylketonuria (PKU)?

(A) PKU is an autosomal dominant disorder.

(B) PKU is a disorder of phenylalanine metabolism.

(C) Untreated PKU leads to severe mental retardation (IQ 50) and seizures.

(D) PKU is not easily recognized in a newborn infant.

(E) Mental retardation because of PKU is rare because of newborn screening.

16. The treatment of PKU is characterized by?

(A) restriction of dietary phenylalanine

(B) must avoid fruits and vegetables that have high phenylalanine content

(C) careful monitoring of phenylalanine and tyrosine metabolism

(D) phenylalanine-free formulas are only needed during the first year of life

(E) A and C

17. Which of the following are true regarding the long-term management of PKU?

(A) Dietary restriction of phenylalanine may be discontinued after 8 years of age.

(B) There is no further loss of IQ in untreated PKU after 6 to 10 years of age.

(C) The outcome of pregnancy in untreated mothers with PKU leads to severe mental retardation, microcephaly, and birth defects in offspring.

(D) Dietary treatment during pregnancy eliminates the risks associated with maternal PKU.

(E) All of the above.

Answers

1. **(E)** The clinical features of hypoglycemia include irritability, pallor, cyanosis, tachycardia, tremors, lethargy, apnea, seizures, diaphoresis, anxiety, headache, tachypnea, weakness, confusion, stupor, ataxia, and coma. When a patient presents with these features, a glucose determination by oxidase reagent strip is indicated while the child is being stabilized and other investigations (such as the other options listed) are being considered and organized.

2. **(B)** Determining the underlying etiology of the hypoglycemia is of utmost importance but should not interfere with the primary goal of treatment with glucose. Prolonged exposure to hypoglycemia may result in irreversible brain damage and eventually death. Patients with symptoms and glucose <45 mg/dL, and/or glucose of 25 to 35 mg/dL irrespective of symptoms, require treatment. Intravenous glucose is the first line of therapy. Glucose is administered in a dose of 0.5 g/kg/dose. Dextrose 25% at a dose 2 to 4 mL/kg is appropriate. In neonates and preterm infants, dextrose 10% at a dose of 5 to 10 mL/kg/dose is used to avoid sudden hyperosmolarity. In older children and adolescents, dextrose 50% at a dose of 1 to 2 mL/kg/dose is used. Patients with mild hypoglycemia who are capable of eating or drinking are treated with orange juice or some other age-appropriate source of oral glucose.

3. **(E)** The differential diagnosis for hypoglycemia includes metabolic diseases, endocrine disorders, poisoning, liver disease, and systemic disorders. The initial laboratory data is crucial in refining the diagnostic possibilities. The endocrine causes of hypoglycemia can be determined by the tests mentioned and are maximally useful when obtained at the time of the hypoglycemia. The metabolic diagnosis leading to hypoglycemia can be categorized based on hepatomegaly, presence or absence of ketones, and studies that reflect fat, protein, and carbohydrate metabolism. The metabolic labs are still useful even if obtained within

Table 81-1. INBORN ERRORS OF METABOLISM AND CHARACTERISTIC LABORATORY FINDINGS

Disorders	Laboratory Findings
Fatty acid oxidation defects (includes MCAD, LCHAD, VLCAD)	Metabolic acidosis; elevated liver transaminases; hyperammonemia; non-ketotic hypoglycemia; carnitine deficiency, abnormal urine organic acids
Galactosemia	Positive urine reducing substances; conjugated hyperbilirubinemia; liver dysfunction with elevated transaminases; hypoglycemia
Glycogen Storage Disorders	Hypercholesterolemia, hyperlipidemia, lactic acidosis, elevated uric acid, hypoglycemia
Organic acidemias (includes MMA, PA, IVA, MCD)	Metabolic acidosis with increased anion gap; elevated plasma and urine ketones; variably elevated plasma ammonia and lactate; abnormal urine organic acids
Urea cycle defects	Variable respiratory alkalosis; no metabolic acidosis; markedly elevated plasma ammonia; elevated orotic acid in OTC; abnormal plasma amino acids
Maple syrup urine disease	Metabolic acidosis with increased anion gap; elevated plasma and urine ketones; abnormal plasma amino acids
Tyrosinemia	Synthetic dysfunction of the liver with normal transaminases; succinylacetone in urine organic acids; abnormal plasma amino acids; generalized aminoaciduria

MCAD, medium chain acyl CoA dehydrogenase; LCHAD, long chain hydroxyacyl CoA dehydrogenase; VLCAD, very long chain acyl CoA dehydrogenase; MMA, methylmalonic acidemia; PA, propionic acidemia; IVA, isovaleric acidemia; MCD, multiple carboxylase deficiency; OTC, ornithine transcarbamylase deficiency.

the first few hours after the hypoglycemia. They can be misleading, however, if done days after recovery; and in some diseases, the diagnostic metabolites will clear with time.

4. **(A)** MCAD is the most common of the fatty acid oxidation disorders, which are characterized by non-ketotic hypoglycemia, with mild acidosis. Other findings may include elevated liver transaminases, mild elevation of lactate, hepatomegaly, elevated creatine phosphokinase (CPK), carnitine deficiency and evidence of medium-chain dicarboxylic aciduria on urine organic acid or acylcarnitine analysis (Table 81-1). Hyperinsulinism typically presents at an earlier age with non-ketotic hypoglycemia, no acidosis or liver abnormalities, and hypoglycemia occurs after a short fast. Salicylate poisoning has an elevated anion gap acidosis. Galactosemia typically has more significant liver abnormalities with conjugated hyperbilirubinemia. Physiologic ketotic hypoglycemia has significant ketosis.

5. **(E)** The risk for hypoglycemia in fatty acid oxidation disorders is highest after a prolonged fast, especially during times of intercurrent viral illness. The symptoms of diaphoresis, lethargy, and vomiting are non-specific and signs of the hypoglycemia or viral illness and not the specific underlying disease. A family history of SIDS should raise the suspicion for an inherited inborn error of metabolism. Many metabolic conditions go unrecognized at the time of presentation and are diagnosed as SIDS or Reye syndrome.

6. **(B)** With few exceptions, inborn errors of metabolism, including fatty acid oxidation defects, are inherited in an autosomal recessive pattern. Therefore, the parents of the affected child should be counseled that there is a 25% (one-fourth) risk of recurrence for the condition with each additional pregnancy, and unaffected children are at a two-thirds risk of being carriers. There are several conditions (Hunter syndrome, ornithine transcarbamylase deficiency, and Lesch-Nyhan syndrome) associated with X-linked inheritance patterns, where boys are typically affected and females may be asymptomatic carriers, but because of X-inactivation patterns, girls may be mildly to severely affected as well.

7. **(D)** There are several types of glycogen storage disorder and they can present with different clinical features, and it is difficult to differentiate be-

tween them on a purely clinical basis. These disorders result in hypoglycemia because of the inability to break down stored glycogen, with resulting medical problems listed in the question. Insulin-induced hypoglycemia would not result in lipid abnormalities or hepatomegaly, and would give non-ketotic hypoglycemia. Growth hormone deficiency will have growth retardation and hypoglycemia, but may be associated with micropenis and does not have the lipid abnormalities or hepatomegaly. Fatty acid oxidation defects were discussed above.

8. **(E)** Galactosemia is an inborn error of carbohydrate metabolism that results from deficiency of galactose-1-phosphate uridyl transferase, and is part of most newborn screening programs. Manifestations (Table 81-1) usually appear within days of the initiation of milk feedings and may have onset prior to newborn screen results. Any newborn patient with liver dysfunction including cirrhosis, hepatomegaly, cataracts, renal Fanconi syndrome (renal tubular glycosuria, generalized aminoaciduria, proteinuria), presence of urine reducing substance and especially *E. coli* sepsis should have consideration for possible galactosemia.

9. **(D)** Treatment of galactosemia involves restriction of galactose in the diet, mostly by exclusion of milk and its products. The earlier the treatment is initiated, the better for the long-term prognosis. Despite treatment, milder manifestations of the symptoms may be present; especially problems in school even with normal IQ levels, and close follow-up of growth and development are indicated. Liver failure may be present in the initial presentation of galactosemia but typically resolves with treatment and is not a long term complication.

10. **(C)** The characteristic findings for organic acidemia (Table 81-1) include significant anion gap acidosis, ketosis, variable elevations in lactate and ammonia, neutropenia, and thrombocytopenia. Urine organic acid analysis will typically reveal the main anion contributing to the acidosis and the diagnosis. All protein feeds should be stopped and the child should be given liberal amounts of intravenous glucose while the results of the laboratory tests are pending. Intravenous bicarbonate

should be administered and because of the ongoing organic acid production may require large amounts. Dialysis should be considered for severely acidotic neonates.

11. **(E)** When an organic acidemia is suspected, vitamin B_{12} and biotin should be given in case the patient has a B_{12} responsive form of methylmalonic acidemia or multiple carboxylase deficiency, which is sometimes responsive to biotin. A multivitamin is not useful in this case, and CoQ10 is typically used for children with forms of mitochondrial defects.

12. **(C)** Hyperammonemia is a common finding in many inborn errors of metabolism including organic acidemias and urea cycle defects. Urea cycle defects are characterized by significant hyperammonemia (typically >1000 μmol/L) and respiratory alkalosis in the early presentation, where organic acidemias usually have severe metabolic acidosis (Table 81-1). Plasma amino acid analysis and urine orotic acid are useful in differentiation of the types of urea cycle defects, which is important to distinguish direct therapies. Synthetic liver dysfunction with normal transaminases suggest tyrosinemia, vomiting, lethargy, and tachypnea, which are non-specific features, and a large spleen and liver with hypercholesterolemia and hypoglycemia suggestive of a glycogen storage disorder.

13. **(C)** Immediate treatment should include removal of all sources of protein, and in cases of severe hyperammonemia hemodialysis (as opposed to peritoneal dialysis, continuous arteriovenous hemoperfusion, and exchange transfusion) is the most efficient way to remove the ammonia. Cerebral edema is common in urea cycle defects and should be treated aggressively. Carnitine is used in the treatment of fatty acid oxidation defects but not in urea cycle defects.

14. **(E)** Tyrosinemia should be considered in any child who presents with liver disease in early infancy and is characterized by elevations of tyrosine and methionine with generalized aminoaciduria (Table 81-1). α_1-Antitrypsin deficiency may present with clinical manifestations similar to neonatal or giant cell hepatitis. Neonatal hemochromatosis is a poorly understood disorder with an associated

fulminating course and hepatic and extrahepatic parenchymal iron deposition.

15. **(A)** Phenylketonuria (PKU) is an inborn error of phenylalanine (phe) metabolism most often because of deficiency of the enzyme phenylalanine hydroxylase, which converts phe into tyrosine. Newborns with PKU have a normal examination and the diagnosis is not evident until 6 to 12 months of age when the symptoms of mental retardation, seizures, spasticity, and hypopigmentation are evident. Screening for PKU is a part of all newborn screening programs and has been successful in early identification and treatment which has virtually eliminated the severe clinical manifestations. PKU is inherited in an autosomal recessive fashion with 25% risk of recurrence for siblings of an affected individual.

16. **(E)** Treatment of PKU involves dietary restriction of phe, and careful monitoring of phe and tyrosine levels. Fruits and vegetables are low in phe while high protein content foods are rich in phe. The use of phe free formulas are needed throughout life to provide adequate calories and other nutrition.

17. **(C)** Previous treatment recommendations suggested that the PKU diet could be safely discontinued at 5 or 6 years of age. Recent studies have shown that there is a uniform and progressive loss of IQ after stopping the diet leading to the current recommendations to continue the diet throughout life. The successful treatment of PKU has allowed affected individuals to become normal, functioning adults. Women with PKU are at risk during pregnancy of having children with severe mental retardation as a result of fetal exposure to high phenylalanine levels throughout pregnancy, even though the children do not typically have PKU themselves. Initiation of the diet prior to conception and continuing throughout pregnancy decreases, but does not eliminate, the potential for retardation, microcephaly and birth defects.

SUGGESTED READING

Burton B: Inborn errors of metabolism in infancy: A guide to diagnosis. *Pediatrics* 102:69, 1998.

Nyhan WL, Ozand PT et al: *Atlas of Metabolic Diseases.* London: Chapman & Hall Medical, 1998.

CASE 82: A NEWBORN WITH A VSD AND A THIN UPPER LIP

A newborn is evaluated for a heart murmur and found to have a ventricular septal defect (VSD). History is notable for lack of prenatal care. At the time of delivery ultrasound evaluation showed intrauterine growth retardation.

On examination the child is noted to have symmetric growth retardation, small palpebral fissures, thin upper lip, and underdeveloped philtrum.

SELECT THE ONE BEST ANSWER

1. The most likely diagnosis to explain these features is?

   (A) diabetic embryopathy
   (B) fetal alcohol syndrome
   (C) sporadic heart defects with familial features
   (D) chromosome anomaly
   (E) maternal smoking

2. Which of the following are common features of fetal alcohol syndrome?

   (A) microcephaly and mid-face hypoplasia
   (B) short palpebral fissures, epicanthal folds, ptosis, strabismus
   (C) hypoplastic philtrum with thin upper lip
   (D) mild to moderate mental retardation
   (E) all of the above

3. A child with VSD, sacral agenesis, rib and vertebral anomalies, femoral hypoplasia, and renal malformation is most likely the result of?

   (A) warfarin embryopathy
   (B) fetal alcohol syndrome
   (C) diabetic embryopathy
   (D) folic acid deficiency
   (E) chromosome abnormality

4. Which of the following are features of the fetal phenytoin sodium (Dilantin) syndrome?

   (A) caudal regression, sacral agenesis, renal defects, cardiac defects
   (B) spina bifida, craniofacial abnormalities
   (C) hypoplasia of midface, low nasal bridge, ocular hypertelorism, cleft lip and palate, and hypoplasia of distal phalanges with small nails

(D) intrauterine growth retardation (IUGR), microcephaly, mental retardation, birth defects such as congenital heart defects, and vertebral anomalies

(E) none of the above

5. A newborn with a severe degree of nasal hypoplasia, choanal atresia, microcephaly, optic atrophy, lag in skeletal maturation, and stippling of epiphyseal growth centers is characteristic of prenatal exposure to?

(A) antihistamine
(B) isotretinoin
(C) heparin
(D) warfarin
(E) hydantoin

6. A newborn is treated for a myelomeningocele. Counseling of the family regarding neural tube defects should include which of the following?

(A) no increased risk of recurrence for future children
(B) use of prenatal vitamins during all subsequent pregnancies
(C) twenty-five percent risk of recurrence for future children and prenatal thiamine
(D) three percent to 4% risk of recurrence for future children and use of 4 mg folate per day starting prior to conception
(E) fifty percent recurrence risk and use of 0.4 mg folate per day during pregnancy

7. Which of the following definitions is incorrect?

(A) Association: Relationship between birth defects and prenatal infections.
(B) Malformation: morphological defect of an organ from an intrinsically abnormal developmental process (congenital heart defect).
(C) Disruption: extrinsic destructive process that interferes with previously normal development (amniotic bands that cause amputation of finger).
(D) Deformation: extrinsic mechanical force that causes asymmetric abnormalities (breech position causing tibial bowing and club foot).
(E) Dysplasia: abnormal cellular organization or function that generally affects only a single tissue type (cartilage abnormalities that result in achondroplasia).

8. Strands of amniotic membrane (amniotic bands) may become dislodged and attach to various body parts and cause which of the following birth defects?

(A) cleft lip and/or palate
(B) ring-like constriction of limbs
(C) amputations of digits
(D) clefts of the face and eye
(E) all of the above

9. Premature closure of a cranial suture (craniosynostosis) can lead to alterations in symmetric head growth. Which of the following head shapes is not matched with the appropriate cranial suture closure?

(A) plagiocephaly: unilateral coronal synostosis
(B) dolichocephaly: sagittal synostosis
(C) turricephaly: bilateral coronal synostosis
(D) plagiocephaly: positional affect
(E) turricephaly: metopic suture synostosis

10. A newborn with vertebral anomalies, anal atresia, tracheoesophageal fistula, radioulnar synostosis, and horseshoe kidney most likely has?

(A) DiGeorge syndrome
(B) VATER association
(C) CHARGE association
(D) MURCS association
(E) Poland anomaly

11. A newborn with coloboma of the eye, heart defect, choanal atresia, and ambiguous genitalia most likely has?

(A) DiGeorge syndrome
(B) VATER association
(C) CHARGE association
(D) MURCS association
(E) Poland anomaly

12. A newborn with evidence of fetal compression leading to a squashed, flat face, clubbing of the feet, pulmonary hypoplasia, and breech presentation should have a detailed evaluation of which of the following organ systems?

(A) genitourinary system
(B) cardiovascular
(C) CNS

(D) dermatologic

(E) peripheral nervous system

13. Long-term management of Beckwith-Wiedemann syndrome includes?

(A) calcium monitoring and replacement

(B) routine renal ultrasounds and AFP measurements

(C) growth hormone replacement

(D) seizure precautions

(E) monitoring for development of cardiomyopathy

14. The most likely diagnosis in a child with hyperphagia resulting in morbid obesity, micropenis, short stature, small hands and feet, and hypotonia is?

(A) Angelman syndrome

(B) Beckwith-Wiedemann syndrome

(C) Prader-Willi syndrome

(D) Bardet-Biedl syndrome

(E) Sotos syndrome

15. The clinical features suggestive of 22q11 deletion (velocardiofacial, DiGeorge syndrome) include all of the following except?

(A) transverse palmar crease

(B) conotruncal heart defects

(C) hypoparathyroidism

(D) immune dysfunction

(E) velopharyngeal insufficiency

16. The best way to diagnose a microdeletion syndrome (e.g., Prader-Willi, Williams, and DiGeorge syndrome) is?

(A) routine karyotype

(B) FISH (fluorescence in situ hybridization)

(C) sequencing

(D) PCR (polymerase chain reaction)

(E) none of the above

Answers

1. **(B)** Most teratogenic drugs exert a deleterious effect in a minority of exposed fetuses. The features described are most consistent with fetal alcohol exposure. Diabetic embryopathy can cause heart defects, but do not lead to the dysmorphic features described or intrauterine growth retardation (IUGR). Sporadic heart defects do not typically have IUGR. All infants with dysmorphic features and heart defect without a specific diagnosis should have chromosome analysis and fluorescence in situ hybridization (FISH) studies for 22q deletion, but the features noted in this case point toward alcohol exposure. Maternal smoking is associated with IUGR but not specific heart defects or dysmorphism.

2. **(E)** All of the features listed are frequent in the fetal alcohol syndrome. Additional features include prominent lateral palatine ridges, micrognathia, flat nasal bridge, short and upturned nose, VSD, atrial septal defect (ASD), pectus excavatum, altered palmar creases, small fifth fingernails, hemangiomas, poor coordination, fine motor impairment, hypotonia, irritability in infancy, and hyperactivity in childhood.

3. **(C)** Congenital malformations occur more frequently in infants of diabetic mothers than in the general population and multiple anomalies may be present. These anomalies include those mentioned and also coarctation, complete transposition, macrosomia, brain malformations (including holoprosencephaly, agenesis of the corpus callosum, and others), and renal malformations.

4. **(C)** The features of the fetal hydantoin syndrome are seen in approximately 7% to 10% of exposed infants and an additional 30% may show lesser effects. In addition to the features listed, the syndrome is characterized by prenatal onset growth failure for weight, length, and head circumference, mental retardation, craniofacial features of wide anterior fontanel, metopic ridging, ocular hypertelorism, broad depressed nasal ridge, short nose with bowed upper lip, major malformations including clefts of the lip and palate, cardiovascular anomalies, and minor limb reduction malformations. The features in answer A are characteristic of maternal diabetes, those in answer B characteristic for valproic acid exposure, and in answer D characteristic for maternal PKU.

5. **(D)** Prenatal exposure to warfarin leads to increase in abortion, stillbirth, and prenatal growth deficiency. The period of greatest risk is

6 to 9 weeks postconception. Developmental delays, mental deficiency, hypotonia, and seizures may occur. After 9 weeks ocular defects and midline CNS malformations may occur. Antihistamine exposure is not known to lead to increased risk of birth defects. Isotretinoin exposure occurs by treatment of acne or other skin disorders, and leads to features reminiscent of the DiGeorge sequence. Heparin exposure leads to 10% to 15% risk of stillbirth and 20% risk for premature birth, but a specific malformation syndrome has not been described. Fetal hydantoin syndrome is reviewed in question 4.

6. **(D)** Neural tube defects occur with an incidence of about 1/1,000 live births. Most cases are inherited in a polygenic or multifactorial pattern with both genetic and environmental factors contributing to the increased recurrence risk. The risk of recurrence after one affected child rises to 3% to 4% and increases to approximately 10% with two previous abnormal pregnancies. Periconceptional use of folic acid supplementation has been shown to decrease the risk of neural tube defects. Folic acid should be started one month prior to conception and continued until at least 12 weeks of gestation. All women considering pregnancy should take 0.4 mg folic acid daily, and women who have previously had a pregnancy with a neural tube defect should take 4 mg folic acid daily.

7. **(A)** All definitions are correct except for an association. See question 10 for definition of association. Structural dysmorphisms are characterized based on the mechanism of injury and are important in defining etiology and recurrence risk.

8. **(E)** All can be seen with amniotic bands. The bands can become adherent to any part of the fetal body and impair vascular supply or interfere with normal tissue growth leading to a variety of malformations. The bands can be swallowed and lead to major disruption and clefts of the face.

9. **(C)** Premature fusion of a cranial suture leads to asymmetric head growth. Positional plagiocephaly is a very common cause of plagiocephaly and does not always imply a craniosynostosis. Craniosynostosis can be part of a genetic syndrome and associated with other dysmorphic features

and/or birth defects, and can also be isolated and occur in an autosomal dominant fashion. Recognition of positional plagiocephaly at an early stage is important in the treatment, as the use of a helmet is very successful before the anterior fontanel closes.

10. **(B)** An association is the nonrandom occurrence of multiple anomalies without a known developmental field defect, sequence initiator, or causal relationship, but with such a frequency that the malformations have a statistical connection. VATER association: Vertebral anomalies, Anal anomalies, Tracheoesophageal fistula, Renal or Radial anomalies.

11. **(C)** CHARGE association: Coloboma of the eye, Heart defects, Atresia of the choanae, Retardation of growth and development, Genital anomalies, Ear anomalies. DiGeorge syndrome is characterized by conotruncal heart defects, immune deficiency, and hypoparathyroidism. MURCS association: Müllerian duct aplasia, Renal aplasia, Cervicothoracic Somite dysplasia. Poland anomaly is characterized by unilateral defect of the pectoralis muscle and syndactyly of the hand.

12. **(A)** The features listed are those of severe oligohydramnios and are commonly referred to as the Potter facies or syndrome. Normal fetal lung development is dependent on the normal production and inhalation of amniotic fluid, and in the absence of amniotic fluid, significant pulmonary hypoplasia occurs and is the cause of death in many affected individuals. The underlying mechanism can be renal agenesis or renal dysplasia and these complications should be investigated in any child with the Potter facies. Additional causes include bladder outlet obstruction or prolonged premature rupture of the membranes.

13. **(B)** Beckwith-Wiedemann syndrome is an overgrowth condition which is a complex, multigenic disorder caused by alterations in growth regulatory genes on chromosome 11p15. Clinical features include macrosomia, hemihyperplasia, macroglossia, abdominal wall defects, embryonal tumors, adrenocortical cytomegaly, ear anomalies, visceromegaly, renal abnormalities, and neonatal hypoglycemia. Children with Beckwith-

Wiedemann have an increased risk for cancer (estimated to be 7.5%) and the two most common tumors are Wilms tumor and hepatoblastoma. Screening includes every three months abdominal ultrasounds until 8 years of age for Wilms tumor and AFP for the first few years as a marker for hepatoblastoma. AFP levels tend to be higher in children with Beckwith-Wiedemann in the first year of life. Calcium levels are typically normal in Beckwith-Wiedemann syndrome but may be abnormal in Williams syndrome and 22q deletion. Growth hormone is not appropriate as this is an overgrowth condition, and there is not an increased incidence of seizures. Structural cardiac abnormalities occur in 9% to 34%, cardiomyopathy has been rarely reported and cardiomegaly of early infancy usually resolves spontaneously.

14. **(C)** Prader-Willi syndrome is a result of genetic abnormalities involving an imprinting region on the long arm of chromosome 15. In addition to the features listed, affected individuals typically have infantile central hypotonia and feeding difficulties with failure to thrive, rapid weight gain between 1 and 6 years, developmental delays and mental retardation, hypopigmentation, thick viscous saliva, skin picking, and high pain threshold. Angelman syndrome is characterized by microcephaly, seizures, ataxia and severe mental retardation. Beckwith-Wiedemann was discussed in question 14, Bardet-Biedl and Sotos syndromes are both overgrowth syndromes. Bardet-Biedl is characterized by polydactyly, retinitis pigmentosa, hypertension, truncal obesity, and developmental delays. Sotos syndrome is characterized by growth greater than the 97th centile, significant macrocephaly, developmental delays, and characteristic facial features.

15. **(A)** Velocardiofacial syndrome and DiGeorge syndrome were clinically distinct syndromes which are now known to be a result of a microdeletion of 22q11. The common clinical features of this microdeletion include: conotruncal heart defects in 70% of patients (TOF, interrupted aortic arch, VSD, truncus arteriosus, vascular ring, ASD, aortic arch anomaly); feeding difficulties in 30%; immune dysfunction in 70% (impaired T-cell production and function, IgA deficiency); hypoparathyroidism leading to hypocalcemia in 50%; palate abnormalities in 70% (velopharyngeal in-

competence [VPI], submucosal or overt cleft palate, bifid uvula, cleft lip/palate); developmental delays and psychiatric abnormalities; growth failure. Transverse palmar crease is a sign of Down syndrome.

16. **(B)** Microdeletion syndromes are caused by deletions of relatively large segments of the genome, 1–3 megabases (Mb) of DNA, which affect multiple genes. The resolution of routine cytogenetics is 3 to 5 Mb of DNA so these microdeletions are not readily detected by routine methods. FISH is a molecular cytogenetic method which combines DNA probes and fluorescence methods to identify specific regions of chromosomes. Each microdeletion syndrome always involves the same region of a specific chromosome and probes directed at these regions can be used to detect the deletions. The syndromes are suspected based on specific clinical features and then FISH with a probe specific for that syndrome can be ordered/done. Sequencing is used to determine the exact sequence of DNA and is used to detect single base pair mutations. Polymerase chain reaction (PCR) is a molecular technique that allows amplification of discrete fragments of DNA and is used in many diagnostic tests.

SUGGESTED READING
Jones KL: *Smith's recognizable patterns of human malformation*. Philadelphia: WB Saunders, 1997.
Aase JM: *Diagnostic Dysmorphology*. New York: Plenum Medical Book Company, 1990.

CASE 83: A 6-MONTH-OLD BOY WITH SHORT STATURE SUGGESTIVE OF SKELETAL DYSPLASIA

A 6-month-old boy comes for evaluation secondary to short stature. The history shows that the child was born after an uncomplicated pregnancy and delivery. He has been well with no medical complications or hospitalizations. The parents do not remember that anyone was concerned about his size at birth but they noted shortly thereafter that he was not growing as they expected and they feel he has short extremities. They also report that recently he has been snoring more at night and has loud breathing during the daytime.

On physical examination growth parameters show: height 60 cm (<5th percentile), head circumference 46 cm (>95th percentile). You note macrocephaly, frontal bossing, flat nasal bridge, hypoplasia of the maxilla, rhizomelic shortening of the extremities, lumbar lordosis, and short hands and feet.

SELECT THE ONE BEST ANSWER

1. Based on the clinical features the most likely diagnosis is?

    (A) achondroplasia
    (B) Turner syndrome
    (C) hypochondroplasia
    (D) osteogenesis imperfecta
    (E) chromosome anomaly

2. Evaluations that could be helpful in establishing the diagnosis might include?

    (A) skeletal survey
    (B) bone age
    (C) genetic testing
    (D) karyotype
    (E) A and C

3. The child is confirmed to have achondroplasia. What are potential medical complications that need to be addressed in this child?

    (A) obstructive or central sleep apnea
    (B) renal malformations
    (C) congenital heart defects
    (D) diabetes mellitus
    (E) fatty liver

4. In regard to the history of the snoring and breathing issues reported, what evaluations should be considered?

    (A) sleep study
    (B) MRI scan of the brainstem
    (C) evaluation for possible tonsillectomy
    (D) counseling regarding weight control
    (E) all of the above

5. How should the parents (who are both of normal height) be counseled about the recurrence risk for another child with achondroplasia?

    (A) No chance of recurrence
    (B) Recurrence risk equals the new mutation rate, the same as all pregnancies.
    (C) Small chance of recurrence but related to paternal age and chance of germline mosaicism.

    (D) Fifty percent chance of another affected child.
    (E) Twenty-five percent chance of an affected child.

6. How should a person who has achondroplasia be counseled about the chance of having an affected child?

    (A) Achondroplasia is an autosomal dominant condition with 50% chance of an affected offspring.
    (B) Achondroplasia is an autosomal recessive condition with 25% chance of an affected offspring.
    (C) Achondroplasia is an X-linked condition and only affects females.
    (D) There is no chance for an affected offspring.
    (E) The chance of an affected offspring is very low.

7. The skeletal survey on a child with short stature shows microcephaly, oval-shaped and hook-shaped vertebral bodies in lateral view of spine, wide iliac flare, irregular diaphyseal modeling, metaphyseal widening, all features of dysostosis multiplex. The most likely diagnosis is?

    (A) warfarin embryopathy
    (B) growth hormone deficiency
    (C) nutritional rickets
    (D) MPS
    (E) chromosome abnormality

8. Clinical features of MPS include all of the following except?

    (A) coarse facial features
    (B) hepatomegaly or splenomegaly
    (C) hypoxic structural heart defects
    (D) developmental delays and/or mental retardation
    (E) restricted joint mobility

9. If an MPS disease is suspected, which of the following investigations should be considered in pursuing the diagnosis?

    (A) skeletal survey
    (B) urine screening for glycosaminoglycan excretion
    (C) enzyme analysis

(D) all of the above

(E) none of the above

10. MPS occurs by which of the following inheritance patterns?

(A) autosomal recessive

(B) X-linked inheritance

(C) autosomal dominant inheritance

(D) A and B

(E) A and C

11. A child with short neck, limited neck motion, and low occipital hair line has cervical spine radiological findings that show cervical vertebral fusion. The most likely diagnosis is?

(A) MPS

(B) achondroplasia

(C) Klippel-Feil syndrome

(D) hypochondroplasia

(E) osteogenesis imperfecta

12. Which of the following malformations is associated with the Klippel-Feil syndrome?

(A) cleft lip and/or palate

(B) congenital heart defects especially VSD

(C) abnormalities of the ribs

(D) congenital deafness

(E) all of the above

13. What are the recommendations regarding evaluation of an individual with Down syndrome with respect to participation in sports?

(A) No specific precautions are needed

(B) Individuals with Down syndrome should be restricted from all sports activities

(C) Lateral cervical radiographs in the neutral, flexed, and extended position in children between 3 and 5 years of age

(D) Routine blood counts

(E) None of the above

14. A child presents with blue sclera, multiple fractures from minimal trauma, bowing of the lower limbs, and opalescent dentin (dentinogenesis imperfecta). The most likely diagnosis is?

(A) achondroplasia

(B) osteogenesis imperfecta

(C) MPS

(D) Ellis-van Creveld syndrome

(E) none of the above

15. Which of the following do not correctly describe the clinical features associated with the specific subtype of OI?

(A) Osteogenesis imperfecta (OI) Type I: Few fractures at birth, deformities of the limbs, mild short stature, dentinogenesis imperfecta, and generalized osteopenia.

(B) OI Type II: Low birthweight and length, crumpled long bones, beaded ribs, soft skull, extremely short, bent and deformed long bones, and early lethality.

(C) OI Type III: Newborn or young infant with mild bowing of extremities, mild scoliosis and no effect on final height.

(D) All are correct.

(E) None are correct.

16. Which of the following medical complications is common in OI?

(A) hearing loss

(B) cleft lip and palate

(C) congenital heart defect

(D) renal abnormality

(E) duodenal atresia

Answers

1. **(A)** Achondroplasia is characterized by abnormal bone growth that results in short stature with disproportionately short arms and legs, a large head, and characteristic facial features. The clinical features include short stature, rhizomelic (proximal) shortening of the arms and legs with redundant skin folds on limbs, limitation of elbow extension, trident configuration of the hands, genu varum (bow legs), thoracolumbar gibbus in infancy, exaggerated lumbar lordosis, which develops when walking begins, large head with frontal bossing, and midface hypoplasia. Turner syndrome is characterized by short stature but not by macrocephaly or the other clinical features noted. Hypochondroplasia is very similar to achondroplasia but is typically less severe and does not have the facial features listed. OI is a disease of bone fractures.

2. (E) Skeletal survey may show findings characteristic of achondroplasia including narrowing of the interpediculate distance of the caudal spine, notchlike sacroiliac groove, and circumflex or chevron seat on the metaphysis. Achondroplasia is a result of mutations in the *FGFR3* gene on chromosome 4p. The common mutation, Gly380Arg, accounts for 98% of all cases and is clinically available.

3. (A) Sleep apnea may be obstructive or central secondary to craniocervical junction cord compression. The other choices are not common problems in achondroplasia. The best predictors of need for suboccipital decompression include lower-limb hyperreflexia or clonus, central hypopnea demonstrated by polysomnography, and reduced foramen magnum size, determined by CT examination of the craniocervical junction. Additional problems include spinal stenosis and obesity.

4. (E) As many as 7.5% of infants with achondroplasia die in the first year of life from obstructive apnea or central apnea. Obstructive apnea may result from mid-face hypoplasia. Brainstem compression is common and may cause abnormal respiratory function, including central apnea. In one study, 10% of infants had craniocervical junction compression with abnormality of the cervical spinal cord. All children undergoing surgical decompression of the craniocervical junction showed marked improvement of neurologic function.

5. (C) The majority of children with achondroplasia are because of new mutations and are not inherited from an affected parent. All new mutations occur on the paternal chromosome and are related to advanced paternal age. There are several reports of normal parents having more than one affected child supporting the hypothesis of germline mosaicism in one of the parents. Fifty percent recurrence risk would be used for counseling a person affected with an autosomal dominant condition with regard to passing the condition on to an offspring. Twenty-five percent recurrence risk is used for normal parents who have a child with an autosomal recessive condition.

6. (A) Achondroplasia is an autosomal dominant disease with only one copy of the *FGFR3* allele being mutated and thus a 50% chance of passing on the mutated allele.

7. (D) The term dysostosis multiplex refers to the specific skeletal findings mentioned and they are specific in the sense that their presence indicates an abnormality of complex carbohydrate degradation or lysosomal transport. The intralysosomal accumulation of partially degraded complex carbohydrates results in a variety of disorders which, depending on the type of stored material, have been classified as mucopolysaccharidoses, oligosaccharidoses and glycoproteinosis. The finding of dysostosis multiplex is specific for one of these classes of disorders but not diagnostic of specific ones.

8. (C) The clinical features of MPS have significant overlap, although there is distinct variations within the different subtypes. The general features that should be suspicious for MPS include those listed as well as microcephaly, corneal opacities, mental retardation with age of onset of developmental issues including neurodegeneration varying from the newborn period to several years of age, short stature, progressive joint contractures, and heart disease (includes valvular disease and cardiomyopathy, but does not include structural lesions causing hypoxia).

9. (D) When MPS is suspected on a clinical basis, a skeletal survey to look for the presence of dysostosis can be helpful. The presence of dysostosis is specific for the MPS as a class of disease but is not specific for a particular subtype. Urine screening tests to look for excretion of glycosaminoglycans can be helpful but are not always diagnostic and can sometimes be normal even though the patient has a form of MPS. Finally, specific enzyme analysis is available for the different subtypes of MPS and can be tested on blood and/or skin fibroblasts depending on the specific subtype in question.

10. (D) Like most metabolic diseases the vast majority of MPS are inherited in an autosomal recessive fashion. When a child is newly diagnosed, the family should be counseled that the parents are carriers of a gene mutation, and their chance of recurrence for future offspring is 25% for each pregnancy. The one exception with regard

to MPS is type II (Hunter syndrome), which is X-linked and mostly affects boys, while females may be asymptomatic carriers.

11. **(C)** Klippel-Feil syndrome is characterized by the triad of clinical features mentioned. There is variability in the degree and amount of cervical fusion. No specific genetic defect has been identified as a cause of the syndrome. Most cases are sporadic but familial recurrence has been reported.

12. **(E)** The high association of malformations in other organ systems warrants careful evaluation of all patients. In addition to the anomalies listed, additional features include: extraocular palsies, microcephaly and hydrocephalus, nystagmus, thoracic scoliosis, spina bifida occulta, Sprengel's deformity, webbing of the neck, and renal agenesis. Treatment consists of correcting the associated anomalies when possible.

13. **(C)** The current recommendations include screening as indicated in answer C. Children with borderline findings or abnormal films should be evaluated with a careful neurological examination to rule out spinal cord compression. Neuroimaging (CT or MRI) is probably indicated. Significant changes in a child's neurological status would necessitate evaluation and possible treatment. Asymptomatic children with instability (5 to 7 mm) should be managed conservatively, with restriction only in those activities which pose a risk for cervical spine injury. Contact sports, such as football, wrestling, rugby, boxing, and recreational activities such as trampolining, gymnastics (tum-

bling), and diving, which require significant flexion of the neck, would best be avoided. It is unnecessary to restrict all activities.

14. **(B)** OI is a result of a disorder of collagen synthesis and is the most prevalent of the osteoporosis syndromes in childhood. OI is characterized by fractures and skeletal deformities and some of the affected die in the newborn period with extreme fragility of bone and numerous fractures, others manifest bone fragility later in life and live a normal life span.

15. **(C)** There is great overlap in the clinical subtypes and all are a result of mutations in collagen. The different clinical severity is a result of different genetic mutations and their severity and effect on collagen synthesis and function. The clinical features of each subtype are all described correctly except for type III. OI type III has severe bone fragility and multiple fractures, which lead to progressive skeletal deformity, and severe short stature.

16. **(A)** In OI type I, hearing loss is rare before the end of the first decade but affects most patients by the fifth decade. Type II is typically lethal so there is little associated hearing loss described. Hearing impairment is not a common feature in OI type III.

SUGGESTED READING
Spranger JW, Brill PW, Poznanski A: *Bone Dysplasias.* New York: Oxford University Press, 2002.

Hematology and Oncology

11

CASE 84: A NEONATE WITH HYPERBILIRUBINEMIA

You are called to evaluate a 4-day-old infant in the nursery for worsening jaundice. The patient is the first child of a 32-year-old mother, who had an uncomplicated full-term pregnancy and normal spontaneous vaginal delivery. The mother is otherwise healthy but has a sister who had her gallbladder removed as a child. The infant has been formula-fed and has been eating and stooling normally. The total bilirubin level is 19.2 mg/dL, with a direct fraction of 0.3 mg/dL.

On physical exam, the infant is jaundiced but otherwise well, with no other significant physical findings.

SELECT THE ONE BEST ANSWER

1. The differential diagnosis of the unconjugated hyperbilirubinemia in this child includes which of the following?

   (A) biliary atresia
   (B) α_1-antitrypsin deficiency
   (C) ABO blood type incompatibility
   (D) Caroli syndrome

2. The laboratory evaluation of this infant's hyperbilirubinemia should include all of the following except:

   (A) complete blood count with smear
   (B) indirect and direct Coombs test
   (C) prothrombin time/partial thromboplastin time
   (D) maternal blood type

3. Which of the following combinations of parents' blood types place an infant at highest risk for hemolytic anemia?

   (A) maternal Rh negative, paternal Rh negative, first child
   (B) maternal Rh negative, paternal Rh positive, second child
   (C) maternal type O, paternal type O, first child
   (D) maternal type AB, paternal type B, second child

4. The differential diagnosis of a neonate with hemolytic anemia includes all of the following except:

   (A) pyruvate kinase deficiency
   (B) ABO incompatibility
   (C) Crigler-Najjar syndrome
   (D) hereditary spherocytosis

5. Erythroblastosis fetalis is characterized by all of the following except:

   (A) elevated amniotic fluid bilirubin levels
   (B) fetal anasarca
   (C) decreased umbilical cord nucleated red blood cells
   (D) fetal hepatosplenomegaly

6. Treatment of the infant with Rh-hemolytic disease could include which of the following?

   (A) red blood cell exchange transfusion with neonatal cross-matched blood
   (B) red blood cell transfusion with maternal cross-matched blood

(C) fresh frozen plasma every 8 hours

(D) intravenous immunoglobulin for the mother prior to delivery

7. The direct Coombs test is an evaluation for which of the following?

(A) antiwhite blood cell antibodies in the serum

(B) antiplatelet antibodies bound to the patient's platelets

(C) antibodies to red blood cells bound to the red blood cell membrane

(D) serum antibodies against all blood cells

8. Physiologic anemia of infancy occurs at what age for healthy, full-term infants?

(A) 1 to 2 days old

(B) 2 to 3 weeks old

(C) 2 to 3 months old

(D) 10 to 12 months old

9. Which of the following is the *best* treatment for physiologic anemia of infancy?

(A) oral ferrous sulfate

(B) careful observation

(C) folic acid supplementation

(D) monthly red blood cell transfusions

10. G6PD (glucose-6-phosphate dehydrogenase) deficiency is *least* common in which of the following ethnic groups?

(A) Northern African

(B) Northern European

(C) Southern Asian

(D) Southern European

11. G6PD deficiency is inherited in what fashion?

(A) X-linked

(B) autosomal recessive

(C) autosomal dominant with variable penetrance

(D) mitochondrial

12. The presence of Heinz bodies on the peripheral blood smear is a feature of which of the following disorders?

(A) G6PD deficiency

(B) autoimmune hemolytic anemia

(C) neonatal alloimmune thrombocytopenia

(D) sickle cell disease

13. Which of the following chemicals, when ingested, is *not* associated with hemolytic crisis in patients with G6PD deficiency?

(A) Primaquine

(B) Trimethoprim-sulfamethoxazole

(C) Methylene blue

(D) Acetaminophen

14. Which of the following is *not* a feature of hemolytic crises in patients with G6PD deficiency?

(A) hemoglobinuria

(B) splenomegaly

(C) pulmonary infiltrates

(D) jaundice

15. Hereditary spherocytosis is *most* commonly caused by a defect in which red blood cell protein?

(A) hemoglobin

(B) spectrin

(C) pyruvate kinase

(D) ankyrin

16. Which of the following laboratory tests would be *most* useful in diagnosing hereditary spherocytosis?

(A) Coombs test

(B) osmotic fragility test

(C) platelet aggregation test

(D) hemoglobin electrophoresis

17. Which of the following is the *most* effective long-term treatment for patients with hereditary spherocytosis?

(A) monthly exchange transfusions

(B) splenectomy

(C) methylprednisolone therapy

(D) intravenous spectrin replacement therapy

18. Postsplenectomy patients are *not* at increased risk for infections from which of the following bacteria?

(A) *Streptococcus pneumoniae*

(B) *Haemophilus influenzae*

(C) *Mycoplasma pneumoniae*

(D) *Escherichia coli*

Answers

1. **(C)** Neonatal jaundice occurs in approximately two-thirds of infants and is defined by bilirubin levels over 5 mg/dL. Bilirubin is generated as one of the products of the breakdown of hemoglobin, and the conjugation of bilirubin to bilirubin glucuronide occurs in the liver. Neonatal unconjugated hyperbilirubinemia is therefore the result of either increased bilirubin production or decreased conjugation. Neonatal hemolytic anemias, with increased bilirubin production, can result in severe unconjugated hyperbilirubinemia in neonates. Blood group mismatches because of ABO or Rh mismatches are common causes of neonatal hemolytic anemia and unconjugated hyperbilirubinemia. Other causes of unconjugated hyperbilirubinemia include hemolytic anemias because of red blood cell membrane or enzyme defects and increased red blood cell turnover associated with polycythemia or internal hemorrhages such as cephalohematomas or intraventricular hemorrhages. Decreased bilirubin conjugation as a result of Crigler-Najjar or Gilbert's syndromes also result in unconjugated hyperbilirubinemia. Biliary atresia, α_1-antitrypsin deficiency and Caroli syndrome are all causes of neonatal conjugated hyperbilirubinemia.

2. **(C)** Evaluation for suspected neonatal hemolytic anemias should include evaluation of the complete blood count along with indirect and direct Coombs tests and maternal and neonatal blood types. In the absence of excessive bleeding or bruising, there is no indication for coagulation studies. The complete blood count will reveal the degree of anemia, if any, and the peripheral smear will demonstrate the morphologic features of the red blood cells that could suggest underlying etiologies. The Coombs tests will evaluate whether or not there are any antibodies that could be contributing to autoimmune or alloimmune hemolysis. Neonatal and maternal blood types are needed to evaluate for ABO and Rh incompatibility.

3. **(B)** Mothers with Rh negative blood type develop antibodies against the Rh antigen after exposure during pregnancy with an Rh-positive fetus or after transfusion with Rh-positive blood. In the presence of an Rh-positive fetus, the mother's an-

tibodies can cross the placenta and destroy fetal red blood cells, resulting in neonatal hemolytic anemia. Rh hemolytic disease can be prevented with high titer Rho(D) immune globulin treatment for Rh-negative mothers who have been exposed to Rh-positive infants. Similarly, mothers with type O blood have antibodies against antigens for blood types A and B that can react to and destroy fetal red blood cells with these blood type antigens. However, a fetus who also possesses type O blood will not be susceptible to hemolysis from these antibodies. A mother with type AB blood has no antibodies to blood group antigens, and therefore the fetus is not exposed to any anti-red blood cell antigen antibodies. Despite the presence of these antibodies, only 33% of infants with ABO "mismatch" will have a positive direct Coombs test, and of those only 20% will develop jaundice from excessive hemolysis.

4. **(C)** Crigler-Najjar syndrome is caused by the absence of glucuronyl transferase and results in severe indirect hyperbilirubinemia. Pyruvate kinase and glucose-6-phosphate dehydrogenase are both red blood cell enzymes that, when deficient, can result in neonatal hemolytic anemia. Hereditary spherocytosis, as well as other syndromes with red blood cell structural abnormalities such as hereditary elliptocytosis and paroxysmal nocturnal hemoglobinuria, can also result in neonatal hemolytic anemia. Maternal-fetal blood type mismatch such as ABO incompatibility results in alloimmune hemolytic anemia, with the mother's antibodies reacting to and destroying the neonatal red blood cells.

5. **(C)** Erythroblastosis fetalis, or hydrops fetalis secondary to Rh hemolytic disease, is characterized by severe fetal hemolytic anemia as a result of anti-Rh antibody from an Rh-negative mother crossing the placenta and attacking fetal Rh-positive red blood cells. The hemolysis results in intrauterine hyperbilirubinemia, which can be detected in amniotic fluid samples. Furthermore, the severe anemia results in fetal high output cardiac failure with anasarca and peripheral edema. Hepatosplenomegaly as a result of extramedullary hematopoiesis also occurs. Nucleated red blood cells, or "erythroblasts," are elevated as a result of fetal marrow hyperproduction to compensate for the anemia.

6. **(B)** Red blood cell transfusions or exchange transfusions are often required for infants suffering from Rh-hemolytic disease, but must be cross-matched against the mother and not the infant, as the mother's antibodies are the source of the hemolytic anemia. Fresh frozen plasma has no role in the management of the hemolytic anemia in the infant. Treatment of the mother with Rho(D) immune globulin prior to delivery can reduce the autoimmune hemolysis, but intravenous immunoglobulin does not have the same beneficial effect.

7. **(C)** The direct Coombs test takes the patient's red blood cells and places them in the presence of complement proteins in an in vitro setting. The occurrence of hemolysis confirms the presence of antibodies directly bound to the patient's red blood cells. The indirect Coombs test evaluates the patient for antibodies to red blood cells that are circulating freely in the serum. The Coombs tests do not evaluate for antibodies against any other types of blood cells.

8. **(C)** Infants in their first few days of life cease producing new red blood cells as a result of the oxygen-rich environment (relative to in utero) and a decreased responsiveness of their bone marrow to erythropoietin. The hemoglobin levels fall to a nadir of 9–10 g/dL at 10–12 weeks of age, at which time erythropoiesis resumes. Premature infants or infants with other causes of neonatal anemia have an earlier onset of physiologic anemia with a lower nadir level of hemoglobin, often down to 6 to 8 g/dL at 4 to 8 weeks of age.

9. **(B)** Careful observation is generally all that is required for physiologic anemia, as the infant's erythropoietic system matures and the anemia resolves. Iron and folic acid supplementation are not indicated for isolated physiologic anemia, and transfusions are only indicated for severe symptomatic anemia, which does not occur with isolated physiologic anemia. Blood transfusions can in fact suppress the endogenous erythropoietin production and delay recovery from physiologic anemia.

10. **(B)** The presence of G6PD deficiency is most common in African populations and populations around the Mediterranean Sea, with increased frequency also seen in Southern Asian populations and American Indians. G6PD deficiency occurs in approximately 12% of African-American males, while in Southeast Asia the incidence is approximately 6%. Northern Europeans have the lowest incidence of G6PD deficiency among the populations listed.

11. **(A)** G6PD deficiency is an X-linked disorder. Affected males have a single mutated copy of the G6PD gene, while affected females are usually compound heterozygotes with two different mutant G6PD gene alleles. Deficiency of G6PD in African Americans is most commonly the result of a mutation that renders the enzyme unstable, leaving new red blood cells with relatively normal enzyme levels but old red blood cells with nearly absent enzyme levels and with increased susceptibility to oxidant stress. The mutations in the G6PD gene that occur in other populations, particularly the Mediterranean and Middle Eastern populations, generally result in absent G6PD expression, and these patients are more susceptible to oxidant-induced red blood cell lysis and are also susceptible to hemolysis induced by fava beans (termed "favism").

12. **(A)** Heinz bodies are intracellular inclusions of oxidized and degenerated hemoglobin seen in red blood cell enzyme deficiencies such as G6PD deficiency. The inclusions are often attached to the red blood cell membrane and can be "eaten" by splenic macrophages, resulting in the characteristic "bite cells" of red blood cell enzyme deficiencies. Autoimmune hemolytic anemia is characterized by microspherocytosis, but there are no intracellular inclusions. Neonatal alloimmune thrombocytopenia has no unusual red blood cell features. Sickle cell disease has sickled red blood cells and often has Howell-Jolly bodies from splenic hypofunction, but is not associated with Heinz bodies.

13. **(D)** Hemolysis in patients with G6PD deficiency is stimulated by oxidative stress, which can be caused by stress from infections, diabetic ketoacidosis, or by medications and chemicals such as primaquine, sulfa drugs, and methylene blue. Other chemicals that can trigger hemolysis include dapsone, nitrofurantoin, trinitrotoluene, naphthalene, and acetanilid, among others. Fava beans can stimulate hemolysis in certain populations with specific

forms of G6PD mutations, such as those that occur in Mediterranean populations. Acetaminophen is not associated with hemolytic crises in patients with G6PD deficiency.

14. **(C)** Hemolytic crises in patients with G6PD deficiency and other hemolytic anemias are characterized by fatigue, pallor, scleral icterus and jaundice, splenomegaly, and hemoglobinuria. Laboratory findings include anemia with increased free plasma hemoglobin and decreased plasma haptoglobin. Pulmonary infiltrates are not associated with hemolytic crises.

15. **(B)** Hereditary spherocytosis is the most common structural red blood cell defect and affects approximately 1 in 5000 people. The most common cause of hereditary spherocytosis is a defect in spectrin, a protein responsible for the structural integrity of the red blood cell membrane. Defects in associated proteins, such as band 3, protein 4.2, and ankyrin, can also play a role in the defect but act via a relative spectrin deficiency. Hereditary spherocytosis is most common in Northern Europeans and is characterized by anemia, jaundice, and splenomegaly. Most cases are inherited in an autosomal dominant fashion, but approximately 10% are inherited as a recessive trait. Hemoglobin deficiencies do not cause spherocytosis, and pyruvate kinase is a red blood cell enzyme that is unrelated to the structural features of the red cell membrane.

16. **(B)** The osmotic fragility test is the most specific test for the diagnosis of hereditary spherocytosis. Red blood cells are incubated in the presence of varying degrees of hypotonic solutions, and the red blood cell lysis is measured. Spherocytes, as a result of their decreased surface area, will be more susceptible to hypotonic lysis compared to normal red blood cells. The Coombs test detects the presence of antibodies in cases of autoimmune hemolytic anemia, which can be associated with prominent spherocytosis on the peripheral blood smear, but will be negative in cases of hereditary spherocytosis. Platelet aggregation studies and hemoglobin electrophoreses are not useful in the diagnosis of spherocytosis.

17. **(B)** Splenectomy should be an option for any patient with hereditary spherocytosis who requires frequent transfusions, has severe symptoms of anemia such as cardiac dysfunction or poor growth, has severe splenomegaly with significantly increased risk of rupture, or has persistent symptoms of hypersplenism such as leukopenia or thrombocytopenia. Splenectomy usually results in a persistently elevated baseline hemoglobin. Patients undergoing splenectomy should receive immunizations against *H. influenzae* and *S. pneumoniae* if possible prior to surgery, and should be started on penicillin prophylaxis as soon as possible after splenectomy. Furthermore, splenectomy should be avoided if possible until patients are over the age of 5 years to reduce the incidence of severe bacterial infections that can occur in younger children. Exchange transfusions are not indicated for treatment of spherocytosis and steroids have no effect. Spectrin replacement is not yet a viable treatment option.

18. **(C)** *S. pneumoniae*, *H. influenzae*, and *E. coli* are all encapsulated organisms, and patients with either splenic hypofunction or after surgical splenectomy are at increased risk for infections from these and other encapsulated organisms. *M. pneumoniae* is not an encapsulated organism and splenectomized patients are not at higher risk of mycoplasma infections. Patients who need splenectomies should receive *H. influenzae* and pneumococcal vaccines prior to the splenectomy, and then should receive penicillin prophylaxis post-splenectomy to reduce the incidence of bacteremia and sepsis from encapsulated organisms.

SUGGESTED READING

Prchal JT, Gregg XT: Red cell enzymopathies. In: Hoffman R, Benz EJ, Shattil SJ, et al (eds): *Hematology: Basic Principles and Practice*, 3rd ed. Philadelphia: Churchill Livingstone, 2000, pp 568–569.

Gallagher PG, Jarolin P: Red cell membrane disorders. In: Hoffman R, Benz EJ, Shattil SJ, et al (eds): *Hematology: Basic Principles and Practice*, 3rd ed. Philadelphia: Churchill Livingstone, 2000, pp 578–585.

Cashore WJ. Neonatal hyperbilirubinemia. In: McMillan JA, DeAngelis CD, Feigin RD et al (eds): *Oski's Pediatrics: Principles and Practice*, 3rd ed. Philadelphia: Lippincott Williams and Wilkins, 1999, pp 202–204.

Committee on Infectious Diseases, American Academy of Pediatrics. Immunization in Special Circumstances. In: Pickering LK (ed): *Red Book*, 26th ed. Elk Grove, IL: American Academy of Pediatrics, 2003, pp 80–81.

Tabbara IA: Hemolytic Anemias: Diagnosis and Management. 1992. *Med Clin North Am* 76(3): 649–68.

CASE 85: AN 18-MONTH-OLD GIRL WITH ANEMIA

An 18-month-old Hispanic girl is brought to your office for routine evaluation. A screening hemoglobin level was noted to be 4.6 g/dL. The child does appear pale and has a "cranky" disposition, according to the parents. On further history, the child's parents inform you that her diet consists of approximately 36 ounces of cow's milk per day. There is no prior history of anemia and no history of pica, trauma, or recent blood loss. The child is the product of a full-term, uncomplicated pregnancy and has been doing well, with no other medical problems and normal growth and development to date. There is no family history of blood disorders.

Her physical exam is notable for mild pallor and a 2/6 systolic ejection murmur at the left sternal border.

SELECT THE ONE BEST ANSWER

1. The *most* likely diagnosis for this child is:

   (A) acute lymphoblastic leukemia
   (B) iron deficiency anemia
   (C) lead poisoning
   (D) anemia of chronic disease

2. The *most* useful diagnostic test at this point would be:

   (A) complete blood count with smear
   (B) serum ferritin level
   (C) hemoglobin electrophoresis
   (D) direct and indirect Coombs

3. The differential diagnosis of a child with microcytic anemia includes all of the following *except*:

   (A) lead intoxication
   (B) folate deficiency
   (C) iron deficiency
   (D) anemia of chronic disease

4. The majority of the body's iron is located in:

   (A) erythrocytes
   (B) splenic histiocytes
   (C) cardiac myocytes
   (D) hepatocytes

5. Which of the following compounds does *not* inhibit iron absorption from the gastrointestinal tract?

   (A) ascorbic acid
   (B) phytates
   (C) phosphates
   (D) sodium bicarbonate

6. Which of the following is the *least* likely cause of iron deficiency in adolescents?

   (A) menorrhagia
   (B) pregnancy
   (C) pubertal growth acceleration
   (D) sedentary lifestyle

7. Which of the following is *not* a complication of iron deficiency anemia?

   (A) geophagia (compulsive dirt eating)
   (B) cognitive delay
   (C) hypertrophic cardiomyopathy
   (D) short stature

8. Which of the following is a laboratory finding associated with iron deficiency?

   (A) serum TIBC (total iron binding capacity), increased
   (B) serum ferritin, increased
   (C) red blood cell MCV, increased
   (D) serum iron, increased

9. Treatment options for children with iron deficiency anemia include all of the following *except*:

   (A) red blood cell transfusion
   (B) oral ferrous sulfate
   (C) intravenous iron dextran
   (D) oral folic acid

10. β-thalassemia is found most commonly in which of the following ethnic groups?

    (A) Southeast Asian
    (B) Northern European
    (C) Ashkenazi Jewish
    (D) American Indian

11. Which of the following is *not* a physical feature found in patients with thalassemia major?

    (A) frontal bossing
    (B) splenomegaly
    (C) scleral icterus
    (D) tibial bowing

12. Hemoglobin H disease is associated with how many α-globin gene deletions?

    (A) 0
    (B) 1
    (C) 2
    (D) 3

13. Which of the following is *not* a complication of transfusion-associated hemochromatosis?

    (A) dilated cardiomyopathy
    (B) diabetes mellitus
    (C) renal insufficiency
    (D) hypogonadism

14. Which of the following is a normal childhood hemoglobin electrophoresis pattern?

    (A) 96% A, 3% A2, 1% F
    (B) 90% A, 8% A2, 2% F
    (C) 90% A, 2% A2, 8% F
    (D) 80% A, 10% A2, 10% F

15. Which of the following statements regarding Diamond-Blackfan anemia is *false*?

    (A) Diamond-Blackfan anemia is usually microcytic.
    (B) Reticulocyte count in patients with Diamond-Blackfan anemia is low.
    (C) Patients with Diamond-Blackfan anemia have abnormalities of their thumbs.
    (D) Diamond-Blackfan anemia is usually diagnosed in patients before their first birthday.

16. Which of the following anemic patients is *most* likely to have transient erythroblastopenia of childhood?

    (A) 2-month-old male with macrocytic anemia
    (B) 11-month-old female with increased fetal hemoglobin levels
    (C) 28-month-old male with a history of upper respiratory infection
    (D) 35-month-old female with failure to thrive

17. Which of the following is *not* a symptom of lead toxicity?

    (A) recurrent emesis
    (B) constipation
    (C) behavioral changes
    (D) polyuria

Answers

1. **(B)** The most likely diagnosis is iron deficiency anemia, based on the patient's age and her history of cow's milk intake. Iron deficiency is a common cause of anemia in children, with a peak incidence between 6 months and 3 years of age. Iron stores initially are accumulated during the last 3 months of pregnancy, and so iron deficiency in neonates and early infancy is due either to prematurity, early blood losses, or hemolysis. In contrast, iron deficiency in older infants and toddlers is usually a result of dietary deficiency, most commonly a result of excessive cow's milk intake. Cow's milk is a poor source of iron, with only 0.5 to 1 mg/L of iron and with only 10% of the iron bioavailable. Furthermore, excessive intake of cow's milk is associated with decreased intake of other, more iron-rich, foods. Cow's milk also frequently causes mucosal irritation in the gastrointestinal tract, leading to chronic low-grade blood loss. As iron deficiency develops slowly, over months to years, even severe anemia is relatively well-tolerated by children with few symptoms. After correction of the iron deficiency, however, parents often note that children are less pale, have more energy, and are less "cranky." Management of dietary iron deficiency involves decreasing or eliminating cow's milk intake and increasing the intake of other iron-rich foods such as meats and leafy green vegetables, in addition to added oral iron supplements as needed.

   Children with acute leukemias usually present with other cytopenias in addition to anemia and are commonly symptomatic from their cytopenias, with fevers, fatigue, petechiae, and bleeding. Anemia of chronic disease occurs in patients with a history of chronic inflammation, such as those with collagen vascular diseases, chronic infections (particularly osteomyelitis and tuberculosis), or renal insufficiency. The anemia of chronic disease is generally mild and of slow onset and is secondary to poor utilization of iron stores and suboptimal bone marrow responsiveness to erythropoietin. Management involves treatment of the underlying disease, as additional iron will not be utilized by the bone marrow nor effective in raising the hemoglobin level. Lead poisoning can be associated with microcytic anemia and is also frequently associated with iron deficiency, which results in increased lead absorption and toxicity. Anemia because of lead poisoning is usually a late finding and, fortunately, is rare in modern times because of the removal of lead from previously common sources such as paint and gasoline.

2. **(A)** The complete blood count with peripheral smear is the single most useful diagnostic test for iron deficiency. The complete blood count not only details the degree of anemia but also describes the red blood cell features, including the MCV and RDW, which will help to differentiate the anemia of iron deficiency (characterized by a low MCV and high RDW) from anemia because of thalassemia (characterized by a low MCV with a normal RDW). Furthermore, the peripheral smear will demonstrate the characteristic microcytosis with hypochromia and poikilocytosis of iron deficiency. The serum ferritin level is normally decreased with iron deficiency but can be falsely normal or high with any concurrent systemic inflammation. A hemoglobin electrophoresis would be useful to diagnose β-thalassemia or other hemoglobinopathies, but is not helpful in the diagnosis of iron deficiency. Electrophoresis in patients with thalassemia can be falsely normal in the presence of iron deficiency. The Coombs tests look for antibodies to red blood cells in the patient's serum (indirect) or bound directly to the patient's red blood cells (direct), and are useful to diagnose autoimmune hemolytic anemias, but would not be useful in this case.

3. **(B)** Folate deficiency is a cause of macrocytic anemia and is also associated with hypersegmentation of neutrophils on the peripheral smear. The differential diagnosis of microcytic anemia in children includes lead poisoning, α- and β-thalassemias, iron deficiency, anemia of chronic disease, and sideroblastic anemia. Iron deficiency is by far the most common, occurring in up to 10% of children in the United States. The anemia of chronic disease is also common, but can be normocytic in over one-half of the cases. Anemias because of hemoglobinopathies such as sickle cell disease, red blood cell enzyme defects or structural defects, and autoimmune hemolytic anemias

are all generally normocytic. Macrocytic anemias can be a result of folate deficiency, vitamin B_{12} deficiency, or myelodysplastic or aplastic anemias.

4. **(A)** The average adult male has approximately 5 g of total body iron, and the majority (60% to 80%) of the body's total iron is bound to erythrocyte hemoglobin. Approximately 10% to 30% of the total body iron stores are located in the reticuloendothelial cells of the liver and spleen. The heart and liver have only minimal amounts of iron under normal conditions, but can contain large amounts of iron in states of iron overload. Only 0.1% of the total body iron stores can be found in the plasma, bound to transferrin. Only 1 mg of the total body iron is lost each day through sloughed skin and enteric mucosal cells and therefore must be replaced through the diet. The human body unfortunately has no other mechanism for selective iron excretion.

5. **(A)** Dietary iron is generally absorbed in the duodenum, and the absorption is regulated both in the form of the dietary iron as well as by the local intestinal environment. At neutral pH, iron is primarily in the ferric (Fe+3) form, which is poorly absorbed. In the stomach and duodenum, the acidic pH converts iron to the ferrous (Fe+2) form, which is more readily absorbed. Furthermore, iron found in heme moieties (from meat sources) is more readily absorbed compared to free elemental iron. Ascorbic acid and citric acid increase the absorption of iron from the intestine by reducing the iron from the ferric to the ferrous state. Phytates (found in soy-based formulas) and phosphates (found in cow's milk) both bind to free iron in the gastrointestinal tract and inhibit its absorption. Bicarbonate increases the gastric pH, which also inhibits conversion of iron to its ferrous form and reduces its absorption.

6. **(D)** The activity level of adolescents is unrelated to their iron stores. However, any cause of chronic blood loss, such as heavy menstrual bleeding, or any period of increased physiologic iron demand, such as pregnancy or growth spurts, can lead to iron deficiency. Dietary causes of iron deficiency are extremely rare in adolescents but can occur with unusual dietary patterns, such as strict vegetarianism or anorexia nervosa.

7. (**C**) Cardiomyopathy is generally not a complication of iron deficiency, although children with severe long-standing anemia of any etiology can have cardiac dysfunction as a result of excessive workload. Geophagia, a form of pica, along with cognitive delays, delayed growth, and irritability are all associated with iron deficiency. The cognitive delays, unfortunately, may not be totally reversible with correction of the iron deficiency. Iron deficiency has also been associated with breath-holding spells, febrile seizures, protein-losing enteropathy (because of the loss of enteric mucosal cells), and, rarely, thromboembolic strokes hypothesized to be secondary to a decrease in red blood cell membrane fluidity and flexibility that occurs with iron deficiency.

8. (**A**) The presence of iron deficiency is associated with a variety of laboratory abnormalities, including abnormalities in the blood count and abnormalities of other serum proteins. The features of iron deficiency in the complete blood count include a low MCV, an elevated RDW, and associated hypochromia and poikilocytosis. Laboratory values consistent with iron deficiency include decreased ferritin, increased TIBC (total iron binding capacity), decreased serum transferrin saturation, increased free erythrocyte protoporphyrin, and decreased serum iron. Anemia of chronic disease, by comparison, is characterized by a decreased TIBC and normal serum ferritin level, while β-thalassemia is generally associated with normal to increased serum iron, normal TIBC, and normal to increased serum ferritin levels.

9. (**D**) Folic acid therapy is not indicated for treatment of iron deficiency except in those cases of combined iron and folate deficiency, such as with severe malnutrition. While oral ferrous sulfate at 3 to 6 mg/kg of elemental iron per day is the usual first option for treatment, intravenous iron therapy is an option for those patients with extremely low iron stores or those who would not absorb or tolerate oral iron. Red blood cell transfusions can be used for patients with very severe anemia, and the iron from the transfused red blood cells can then be recycled by the body for future red blood cell production as well. Responses to treatment for iron deficiency anemia are generally rapid, with an increase in reticulocytes seen within 7 days and increased hemoglobin levels by 1 month.

Iron deficiency anemia develops slowly over time, and progresses through several stages. Initially, depletion of the total body iron stores results in low serum ferritin levels but unchanged hemoglobin and serum iron levels. Upon complete iron store depletion, the serum iron level will drop, associated with an increase in the serum TIBC. Further loss of iron will then result in "iron deficiency anemia," with development of the microcytic, hypochromic anemia characteristic of iron deficiency. Repletion of iron, either by oral, intravenous, or transfusion therapy, will initially replace the red blood cell iron, with normalization of the hemoglobin level and red blood cell MCV. However, in the absence of further aggressive iron repletion, the serum iron and ferritin levels will remain low, and the patient will remain in a state of "iron-limited erythropoiesis." Therefore, it is crucial that iron replacement therapy be continued for several months after the normalization of the red blood cell parameters in order to ensure adequate replacement of the total body iron stores.

10. (**A**) Thalassemias are blood disorders characterized by decreased α- or β-globin chain production, and they have a wide spectrum of clinical symptoms based on the relative levels of the α- and β-globin chains. β-thalassemia is most commonly found in persons of Mediterranean, Northeast African, Indian, Indonesian, and Southeast Asian descent. The gene frequency can be as high as 20% in these populations. In contrast, β-thalassemia is extremely rare in populations from Northern Europe and the far East (Korea, China, and Japan). α-Thalassemia can be found primarily in Mediterranean, West African, and Southwestern Pacific populations, with a gene frequency of up to 70% in some Southwestern Pacific populations, and is extremely rare in populations from Great Britain, Iceland, and Japan.

11. (**C**) β-Thalassemia patients are subdivided based on clinical severity into those with thalassemia carrier, thalassemia trait, thalassemia intermedia, and thalassemia major. β-Thalassemia carriers are asymptomatic, with only mild microcytosis, while patients with thalassemia trait have a mild micro-

cytic anemia but generally are otherwise well. Thalassemia intermedia and thalassemia major both have moderate to severe anemia and require transfusion therapy. Red blood cells produced by the bone marrow in patients with more severe thalassemia are poorly functional, stimulating further red blood cell production. This ineffective erythropoiesis eventually results in bone marrow hyperplasia and extramedullary hematopoiesis, which cause the clinical features of thalassemia major (also called Cooley's anemia) that occur in the absence of regular transfusions. These features of thalassemia major include severe anemia with massive hepatosplenomegaly and growth failure. Bone marrow hyperplasia results in frontal bossing, maxillary prominence, a "hair-on-end" appearance of the skull on radiograph, and long bone changes including severe osteoporosis and cortical thinning from medullary expansion. The thin bony cortices leave the bones susceptible both to bowing and to fractures. Scleral icterus and jaundice are not features of thalassemia.

Laboratory features of β-thalassemia include elevated hemoglobin A2, although hemoglobin F, or fetal hemoglobin, is usually normal. The red blood cells in patients with thalassemia are microcytic, with hypochromia and basophilic stippling. The presence of target cells and ovalocytes is also consistent with thalassemia.

12. **(D)** The α-globin chains in hemoglobin are produced by four separate α-globin gene alleles. A single allele deletion results in an asymptomatic carrier state, with microcytosis but no anemia. Two α-globin allele deletions cause α-thalassemia trait, with mild anemia but marked hypochromia and microcytosis. Deletion of three alleles results in more severe hemoglobin H disease, characterized by moderate anemia, with hemoglobin levels of 7 to 10 g/dL, associated with jaundice and hepatosplenomegaly. Hemoglobin H is composed of four β-globin chains and comprises 5% to 30% of the total hemoglobin in hemoglobin H disease patients. Hemoglobin H unfortunately has no oxygen delivering capacity and precipitates within the red blood cell, forming Heinz bodies and inducing splenic sequestration and destruction.

Deletion of all four α-globin alleles results in hydrops fetalis with severe intrauterine microcytic anemia and hepatosplenomegaly. The hemoglobin present is exclusively Bart's hemoglobin, or γ4, which is composed of four fetal γ-globin chains. Bart's hemoglobin, like hemoglobin H, has no oxygen delivering capacity and so hydrops fetalis is invariably fatal (either in utero or perinatally) in the absence of transfusion therapy.

13. **(C)** Transfusion therapy for patients with thalassemia frequently results in hemochromatosis, or "iron overload." While many organs are affected by iron overload, the kidneys are relatively spared. Iron overload is associated with dilated cardiomyopathy because of excessive iron deposition in cardiac myocytes, diabetes mellitus because of pancreatic iron deposition, and hypogonadism from pituitary failure secondary to iron deposition. Other complications of iron overload include growth failure, hypothyroidism, hypoparathyroidism, and hepatic fibrosis with an increased risk of hepatocellular carcinoma.

Treatment of iron overload in cases of hereditary hemochromatosis consists of regular phlebotomy to withdraw iron and reduce the body's iron stores. In cases of transfusion-induced iron overload, iron reduction is accomplished with desferrioxamine chelation. Desferrioxamine, which must be given either intravenously or subcutaneously, binds to iron in the bloodstream and is then excreted in the urine. The success of chelation can be measured by serum ferritin levels or by liver biopsy, the most sensitive measure of total body iron stores.

14. **(A)** Normal red blood cells have a mixture of predominantly hemoglobin A (α2β2), with small amounts of hemoglobins A2 (α2δ2) and F (α2γ2). Normally hemoglobin A comprises at least 95% of the total hemoglobin, with hemoglobin A2 ranging from 2% to 4% and hemoglobin F 0.5% to 1%. Increasing amounts of hemoglobin F relative to hemoglobin A are found in fetuses and neonates, prior to the conversion of the erythrocyte precursors to adult hemoglobin A production. Increased levels of hemoglobin F can be found in cases of hereditary persistence of fetal hemoglobin, while increased levels of hemoglobin A2 are found in patients with β-thalassemia.

15. **(A)** Diamond-Blackfan anemia (DBA) is a congenital form of pure red blood cell aplasia that

usually presents in infancy. The incidence of DBA is approximately 5/1,000,000 births, with 80% of the cases being sporadic. 90% of the cases initially present in the first 6 months of life. DBA does not have any race or sex predilection. Physical features of DBA, which occur in approximately one-third of cases, include craniofacial abnormalities such as microcephaly, microphthalmia, hypertelorism, micrognathia, growth failure (either intrauterine or postnatal), and abnormal thumbs, which can be bifid, duplicated, subluxed, hypoplastic, absent, or triphalangeal. The laboratory features include macrocytic anemia, decreased or absent reticulocytes, and an otherwise normal blood count. DBA is also characterized by an increase in hemoglobin F and the presence of i antigen on red blood cells, which is normally only found on fetal red blood cells. Treatment of DBA involves blood transfusions as needed, but approximately 25% of patients will respond to steroid treatment with an increased hemoglobin level. Bone marrow transplantation is often required, particularly in cases that do not respond to steroid therapy, and is the only currently available curative therapy.

16. **(C)** TEC, or transient erythroblastopenia of childhood, is most frequently confused with other forms of congenital anemia such as Diamond-Blackfan anemia. The features most consistent with TEC include a normocytic anemia in a patient over 2 years of age, often with a history of a preceding viral upper respiratory infection. Reticulocytes are also decreased in patients with TEC, as are the red blood cell precursors in the bone marrow. Features that would suggest Diamond-Blackfan anemia include age of onset less than one year, abnormal physical features (particularly abnormal thumbs) or growth failure, and elevations in MCV, adenosine deaminase levels, fetal hemoglobin, and i antigen (a red blood cell antigen normally only found on fetal red blood cells). The most significant characteristic feature of TEC is spontaneous recovery in the absence of treatment, while anemias because of DBA or other congenital red cell aplasias will not resolve without other therapy.

17. **(D)** Lead toxicity is a cause of microcytic anemia in children that must be ruled out with initial screening because of potentially severe and irreversible complications. Sources of lead poisoning include leaded gasoline, lead smelters, paint chips from houses with lead-based paint, old batteries, magazine color pages, and lead-glazed pottery. Lead toxicity is associated with abdominal pain, emesis, constipation, peripheral neuropathy, renal disease, and can eventually result in encephalopathy with decreased IQ, altered behavior, ataxia, and seizures. Decreased hemoglobin levels from lead toxicity are a product of inhibition of heme synthesis, resulting in accumulation of heme precursors and causing an elevation in the serum-free erythrocyte protoporphyrin levels.

SUGGESTED READING

Recht M, Pearson HA: Nutritional anemias. In: McMillan JA, DeAngelis CD, Feigin RD, et al (eds): *Oski's Pediatrics: Principles and Practice*. 3rd ed. Philadelphia: Lippincott Williams and Wilkins, 1999, pp 1447–1448.

Martin PL, Pearson HA: Hypoplastic and aplastic anemias. In: McMillan JA, DeAngelis CD, Feigin RD, et al (eds): *Oski's Pediatrics: Principles and Practice*. 3rd ed. Philadelphia: Lippincott Williams and Wilkins, 1999, pp 1457–1460.

Chisolm JJ Jr: Lead poisoning. In: McMillan JA, DeAngelis CD, Feigin RD, et al (eds): *Oski's Pediatrics: Principles and Practice*. 3rd ed. Philadelphia: Lippincott Williams and Wilkins, 1999, pp 629–635.

Brittenham GM: Disorders of iron metabolism: Iron deficiency and overload. In: Hoffman R, Benz EJ, Shattil SJ, et al (eds): *Hematology: Basic Principles and Practice*, 3rd ed. Philadelphia: Churchill Livingstone, 2000, pp 412–417.

Forget BG: Thalassemia syndromes. In: Hoffman R, Benz EJ, Shattil SJ, et al (eds): *Hematology: Basic Principles and Practice*, 3rd ed. Philadelphia: Churchill Livingstone, 2000, pp 485–506.

Abshire TC: Sense and sensibility: approaching anemia in children. *Contemp Pediatr* 18(9):104–113, 2001.

Lo L, Singer ST: Thalassemia: current approach to an old disease. *Pediatr Clin North Am* 49:1165–91, 2002.

Walters MC, Abelson HT: Interpretation of the complete blood count. *Pediatr Clin North Am* 43(3):599–622, 1996.

CASE 86: A 16-YEAR-OLD WITH SICKLE CELL DISEASE AND RESPIRATORY DISTRESS

A mother brings her 16-year-old son, who is known to have sickle cell disease, to the emergency room with "difficulty breathing." He was well until approximately 1 week ago when he began having bilateral leg and arm pain, which are his usual sites for sickle cell pain. He was taking ibuprofen and codeine at home with some relief. The past evening the pain worsened, and he also began having fevers to 101.6°F (38.6°C). This morning he also began having some chest pain and difficulty taking deep breaths and so his mother brought him to the emergency room. The patient has had several past admissions for his sickle cell disease for vaso-occlusive crisis pain management. He has never received a blood transfusion.

On physical exam, the patient is awake and alert, but clearly in pain. His sclerae are icteric bilaterally. He has a 3/6 systolic ejection murmur, and he has decreased breath sounds in his right lung base. The remainder of his exam is noncontributing.

His blood count reveals a white blood cell count of 16,500/μl, with a hemoglobin of 6.5g/dL and a platelet count of 426,000/μl. His differential has 65% neutrophils, 25% lymphocytes, 8% monocytes, and 2% eosinophils, and his reticulocyte count is 18.6%. A chest radiograph reveals a small fluffy infiltrate in the right lung lower lobe.

SELECT THE ONE BEST ANSWER

1. At this time, the patient *most* likely has which of the following complications of sickle cell disease?

    (A) splenic sequestration
    (B) aplastic crisis
    (C) priapism
    (D) acute chest syndrome

2. The most common symptoms associated with acute chest syndrome in pediatric patients with sickle cell disease include all of the following *except*:

    (A) hemoptysis
    (B) temperature >101.3°F (38.5°C)
    (C) O$_2$ saturation <90%
    (D) chest pain

3. The management of acute chest syndrome should include all of the following *except*:

    (A) opioids for pain control
    (B) broad spectrum antibiotics
    (C) aerosolized nitrous oxide
    (D) incentive spirometry

4. Which of the following antibiotics is the *best* initial choice in the management of a patient with sickle cell disease and fever?

    (A) ceftriaxone
    (B) clindamycin
    (C) vancomycin
    (D) metronidazole

5. Which of the following is *not* a side effect of the opioids used for pain management in children with sickle cell disease?

    (A) constipation
    (B) nausea
    (C) pruritus
    (D) hematuria

6. Acute chest syndrome is *most* common in patients with which of the following hemoglobin genotypes?

    (A) AS
    (B) SS
    (C) SC
    (D) β-thalassemia

7. Recurrent acute chest syndrome is associated with all of the following complications *except*:

    (A) chronic hypoxia
    (B) pulmonary hypertension
    (C) emphysema
    (D) cor pulmonale

8. Which of the following is the *most* likely result of neonatal hemoglobin electrophoresis for patients with sickle cell trait?

    (A) FS
    (B) FSC
    (C) FA
    (D) FAS

9. Which of the following is the approximate hemoglobin S gene carrier frequency in the United States' African-American population?

    (A) 4%
    (B) 8%
    (C) 16%
    (D) 32%

10. Which of the following findings on the peripheral blood smear is a feature of decreased splenic function in patients with sickle cell disease?

(A) Auer bodies
(B) basophilic stippling
(C) Howell-Jolly bodies
(D) polychromasia

11. Renal complications of patients with sickle cell anemia include all of the following *except*:

(A) hyposthenuria
(B) hematuria
(C) proteinuria
(D) glucosuria

12. Gallstones found in patients with sickle cell anemia are composed primarily of which of the following compounds?

(A) calcium oxalate
(B) calcium bilirubinate
(C) calcium carbonate
(D) xanthine oxide

13. Acute hemiparesis in patients with sickle cell disease is *best* managed by which of the following?

(A) red blood cell transfusion
(B) red blood cell exchange transfusion
(C) non-steroidal anti-inflammatory agents
(D) hyperbaric oxygen

14. All of the following are neurologic complications of strokes in pediatric patients with sickle cell disease *except*:

(A) recurrent stroke
(B) cognitive delay
(C) optic neuritis
(D) seizure disorder

15. Which of the following has been shown to be *most* effective in preventing recurrence of strokes in patients with sickle cell disease?

(A) aspirin
(B) low-molecular-weight heparin
(C) folic acid
(D) regular red blood cell transfusions

16. Aplastic crises in patients with sickle cell disease are *most* commonly associated with which of the following infections?

(A) Epstein-Barr virus
(B) adenovirus
(C) *S. pneumoniae*
(D) parvovirus B19

17. Which of the following complications of sickle cell disease is *most* likely to occur during infancy?

(A) priapism
(B) transient ischemic attack
(C) acute chest syndrome
(D) dactylitis

18. Which of the following antibiotics is *most* effective for prophylaxis against *S. pneumoniae* in patients with sickle cell disease?

(A) trimethoprim-sulfamethoxazole
(B) penicillin
(C) rifampin
(D) fluconazole

Answers

1. (D) Sickle cell disease is characterized by a mutation in the hemoglobin β chain, where a valine is substituted for a glutamic acid at the β6 position. This amino acid substitution predisposes the hemoglobin molecule to polymerization, particularly under hypoxic or acidic conditions, with hemoglobin polymerization resulting in "sickling" of the red blood cell. Symptoms of sickle cell disease can occur with hemoglobin genotypes including homozygous hemoglobin SS and combinations of hemoglobin S with other mutant β-globin chains, such as hemoglobin SC, Sβ⁰ thalassemia, or Sβ+ thalassemia. The disease severity varies to some degree with the genotype, as patients with SS and Sβ⁰ genotypes tend toward more severe disease. Red blood cell sickling and the resulting microvascular obstruction is the cause of the wide range of complications associated with sickle cell disease.

In a patient with sickle cell disease of any genotype, the combination of respiratory symptoms, fever, chest pain, and an infiltrate on chest radiograph after an episode of vaso-occlusive pain are all consistent with the diagnosis of acute chest syndrome. Acute chest syndrome occurs at least once in up to 50% of patients with sickle cell disease. The etiology of acute chest syndrome in patients with sickle cell disease is unclear, but may include components of both pulmonary infection and infarction in addition to fat embolism from infarcted bone marrow. Therefore, any combination of the above symptoms should be treated as acute chest syndrome. Patients who have had prior episodes of acute chest syndrome are more likely to have recurrent episodes.

2. **(A)** The most common symptoms in pediatric acute chest syndrome are fever and cough, with approximately 70% also having some degree of hypoxia. Chest pain, dyspnea, and wheezing can be seen less commonly. Up to 60% of patients, however, will have a normal pulmonary exam. While hemoptysis occurs frequently in adult sickle cell patients with acute chest syndrome, it is rare in pediatric sickle cell patients. Other associated findings with acute chest syndrome include a drop in hemoglobin and an elevation in the baseline white blood cell count. Acute chest syndrome, if not appropriately treated, can rapidly progress to respiratory insufficiency and acute respiratory distress syndrome (ARDS) and can be fatal.

3. **(C)** The management of acute chest syndrome requires multiple interventions for the best outcome. Pain control to prevent respiratory "splinting" is important, as the inability to take deep breaths will lead to further lung collapse and worsening of the acute chest syndrome. However, oversedation with respiratory depression should also be avoided and so the opioid dose in patients with acute chest syndrome must be carefully titrated. IV hydration is also important, as dehydration contributes to further intravascular sickling. Overhydration with potential pulmonary edema and worsening symptoms must also be avoided. Antibiotics to cover the possible infectious etiologies (which include *S. pneumoniae*, *H. influenzae*, *N. meningitidis*, *C. pneumoniae* and *M. pneumoniae*, as well as many other bacteria and viruses) are important in the management of acute chest syndrome. Incentive spirometry to maintain alveolar patency is also important, and bronchodilator therapy can be a useful adjunct as well. Intubation for severe respiratory distress may also be required. Nitrous oxide therapy is not recommended for the management of acute chest syndrome.

Red blood cell transfusions are the most effective therapy for acute chest syndrome. Patients with sickle cell disease generally have baseline hemoglobin values of 7 to 9 g/dL and transfusions that raise the hemoglobin well above this range can lead to hyperviscosity and further sickle cell complications such as strokes. Those patients with baseline hemoglobin values over 10 g/dL should undergo exchange transfusion rather than simple transfusion to avoid hyperviscosity complications. The goal for blood transfusion or exchange transfusion should be to lower the percentage of sickled cells in the blood while avoiding further complications.

4. **(A)** Children with sickle cell disease are at increased risk for severe bacterial infections because of splenic hypofunction, secondary to slowly progressive autoinfarction of splenic tissue. The average age of complete splenic infarction is approximately 2 to 4 years old in patients with hemoglobin SS, but can be delayed to 6 to 8 years of age in patients with hemoglobin SC or Sβ+ thalassemia. Even prior to this age, however, children with sickle cell disease are more susceptible to encapsulated organism infection and rapidly progressive sepsis in the absence of treatment. Potential organisms include *S. pneumoniae*, *S. pyogenes*, *H. influenzae*, *N. meningitidis*, *Salmonella* species, and *E. coli*. Therefore, children with sickle cell disease should receive all of the recommended vaccines on time, and those who have fevers should always be evaluated by a physician and should undergo laboratory evaluation including complete blood count with reticulocyte count, blood culture, urinalysis and urine culture, and chest radiograph.

Ceftriaxone, a broad-spectrum third-generation cephalosporin, is the antibiotic most likely to cover the majority of potential pathogens in children with sickle cell disease, and particularly *S. pneumoniae*, the most common cause of infections and infectious morbidity in sickle cell patients. Other second- and third-generation cephalosporins are also acceptable options. Macrolides are frequently added to cover possible Chlamydia and Mycoplasma pulmonary infections. Although clindamycin and vancomycin are effective against most gram-positive bacteria, including *S. aureus*, they are not effective against the encapsulated gram-negative bacteria that are potential causes of infections and therefore are not appropriate choices for initial management. Anaerobic infections are also not significantly increased in patients with sickle cell disease and so metronidazole is not an appropriate initial choice.

5. (**D**) Opiates have several common side effects, including impaired gastrointestinal motility and constipation, nausea and vomiting, hypotension, respiratory depression, lowered seizure threshold, and pruritus, which must be managed in order to maximize the pain management in children with sickle cell crises. Hematuria is not a side effect of opiates, but does commonly occur in patients with sickle cell disease.

6. (**B**) Patients with hemoglobin SS and $S\beta^0$ thalassemia tend to have the most severe complications from sickle cell disease, including more frequent episodes of acute chest syndrome. Patients with hemoglobins SC and $S\beta^+$ thalassemia generally have milder symptoms, although the range of severity is wide and patients with hemoglobins SC or $S\beta^+$ thalassemia can have very severe complications. Patients with β-thalassemia do not have complications from red blood cell sickling, such as acute chest syndrome. Other factors, such as the amount of fetal hemoglobin (hemoglobin F) or the presence of coexisting α-thalassemia or other unknown factors may play a role in modifying sickle cell disease severity. People with hemoglobin AS, or sickle cell trait, do not experience acute chest syndrome and have virtually no symptoms, but should receive genetic counselling regarding the risks of sickle cell disease in their offspring.

7. (**C**) Recurrent acute chest syndrome results in pulmonary injury with intimal hyperplasia and fibrosis, with the development of chronic pulmonary infiltrates, chest pain, and hypoxia and the eventual development of pulmonary hypertension and cor pulmonale. Emphysema does not occur as a result of recurrent acute chest syndrome.

8. (**D**) The results of neonatal hemoglobin electrophoresis are reported in order of decreasing amounts of the expressed hemoglobin molecules. For example, patients with normal hemoglobin, or hemoglobin AA, will have more fetal hemo-

globin (hemoglobin F) than hemoglobin A at birth, and will have a neonatal hemoglobin electrophoresis result of "FA." Patients with homozygous hemoglobin SS will still have more fetal hemoglobin at birth than sickle hemoglobin, and so their neonatal electrophoresis result will be "FS." Patients with hemoglobin SC disease will have a neonatal electrophoresis result of "FSC." Patients with sickle cell trait have more hemoglobin A than hemoglobin S, as A is more stable than S, and so the correct result for patients with sickle trait is "FAS." Patients with hemoglobin $S\beta^+$ thalassemia will have some hemoglobin A, but not as much as the hemoglobin S, and therefore the result will be "FSA."

9. (**B**) Approximately 8% of U.S. African Americans carry the hemoglobin S gene, resulting in a sickle cell disease frequency of approximately 1/600 African Americans. By comparison, approximately 4% of African Americans in the United States carry the hemoglobin C gene, 1% carry a gene mutation for β-thalassemia, and 1% to 3% carry a gene mutation for α-thalassemia. Sickle cell disease can also be found in Middle Eastern, Indian, and Central and South American populations, while the hemoglobin S gene mutation is extremely rare in Caucasians. The prevalence of sickle cell disease has been linked to protection from malaria infection, with those patients with sickle cell trait or disease being relatively spared from the severe complications of malaria.

10. (**C**) Howell-Jolly bodies are intracellular collections of precipitated hemoglobin that, under normal circumstances, cause the red blood cell to be trapped in the spleen, either to be totally destroyed or to have the Howell-Jolly body "removed" by splenic macrophages, resulting in smaller, more fragile red blood cells that leave the spleen. The presence of red blood cells with these bodies in the peripheral circulation suggests the loss of the splenic filtration function, either because of surgical splenectomy or functional splenectomy from progressive infarction that occurs in patients with sickle cell disease. The average age of complete splenic infarction is approximately 2 to 4 years old for patients with hemoglobin SS, but is delayed to 6 to 8 years of age in patients with hemoglobin SC. Auer bodies

are white blood cell inclusions found in patients with acute promyelocytic leukemia. Basophilic stippling is seen in lead poisoning and represents residual ribosomal material within the red blood cells precipitated as a result of the presence of toxins. Polychromasia refers to the presence of reticulocytes on the peripheral smear, which appear more purplish than the mature red blood cells. While patients with sickle cell disease do have an increase in reticulocytes and have significant polychromasia on their peripheral smears, it is not associated with their splenic function.

11. **(D)** Renal disease is a common complication of patients with sickle cell disease. The kidney is particularly susceptible to injury in patients with sickle cell disease because of the relatively hypoxic environment of the renal medulla and the high oxygen requirements of the renal parenchyma. Renal disease occurs in up to 25% of adolescents with sickle cell disease, and up to 40% of adults with sickle cell disease will have renal insufficiency, with many progressing to end-stage renal disease requiring dialysis and possibly renal transplant. Components of "sickle cell nephropathy" include hyposthenuria, hematuria, proteinuria, renal cortical infarction, papillary necrosis, pyelonephritis, and, rarely, renal cell carcinoma. Glucosuria is not a complication seen in patients with sickle cell disease.

Hyposthenuria refers to the inability of patients with sickle cell disease to concentrate their urine, because of the infarction of and damage to the renal medulla. The presence of hyposthenuria can be found in sickle cell patients by 5 to 10 years of age and becomes irreversible by 15 years of age. Hyposthenuria can cause significant dehydration, particularly in patients experiencing complications of their sickle cell disease. Hematuria can be microscopic or gross and primarily arises from the left kidney (80% of cases), although in approximately 10% of cases, hematuria will arise from both kidneys. Proteinuria can range from microalbuminuria to nephrotic syndrome.

12. **(B)** The gallstones of patients with chronic hemolytic anemias (including sickle cell disease) are composed of bilirubin, a breakdown product of hemoglobin. Cholelithiasis with or without associated cholecystitis occurs in up to 70% of patients with sickle cell disease, and can occur in

children as young as 4 years of age. Approximately one-third of children with gallstones have an underlying hemolytic anemia. Recurrent or severe abdominal pain is common in patients with sickle cell disease and frequently is a result of cholelithiasis or cholecystitis, although hepatitis, pancreatitis, and other intra-abdominal processes must be considered, in addition to abdominal vaso-occlusive pain crises. Recurrent or severe abdominal pain in sickle cell patients with gallstones or episodes of acute cholecystitis are indications for cholecystectomy.

13. **(B)** Acute stroke in patients with sickle cell disease is one of the indications for emergent exchange transfusion. Approximately 10% of children with sickle cell disease have at least one stroke episode by the mean age of 7 to 8 years. Symptoms can range from headaches, changes in vision or other cranial nerve palsies to hemiparesis, seizures, coma, and death. The diagnosis generally can only be made with an MRI, although urgent CT scanning to rule out intracranial hemorrhage (rare in children, but more common in adults with sickle cell disease) should be performed. The use of emergent exchange transfusion in any patient with sickle cell disease and acute neurological symptoms is required to reduce the percentage of hemoglobin S to <30% and results in decreased symptom severity and reduced incidence of long-term complications. Simple red blood cell transfusions are not effective in the treatment of stroke in patients with sickle cell disease, and non-steroidal anti-inflammatory agents and hyperbaric oxygen have no role in stroke management in these cases.

14. **(C)** Patients with sickle cell disease who have strokes have similar symptoms to other patients with acute cerebrovascular injuries, including the acute onset of cranial nerve palsies, hemiparesis, and possibly seizures or coma. While most sickle cell patients will have a complete neurologic recovery from their strokes, complications such as residual neurologic dysfunction, persistent seizure disorder, cognitive delay, behavioral changes, and recurrent strokes can occur. Optic neuritis is not a neurologic complication of strokes in patients with sickle cell disease. Stroke recurrence in patients with sickle cell disease can occur in up to

60% of patients within 3 years of the initial stroke in the absence of treatment. Slowly progressive cognitive delay because of recurrent, otherwise asymptomatic strokes is a common problem in children with sickle cell disease and requires early identification and intervention.

15. **(D)** Regular blood transfusions to maintain a baseline hemoglobin level between 8 and 10 g/dL and a hemoglobin S fraction of <30% is the only proven therapy that can prevent stroke recurrence in children with sickle cell disease. The incidence of stroke recurrence can be decreased from 60% within 3 years of an initial stroke without treatment to <10% with regular blood transfusions. However, the hemoglobin should be maintained below 10 g/dL to avoid hyperviscosity associated with higher hemoglobin levels and an increase in stroke risk.

16. **(D)** Parvovirus B19 infections are associated with aplastic crises in any patient with shortened red blood cell lifespan. Therefore, patients with sickle cell disease, red blood cell enzyme deficiencies, or red blood cell structural defects are susceptible to aplastic crises from parvovirus B19. Parvovirus infects the erythroid precursors within the bone marrow, temporarily halting new red blood cell production. The otherwise normal patient, with a red blood cell lifespan of 120 days, will suffer a small, likely asymptomatic fall in his total hemoglobin, followed by bone marrow recovery and new red blood cell production. Patients with a decreased red blood cell lifespan, because of the inability of the marrow to produce new red blood cells appropriately, will have severe, possibly life-threatening falls in hemoglobin levels. Infections with bacteria and other viruses, such as EBV or adenovirus, do not commonly have bone marrow toxicity and generally do not cause aplastic crises.

17. **(D)** Dactylitis, or hand-foot syndrome, is a complication of sickle cell disease that most commonly occurs in infants younger than 1 year of age. Dactylitis is characterized by painful non-pitting edema of the dorsal surfaces of the hands and feet bilaterally, without other locations of pain or swelling. Dactylitis also frequently is accompanied by low-grade fevers. The etiology is not completely understood but most likely in-

volves vaso-occlusion within the distal extremities, and management is similar to other types of vaso-occlusive pain crises. Priapism is a condition of prolonged, painful erection that occurs in up to 40% of adolescent males with sickle cell disease and requires urgent intervention with intravenous fluids, pain control, and either medical or surgical interventions to reduce the erection. Priapism rarely occurs in children until 10 years of age and never in infancy. The erections of priapism can last for 30 minutes to several days, and recurrence can lead to eventual impotence. Acute chest syndrome and transient ischemic attacks both can occur in infancy, but are more common in older children and adults. The average age of initial cerebral vascular accidents in children with sickle cell disease is 7 to 8 years of age.

18. **(B)** Penicillin is the first choice for pneumococcal prophylaxis in patients with sickle cell disease, which is required because of the decreased splenic function and increased risk of sepsis from encapsulated organisms. Trimethoprim-sulfamethoxazole, rifampin, and fluconazole are agents not generally effective against *S. pneumoniae*. In patients who are allergic to penicillin, erythromycin would provide a second option for prophylactic therapy.

SUGGESTED READING

Embury SH, Vichinsky EP: Sickle cell disease. In: Hoffman R, Benz EJ, Shattil SJ, et al (eds): *Hematology: Basic Principles and Practice*, 3rd ed. Philadelphia: Churchill Livingstone, 2000, pp 510–543.

Lane PA: Sickle cell disease. *Pediatr Clin North Am* 43(3): 639–662, 1996.

American Academy of Pediatrics. Health supervision for children with sickle cell disease *Pediatrics* 109(3): 526–535, 2002.

CASE 87: A 14-YEAR-OLD BOY WITH A PAINFUL LEFT THIGH

A 14-year-old boy is brought to your office by his father for left leg pain. He had injured his left leg several weeks earlier playing football. He was not seen by a physician at the time of injury. The pain has persisted despite minimal activity since that time, and the pain has not been relieved with the use of ibuprofen.

He has been seen in your office since he was an infant, and he has no history of any medical problems.

The family history is also negative for any significant medical problems. He has been doing well in school and had been active in sports prior to this injury, with no history of prior leg injuries.

On physical exam, he is well-appearing with normal vital signs. His left leg appears grossly normal, but is tender above the left knee. Radiographs reveal a lytic bone lesion in the distal left femur, with no fracture.

SELECT THE ONE BEST ANSWER

1. The differential diagnosis of painful bony lesions in children includes all of the following *except*:

   (A) osteosarcoma
   (B) Ewing's sarcoma
   (C) osteoid osteoma
   (D) non-ossifying fibroma

2. Which of the following sites within bones is the *most* common primary site for osteosarcoma?

   (A) metaphysis
   (B) diaphysis
   (C) bone marrow
   (D) epiphysis

3. The peak incidence of osteosarcoma occurs in which age range?

   (A) 1 to 4 years
   (B) 5 to 8 years
   (C) 9 to 12 years
   (D) 13 to 17 years

4. Which of the following is *not* a risk factor for osteosarcoma?

   (A) history of bilateral retinoblastoma
   (B) history of prior radiation exposure
   (C) Down syndrome
   (D) family history of leukemia

5. Which of the following is the peak age range for diagnosis of patients with Ewing's sarcoma?

   (A) 1 to 5 years
   (B) 5 to 10 years
   (C) 10 to 20 years
   (D) 20 to 30 years

6. Which of the following is the *least* common site of Ewing's sarcoma?

   (A) femur
   (B) ilium
   (C) rib
   (D) skull

7. Which of the following clinical features is *least* likely to distinguish osteosarcoma from Ewing's sarcoma?

   (A) fever
   (B) tumor location
   (C) radiographic appearance
   (D) age of onset

8. Which of the following is *not* a clinical feature of Langerhans cell histiocytosis?

   (A) diabetes mellitus
   (B) seborrheic dermatitis
   (C) lytic bone lesions
   (D) pancytopenia

9. Which of the following is the *least* likely laboratory finding in patients with hemophagocytic lymphohistiocytosis?

   (A) thrombocytopenia
   (B) elevated alkaline phosphatase
   (C) elevated serum triglycerides
   (D) low serum fibrinogen

10. Which of the following blood products should *not* be used in pediatric patients with malignancies who are receiving chemotherapy?

    (A) platelet apheresis units
    (B) blood-type matched fresh frozen plasma
    (C) packed red blood cells obtained from the patient's siblings
    (D) leuko-reduced or leuko-filtered red blood cells

11. In which of the following clinical situations is a platelet transfusion *least* likely to be effective?

    (A) correction of thrombocytopenia in a patient with acute ITP
    (B) control of bleeding in a patient with Fanconi's anemia
    (C) preparation for a lumbar puncture in a patient recently diagnosed with leukemia
    (D) treatment of an intracranial hemorrhage in a patient with Wiskott-Aldrich syndrome

12. In which of the following clinical situations is the use of fresh frozen plasma (FFP) the *most* effective treatment option?

 (A) persistent hemorrhage in a patient with hepatic insufficiency
 (B) presurgical prophylaxis in a patient with hypofibrinogenemia
 (C) correction of prolonged partial thromboplastin time in a patient receiving heparin therapy
 (D) treatment of a hemarthrosis in a patient with hemophilia A

13. Infections from which of the following viruses are *not* acquired via blood product transfusions?

 (A) cytomegalovirus
 (B) hepatitis B virus
 (C) influenza virus
 (D) human immunodeficiency virus

14. Features of patient reactions to red blood cell transfusions include all of the following *except*:

 (A) temperature >101.3°F (38.5°C)
 (B) myoglobinuria
 (C) hyperbilirubinemia
 (D) dyspnea

15. Long-term complications of radiation therapy include all of the following *except*:

 (A) diabetes mellitus
 (B) secondary amenorrhea
 (C) coronary artery disease
 (D) restrictive lung disease

16. Which of the following types of chemotherapy is *not* matched correctly with one of its side effects?

 (A) doxorubicin   pulmonary fibrosis
 (B) cisplatin   high frequency hearing loss
 (C) cyclophosphamide   hemorrhagic cystitis
 (D) corticosteroids   avascular necrosis

Answers

1. **(D)** Osteosarcoma and Ewing's sarcoma are both primary bone malignancies that occur in children and young adults and most commonly present with pain localized to the tumor site. Osteosarcoma (also known as osteogenic sarcoma) is a relatively common pediatric malignancy, with approximately 400 cases per year in children younger than 20 years of age in the United States. Ewing's sarcoma and a related tumor, peripheral primitive neuroectodermal tumor (PPNET), are similar entities with similar tissues of origin that can arise within either bone or soft tissues and are members of a group of tumors called the "small round blue cell tumors of childhood," a group that also includes neuroblastoma, lymphoma, and rhabdomyosarcoma. Ewing's sarcoma accounts for approximately 100 cases of pediatric malignancy per year in the United States. Osteoid osteoma is a common benign bony lesion that generally occurs in the lower extremities and presents with nighttime pain that is relieved with nonsteroidal anti-inflammatory medications. Non-ossifying fibromas (also called fibrous cortical defects) are benign developmental defects in ossification that are painless, usually only detected incidentally, and require no therapy.

2. **(A)** Osteosarcoma most commonly occurs in the metaphyses of long bones, but can spread into the diaphyses and epiphyses via local invasion. Bone marrow involvement with osteosarcoma is extremely rare.

   The most common sites of osteosarcoma are at those sites with the most rapid bone growth: the distal femur, proximal tibia, and proximal humerus. Approximately 65% of all osteosarcomas occur in the femur, and over 80% of femoral osteosarcomas occur in the distal end. The second most common site is the proximal tibia, while the third most common site is the proximal humerus. Approximately 20% of osteosarcomas occur in the arms, primarily in the proximal humerus. In general, the outcomes for localized osteosarcoma are good, with 60% to 80% long-term survival with current treatments. Children with metastatic osteosarcoma, however, do significantly worsen, with only a 20% to 30% survival rate. Osteosarcoma can also rarely occur in flat bones such as the skull, ribs, and pelvis, where it also has a much poorer outcome.

3. **(D)** The peak incidence of osteosarcoma occurs in the second decade of life, particularly during the pubertal growth spurt, and tends to occur

slightly earlier in girls (who have an earlier onset of puberty). The development of osteosarcoma may in part be associated with the rapid bone growth that occurs during these times. Osteosarcoma is very rare in children younger than 5 years of age and uncommon in adults older than 30 years of age.

4. **(C)** Down syndrome is associated with an increased incidence of hematologic malignancies but does not have an increased incidence of osteosarcoma or other sarcomas. Children with cases of bilateral retinoblastoma almost always have germline mutations in the *Rb* gene, which are also associated with an increased incidence of secondary malignancies, approximately 50% of which are osteosarcomas. The risk of osteosarcoma in patients with *Rb* gene mutations is approximately 500 times that of the general population.

Prior radiation exposure, including radiation therapy for childhood malignancies, is also associated with an increased incidence of osteosarcoma. Radiation exposure has been linked to up to 5% of osteosarcoma cases, and osteosarcoma can occur up to 40 years after exposure to radiation.

A family history of sarcomas, leukemias, adrenocortical carcinomas, and breast and bone cancers can be found in families with hereditary mutations in the *p53* gene, termed the Li-Fraumeni syndrome, which also is associated with an increased incidence of osteosarcoma. Other syndromes associated with increased osteosarcoma incidence include Paget's disease and Ollier's disease (enchondromatosis), both of which more commonly are associated with adult-onset osteosarcoma.

5. **(C)** Ewing's sarcoma is most common during the second decade of life but can occur both in younger and older populations as well. Seventy percent of the cases occur in children younger than 20 years of age, and one-half of the cases occur between 10 and 20 years of age. Ewing's sarcoma is extremely rare in adults older than 30 years of age. Ewing's sarcomas are also extremely rare in African Americans and Asians, occurring most commonly in Caucasian populations. There is no apparent connection between the onset of Ewing's sarcoma and the occurrence of puberty, and there are no associated syndromes or exposures that increase the risk of Ewing's sarcoma.

6. **(D)** Ewing's sarcoma can present in a wide variety of locations, and, although most arise from within the skeleton, some Ewing's sarcomas can arise in soft tissues as well. The primary sites for Ewing's sarcoma are the pelvis and lower extremities, with approximately 20% of cases in the pelvis, 20% in the femurs, and 10% each in the tibias and fibulas. Approximately 9% of cases occur in the chest wall and are sometimes known as Askin tumors. Ewing's sarcomas are more common in the axial skeleton than osteosarcomas, but only approximately 3% of cases occur in the skull.

7. **(D)** Ewing's sarcoma and osteosarcoma both occur predominantly in the same age range of patients (between 10 and 20 years of age). However, Ewing's sarcoma and osteosarcoma have distinct features that can assist in the diagnosis prior to biopsy. Ewing's sarcoma tends to be associated with systemic symptoms such as fever and weight loss, while osteosarcoma usually only presents with local symptoms such as pain and swelling. Ewing's tumors are more commonly located in the axial skeleton and are usually diaphyseal, as opposed to osteosarcomas which are more commonly metaphyseal and more likely to occur in the extremities. Furthermore, Ewing's sarcoma classically demonstrates reactive bone formation (described as "onion skin" or "hair-on-end" periosteal reaction visible on x-rays) that is not usually found in osteosarcomas, which typically present with lytic bony lesions. A family history of other sarcomas, leukemias, breast cancers, or adrenal cancers suggests the possibility of Li-Fraumeni syndrome. Li-Fraumeni syndrome, a tumor predisposition syndrome as a result of mutations in the *p53* gene, is associated with an increase in osteosarcoma incidence, but is not associated with Ewing's sarcoma.

8. **(A)** Langerhans cell histiocytosis (LCH) is a monoclonal disorder of histiocytes with a wide variety of clinical presentations that affects approximately 4 children per million per year. Previously recognized entities such as histiocytosis X, Letterer-Siwe disease, Hand-Schüller-Christian Syndrome, and eosinophilic granuloma are now all classified as subtypes of LCH. The most benign form of LCH is eosinophilic granuloma, which consists of isolated lytic bony lesions, most

commonly in the skull but also occurring in the vertebrae, mandible, ribs, ilium, scapula, and long bones. The bony lesions can be asymptomatic or can cause localized pain or swelling. Hand-Schüller-Christian disease is multifocal LCH characterized by skull lesions, diabetes insipidus, and exophthalmos. Other less common features include other pituitary hormonal abnormalities, gingival ulcerations with premature tooth eruption, chronic otitis media, and persistent seborrheic rashes. Letterer-Siwe disease is the most severe form of LCH, and usually occurs before 2 years of age. Letterer-Siwe disease is characterized by more severe visceral involvement, including lung, liver, intestinal, and marrow disease, with persistent fevers, irritability, failure to thrive, malabsorption, pancytopenia, and other symptoms related to diffuse organ involvement. Letterer-Siwe disease only accounts for 15% of LCH cases, but has the worst prognosis and is the least responsive to therapy.

9. **(B)** Hemophagocytic lymphohistiocytosis (HLH) is a histiocytic syndrome that can be either primary or secondary to infection or neoplasia. Proliferation of activated macrophages results in the symptoms of HLH, which can involve the liver, spleen, bone marrow, and central nervous system. Symptoms include fever, hepatosplenomegaly, skin rashes, and meningeal inflammation with meningismus and, potentially, seizures. Laboratory features include pancytopenia, hypertriglyceridemia, hypofibrinogenemia, hyperferritinemia, and hypoproteinemia. Depressed T cell and NK cell activity can also be demonstrated. Alkaline phosphatase levels are generally normal. Diagnosis of HLH requires the presence of fever, splenomegaly, peripheral cytopenias of at least two cell lines, hypertriglyceridemia or hypofibrinogenemia, and evidence of hemophagocytosis seen either in the bone marrow or in a lymph node biopsy specimen.

10. **(C)** Blood products for patients receiving chemotherapy should be leuko-reduced and irradiated to reduce the transmission rate of cytomegalovirus (carried by donor white blood cells) and to reduce the incidence of graft-versus-host disease (mediated by viable donor lymphocytes). Exposure of the patient to blood products from relatives should be avoided in order to prevent alloimmunization of the patient to potential bone marrow donor antigens. Furthermore, patients receiving chemotherapy often require frequent blood product transfusions, and so exposure to unrelated donors should be minimized as much as possible. Therefore, platelet apheresis units, which are isolated from single donors, are preferred over units pooled from multiple donors. Fresh frozen plasma should be given to replace coagulation factors when needed and should be blood-type matched to reduce the incidence of immune-mediated reactions from the antibodies carried in the transfused plasma.

11. **(A)** Platelet transfusions are necessary both for control of active bleeding and for prevention of spontaneous hemorrhages in patients with decreased or dysfunctional platelets. Platelet transfusions should be given to prevent spontaneous hemorrhages when the platelet count is below 10,000/μL. In most cases, lumbar punctures can be performed safely with platelet counts >10,000/μL, and intramuscular injections should be avoided when platelet counts are below 20,000/μL. To prevent intracranial hemorrhages in patients with brain tumors, the platelet count should be maintained over 30,000–50,000/μL.

Platelet transfusions are most useful in states of platelet hypo-production, such as in patients receiving chemotherapy or in conditions of bone marrow hypoplasia such as Fanconi's anemia or aplastic anemia, and in conditions with intrinsic platelet dysfunction, such as Wiskott-Aldrich syndrome, Bernard-Soulier syndrome, or Glanzmann's thrombasthenia. Platelet transfusions are less likely to increase platelet counts in cases of increased platelet consumption, such as immune thrombocytopenic purpura (ITP), disseminated intravascular coagulation (DIC), or Kasabach-Merritt syndrome, or in cases of platelet sequestration from hypersplenism. The transfused platelets in cases of increased consumption or sequestration will be rapidly consumed or sequestered. Correction of thrombocytopenia in these cases requires treatment for the underlying condition rather than platelet transfusions.

12. **(A)** Fresh frozen plasma (FFP) is a plasma product isolated from whole blood by centrifugation.

Rapid freezing is used to preserve the plasma proteins, which include clotting factors II, V, VII, VIII, IX, X, XI, XII, and other proteins such as protein C, protein S, antithrombin III, complement factors, and immunoglobulins. FFP contains small amounts of fibrinogen, factor XIII, and von Willebrand factor, but these factors can be found in higher concentrations in cryoprecipitate, generated from rapid thawing of FFP.

Clotting factors are predominantly synthesized in the liver, and so hepatic insufficiency is associated with clotting factor deficiencies that result in prolongation of the prothrombin and partial thromboplastin times. Replacement of these factors with FFP is frequently necessary to control bleeding. Because FFP is a poor source of fibrinogen, FFP should not be used as a source of fibrinogen replacement in a patient with hypofibrinogenemia; instead, cryoprecipitate should be used as needed. For patients with single factor deficiencies, such as in patients with hemophilia, replacement of factor with FFP would require large volumes and exposures to large numbers of donors, each with added risk of transfusion-related infections. Therefore, factor replacement with purified or recombinant products, which have lower risks of transmission of viral infections because of postsynthetic processing, is preferred for treatment of any bleeding episodes in these patients.

In patients receiving anticoagulant therapy, reversal of the anticoagulant action is frequently required, either to control excessive bleeding or prior to surgical procedures. Heparin functions as an anticoagulant by inhibiting serine proteases in the coagulation cascade, including thrombin-mediated generation of fibrin. The effects of heparin can be reversed rapidly by administration of protamine, a mixture of polypeptides that binds to heparin and neutralizes its inhibitory effect on the coagulation proteases. FFP is less effective in reversing the effects of heparin, as the excess heparin will inhibit FFP-derived factors as well. In patients being treated with warfarin sodium (Coumadin), the vitamin K-dependent clotting factors (factors II, VII, IX, and X) are depleted, and can be replaced on an emergent basis for severe bleeding with FFP. However, for control of non-emergent bleeding or to reverse the effects of warfarin sodium (Coumadin), vitamin K replacement is the preferred method of treatment, with rapid synthesis of the factors by the liver occurring in the presence of vitamin K to correct the deficiency.

13. **(C)** Blood transfusions are associated with a small risk of viral transmission and infection, with potential blood-borne pathogens including human immunodeficiency virus (HIV), hepatitis B and C viruses, cytomegalovirus (CMV), and Epstein-Barr virus (EBV). Other viruses that are primarily spread via respiratory droplets, such as influenza, respiratory syncytial virus, and varicella zoster, are not spread by blood transfusions. Blood products are aggressively screened, both by donor history and serological testing, to reduce the chances of a transfusion-related infection. Non-blood cell containing blood products are treated further to reduce the transmission rate of viruses. The current risks of viral transmission (per units of blood transfused) are approximately 1/2,000,000 units for HIV and 1/500,000 units for hepatitis C. Approximately one-third of packed red blood cell units are CMV positive, and can cause CMV infection in recipients who are CMV negative. The viral transmission rates for products such as fresh frozen plasma and cryoprecipitate are much lower, because of the extra treatment, but are still not completely risk free.

14. **(B)** Reactions to blood product transfusions occur in 1% to 10% of transfusions, and can range from mild fever and chills to anaphylaxis and shock. Reactions occur more commonly in patients who have received prior transfusions. Acute reactions occur within 24 hours of the transfusion, and can have a variety of presentations. Acute hemolytic transfusion reactions because of ABO blood type mismatch are generally the most severe, with symptoms that include fevers, chills, anxiety, nausea, vomiting, shortness of breath, hypotension, hemoglobinemia, hemoglobinuria, renal failure, and disseminated intravascular coagulation. Simple febrile reactions to the presence of donor cytokines can also have fevers, chills, nausea, vomiting, and headaches, but do not have hemoglobinemia or hemoglobinuria. Allergic reactions because of host antibodies to donor plasma proteins can also occur, and can range from minor urticaria to anaphylaxis.

Chronic transfusion reactions can also occur from 4 to 7 days to several weeks posttransfusion. Delayed hemolytic reactions are usually a result of alloimmunization to minor blood group antigens from prior blood transfusions, and are usually less severe than acute reactions. Delayed transfusion reactions usually have only mild fevers, fatigue, and weakness and associated laboratory features of hemolysis such as increased reticulocytes, increased indirect bilirubin, decreased haptoglobin, and peripheral spherocytosis. Hemoglobinuria is rare in delayed transfusion reactions. Myoglobinuria is not a feature of either acute or chronic transfusion reactions.

15. (A) Radiation therapy is associated with a wide range of complications, which vary depending on the radiation site and dose. CNS radiation is associated with cognitive delays, hormonal abnormalities (such as growth hormone deficiency and thyroid dysfunction), and increased risk of cerebrovascular disease. Thoracic radiation is associated both with cardiac damage (ranging from cardiomyopathy to restrictive pericarditis to myocardial infarction from increased atherosclerosis) and with lung damage (with fibrosis and restrictive lung disease). Abdominal irradiation is associated with injury to abdominal organs, primarily gonadal failure and infertility. Furthermore, radiation therapy is associated with an increased risk of secondary malignancies at the sites of radiation. Diabetes mellitus is not a common complication of radiation therapy.

16. (A) Anthracyclines such as doxorubicin are associated with cardiac toxicity and can cause both acute and delayed cardiomyopathy with congestive heart failure. Anthracyclines are not associated with any pulmonary complications. Platinum compounds such as cisplatin are associated with renal toxicity and ototoxicity with high frequency hearing loss. Cyclophosphamide, a commonly used alkylating agent, is also associated with renal toxicity, and its metabolites can irritate the bladder wall, resulting in hemorrhagic cystitis. High-dose steroid therapy has a long list of side effects and complications, including hypertension, hyperglycemia, behavioral changes, and growth delay, but can also cause avascular necrosis, particularly in the hip joint.

SUGGESTED READING

Chintagumpala MM, Mahoney DH Jr: Malignant bone tumors. In: McMillan JA, DeAngelis CD, Feigin RD, et al (eds): *Oski's Pediatrics: Principles and Practice*, 3rd ed. Philadelphia: Lippincott Williams and Wilkins, 1999, pp 1527–1530.

Copley L, Dormans JP: Benign pediatric bone tumors. *Pediatr Clin North Am* 43(4):949–66, 1996.

Himelstein BP, Dormans JP: Malignant bone tumors of childhood. *Pediatr Clin North Am* 43(4):967–984, 1996.

Arico M, Egeler RM: Clinical aspects of Langerhans cell histiocytosis. *Hematol Oncol Clin North Am* 12(2): 247–258, 1998.

Quirolo KC: Transfusion medicine for the pediatrician. *Pediatr Clin North Am* 49:1211–1238, 2002.

CASE 88: A 6-YEAR-OLD WITH FEVERS, FATIGUE, AND BRUISING

A 6-year-old child is brought to your clinic by her parents for recurrent fevers, extreme fatigue, and bruising on her legs. She was a previously well child with no past medical history but was noted by her parents to be "very tired" starting about 1 week ago. Her activity level dropped significantly and she seemed to be "sleeping all the time," according to her mother. She also began having daily fevers 3 days ago, and yesterday was noted to have large bruises on her legs bilaterally, despite no history of trauma. Her parents deny any medication use or any ingestions. The family history is negative for any significant medical problems. Prior to the past week she had been going to school and doing well.

On physical exam, the child is pale and tired-appearing. Her temperature is 102°F (38.9°C) orally. She has a few petechiae in her oropharynx and diffuse cervical lymphadenopathy. She has a 2/6 systolic ejection murmur. Her liver and spleen are both palpable 1 cm below the costal margin. Her legs have multiple large ecchymoses.

Her complete blood count revealed a white blood cell count of 65,000/μL, a hemoglobin of 6.4 g/dL, and a platelet count of 18,000/μL. The differential has 84% large white blood cells with minimal agranular pale blue cytoplasm and large nuclei with very fine chromatin and large nucleoli.

SELECT THE ONE BEST ANSWER

1. The patient's *most* likely diagnosis is which of the following?

   (A) aplastic anemia
   (B) acute lymphoblastic leukemia

(C) immune thrombocytopenic purpura

(D) hemolytic-uremic syndrome

2. Which of the following studies is *not* indicated for this patient at this time?

(A) chest radiograph

(B) bone marrow aspirate

(C) lumbar puncture

(D) spinal MRI

3. Which of the following interventions is indicated for this patient at this time?

(A) intravenous antibiotic therapy

(B) intravenous erythropoietin

(C) oral diuretic therapy

(D) subcutaneous heparin treatment

4. Which of the following features of this patient's presentation places her at highest risk for treatment failure?

(A) her sex

(B) her white blood cell count

(C) her age

(D) her physical exam

5. What is the likelihood of a child with standard-risk acute lymphoblastic leukemia entering remission after the first month of induction therapy?

(A) 5% to 10%

(B) 20% to 30%

(C) 50% to 60%

(D) 90% to 95%

6. Which of the following is *not* a feature of tumor lysis syndrome?

(A) elevated serum uric acid

(B) elevated serum calcium

(C) elevated serum creatinine

(D) elevated serum potassium

7. Measures to prevent the complications of tumor lysis syndrome include all of the following *except*:

(A) intravenous hydration

(B) urine alkalinization

(C) xanthine oxidase inhibition

(D) intravenous potassium phosphate

8. Which of the following is *not* a risk factor for development of childhood leukemia?

(A) previous treatment with chemotherapy

(B) ataxia-telangiectasia

(C) maternal cocaine use during pregnancy

(D) Down syndrome

9. Which of the following is the *least* likely site of leukemia relapse?

(A) bone marrow

(B) CSF

(C) testes

(D) liver

10. The *best* option for *Pneumocystis carinii* prophylaxis in this patient is which of the following?

(A) intravenous dapsone

(B) intravenous pentamidine

(C) oral trimethoprim-sulfamethoxazole

(D) intramuscular penicillin

11. Which of the following immunizations is contraindicated in patients receiving chemotherapy?

(A) measles-mumps-rubella (MMR)

(B) tetanus-diphtheria (Td)

(C) *H. influenzae* type b

(D) inactivated poliomyelitis vaccine (IPV)

12. With which of the following blood counts is neutropenia present?

(A) WBC 8500; 51% neutrophils

(B) WBC 2000; 89% neutrophils

(C) WBC 16,000; 10% neutrophils

(D) WBC 5000; 15% neutrophils

13. Which of the following antibiotic regimens is *least* effective for febrile patients with neutropenia?

(A) intravenous ceftazidime

(B) intravenous vancomycin

(C) intravenous nafcillin and gentamicin

(D) intravenous meropenem

14. Which of the following is the *least* common type of infection in patients with an absolute neutrophil count <500?

(A) gingivitis

(B) cellulitis

(C) bacterial pneumonia

(D) bacterial meningitis

15. Features of Shwachman-Diamond syndrome include all of the following *except*:

(A) protein malabsorption

(B) cyclic neutropenia

(C) metaphyseal dysostosis

(D) elevated risk of aplastic anemia

16. Which of the following procedures is contraindicated in patients with severe neutropenia?

(A) lumbar puncture

(B) peripheral venous blood sampling

(C) throat culture

(D) rectal temperature

17. Which of the following is *not* an acceptable treatment option for the management of a varicella-naive patient receiving chemotherapy who develops a new varicella infection?

(A) intravenous immunoglobulin

(B) acyclovir

(C) ribavirin

(D) varicella-zoster immune globulin

Answers

1. **(B)** The presence of cytopenias with blast forms on the peripheral smear is characteristic of acute leukemia. Leukemias are the most common form of childhood cancer and account for approximately one-third of all pediatric malignancies. There are approximately 3000 new cases of pediatric leukemia each year in the United States, which occur in all races and equally in boys and girls. Approximately 75% of new leukemias are acute lymphoblastic leukemia, while approximately 20% are acute myeloid leukemia. The peak age of onset of acute leukemia in children is between 2 and 5 years of age. The underlying etiology of acute leukemias in children is generally unknown, although there is an increased risk of acute leukemia in children with syndromes such as Down syndrome, Bloom syndrome, Fanconi syndrome and ataxia-telangiectasia. Symptoms of acute leukemias in children are generally related to their cytopenias with bleeding, easy bruising and petechiae from thrombocytopenia, pallor and fatigue from anemia, and fevers and infections from functional neutropenia. Children with acute leukemia also frequently have diffuse lymphadenopathy, hepatosplenomegaly, and bone pain with limping or refusal to walk.

Aplastic anemia can present with the acute onset of pancytopenia, but does not have associated peripheral white blood cell blasts. Aplastic anemia can be either acquired or congenital, such as with Fanconi syndrome. Potential causes of acquired aplastic anemia include environmental toxins, infections, and prior radiation therapy or chemotherapy, and treatment requires either immunosuppression or bone marrow transplantation. Immune thrombocytopenic purpura, or ITP, is characterized by isolated thrombocytopenia with no other blood count abnormalities, while hemolytic uremic syndrome, or HUS, is usually secondary to a prodromal diarrheal illness, with associated renal failure, anemia, and thrombocytopenia.

2. **(D)** The initial work-up of a patient with leukemia includes a chest radiograph to rule out an underlying mediastinal mass with the possibility of airway compromise. Furthermore, bone marrow evaluation and a lumbar puncture are required for evaluation of the patient's disease status. In general, the bone marrow in cases of acute leukemia is filled with over 80% leukemic blasts and severely decreased numbers of precursors for other types of blood cells. In the absence of peripheral neurologic symptoms, a spinal MRI is not indicated. Approximately 5% to 10% of new cases of acute leukemia will have leukemic blasts present in the CSF at diagnosis and rarely can have symptoms such as headache or cranial nerve palsies; but the presence or absence of leukemic blasts in the spinal fluid cannot be determined by imaging.

3. **(A)** Any patient with fever and neutropenia requires urgent intravenous antibiotic therapy. A patient with new acute leukemia, while potentially having a normal absolute neutrophil count, likely has few functional neutrophils and is therefore functionally neutropenic and at high risk for serious bacterial infections. While this patient would benefit from blood and platelet transfusions at this time, there is no indication for starting erythropoietin. Furthermore, diuresis and anticoagulation are not indicated at this time.

4. **(B)** Initial risk groups for pediatric leukemia are based on patient age and total white blood cell count. The patient's white blood cell count of >50,000/μL places her in the high-risk category for acute lymphoblastic leukemia (ALL). Girls with ALL tend to have a slightly higher survival rate than boys, although sex is not a feature used to determine the initial risk groups for treatment purposes. Patients between 1 and 10 years old are considered "standard risk," while those patients younger than 1 year of age or older than 10 years of age are considered "high risk" and require more intensive therapy. Physical exam features have no prognostic significance for ALL outcomes. Other prognostic features include cellular ploidy (with hypodiploid leukemias having a worse outcome) and other chromosomal abnormalities, such as the Philadelphia chromosome [t(9;22) bcr-abl translocation], which are associated with a worse outcome.

5. **(D)** The likelihood of remission after induction therapy for standard risk ALL in a child is over 90%. The current likelihood of a long-term "cure" is approximately 70% to 80%, with lower survival for higher risk patients, patients with relapsed disease and for those with acute myeloid leukemia.

6. **(B)** Tumor lysis syndrome, which most commonly occurs in leukemias and rapidly growing lymphomas, can occur both before and after therapy is initiated. The rapid cellular turnover in these types of tumors results in the release of large amounts of intracellular breakdown products and electrolytes into the blood. Features of tumor lysis include elevations in uric acid, potassium, phosphorus, lactate dehydrogenase (LDH), and aspartate aminotransferase (AST). Calcium levels are frequently low, because of the elevated phosphorus levels, and can result in anorexia, vomiting, muscle cramps or spasms, tetany, and seizures. The uric acid and calcium phosphate can then precipitate in renal tubules and cause renal insufficiency or even failure, resulting in elevations of the serum creatinine levels.

7. **(D)** The management of tumor lysis syndrome includes aggressive hydration with intravenous fluids, urine alkalinization, and reduction of uric acid levels. The goals of hydration and alkalinization are to maintain good urine output and prevent precipitation of uric acid within the renal tubules. Inhibition of xanthine oxidase (which generates uric acid from nucleic acid metabolism) with allopurinol or direct metabolism of uric acid with intravenous urate oxidase decreases the serum levels of uric acid and reduces the risk of renal obstruction. Treatment of elevations in potassium and phosphorus with diuretics or medications such as insulin, calcium gluconate, or Kayexalate are also indicated as needed. Potassium and phosphorus should not be added to intravenous fluids, because of the already increased levels frequently seen in patients with tumor lysis syndrome and the potential for associated renal insufficiency. Dialysis for severe renal insufficiency may be required in some cases.

8. **(C)** Risk factors for the development of childhood leukemia include prior chemotherapy with either alkylating agents or topoisomerase inhibitors, both of which increase the incidence of secondary malignancies. Alkylating agents such as cyclophosphamide are associated with an increased risk of leukemias, usually within 5 years of exposure. Topoisomerase inhibitors such as etoposide are associated with an increased risk of myeloid malignancies, usually within 2 years. Ataxia-telangiectasia is a tumor predisposition syndrome associated with an increased risk of leukemias. Down syndrome is associated with a risk of transient myeloproliferative disorder (TMD), a neonatal leukemia-like proliferation of white blood cells that will spontaneously resolve without therapy. Unfortunately, in 20% of cases of TMD, true leukemia develops later in childhood, and patients with Down syndrome have a 500-fold increased risk of the M7 subtype of acute myelogenous leukemia compared to normal children. No linkage has been demonstrated between maternal illicit drug use during pregnancy and any increased incidence in childhood leukemia.

9. **(D)** Leukemia relapses most commonly occur in the bone marrow, but can also occur in the CSF and testes, both sanctuary sites where chemotherapy penetration is limited by the blood-brain and blood-testes barriers, respectively. Leukemia relapses can occur in solid organs such as the liver or spleen, but are extremely rare.

10. **(C)** *Pneumocystis carinii* infections are common in patients with malignancies receiving chemotherapy and occur in up to 50% of these patients in the absence of prophylactic therapy. *Pneumocystis carinii* pneumonia (PCP) is characterized by fever, non-productive cough, tachypnea, hypoxia, and bilateral diffuse interstitial infiltrates seen on chest radiograph. Acute, fulminant PCP is more common in patients with malignancies than in patients with other forms of immunodeficiency, where PCP is a more chronic, indolent infection. Diagnosis of PCP requires either sputum cultures or bronchoalveolar lavage to look for characteristic cysts and trophozoites of *Pneumocystis carinii*.

Oral trimethoprim-sulfamethoxazole is the most effective prophylactic agent for *Pneumocystis carinii* pneumonia, with a <5% failure rate. Side effects of the trimethoprim-sulfamethoxazole include neutropenia and skin rashes, which can progress to Stevens-Johnson syndrome. Dapsone and aerosolized pentamidine are secondary options for PCP prophylaxis, with approximately 20% failure rates each. Intravenous pentamidine has not been demonstrated to be an effective prophylactic regimen. Penicillin has no role in PCP prophylaxis. Patients with new diagnoses of hematologic malignancies and all patients receiving chemotherapy should receive some form of prophylactic therapy. Furthermore, prophylaxis should continue for up to 6 months after therapy has finished, as the immune system requires several months for full recovery.

11. **(A)** Live virus vaccines such as oral polio (OPV) and measles-mumps-rubella (MMR) are contraindicated in patients receiving chemotherapy. Varicella vaccines, although also composed of live viruses, have been shown to be safe and somewhat effective in patients receiving chemotherapy. Furthermore, although other vaccines are not strictly contraindicated, the relative immunodeficiency in patients receiving chemotherapy will impede the development of productive immunity from vaccines given, and so titers must be checked after completion of chemotherapy to determine whether booster immunizations are needed. In general, vaccinations should be withheld during chemotherapy and should be restarted approximately 3 to 6 months after chemotherapy treatment has been completed.

12. **(D)** Neutropenia is defined as an absolute neutrophil count (ANC) of <1500, with the ANC calculated by multiplying the total white blood cell count by the percentage of neutrophils. Mild neutropenia, with an ANC between 1000 and 1500, is associated with an increased risk of bacterial infections, while moderate (between 500 and 1000) and severe (<500) neutropenias are associated with much higher risks of infections. Decreased numbers of neutrophils will also reduce or eliminate the signs and symptoms associated with infections and inflammation, with reduced or absent pyuria, minimal CSF pleocytosis, normal chest radiographs, and minimal redness or swelling of skin. Fever is often the only sign of infection in these patients, and should be treated urgently.

Pseudoneutropenia is a condition common in African Americans in the United States, characterized by an ANC between 1000 and 1500, but with no increased risk of infections. Neutrophils are generally present within the blood stream or attached to the vascular endothelial surfaces (a process called margination). Neutrophils can be induced to release from the vascular endothelial cell surfaces by treatment with corticosteroids or epinephrine. Pseudoneutropenia is a result of increased margination of neutrophils, and therefore the true neutrophil count is normal and the patient will have normal responses to infections.

13. **(B)** Antibiotic coverage for patients with fevers and neutropenia needs to account for the most common and the most serious infections. Historically, gram-negative bacterial infections predominated in patients with neutropenia and were frequently rapidly fatal. More recently, with the increased use of central venous catheters, there has been a dramatic increase in the prevalence of gram-positive bacterial infections as well.

Gram-negative infections most commonly arise from endogenous enteric bacteria that are able to penetrate mucosal barriers as a result of the neutropenia, and they are both common and serious and can cause rapid decompensation and death if not treated. Treatment regimens for patients with fevers and neutropenia must therefore include broad-spectrum gram negative coverage. Infections because of *Pseudomonas aeruginosa* are particularly dangerous in neutropenic patients, and any antibiotic regimen used must provide some anti-pseudomonal coverage. For patients with fever and neutropenia, vancomycin, which only covers gram-positive organisms, is therefore not a good option for monotherapy. Gram-positive organisms from either endogenous skin flora or endogenous enteric flora can also frequently cause infections, but are less likely to be rapidly fatal. Therefore, broad spectrum gram-positive coverage is generally not required for initial therapy. The other antibiotics or antibiotic combinations provide adequate gram-negative and gram-positive coverage for initial therapy.

14. **(D)** Patients with absolute neutrophil counts <500 are most susceptible to infections from endogenous flora, which are prominent in the gastrointestinal tract and mucous membranes. The neutropenia results in impaired mucosal barrier defenses, allowing for infections to develop. Therefore, the most common infections include skin infections (cellulitis), respiratory infections (upper and lower), and GI infections (oral infections such as stomatitis or gingivitis and rectal infections such as perirectal abscesses). Bacterial meningitis does not occur more frequently in patients with neutropenia, although it can be more severe.

15. **(B)** Features of Shwachman-Diamond syndrome include persistent neutropenia with recurrent skin and respiratory bacterial infections, pancreatic insufficiency with malabsorption and failure to thrive, and metaphyseal chondrodysplasia (most commonly at the hips, knees, shoulders, and wrists). Pancreatic insufficiency and recurrent infections generally begin before the patient reaches 10 years of age. Aplastic anemia occurs in up to 25% of cases of Shwachman-Diamond syndrome, as well as short stature, cleft palate, microcephaly, and thrombocytopenia. There is also an associated increased risk of progression to acute leukemia.

16. **(D)** Rectal temperatures and any procedures that involve potential injury to the perirectal tissues such as administration of rectal contrast, should be avoided in patients with neutropenia, because of the risk of mucosal surface disruption and localized or disseminated infection. Other procedures such as peripheral blood sampling and placement of intravenous lines or lumbar punctures, if performed with sterile technique, are acceptable to perform in patients with neutropenia. Oral procedures such as tooth brushing or throat cultures, are also acceptable but should be done carefully to avoid mucosal injury. Extensive dental work, however, should be avoided if possible.

17. **(C)** Urgent management of varicella exposure in a patient receiving chemotherapy is crucial to avoid potentially life-threatening complications associated with active varicella infections. Primary varicella infections in particular have a mortality rate of up to 20% in patients receiving chemotherapy, with disseminated varicella affecting the lungs, liver, and central nervous system. Varicella-naive children who are exposed to varicella while on chemotherapy should receive varicella immune globulin within 72 hours of exposure, although in the absence of varicella immune globulin, intravenous immune globulin can be used instead. Furthermore, high-dose intravenous acyclovir should also be given for those patients who develop symptoms of varicella. Ribavirin is not efficacious against varicella and should not be used.

SUGGESTED READING

Mahoney DH Jr: Acute lymphoblastic leukemia. In: McMillan JA, DeAngelis CD, Feigin RD, et al (eds): *Oski's Pediatrics: Principles and Practice*, 3rd ed. Philadelphia: Lippincott Williams and Wilkins, 1999, pp 1493–1500.

Mahoney DH Jr: Quantitative granulocyte disorders. In: McMillan JA, DeAngelis CD, Feigin RD, et al (eds): *Oski's Pediatrics: Principles and Practice*, 3rd ed. Philadelphia: Lippincott Williams and Wilkins, 1999, pp 1461–1464.

Pui C-H, Campana D, Evans WE: Childhood acute lymphoblastic leukaemia: current status and future perspectives. *Lancet* 2:597–607, 2001.

Viscoli C, Castagnola E: Treatment of febrile neutropenia: what is new? *Curr Opin Infect Dis* 15:377–382, 2002.

Jeha S: Tumor lysis syndrome. *Semin Hematol* 38(4 supp 10):4–8, 2001.

CASE 89: A 5-YEAR-OLD CHILD WITH PETECHIAE

A 5-year-old boy was brought to the emergency room for evaluation of a new rash. The patient awoke this morning covered in "red dots," according to his mother. He had a "cold" approximately 2 weeks previously, but otherwise has been well. He takes no medications and has had no sick contacts. There is no history of toxin ingestions. The family history is non-contributory.

On physical exam, the child is well-appearing and afebrile. He has diffuse petechiae covering his face, neck, chest, back, stomach, arms and legs. He also has large bruises on his forearms and upper and lower legs. He has no palpable lymphadenopathy or hepatosplenomegaly.

A complete blood count done in the emergency room is within normal limits except for a platelet count of 8,000/μL.

SELECT THE ONE BEST ANSWER

1. The differential diagnosis for a petechial rash of acute onset includes all of the following *except*:

   (A) immune thrombocytopenic purpura (ITP)
   (B) Rocky Mountain spotted fever
   (C) infectious mononucleosis
   (D) acute lymphoblastic leukemia

2. Which of the following laboratory abnormalities is *most* commonly associated with the development of petechiae?

   (A) thrombocytopenia
   (B) prolonged prothrombin time
   (C) elevated fibrin degradation products
   (D) low factor VIII level

3. The *most* likely diagnosis for this child is:

   (A) acute lymphoblastic leukemia
   (B) ITP
   (C) von Willebrand disease (vWD)
   (D) thrombocytopenia with radii (TAR) syndrome

4. Which of the following tests is *not* indicated in the initial evaluation of a patient with a suspected bleeding disorder?

   (A) platelet function analysis
   (B) direct Coombs test
   (C) partial thromboplastin time
   (D) complete blood count

5. Which of the following medications is *not* associated with immune-mediated thrombocytopenia?

   (A) erythromycin
   (B) penicillin
   (C) trimethoprim-sulfamethoxazole
   (D) chloroquine

6. Which of the following is *not* an indication for a bone marrow evaluation in cases of thrombocytopenia?

   (A) fever
   (B) concurrent neutropenia
   (C) hepatosplenomegaly
   (D) history of upper respiratory infection

7. The *most* common age range for the presentation of acute ITP is:

   (A) 0 to 1 years
   (B) 2 to 10 years
   (C) 10 to 15 years
   (D) 15 to 20 years

8. Which of the following is the *least* common complication of ITP?

   (A) intracranial hemorrhage
   (B) epistaxis
   (C) intra-articular hemorrhage
   (D) melena

9. Which of the following is the *best* initial treatment for patients with ITP?

   (A) intravenous immune globulin
   (B) ibuprofen
   (C) splenectomy
   (D) platelet transfusion

10. Which of the following is *not* a feature of Wiskott-Aldrich syndrome?

    (A) eczematous rash
    (B) thrombocytopenia
    (C) anemia
    (D) recurrent infections

11. Which of the following syndromes is *not* associated with an increased incidence of neonatal thrombocytopenia?

    (A) Glanzmann's thrombasthenia
    (B) Kasabach-Merritt syndrome
    (C) Down syndrome
    (D) Fanconi's anemia

12. What is the inheritance pattern for factor VIII deficiency?

    (A) autosomal recessive
    (B) autosomal dominant
    (C) X-linked
    (D) mitochondrial

13. Which of the following procedures is contraindicated in a patient with uncorrected severe factor IX deficiency?

    (A) peripheral intravenous line placement
    (B) femoral central line placement
    (C) antecubital venous blood draw
    (D) brain CT scan

14. Laboratory findings associated with hemophilia A include which of the following?

    (A) prolonged prothrombin time (PT)
    (B) prolonged partial thromboplastin time (PTT)
    (C) prolonged thrombin time
    (D) prolonged fibrin time

15. Which of the following is *not* a useful treatment option for control of bleeding in a patient with hemophilia B?

    (A) recombinant factor IX
    (B) recombinant factor VIII
    (C) activated factor VII
    (D) aminocaproic acid

16. Which of the following is the *least* likely to occur in patients with vWD?

    (A) gingival hemorrhage
    (B) menorrhagia
    (C) prolonged epistaxis
    (D) hemarthrosis

17. Which of the following is the *best* treatment for a patient with severe bleeding and type I vWD?

    (A) intranasal ddAVP
    (B) fresh frozen plasma
    (C) recombinant factor VIII
    (D) platelet transfusion

18. Which of the following statements regarding vWD is *true*?

    (A) Incidence of vWD is higher in males than in females.
    (B) vWD is the most common hereditary bleeding disorder in the United States.
    (C) vWD is characterized by frequent bleeding into joints.
    (D) Type 3 vWD is the most common subtype.

Answers

1. **(C)** Petechial rashes are uncommon in pediatrics but frequently are a presenting symptom of severe systemic illness. The differential diagnosis of acute onset petechiae includes both infectious and non-infectious causes. Infections with meningococcus, rickettsia, and TORCH (toxoplasmosis, other agents, rubella, cytomegalovirus, herpes simplex) organisms, along with sepsis from any organism causing disseminated intravascular coagulation (DIC) can be associated with petechial rashes. Infectious mononucleosis is generally not associated with petechiae. Non-infectious causes of petechial rashes include ITP, a common cause of acute thrombocytopenia and petechiae, as well as drug-induced immune thrombocytopenia, hemolytic-uremic syndrome, and Henoch-Schönlein purpura. Bone marrow suppression of platelet production in diseases such as acute lymphoblastic leukemia and aplastic anemia also can be associated with thrombocytopenia and petechiae.

2. **(A)** Petechiae are the result of capillary hemorrhages and abnormal platelet function, caused by either decreased platelet number or intrinsic platelet dysfunction. Abnormal platelet function or number can also be associated with purpura, easy bruising, and mucocutaneous bleeding such as epistaxis and menorrhagia. Therefore, in the patient with petechiae, the most likely abnormality is thrombocytopenia. While abnormal prothrombin times and partial thromboplastin times are associated with bleeding disorders, the symptoms generally do not include petechiae. Low factor VIII or IX levels in particular are associated with intra-articular and deep muscle hemorrhages rather than petechiae. Elevated fibrin degradation products are associated with activation of the coagulation cascade, such as that which occurs in deep venous throm-

boses or DIC, and are not directly related to the presence or absence of petechiae.

3. **(B)** The most likely diagnosis for an otherwise healthy child with the acute onset of petechiae with thrombocytopenia is ITP, particularly in toddlers with a history of a recent upper respiratory infection and no family history of other disorders. ITP is generally associated with a history of a viral illness 1 to 3 weeks prior to the onset of thrombocytopenia. Characteristically children have diffuse petechiae with purpura and ecchymoses, but are otherwise well, with no fevers, weight loss, bone pain, organomegaly, and with an otherwise normal physical exam and no history of medication use. Other less common bleeding complications of ITP include epistaxis, gastrointestinal bleeding, and hematuria. Less than 1% of cases experience an intracranial hemorrhage, but the associated morbidity and mortality from intracranial hemorrhage is significant. The peripheral smear will show characteristic scant but large platelets, with the remainder of the complete blood count and peripheral smear being normal.

Acute lymphoblastic leukemia occurs in children in the same age range as ITP, but is associated with other findings such as fevers, organomegaly, and other abnormalities in the complete blood count. vWD generally is not associated with petechiae, although type 2B, a rare subtype, is associated with thrombocytopenia and can present with petechiae. In general, vWD does not have an acute onset and most commonly is associated with a positive family history. TAR syndrome is a rare autosomal recessive syndrome characterized by congenital thrombocytopenia, with neonatal onset of petechiae and purpura and associated limb anomalies, including absent radii bilaterally but with normal thumbs. The normal thumbs distinguish TAR syndrome from Fanconi's anemia, which can also have cytopenias and limb anomalies but is associated with abnormal thumbs.

4. **(B)** The initial evaluation of a child with easy bruising, bleeding, and/or petechiae should include a complete blood count with differential and evaluation of the peripheral smear to assess the platelet count and morphology. In addition, the prothrombin time and partial thromboplastin time should be performed to assess the function of the coagulation cascade, and a screening test for platelet function such as a platelet function analysis is also indicated. Bleeding times should not be performed as a screening test in children for possible bleeding disorders, because of the limited expertise in correctly performing the test and the poor sensitivity and specificity of the results. The thrombin time can be useful in addition for evaluating a patient for a fibrinogen defect. A direct Coombs test will not be helpful in assessing the status of the coagulation system. Further testing can then focus on any abnormalities found in the initial screen, such as testing factor levels in patients with prolonged prothrombin or partial thromboplastin times or platelet aggregation studies for patients with abnormal platelet function analyses.

5. **(A)** Many different types of medications, including many antimicrobials, can induce immune-mediated thrombocytopenia. Some medications, such as valproic acid and chemotherapeutic agents, cause thrombocytopenia via myelosuppression in a dose-dependent fashion. Other types of medications, including antibiotics such as the penicillins, sulfonamides, and quinines, as well as non-steroidal anti-inflammatory medications, anti-convulsants, diuretics, and acetaminophen are associated with immune-mediated thrombocytopenias. Macrolides such as erythromycin do not generally cause these immune-mediated reactions. Other medications associated with immune-mediated thrombocytopenia include heparin and gold, which both can be associated with the development of anti-platelet antibodies.

Medications that induce immune-mediated thrombocytopenia can do so via two different mechanisms. Heparin and gold induce antibodies in 1% to 3% of cases, and the antibodies act through platelet activation, leading to platelet consumption and a combination of thrombosis from platelet activation and bleeding from thrombocytopenia. Other medications, such as chloroquine, can induce antibodies that bind to platelet surface proteins only in combination with the drug itself. These antibody-drug coated platelets could then be sequestered in the reticuloendothelial system, resulting in severe thrombocytopenias and potentially severe bleeding.

6. **(D)** The history of an upper respiratory infection is most consistent with the diagnosis of acute

ITP, and a bone marrow evaluation is not required for those patients with characteristic features of ITP. The presence of fever, other cytopenias, lymphadenopathy, or organomegaly are more likely to be associated with other diagnoses, such as acute leukemia, and therefore patients with these features should undergo bone marrow evaluations.

7. (**B**) The peak age of onset of ITP is between 2 and 6 years old, and is much less common in infants younger than 1 year of age and in adolescents. Eighty percent to ninety percent of pediatric ITP cases are self-limited and have complete recovery of platelet counts within 6 months, independent of the type of treatment used. ITP that occurs in patients younger than 1 year of age or in those older than 10 years of age is more likely to be chronic, with persistent and possibly lifelong thrombocytopenia that is often less responsive to treatment. Children with chronic ITP can also have other associated autoimmune diseases or immunodeficiencies, such as systemic lupus erythematosus or common variable immunodeficiency, with immune-mediated thrombocytopenia as the presenting symptom.

8. (**C**) Platelet disorders with thrombocytopenia or platelet dysfunction are associated with petechiae, purpura, and mucocutaneous bleeding, including epistaxis, gingival hemorrhage, and gastrointestinal bleeding. Spontaneous intracranial hemorrhage is a rare, but severe, complication of ITP, with an estimated incidence of between 0.1% to 0.5% of ITP cases. Joint bleeding is a common complication of clotting factor deficiencies such as factor VIII or factor IX deficiency (hemophilia A or B, respectively) but is almost never seen in patients with platelet disorders.

9. (**A**) The most frequently used initial treatments for ITP are either intravenous immune globulin (IVIG) or anti-Rho-D immune globulin (WinRho). Corticosteroids can also be effective, but bone marrow evaluation should be performed prior to steroid use to rule out the presence of underlying leukemia. Platelet transfusions are generally not indicated for ITP treatment, as the platelets will be rapidly destroyed by the immune-mediated platelet consumption occurring in ITP. Non-steroidal anti-inflammatory medications such as ibuprofen should also be avoided, as they inhibit platelet function. Anti-Rho-D immune globulin acts via binding to red blood cells and inducing red blood cell sequestration in the spleen, thereby displacing platelets to be released back into the bloodstream. Therefore, one of the side effects of anti-Rho-D treatment is anemia, and its use should be avoided in patients who are anemic prior to treatment. The mechanism of IVIG action is poorly understood.

The use of either IVIG, anti-Rho-D, or corticosteroids will not have any effect on the natural course of the disease, but can temporarily increase the platelet count to reduce the incidence of bleeding complications. Since approximately 80% to 90% of cases of ITP will spontaneously resolve regardless of the treatment used, careful observation can also be a therapeutic option, with later intervention as needed. For emergent cases with severe bleeding unresponsive to other therapies, splenectomy can reduce platelet consumption and sequestration and lead to an increased platelet count, but should not be used as the primary therapy. Splenectomy is generally reserved for cases of chronic ITP unresponsive to other therapies and with reduced quality of life because of bleeding complications.

10. (**C**) Wiskott-Aldrich syndrome is a rare, X-linked disorder that is characterized by neutropenia, thrombocytopenia, and an eczematous skin rash. Anemia is not a feature of the syndrome. The immune deficiency of Wiskott-Aldrich syndrome results in increased infections of all types, including viral, bacterial, and fungal infections. The thrombocytopenia is characterized by small platelets and an increased risk of bleeding, with a significant risk of intracranial hemorrhage. Wiskott-Aldrich syndrome can also be associated with other autoimmune disorders such as Coombs positive hemolytic anemia, arthritis, and vasculitis. Patients with Wiskott-Aldrich syndrome have an over 100-fold increased risk of malignancies, including lymphomas and brain tumors. Splenectomy can result in an increased platelet count, reduced risk of bleeding complications, and increased patient survival, but bone marrow transplantation is the only currently available curative therapy.

11. **(A)** Neonatal thrombocytopenia is a relatively common finding and can be the result of a variety of underlying conditions. Maternal antibodies can cross the placenta to cause alloimmune thrombocytopenia in the fetus, and maternal use of certain medications can also cause neonatal thrombocytopenia. Neonatal infections, sepsis, DIC, and thrombosis can all also be associated with thrombocytopenia.

Neonates with large hemangiomas or vascular malformations can have associated consumptive coagulopathy with DIC and thrombocytopenia, termed the Kasabach-Merritt syndrome. Other congenital causes of thrombocytopenia include syndromes such as thrombocytopenia-absent radius (TAR) syndrome, congenital amegakaryocytic thrombocytopenia, Bernard-Soulier syndrome, and Wiskott-Aldrich syndrome.

Fanconi's anemia is an autosomal recessive aplastic disorder associated with chromosomal instability that can have isolated neonatal thrombocytopenia or pancytopenia as well as skeletal anomalies. However, the most common age of onset of cytopenias in patients with Fanconi's anemia is between 3 and 14 years of age, with only 5% of cases diagnosed in infancy. Neonates with chromosomal disorders such as trisomies 13, 18, or 21 can also frequently have isolated thrombocytopenia of unknown etiology. Glanzmann's thrombasthenia is a rare, autosomal recessive disorder associated with defective platelet adhesion and bleeding but with normal platelet counts.

12. **(C)** Factor VIII deficiency, or hemophilia A, is inherited in an X-linked pattern. Factor IX deficiency, or hemophilia B, is also X-linked, while factor XI deficiency (sometimes called hemophilia C) is inherited in an autosomal recessive manner.

Hemophilia A occurs in approximately 1 in 4000 newborn males, while hemophilia B occurs in approximately 1 in 30,000. Both are associated with an increased risk of bleeding. Possible neonatal complications include umbilical stump bleeding, bleeding from circumcision sites, and intracranial hemorrhage. Children with hemophilia can have mucocutaneous bleeding and purpura, but deep soft tissue hemorrhages and intra-articular joint hemorrhages (termed hemarthroses) are the hallmarks of the disease. Hemarthrosis

can occur at any age, but most commonly occurs with the increased (but still uncoordinated) ambulation seen in late infancy and early toddlerhood. Hemarthroses are characterized by acute joint warmth, swelling, and tenderness, and if recurrent, can result in chronic arthritis and eventual joint destruction. Other bleeding complications seen in patients with hemophilia include oral hemorrhages (particularly after dental procedures), gastrointestinal bleeding, and hematuria.

The severity of bleeding symptoms is related to the level of factor in the blood, with mild cases having >5% of factor, moderate cases having 1% to 5% factor levels, and severe cases having <1% factor levels. Normal factor levels range from 60% to 150%, with female heterozygotes having levels between 20% to 50% and having no bleeding symptoms.

13. **(B)** Placement of central lines or arterial lines, lumbar punctures, intramuscular injections, and any surgical procedures should be avoided in patients with hemophilia (severe factor VIII or IX deficiency) until after factor replacement therapy has been given. Peripheral venipuncture can be done, although repeated traumatic efforts should be avoided. Hemophilia patients who have suffered head trauma should receive factor replacement therapy *before* any brain imaging is performed, as any intracranial hemorrhage that has occurred will continue bleeding until factor replacement is given.

14. **(B)** Factor VIII deficiency results in a prolonged PTT, with a normal PT and thrombin time. Fibrin time is not a true test. Factor VIII is involved in the intrinsic coagulation cascade, which is initiated by factor XII interaction with high molecular weight kinins or kallikrein and resulting in serial activation of factors XI and IX, with factor VIII acting as a cofactor with activated factor IX for activation of factor X. The PTT measures the function of the intrinsic cascade, and is therefore prolonged in cases of factor VIII or IX deficiency. The PT measures the extrinsic clotting cascade, with factor VII interacting with tissue factor to activate factor X. Activated factor X can then activate factor V, which then activates thrombin (factor II), which then

cleaves fibrinogen to form fibrin. Factor XIII is then required for fibrin cross-linking to form a stable blood clot.

15. **(B)** Therapy for bleeding in a patient with hemophilia B, or factor IX deficiency, includes local control measures such as ice and direct pressure, but also can include topical thrombin and oral aminocaproic acid, an anti-fibrinolytic agent. For more severe bleeding, replacement of the deficient factor is required. With mild mucocutaneous bleeding, the goal of factor replacement should be to increase the factor level to approximately 20% to 30%. With more severe bleeding, the target factor level is much higher. Patients with hemarthroses should receive factor replacement to attain a 60% to 80% factor level, while patients with suspected or documented intracranial hemorrhages should attain a 100% factor level. The replacement factor used is specific for the underlying defect, as factor VIII will not suffice for treatment of patients with factor IX deficiency and vice versa. However, in hemophilia patients who have developed inhibitory antibodies against the replacement factor treatments, the need for replacement factor can be bypassed with the use of preactivated downstream clotting proteins, such as activated factor VII, which directly activates factor X and promotes clot formation in the absence of either factors VIII or IX.

16. **(D)** von Willebrand disease (vWD) is characterized by deficiencies or dysfunction of von Willebrand factor, a large serum protein involved in platelet interactions with each other and with the forming blood clot. vWD can be divided into three types, depending on the underlying defect in von Willebrand factor. Type I vWD is caused by decreased amounts of von Willebrand factor, while type III is caused by a complete absence of von Willebrand factor. Type II is composed of four subtypes, each a result of different mutations that affect the function of the protein. Each type of vWD is associated with increased bleeding, particularly bleeding from mucous membranes (epistaxis and menorrhagia) and postoperative bleeding after surgical procedures such as dental extraction or tonsillectomy/adenoidectomy. Chronic blood loss can be severe enough to cause iron deficiency anemia, and vWD should always be suspected in older children or adolescents who develop iron deficiency anemia.

17. **(A)** Type I vWD is caused by decreased production of von Willebrand factor. vWF is produced and stored in both platelets and vascular endothelial cells, and ddAVP (or desmopressin) can stimulate the release of available von Willebrand factor in most patients to increase the serum levels and assist in clot formation. Side effects of ddAVP include hyponatremia, and serum sodium levels should be monitored in patients receiving frequent ddAVP doses to control bleeding. Fresh frozen plasma has only very small amounts of von Willebrand factor and would not be effective therapy for severe bleeding. Cryoprecipitate, however, contains large amounts of von Willebrand factor and can be used for replacement. Endogenous von Willebrand factor in the bloodstream is bound to factor VIII and protects factor VIII from degradation, and so the best treatment option for bleeding patients with reduced von Willebrand factor or for those who do not respond to ddAVP is replacement with partially purified factor VIII products, which also contain large amounts of von Willebrand factor. Recombinant factor VIII products are composed solely of purified factor VIII and do not contain any von Willebrand factor. Except in cases of type IIB vWD that are associated with thrombocytopenia, platelet counts are generally normal in vWD patients, and so transfusions would not be of any benefit to control bleeding.

18. **(B)** vWD is a group of heterogenous disorders with an underlying defect in von Willebrand factor amount or function. vWD is an autosomal dominant disorder that occurs equally in males and females, and occurs in approximately 1% of the general population, making it the most common inherited bleeding disorder in the United States. Type I vWD, due to decreased von Willebrand factor production, is the most common subtype of vWD, accounting for approximately 80% of cases. Types 2 and 3 vWD are much less common, the result of either a defect in the von Willebrand factor protein or absent von Willebrand factor production, respectively. Bleeding symptoms in patients with vWD are generally mild to moderate, and predominantly involve mucocutaneous sites, with

prolonged epistaxis, menorrhagia, and prolonged bleeding after dental procedures being common. Deep soft tissue hemorrhages and hemarthroses (intra-articular joint hemorrhages) that characterize patients with hemophilia are extremely rare in patients with vWD.

SUGGESTED READING

DiMichele D, Neufeld EJ: Hemophilia: a new approach to an old disease. *Hematol Oncol Clin North Am* 12(6): 1315–1342, 1998.

Casella JF, Bowers DC, Pelidis MA: Disorders of coagulation. In: McMillan JA, DeAngelis CD, Feigin RD, et al (eds): *Oski's Pediatrics: Principles and Practice*, 3rd ed. Philadelphia: Lippincott Williams and Wilkins, 1999, pp 1475–1489.

Furie B, Furie BC: Molecular basis of blood coagulation. In: Hoffman R, Benz EJ, Shattil SJ, et al (eds): *Hematology: Basic Principles and Practice*, 3rd ed. Philadelphia: Churchill Livingstone, 2000, pp 1783–1804.

Allen GA, Glader B: Approach to the bleeding child. *Pediatr Clin North Am* 49:1239–1256, 2002.

DiPaola JA, Buchanan GR: Immune thrombocytopenic purpura. *Pediatr Clin North Am* 49:911–928, 2002.

Ewenstein BM: von Willebrand's disease. *Annu Rev Med* 48:525–542, 1997.

CASE 90: A 3-YEAR-OLD GIRL WITH AN ABDOMINAL MASS

A mother brings in her 3-year-old daughter for evaluation after feeling a "lump" in her abdomen while giving her a bath. The child has been healthy and has no significant past medical history. She has had normal growth and development to date. There is no family history of significant medical problems.

On physical exam, the child is well-appearing, laughing and playing on her mother's lap. Her physical exam is notable for a large, firm mass palpable on the left side of her abdomen.

SELECT THE ONE BEST ANSWER

1. Which of the following is the *least* likely cause of abdominal masses in children?

   (A) teratoma
   (B) neuroblastoma
   (C) Wilms' tumor
   (D) renal cell carcinoma

2. Which of the following clinical features is *not* associated with an increased incidence of Wilms' tumor?

   (A) hemihypertrophy
   (B) renal insufficiency
   (C) aniridia
   (D) atrial septal defect

3. Children with Beckwith-Wiedemann syndrome are at increased risk for which of the following pediatric malignancies?

   (A) medulloblastoma
   (B) hepatoblastoma
   (C) acute lymphoblastic leukemia
   (D) retinoblastoma

4. Which of the following is the *most* common extracranial solid tumor in children?

   (A) Wilms' tumor
   (B) hepatoblastoma
   (C) neuroblastoma
   (D) rhabdomyosarcoma

5. Which of the following age ranges has the *highest* incidence of Wilms' tumor?

   (A) 0 to 1 months
   (B) 6 to 12 months
   (C) 1 to 5 years
   (D) 10 to 15 years

6. Which of the following is the *most* common presentation of children with Wilms' tumor?

   (A) asymptomatic abdominal mass
   (B) hypertensive crisis
   (C) gross hematuria
   (D) unilateral headache

7. What percentage of Wilms' tumors are bilateral (i.e., present in both kidneys) at initial diagnosis?

   (A) 1%
   (B) 10%
   (C) 50%
   (D) 90%

8. Presenting features of children with neuroblastoma can include all of the following *except*:

   (A) periorbital ecchymoses
   (B) unilateral miosis
   (C) rapid, irregular eye movements
   (D) elevated α-fetoprotein levels

9. Which of the following laboratory values is *most* likely to be abnormal in children with neuroblastoma?

   (A) white blood cell count
   (B) serum ALT and AST (alanine/aspartase aminotransferase) levels
   (C) urine catecholamines
   (D) prothrombin time

10. Stage 4S neuroblastoma is characterized by the presence of disease at all of the following sites *except*:

    (A) liver
    (B) bone marrow
    (C) long bones
    (D) skin

11. Which of the following is the *least* common site of neuroblastoma metastatic disease?

    (A) bones
    (B) bone marrow
    (C) central nervous system
    (D) liver

12. Which of the following syndromes is *not* associated with an increased risk of pediatric malignancies?

    (A) ataxia-telangiectasia
    (B) Li-Fraumeni syndrome
    (C) Bloom syndrome
    (D) osteogenesis imperfecta

13. Which of the following neoplasms does *not* have an increased incidence in patients with type I neurofibromatosis?

    (A) plexiform neurofibroma
    (B) pheochromocytoma
    (C) medulloblastoma
    (D) optic glioma

14. Which of the following is the *most* common neonatal solid tumor?

    (A) teratoma
    (B) hepatoblastoma
    (C) germinoma
    (D) medulloblastoma

15. Which of the following tumors is *least* likely to arise in the anterior mediastinum?

   (A) non-Hodgkin's lymphoma
   (B) germ cell tumor
   (C) thymoma
   (D) neuroblastoma

16. Which of the following pediatric tumors is associated with increased β-hCG levels?

   (A) neuroblastoma
   (B) seminoma
   (C) choriocarcinoma
   (D) teratoma

Answers

1. **(D)** The differential diagnosis of pediatric abdominal masses includes both neoplastic and non-neoplastic causes. Potential pediatric neoplasms that can present as abdominal masses include germ cell tumors, neuroblastomas, Wilms' tumors, lymphomas, and rhabdomyosarcomas, among others. Renal cell carcinoma can occur in children but is extremely rare. Other non-neoplastic causes of palpable pediatric abdominal masses to be considered include impacted stool, distended bladder, intra-abdominal abscesses, ovarian cysts, pyloric stenosis, and enlarged kidneys secondary to polycystic kidney disease, hydronephrosis, or renal vein thrombosis.

2. **(D)** Several syndromes and physical features are associated with increased incidence of Wilms' tumor. Beckwith-Wiedemann syndrome, WAGR syndrome (*W*ilms' tumor, *A*niridia, *G*enitourinary malformations, and mental *R*etardation), and Denys-Drash syndrome (renal failure, pseudohermaphroditism, and Wilms' tumor) are associated with an increased incidence of Wilms' tumor. Patients with hemihypertrophy or aniridia also have an increased risk and should be screened regularly for abdominal malignancies. Patients with aniridia associated with chromosome 11p13 deletion have up to a 50% incidence of Wilms' tumor by 4 years of age. There is no increased incidence in Wilms' tumor associated with the presence of cardiac defects.

   Nephrogenic rests are sites of abnormal persistent embryonal nephroblastic tissue that are more commonly found in patients with syndromes that predispose patients to Wilms' tumor, such as WAGR syndrome, Beckwith-Wiedemann syndrome, and Denys-Drash syndrome. Nephrogenic rests are renal parenchymal lesions that are precursors to Wilms' tumor development. They occur in 1% of the general population, but in 35% of patients with unilateral Wilms' tumors and in nearly 100% of patients with bilateral Wilms' tumors. If present, particularly if multiple (called nephroblastomatosis), patients should undergo regular abdominal screening to monitor for progression of the lesions to Wilms' tumor.

3. **(B)** Beckwith-Wiedemann syndrome occurs in approximately 1 in 15,000 infants and is associated with abnormal imprinting on chromosome 11p15. The normally imprinted (and thus inactive) maternal allele is lost, resulting in uni-paternal disomy and Beckwith-Wiedemann syndrome. Beckwith-Wiedemann syndrome is characterized by macrosomia, macroglossia, organomegaly, neonatal hypoglycemia, and abdominal wall defects such as omphalocele, diastasis recti, and umbilical hernia. Other common features include linear earlobe creases, microcephaly, advanced bone age, and absent gonads. Beckwith-Wiedemann syndrome is also associated with an increased risk of hepatoblastoma, gonadoblastoma, Wilms' tumor, and adrenal tumors, but not leukemias. Children with Beckwith-Wiedemann syndrome should be followed with abdominal ultrasounds and serum α-fetoprotein levels every 6 months until they are at least 6 years of age to monitor for these tumors.

4. **(C)** Neuroblastoma is the most common extracranial solid tumor in children and the third most common overall (after leukemias and brain tumors), with approximately 600 new cases in the United States each year. Wilms' tumor is the fifth most common (with approximately 450 new United States' cases each year), while rhabdomyosarcoma and other soft tissue sarcomas are the sixth most common. Hepatoblastoma accounts for approximately 100 cases per year in the United States.

5. **(C)** Wilms' tumor in children occurs most commonly between 2 and 4 years of age, and over 80% of cases present before 5 years of age with 98% of cases by the age of 7 years. Bilateral and familial cases of Wilms' tumor and those associated with tumor-predisposition syndromes tend to occur earlier than sporadic cases. Wilms' tumor can occur both in infants and in adolescents, but infants have a higher incidence of other renal tumors such as congenital mesoblastic nephroma and rhabdoid kidney tumors, while adolescents have a higher incidence of renal cell carcinomas.

6. **(A)** Wilms' tumor most commonly presents as an asymptomatic abdominal mass, with over two-thirds of children with Wilms' tumor having masses detected incidentally by parents or physicians. Symptoms of Wilms' tumor can include abdominal pain, which occurs in approximately 33% of cases; hypertension, which occurs in approximately 25% of cases and is rarely emergent; hematuria (gross or microscopic), which occurs in 20% of cases and other symptoms of abdominal mass compression such as intestinal obstruction. Furthermore, anemia because of intratumoral hemorrhage can occur, although usually the onset of anemia is acute and associated with a rapid increase in apparent tumor size because of the hemorrhage. Constitutional symptoms such as fevers, fatigue, and weight loss are rare in cases of Wilms' tumor, while headaches are not a symptom generally associated with Wilms' tumor.

7. **(B)** Approximately 5% to 10% of Wilms' tumor cases are bilateral at diagnosis, although the frequency is much higher among those Wilms' tumor cases associated with genetic syndromes.

Approximately 10% to 15% of Wilms' tumor cases are metastatic at diagnosis, and Wilms' tumor most commonly metastasizes to lungs, lymph nodes, and the contralateral kidney. Brain, bone, and liver metastases do occur, but they are rare. Local invasion into the renal vasculature, which can progress up the inferior vena cava to the right atrium, can also occur and can lead to hypertension and abdominal vein distention. Evaluation of any child with a suspected Wilms' tumor should always include either a chest radiograph or a chest CT scan to rule out pulmonary metastatic disease.

The survival of children with localized Wilms' tumor is good, with a >90% long-term expected survival rate. Children with metastatic Wilms' tumor, however, have only a 50% long-term survival rate.

8. **(D)** Neuroblastoma is a relatively common pediatric neoplasm and the most common extracranial solid tumor in children. Approximately 75% of cases occur in children under 2 years of age, and over 90% occur in children younger than 5 years of age.

Neuroblastoma arises from primordial neural crest cells, and its primary sites are either abdominal or thoracic. Presenting symptoms of neuroblastoma can include bilateral periorbital ecchymoses ("raccoon eyes"), Horner's syndrome (unilateral ptosis, miosis, and anhidrosis), or rapid eye movements (opsoclonus-myoclonus syndrome). Elevated α-fetoprotein levels are more commonly found in hepatoblastomas and some germ cell tumors and are not found in patients with neuroblastoma. Other presenting symptoms of neuroblastoma include fevers, palpable abdominal mass, hypertension, respiratory distress, SVC syndrome, spinal cord compression, weight loss, bone pain, watery diarrhea as a result of vasoactive intestinal peptide secretion, and paraneoplastic ataxia.

9. **(C)** Elevation of urine catecholamines homovanillic acid (HVA) and vanillylmandelic acid (VMA) are found in almost all (~95%) cases of neuroblastoma, and are also elevated in most cases of pheochromocytoma. HVA and VMA are byproducts of catecholamine metabolism, and are increased in cases of neuroblastoma as a result of excessive production from adrenergic tissue. While neuroblastoma can metastasize to the bone marrow in some cases, blood cell production is rarely impaired, although anemia and thrombocytopenia are more common than leukopenia. Furthermore, neuroblastoma that involves the liver can also cause elevated liver enzyme (AST and ALT) levels and prolonged coagulation tests, but much less commonly than elevations in urine catecholamines.

10. **(C)** Stage 4S neuroblastoma is a form of neuroblastoma that occurs only in infants younger than 1 year of age, with metastatic disease limited exclusively to the liver, bone marrow (with <10% involvement), and skin. Bony disease is a feature of stage 4 neuroblastoma, but not stage 4S. Outcomes for stage 4S neuroblastoma, as opposed to stage 4 disease, are extremely good, and can include complete disease resolution in the absence of any therapy.

11. **(C)** Neuroblastoma can metastasize almost anywhere in the body, but is most commonly found in the bone marrow, bones, and liver. Lung and CNS metastases can occur, but are very rare and tend to portend worse outcomes.

The presence of metastatic disease defines stage 4 neuroblastoma, which has the worst prognosis of all stages and requires multi-agent high-dose chemotherapy combined with surgery and radiation therapy for treatment. Stages 1 through 3 have localized disease, with the treatment used and overall prognosis determined by other biologic features, while stage 4S is a unique form of metastatic disease with a good outcome that occurs only in infants.

12. **(D)** Osteogenesis imperfecta is not associated with any increase in pediatric malignancies, while each of the other listed syndromes involve increased incidence of pediatric cancers. Ataxia-telangiectasia is a syndrome characterized by DNA repair defects and presents with cerebellar ataxia and oculocutaneous telangiectasias. Malignancies occur in approximately 15% of cases and include non-Hodgkin's lymphomas and carcinomas. Li-Fraumeni syndrome is a syndrome associated with mutations in the *p53* gene, which is important in cell cycle regulation. Patients with Li-Fraumeni syndrome are predisposed to a variety of malignancies, including soft tissue sarcomas, leukemias and lymphomas, adrenocortical carcinomas, and breast and bone cancers. Bloom syndrome is a rare syndrome most commonly found in patients of Ashkenazi Jewish heritage and is characterized by intrauterine growth reduction, abnormal facies, and facial telangiectasias and other skin lesions. Bloom syndrome patients are predisposed to all types of leukemias, which occur in approximately one-fourth of patients.

13. **(C)** Neurofibromatosis is an autosomal dominant syndrome with an incidence of approximately 1 in 2500 children in the United States. Mutations in the neurofibromin gene are responsible for neurofibromatosis, and the features include café-

au-lait spots, cutaneous neurofibromas, axillary and inguinal freckling, Lisch nodules, sphenoid dysplasia, tibial bowing, and other skeletal anomalies such as short stature and scoliosis. Other features also can include renovascular hypertension, seizures, and developmental delay. Type I neurofibromatosis is also associated with an increased incidence of malignancies, including plexiform neurofibromas and neurofibrosarcomas, pheochromocytomas, and brain tumors such as meningiomas, astrocytomas, acoustic neuromas, and optic gliomas. Patients with neurofibromatosis are not at increased risk for the development of medulloblastoma.

14. **(A)** Teratomas are the most common neonatal solid tumor, accounting for up to one-third of all neonatal tumors. Teratomas are generally benign masses composed of tissues from at least two of the three embryonic germ layers—endoderm, mesoderm, and ectoderm. The tissues within a teratoma can be fully differentiated (resulting in a "mature" teratoma), partially differentiated (resulting in an "immature" teratoma), or malignant. Immature teratomas account for 30% of neonatal teratomas, while malignant teratomas account for <10% (but up to 50% of teratomas in older children). The primary sites include the sacrococcygeal region, the anterior mediastinum, and the central nervous system. Treatment of teratomas is complete surgical excision, and metastases in mature and immature cases are extremely rare. Malignant teratomas require excision and chemotherapy to treat the type of malignant tissue present within the mass.

15. **(D)** The anterior mediastinum is a common site of pediatric tumors, with presenting symptoms ranging from cough or dysphagia to hoarseness, wheezing, dyspnea, or SVC syndrome. The most common anterior mediastinal tumors include lymphomas (particularly T-cell lymphomas), teratomas and other germ cell tumors, and thymic tumors. Neuroblastomas generally arise from sympathetic ganglia and cases of thoracic neuroblastoma are more likely to be located in the posterior mediastinum. Cases of thoracic neuroblastoma are adjacent to the spinal cord and often are associated with spinal canal invasion and spinal cord compression, requiring urgent medical and/or surgical intervention. Over 50% of thymomas are asymptomatic, but approximately one-third are associated with myasthenia gravis.

16. **(C)** Tumors which contain components of syncytiotrophoblastic tissue, such as choriocarcinomas, express high amounts of β-hCG protein. Other germ cell tumors more commonly express high levels of α-fetoprotein (AFP), but not β-hCG, and neuroblastomas express high levels of catecholamines, but neither AFP nor β-hCG. Mature teratomas also do not express either AFP or β-hCG, and so the presence of elevated AFP or β-hCG levels indicates a malignant component to a teratoma.

SUGGESTED READING

Chintagumpala MM, Steuber CP: Wilms tumor. In: McMillan JA, DeAngelis CD, Feigin RD, et al (eds): *Oski's Pediatrics: Principles and Practice*, 3rd ed. Philadelphia: Lippincott Williams and Wilkins, 1999, pp 1515–1516.

Dreyer ZE, Fernbach DJ: Neuroblastoma. In: McMillan JA, DeAngelis CD, Feigin RD, et al (eds): *Oski's Pediatrics: Principles and Practice*, 3rd ed. Philadelphia: Lippincott Williams and Wilkins, 1999, pp 1517–1519.

Golden CB, Feusner JH: Malignant abdominal masses in children: quick guide to evaluation and diagnosis. *Pediatr Clin North Am* 49:1369–1392, 2000.

Infectious Disease

12

CASE 91: A 12-MONTH OLD CHILD WITH DELAYED IMMUNIZATIONS

A 12-month-old boy is brought to your office for evaluation of a cough and runny nose. You note that this is the child's first visit to your office. On questioning the child's mother, she informs you that the child has been seen by another physician three times since birth but has changed health care providers since moving to a new city. After review of the child's immunization record, you note that the child has only received one DTaP, IPV, Hepatitis B, and Hib conjugate vaccine at age 4 months. Two days later, he had fever recorded by the mother at 102.2°F (39°C). The mother is aware that her son is behind with immunizations, based on his age. She tells you that except for the four-month-old visit, her son always had cold symptoms like today's symptoms, so immunizations were not administered.

On physical examination the child is alert and active. His height and weight are at the 10th percentile. The temperature is 100.4°F (38°C). Examination of the ears is normal. Clear rhinorrhea is present. Examination of both lungs and heart is normal. No hepatosplenomegaly exists.

SELECT THE ONE BEST ANSWER TO THE FOLLOWING QUESTIONS

1. The most likely reason the infant is behind for age with immunizations is:

   (A) Minor illness with fever does not contraindicate immunization.

   (B) Fever alone is a contraindication to immunization.

   (C) Infant has an undefined immunodeficiency.

   (D) Fever to 102.2°F (39°C) after the first set of immunizations.

2. The infant receives DTaP-Hepatitis B-IPV, Hib conjugate, pneumococcal conjugate vaccine and MMR vaccine. The minimum interval to the next administration of the third dose of DTaP-IPV-Hep B vaccines needed is:

   (A) 2 weeks
   (B) 4 weeks
   (C) 6 weeks
   (D) 8 weeks

3. The infant's mother asks you whether her infant should receive influenza vaccine. All of the following children are recommended to receive influenza vaccine during the autumn of each year before the start of influenza season except:

   (A) a 5-year-old girl with asthma
   (B) an 18-month-old healthy boy
   (C) a 3-year-old girl with allergic rhinitis
   (D) an 8-year-old boy with diabetes mellitus

4. The mother also asks you about meningococcal vaccine, which she remembers her older brother receiving prior to travel outside the country and wonders whether her infant should also receive that vaccine. You tell her that men-

ingococcal vaccine is indicated for the following circumstances:

(A) a 20-month-old child traveling to sub-Saharan Africa

(B) a 5-year-old child whose classmate in kindergarten developed meningococcemia

(C) a college student living in an apartment rather than on-campus housing

(D) a 2-year-old child with sickle cell disease

5. The mother tells you that she had never heard of the pneumococcal conjugate vaccine (Prevnar) that you also are recommending for her infant. The following statement about Prevnar is true:

(A) Vaccine can protect children against up to 23 different serotypes of *Streptococcus pneumoniae*.

(B) The 12-month-old infant only needs to receive a single dose of the vaccine.

(C) Infants of very low birth weight (less than or equal to 1500 g) should be immunized at a chronological age of 6 to 8 weeks.

(D) The serotypes in the vaccine account for approximately two-thirds of the serotypes that cause invasive disease in children younger than 6 years of age in the United States.

6. Management of a preterm infant lighter than 2000 g at birth who is born to a mother who is HBsAg positive includes all but:

(A) hepatitis B vaccine and HBIG (within 12 hours of birth)

(B) immunization with 3 vaccine doses at 0, 1, and 6 to 7 months chronological age

(C) check anti-HBs and HBsAg at 9 to 15 months of age

(D) reimmunize with three doses of hepatitis B vaccine at 2 month intervals if HBsAg and anti-HBs are negative

7. Hepatitis A vaccine is recommended for the following situation:

(A) an 11-month-old girl traveling with family to India

(B) a 4-year-old girl from Oklahoma entering preschool

(C) a 12-year-old adolescent boy receiving peritoneal dialysis

(D) an 18-year-old adolescent male applying for a job as a food handler

8. An 8-year-old girl sustains a large laceration contaminated with dirt after falling from her bike. Her mother can't recall how many doses of tetanus toxoid her daughter has received. Management of tetanus prophylaxis in this situation of unknown history of prior doses of tetanus toxoid includes:

(A) adult-type dT

(B) TIG

(C) dT and TIG

(D) *Haemophilus influenzae* type b conjugate vaccine containing tetanus toxoid and TIG

9. There are a number of different licensed acellular pertussis vaccines which contain one or more immunogens derived from *Bordetella pertussis* organisms. The antigen that is common to all of the different acellular pertussis vaccines includes:

(A) pertussis toxin

(B) FHA

(C) fimbrial protein (agglutinogens)

(D) pertactin (outer membrane 69-kd protein)

10. Acellular pertussis vaccine in the form of DTaP is appropriate to administer in the following circumstance:

(A) a 5-year-old girl who has received DT vaccine at 2, 4, and 6 months of age and DTaP vaccine at 12, 18, and 24 months of age

(B) a 24-year-old adult working in a hospital experiencing a pertussis outbreak

(C) a 3-year-old boy with documented pertussis disease at age 2½ years

(D) a 6-month-old infant girl with seizures poorly controlled with anti-convulsant therapy

11. An outbreak of measles is occurring in a large urban city in the United States. Measles vaccine can be administered to children as young as:

(A) 4 weeks

(B) 4 months

(C) 6 months

(D) 9 months

12. The following is a contraindication to the administration of the (live virus) measles vaccine:

    (A) history of egg allergy
    (B) history of allergy to chickens or feathers
    (C) an 8-year-old girl with HIV with evidence of moderate immunosuppression with a CD4% of 16
    (D) IVIG given 6 months ago for treatment of Kawasaki disease

13. A mother of a 2-year-old child receives MMR vaccine and subsequently finds out that she was pregnant when the vaccine was administered. The following statement about rubella vaccine and pregnancy is true:

    (A) Receipt of rubella vaccination during pregnancy is an indication to terminate the pregnancy.
    (B) Immune globulin should be administered to the pregnant woman.
    (C) Immunizing the mother's 2-year-old child places the mother at risk for rubella infection.
    (D) No cases of congenital rubella syndrome have been reported in women who have received rubella vaccine during pregnancy.

14. All of the following groups do not require rubella immunization except:

    (A) a woman in the third trimester of pregnancy
    (B) a woman born in 1953 with no history of previous rubella vaccine
    (C) a 13-year-old adolescent female with a previous clinical diagnosis of rubella
    (D) a 6-year-old boy who received 2 doses of MMR vaccine at age 2 and 3 years

15. Exposure to all of the following animal types is an indication of postexposure prophylaxis with rabies vaccine and RIG except:

    (A) raccoons
    (B) woodchucks
    (C) skunks
    (D) squirrels

16. You are asked about the safety of poliovirus vaccine by the mother of a 12-month-old infant. You should tell her that:

    (A) OPV can cause VAPP and the risk is highest after the third dose of vaccine.
    (B) Severe egg allergy (anaphylaxis) is a contraindication to poliovirus vaccine.
    (C) IPV is recommended for household contacts for people with immunodeficiency disorders.
    (D) Fever occurs in approximately 40% of infants who receive IPV vaccine.

17. A 2-month-old infant receives a dose of *H. influenzae* type b conjugate vaccine PRP-OMP (outer membrane protein complex) in ComVax. Then at 4 months he receives a different *H. influenzae* type b conjugate vaccine PRP-T (tetanus toxoid conjugate).

    The next dose should be administered at age:

    (A) 6 months
    (B) 9 months
    (C) 12 months
    (D) 15 months

18. Compared with natural infection with varicella, varicella vaccine is:

    (A) more likely to result in herpes zoster
    (B) more likely to result in transmission of virus to contacts
    (C) more likely to result in mild varicella disease if breakthrough varicella occurs
    (D) more likely to result in the serious adverse event of encephalitis

Answers

1. (**A**) Minor illnesses, e.g., upper respiratory infection or gastroenteritis, with or without fever are not a contraindication to any of the routine childhood vaccines. Temperature of 104.9°F (40.5°C) within 48 hours after immunization with a previous dose of diphtheria and tetanus toxoids and acellular pertussis vaccine (DTaP) is considered a precaution, not a definite contraindication, to subsequent administration of DTaP vaccine.

2. (**B**) The recommended interval to the second dose of vaccine is 2 months. However, for children 4 months through 6 years of age who start late or are greater than 1 month behind, the minimum interval between doses 2 and 3 is 4 weeks

Table 91-1. ESTIMATED RATES OF INFLUENZA-ASSOCIATED HOSPITALIZATIONS/100,000 PERSONS

Study years	Age group	High-risk	Healthy
1973–1993	0–11 mos	1,900	496–1,038[†]
	1–2 yrs	800	186
	3–4 yrs	320	86
	5–14 yrs	92	41

[†]The low estimate is for infants 6–11 months, and the high estimate is for infants age 0–5 months.
Source: Neuzil KM, Mellen BG, Wright PF, et al: Effect of influenza on hospitalizations, outpatient visits, and courses of antibiotics in children. *New Engl J Med* 342:225, 2000.

for DTaP and IPV vaccines and 3 weeks for hepatitis B. The third dose of hepatitis B vaccine should be at least 16 weeks after the first dose.

3. **(C)** Influenza vaccine should be administered to children with specific risk factors such as asthma and diabetes. However, the Advisory Committee on Immunization Practices (ACIP) have now recommended routine influenza vaccine for healthy children between 6 and 23 months old. Hospitalization rates are highest for complicated influenza in the first 2 years of life (see Table 91-1). Rates of hospitalization are comparable with adults older than 65 years of age.

4. **(D)** Meningococcal quadrivalent polysaccharide vaccine can be administered at the age of 2 years and older. Children with sickle cell disease should receive meningococcal vaccine because of functional asplenia. College students who will be living in a dormitory for the first time are at increased risk of developing invasive meningococcal disease. Immunization should be discussed with college students and their parents and offered to those who request the vaccine. The CDC's Advisory Committee on Immunization Practices (ACIP) has now recommended the newly licensed meningococcal conjugate vaccine (MCV4, Menactra) for adolescents (11 to 12 years and 15 years) and college freshmen living in dormitories as well as the four groups at high risk.

5. **(C)** The current pneumococcal conjugate vaccine contains seven serotypes that account for approximately 85% of the serotypes causing invasive pneumococcal infections (including bacteremia and meningitis) in children younger than 6 years of age in the United States. The 12-month-old infant should receive two doses of vaccine 6 to 8 weeks apart.

6. **(B)** Management of preterm infants lighter than 2000 g at birth if the mother is HBsAg positive should include HBIG within 12 hours after birth along with four doses of hepatitis B vaccine at 0, 1, 2 to 3, and 6 to 7 months of chronological age. The first dose of hepatitis B vaccine should also be administered within 12 hours after birth.

7. **(B)** There are certain states in which the average annual reported incidence of hepatitis A has been greater than or equal to twice the national average. In all states, which include Oklahoma, routine immunization of children 1 year of age or older is now recommended.

8. **(C)** Tetanus immune globulin should be administered if there is a history of less than three doses of tetanus toxoid administered or unknown history, and there is not a clean minor wound. Clean minor wounds do not require TIG. Other wounds such as those contaminated with dirt, puncture wounds, avulsions, penetrating wounds, burns, crush wounds and frostbite would require TIG.

9. **(A)** There are five licensed DTaP-containing vaccines available for use in the United States for children. There is no serologic correlate for the efficacy of pertussis vaccine. All of the licensed acellular pertussis vaccines contain pertussis toxin, also termed lymphocytosis promoting factor (LPF).

10. **(C)** Children with well-documented pertussis disease likely have some immunity to *Bordetella pertussis* but the duration of immunity is unknown. Natural disease does not provide complete or lifelong immunity against reinfection. Therefore completing the immunization series with DTaP is recommended. When administering DTaP vaccine to children who have previously received DT vaccine, the total number of doses of diphtheria and tetanus toxoids should not exceed six before the child reaches age 7 years.

11. **(C)** For outbreak control of measles, monovalent vaccine can be administered to infants as young as 6 months of age. These infants should be re-immunized with MMR vaccine at 12 to 15 months of age and again at age 4 to 6 years.

12. **(D)** The usual dose of IGIV for treatment of Kawasaki disease is 2000 mg/kg. The administration of MMR vaccine should be deferred for 11 months after the administration of IGIV. Children with egg allergy are at low risk of anaphylactic reactions to MMR vaccine. Skin testing of children for egg allergy is not predictive of reactions to MMR vaccine. Most anaphylactic reactions are related to other vaccine components. Children with a history of anaphylactic reactions to gelatin or neomycin should only be vaccinated with MMR in settings where anaphylactic reactions can be properly managed. Children with HIV infection should receive MMR vaccine unless there is evidence of severe immunocompromise (CD4% <15).

13. **(D)** Rubella vaccine is contraindicated during pregnancy. However, no cases of congenital rubella syndrome have occurred in the situation in which susceptible women received rubella vaccine within 3 months of conception and delivered infants at term. There also has been no evidence of transmission of vaccine virus from immunized children to household contacts.

14. **(C)** The clinical diagnosis of rubella is not reliable to determine if one is susceptible to rubella. Rubella immunity must be documented by serologic testing. For children who receive their first dose of rubella vaccine, a second dose is not necessary but is given because of the recommendations for two-dose routine measles immunization. The second dose of MMR vaccine can be given as early as 4 weeks after the first dose as long as the first dose is administered at or after the age of 12 months.

15. **(D)** The bites of squirrels, hamsters, guinea pigs, gerbils, chipmunks, rats, mice, rabbits and hares almost never require rabies postexposure prophylaxis. An exception for a rodent bite that does require prophylaxis is the bite of a woodchuck.

16. **(C)** The risk of VAPP is highest after the first dose of oral poliovirus vaccine, occurring in 1/700,000 recipients. OPV vaccine is contraindicated for household contacts of people with immunodeficiency disorder because of the risk spread of OPV to the affected person.

17. **(A)** The recommended dosing schedule for the PRP-OMP vaccine (the one contained in Comvax) is 2, 4, and 12 months. If the PRP-OMP vaccine is only administered for part of the primary series, the number of doses needed to complete the primary schedule for the series is determined by the recommended schedule for the other Hib conjugate vaccine. All other licensed Hib conjugate vaccines require 3 doses for the primary series (2, 4, 6 months) plus a fourth dose as a booster at 12 months of age.

18. **(C)** Varicella occurring in vaccine recipients is milder than in unimmunized children, with fewer vesicles, lower rates of fever and more rapid recovery. Transmission of vaccines virus from one person to another is extremely rare.

SUGGESTED READING

Pickering LK, Baker CJ, Overturf GD, et al: *Red Book 2003 Report of the Committee on Infectious Diseases,* 26th ed. Elk Grove Village, IL: American Academy of Pediatrics, 2003.

Hadler SC, Orenstein WA: Active immunization. In: Long SS, Pickering LK, Prober CG (eds): *Principles and Practices of Infectious Diseases,* 2nd ed. Philadelphia, PA: Churchill Livingstone, 2003, p 45.

CASE 92: A 4-YEAR-OLD IMMUNOCOMPROMISED GIRL WITH AN EXPOSURE TO VARICELLA

A 4-year-old girl, whom you have followed in your practice since birth, was recently diagnosed with acute lymphoblastic leukemia. You had considered the diagnosis after she developed persistent fever, fatigue, back pain, and pallor. She had completed induction chemotherapy and is now in remission. The child's mother calls your office to inform you that she had received a phone call from her daughter's preschool teacher. Two days ago another child developed a rash and was sent home. That child's mother called today to inform the teacher that the child was seen by their pediatrician and diagnosed with chicken pox. The teacher then called your patient's mother to let her know of the other child in the classroom who was diagnosed with chickenpox.

The preschool class that your patient attends has class Monday through Friday for 4 hours per day. Your patient was present in the class for the 4-hour period on the day that the other child developed the rash. Both children were also present in class on the previous day.

SELECT THE ONE BEST ANSWER TO THE FOLLOWING QUESTIONS

1. The first step in the management of varicella exposure in a child with leukemia is:

   (A) Obtain a history of whether or not the child has had varicella.
   (B) Administer the varicella vaccine to the child.
   (C) Contact the pediatrician of the preschool classmate to verify the diagnosis of varicella.
   (D) Draw blood for serologic testing on the child with leukemia.

2. The child with leukemia has no history of varicella. It is next important to determine if:

   (A) the child with leukemia has developed any other skin lesions
   (B) the child with leukemia has had serologic test results to determine his immune status regarding varicella
   (C) the child with leukemia and her classmate played together in the same classroom with face-to-face contact
   (D) the child with leukemia has received IVIG in the past 3 weeks

3. An immunocompromised child who is susceptible to varicella and at high risk for developing severe varicella should receive VZIG within what time period after exposure:

   (A) 48 hours
   (B) 72 hours
   (C) 96 hours
   (D) 120 hours

4. All of the following types of exposure to zoster (shingles) are an indication for VZIG in susceptible people at higher risk for developing severe varicella except:

   (A) residing in one household
   (B) face-to-face indoor play

   (C) intimate contact (touching or hugging) with a person who has zoster
   (D) newborn infant: onset of zoster in the mother 5 days or less before delivery or within 48 hours after delivery

5. Candidates for VZIG, provided an important exposure to varicella has occurred include:

   (A) a term newborn infant whose mother developed varicella 7 days prior to delivery of the infant
   (B) a 21-year-old pregnant woman who has a history of varicella at age 5 years
   (C) hospitalized premature infant (less than 28 weeks gestation), regardless of maternal history of varicella or serologic varicella virus serostatus
   (D) an 8-year-old girl with asymptomatic HIV infection with a history of varicella at age 2 years

6. A healthy term infant is born to a mother who develops varicella 72 hours after delivery. VZIG is not indicated in the infant for the following reason:

   (A) The absolute CD4 and CD4 percentage of the newborn infant are high enough to prevent infection.
   (B) Natural killer cell cytotoxicity prevents neonatal infection.
   (C) The infant will not be at risk of exposure to viremia with varicella zoster.
   (D) Acyclovir should be administered to prevent clinical varicella from occurring in the newborn.

7. VZIG is indicated in all of the following situations in which significant exposure to varicella occurs except:

   (A) a 25-week premature female infant whose mother has a history of varicella during childhood
   (B) a 12-month-old girl with AIDS
   (C) a 15-year-old male with asthma who completed 10 days of a tapering course of steroids
   (D) a 10-month-old male infant receiving immunosuppressive therapy after renal transplant

8. The incidence of minor adverse events associated with the administration of IVIG such as fever,

headache, myalgias, chills, and vomiting are primarily related to:

(A) the concentration of IVIG administered
(B) the rate of infusion of IVIG
(C) the lot number of IVIG administered
(D) the age of the patient receiving IVIG

9. An example of an infrequent serious reaction of IGIV therapy includes:

(A) aplastic anemia
(B) acute renal failure
(C) HIV transmission
(D) Guillain-Barré syndrome

10. IVIG is recommended for use in all of the following disorders except:

(A) a 2-year-old boy with Kawasaki disease
(B) a 3-year-old girl with severe combined immunodeficiency disorder
(C) an 800-g premature infant
(D) a 24-year-old man with chronic B-cell lymphocytic leukemia

11. IGIV is recommended for an HIV-infected child in the following circumstance:

(A) one episode of bacteremic pneumococcal pneumonia in the previous 12 months
(B) serum IgG level of less than or equal to 500 mg/dL [5.0g/L]
(C) chronic Parvovirus B19 infection
(D) chronic diarrhea caused by cryptosporidium

12. The risk of anaphylaxis is highest with IGIV administration in children with which of the following type of deficiency:

(A) IgA
(B) IgD
(C) IgE
(D) Properdin

13. A 10-month-old healthy male infant traveling with his family to Africa was exposed 4 days ago to his 4-year-old native African cousin who was ill at the time with fever, cough, coryza and conjunctivitis. The 4-year-old cousin was diagnosed with measles as have a number of children in the city where the family is visiting. The mother of the 10-month-old child makes an overseas phone call to your office asking your advice. Appropriate management of the 10-month-old includes:

(A) MMR vaccine administration
(B) measurement of serum measles of IgG antibody
(C) immune globulin 0.25 mL/kg by IM route
(D) immune globulin 0.25 mL/kg by IV route

14. IG can be given to prevent or modify measles in a susceptible person within how many days of exposure?

(A) 1
(B) 4
(C) 6
(D) 10

15. A 10-month-old child attending daycare comes to your office. The child is healthy, but his mother is concerned because another child of 2½ years who attends the same daycare center was diagnosed with hepatitis A infection about 1 week ago. Appropriate management of the 15-month-old child includes:

(A) administer IG at dose of 0.02 mL/kg IM
(B) administer IG at dose of 0.02 mL/kg IM plus hepatitis A vaccine IM at a different site
(C) measure hepatitis A virus IgM in order to check for evidence of asymptomatic current infection
(D) measure hepatitis A virus IgG in order to check for evidence of past infection and immunity

16. IG for IM administration should be given within what time period after exposure to have greater than 85% efficacy in preventing symptomatic hepatitis A infection?

(A) 3 days
(B) 7 days
(C) 14 days
(D) 21 days

17. A major limitation of IG for replacement therapy in antibody deficiency disorders is the need for deep IM injections. An alternative is slow subcutaneous administration of IG. Characteristics of

this method of administration include all of following except:

(A) less expensive than IGIV
(B) suitable for home therapy
(C) systemic allergic reactions occurring in 5% of recipients
(D) ability to deliver relatively large volumes of IG

18. A 13-year-old adolescent female with no prior history of hepatitis B immunization accidentally sticks herself with an insulin syringe that belongs to her uncle who has diabetes but also is a known to be an HBsAg-positive person. Appropriate management of the adolescent would include:

(A) Initiate hepatitis B vaccine series.
(B) Initiate hepatitis B vaccine series and HBIG 0.06 mL/kg.
(C) Administer HBIG 0.06 mL/kg.
(D) Administer IGIV 400 mg/kg and initiate hepatitis B vaccine series.

Answers

1. **(A)** Immunocompromised children are candidates for varicella zoster immune globulin (VZIG) if there is no prior history of varicella.

2. **(C)** A carefully obtained history of varicella should be the most important determinant of immunity in immunocompromised children. Immunocompromised patients with no history of varicella and low levels of antibody detected by sensitive antibody assays, have developed varicella. Face-to-face contact indoors with a playmate for greater than one hour is considered an exposure that should warrant administration of VZIG.

3. **(C)** Susceptible individuals at high risk for developing severe varicella should receive VZIG within 96 hours of exposure.

4. **(D)** VZIG is not indicated if the mother has zoster. In this case the mother has had varicella in the past so the infant would have transplacentally acquired varicella zoster antibody. VZIG would be indicated for the newborn in the example above if the mother had developed varicella (chickenpox).

5. **(C)** VZIG would be indicated for the premature infant greater than 28 weeks gestation if the mother lacks a reliable history of varicella or serologic evidence of protection. Premature infants (less than 28 weeks gestation or less than equal to 1000 g birth weight) should receive VZIG regardless of maternal history of varicella. The term newborn infant whose mother developed varicella 5 or more days before delivery will have received transplacental antibody from the mother.

6. **(C)** Newborn infants whose mother had onset of varicella within 5 days before delivery or within 48 hours after delivery should receive VZIG. If the onset of the mother's rash is within 5 days of delivery, the infant has been exposed to maternal viremia in the absence of transplacental VZ antibody. If onset of the mother's rash is within 48 hours after delivery, the infant may be exposed to maternal viremia without the possible protective effect of transplacental antibody. If mother has onset of rash 3 or more days after delivery, the route of infection will be the respiratory route and not via the bloodstream.

7. **(C)** A 10 day course of tapering steroids would not be considered an immunosuppressive dose and therefore VZIG is not indicated. Children who receive high doses of corticosteroids (greater than or equal to 2 mg/kg/day of prednisone or its equivalent) given daily or on alternate days for 14 days or more should not receive live-virus vaccines until corticosteroids have been stopped for at least 1 month.

8. **(B)** The cause of these minor reactions may be related to the formation of IgG aggregates during manufacture or storage. Most reactions will subside when the rate of infusion is decreased.

9. **(B)** Patients greater than or equal to 65 years, patients receiving concomitant nephrotoxic agents, patients with diabetes mellitus, pre-existing renal disease, hypovolemia, and sepsis are at increased risk for acute renal failure and renal insufficiency. Most reports of adverse renal events have involved IGIV preparations containing sucrose.

10. **(C)** IGIV is not recommended for routine use in preterm infants with birth weights less than or equal to 1500 g to prevent late-onset infection.

11. **(C)** Other indications for IGIV therapy in HIV-infected children include: hypogammaglobulinemia (IgG level less than 400 mg/dL), two or more serious bacterial infections (bacteremia, pneumonia, meningitis) in a 1-year period and failure to form antibodies to common antigens.

12. **(A)** Anaphylactic reactions are induced by anti-IgA and can occur in children with absence of circulating IgA but have IgG antibodies to IgA. In these situations with IgA deficiency and hypersensitivity reactions, IGIV with extremely low IgA content is available. Screening for IgA deficiency is not recommended.

13. **(C)** IG can be given to prevent or modify measles in susceptible individuals, particularly children younger than 1 year of age, pregnant women, and immunocompromised children who are household contacts of a person with measles. The dose of 0.5 mL/kg is for immunocompromised children (see Table 92-1).

Table 92-1. INDICATIONS FOR THE USE OF IMMUNE GLOBULIN (IG)

Indication	Comment
Replacement therapy in antibody deficiency disorders	Usual dose 100 mg/kg per month by IM route
	Mostly replaced by IGIV
	Slow subcutaneous administration is safe.
Hepatitis A prophylaxis	International travel by children younger than 1 year (< 3 mos stay, 0.02 ml/kg IM; 3–5 mos stay, 0.06 ml/kg IM; long-term stay, 0.06 ml/kg IM every 5 mos.)
	Postexposure, 0.02 ml/kg IM if <2 weeks since last exposure; if future exposure to HAV likely and age ≥2 years, also HAV vaccine.
Measles prophylaxis	Postexposure, 0.25 ml/kg IM within 6 days of exposure, 0.50 ml/kg IM if immunocompromised.
	Target groups: children <1 yr, older children not vaccinated, immunocompromised children, pregnant women.

IGIV, immune globulin intravenous; HAV, hepatitis A virus.

14. **(C)** IG can be given to prevent or modify measles in a susceptible person if given within 6 days of exposure.

15. **(A)** The appropriate management is administration of IG alone. The child is too young for hepatitis A vaccine. Although most infected children in child care settings are asymptomatic or have non-specific symptoms, serologic testing is not recommended. Testing adds unnecessary cost and may delay administration of IG.

16. **(C)** For postexposure immunoprophylaxis of hepatitis A, IG should be administered within 2 weeks after exposure to HAV (see Table 92-1).

17. **(C)** If IG is administered by the subcutaneous route, systemic allergic reactions occur in less than 1% of infusions and local tissue reactions are generally mild.

18. **(B)** In this clinical situation, the prophylaxis is driven primarily by the exposed adolescent not being immunized with hepatitis B vaccine and the source if HBsAg positive. If the adolescent was unimmunized and source is unknown or not tested, the recommendation is to initiate the hepatitis B vaccine series alone.

SUGGESTED READING

Pickering LK, Baker CJ, Overturf GD, et al: *Red Book: 2003 Report of the Committee on Infectious Diseases*, 26th ed. Elk Grove Village, IL: American Academy of Pediatrics, 2003.

Finlayson JS: Passive immunization. In: Long SS, Pickering LK, Prober CG (eds): *Principles and Practices of Infectious Diseases*, 2nd ed. Philadelphia: Churchill Livingstone, 2003, p 37.

CASE 93: A 2-YEAR-OLD CHILD AT DAY CARE WITH FEVER, ANOREXIA, AND NAUSEA

A 2-year-old boy is brought to your office with a 4-day history of fever followed by decreased appetite. His mother denies vomiting or diarrhea, but she thinks that he may be nauseated after eating or drinking. She also indicates that his stool pattern has changed in that for the past 3 days he has only had two stools. The last stool was firm in consistency. The child has attended daycare for the past 8 weeks. His immunizations, including the pneumococcal conjugate vaccine (Prevnar) have been documented to be complete.

On physical examination the child appears to be ill. The temperature is 101.8°F (38.8°C). The child's weight is 0.1 kg less than when seen approximately 2 months ago for a physical examination prior to entering daycare. There is no rash. The examination of the lungs and heart is normal. There is epigastric fullness and mild right upper quadrant pain with examination of the abdomen.

SELECT THE ONE BEST ANSWER TO THE FOLLOWING QUESTIONS

1. The diagnostic test most likely to be helpful in establishing the diagnosis in this child is:

    (A) serologic test for hepatitis A IgM antibody
    (B) stool culture for *Salmonella, Shigella, Campylobacter*
    (C) enzyme immunoassay of stool for *Giardia* antigen
    (D) serologic test for hepatitis E IgM antibody

2. Hepatitis A infection is identified in an employee of the day care center. This is the second outbreak of hepatitis A in the center in the past year. The appropriate management of a 3-year-old child who also attends the day care is:

    (A) immune globulin 0.02mL/kg IM
    (B) immune globulin 0.06mL/kg IM
    (C) immune globulin 0.02mL/kg IM and hepatitis A vaccine
    (D) hepatitis A vaccine

3. How long should the employee be excluded from the daycare center in relation to the onset of the illness?

    (A) 1 week
    (B) 2 weeks
    (C) 3 weeks
    (D) 4 weeks

4. A 3-year-old child sustains a puncture to the right hand after a bite. Within 24 hours the hand is swollen, erythematous, and tender. There is scant serous discharge at the site of the wound. The source of the puncture wound is most likely a

    (A) ferret

    (B) cat
    (C) iguana
    (D) human

5. A 9-year-old girl who has gone hiking in the woods with her father is found to have a tick attached to her neck. A number of tick-borne diseases can occur after a tick bite. These would include all of the following except:

    (A) Lyme disease
    (B) tularemia
    (C) ehrlichiosis
    (D) leptospirosis

6. In a child care setting, the use of prophylactic antibiotics would be most appropriate for:

    (A) child care contacts of a child who has streptococcal toxic shock syndrome
    (B) child care contacts of an infant who has pertussis
    (C) child care contacts of an infant who has influenza A
    (D) child care contacts of a child who has invasive *H. influenzae* type f disease

7. An outbreak of diarrhea has occurred in a day care center. Important infection control measures in the setting include all but:

    (A) written procedures for handwashing
    (B) diaper changing areas should not be located in food preparation areas
    (C) exclusion of children with diarrhea or stools that contain blood or mucus
    (D) removal of all toys from rooms where children eat and play

8. The mother of a 3-year-old girl with HIV infection is considering enrolling her child in a nearby day care center. You inform her that:

    (A) The child should not be placed in the day care center because of the potential risk of transmission to others.
    (B) The child care providers at the day care center will need to be informed of the child's HIV status.
    (C) The child should not attend the day care center because of the risk of exposure to varicella.

(D) The day care providers should use standard precautions for handling spills of blood and blood-containing body fluids.

9. The mother of a 14-year-old adolescent boy calls you in order to inform you that a 16-year-old girl at her son's high school died of meningitis. The mother's son is a close friend of the girl's boyfriend. You had just heard the same day from one of your colleagues about this adolescent girl who died of meningococcal meningitis. You tell the mother:

(A) Her son should have a throat specimen sent for *Neisseria meningitidis* culture.
(B) Her son should receive a single dose of ceftriaxone.
(C) Her son should receive a single dose of ciprofloxacin.
(D) Her son should be observed closely for a febrile illness.

10. An 18-month-old boy who attends daycare has fever, vomiting, and hematochezia. A stool culture sent grows *Salmonella*, serotype Newport. Methods recommended to limit the spread of this organism include:

(A) stool cultures performed for all attendees and staff members
(B) frequent handwashing measures with staff training
(C) exclusion of asymptomatic children shedding *Salmonella* in the stool
(D) antibiotic therapy for all children in the daycare with diarrhea

11. A 3-year-old girl who attends childcare develops fever, abdominal cramps, and mucoid stools with blood. A stool culture sent grows *Shigella sonnei*. Correct management would include:

(A) stool cultures on all childcare attendees and staff members of the child care facility
(B) administration of an anti-diarrheal compound to shorten the duration of diarrhea
(C) treatment with antibiotic therapy of children with mild symptoms to prevent spread
(D) exclusion of the 3-year-old child from child care for 5 days after the onset of diarrhea

12. There are three neonates in a newborn intensive care unit who are diagnosed with RSV infection in a span of 2 days. All of the following are important methods of preventing the further spread of RSV except:

(A) cohorting infected infants
(B) excluding staff with respiratory illness from the NICU
(C) respiratory isolation of all infants positive for RSV
(D) laboratory screening of all infants in the NICU for RSV

13. A 13-year-old boy has a 2-week history of fever, cough productive of sputum, night sweats, and fatigue. A chest radiograph performed shows a right lower lobe infiltrate and a Mantoux test is placed. The test shows 16 mm of induration. Methods to prevent spread of tuberculosis in this patient in the hospital setting include:

(A) droplet precautions
(B) use a mask within 3 feet of the patient
(C) provide a patient with private room using negative air-pressure ventilation
(D) use gown and gloves with each patient encounter

14. A mother of one of your 13-year-old adolescent female patients calls you because she suspects one of her daughter's classmates may have HIV infection. You counsel her that:

(A) HIV is acquired through contact with tears
(B) HIV in a school-age child must be reported to school personnel
(C) HIV status of a school-age child may only be known by the child's parents, other guardians, and physician
(D) HIV infection in adolescents is primarily acquired perinatally from mothers with HIV infection

15. A 12-year-old boy from China with normal growth and development is known to have hepatitis B infection: hepatitis B surface antigen positive, antibody to hepatitis B core antigen positive and antibody to hepatitis B surface antigen negative. A mother of one of your patients who is in the same classroom is concerned, because her

son has only received one dose of hepatitis B vaccine 1 year ago. You recommend that her child:

(A) begin the three-dose series of hepatitis B vaccine again immediately
(B) complete the three-dose series of hepatitis B vaccine with 2 more doses
(C) receive hepatitis B immune globulin and hepatitis B vaccine
(D) have blood drawn for hepatitis B serology and be given hepatitis B vaccine, if seronegative

16. A pediatric resident sustains a needle stick injury while starting a peripheral intravenous line on a 3-year-old child. The resident is concerned about possible HIV infection. You counsel the resident that:

(A) The transmission risk from a single percutaneous needle stick involving HIV-contaminated blood is 0.3%.
(B) Solid needles carry the highest risk of transmission of HIV.
(C) Anti-retroviral agents should be strongly considered with a needle stick injury from an unknown occupational source.
(D) HIV and HBV are the only viruses that can be transmitted by needle-stick injury.

17. A 15-year-old adolescent female is diagnosed with meningococcemia. She has a 4-year-old brother and an 11-month-old sister at home. Appropriate management of her siblings includes:

(A) nasopharyngeal cultures for *N. meningitidis*
(B) meningococcal quadrivalent vaccine
(C) single dose of azithromycin to both children
(D) rifampin given every 12 hours for 2 days

18. A 2-year-old child living in a residential institution for developmentally disabled children should receive all of the following vaccinations for prevention of infection except:

(A) pneumococcal conjugate vaccine
(B) hepatitis A vaccine
(C) hepatitis B vaccine
(D) meningococcal vaccine

Answers

1. **(A)** This child most likely has acute hepatitis A infection. Diagnosis is confirmed by measuring immunoglobulin (Ig) M antibodies to hepatitis A. This antibody usually disappears within 4 months but can persist longer. The serum IgM anti-HAV antibody is usually present at the onset of clinical illness.

2. **(C)** Immune globulin (IG) is indicated if the exposure has been within the previous 2 weeks. In this clinical situation, hepatitis A vaccine should be administered to the child since future exposure seems likely (this was the second outbreak at the day care center within 1 year).

3. **(A)** Children and adults with acute hepatitis A infection who attend or work in child care settings should be excluded for one week after onset of illness.

4. **(B)** This child has a wound infection occurring within 24 hours of a bite. The description is typical of an infection caused by *Pasteurella* species. Transmission occurs most commonly from the bite or scratch of a cat or dog. Infection can also occur after bite injuries from lions, tigers, rats, and rabbits.

5. **(D)** Leptospirosis is caused by spirochetes of the genus *Leptospira*. Humans become infected through contact of mucosal surfaces on abraded skin with contaminated soil, water, or animal tissues. In the United States, dogs and farm animals are important reservoirs in addition to rats.

6. **(B)** Chemoprophylaxis is indicated for childcare contacts of a child with pertussis infection. Chemoprophylaxis in child care settings is also recommended for meningococcal disease. Chemoprophylaxis is also recommended when two or more cases of invasive *H. influenzae* type b disease have occurred within 60 days. No chemoprophylaxis, however, is recommended for people exposed to a patient with serotype f disease.

7. **(D)** All frequently touched toys in rooms where infants and toddlers stay should be cleaned and disinfected daily but it is not necessary to remove them. For older children who are toilet trained, toys should be cleaned weekly and when soiled.

8. **(D)** Children with HIV infection do not need to be excluded from child care. Standard precautions

Table 93-1. CHEMOPROPHYLAXIS FOR CONTACTS OF INDIVIDUALS WITH INVASIVE MENINGOCOCCAL DISEASE

High risk (recommended)	Low risk (not recommended)	Regimens
Household contact	Casual contact (no exposure to oral secretions)	Rifampin (2 days)
Childcare contact ≤7 days before illness	Indirect contact (only contact is high-risk contact)	Ceftriaxone (single dose)
Direct exposure to index patient's secretions (kissing, sharing toothbrush or utensils)	Health care professional with no direct exposure to patient's oral secretions	Ciprofloxacin (single dose)
Mouth-to-mouth resuscitation, intubation, suctioning		
Frequently slept/ate in same dwelling during 7 days before onset of illness		

should be adopted by the child care center for handling spills of blood and blood-contaminated body fluids and wound drainage of all children. Transmission of HIV has not occurred through day-to-day contact in child care centers. Child care providers do not need to be informed of the HIV status of any child attending child care.

9. **(D)** In this scenario, there is only indirect contact, that is the only contact is with a high-risk contact but no direct contact with the index patient. This is a low-risk situation and chemoprophylaxis is not recommended (see Table 93-1).

10. **(B)** Children with *Salmonella* gastroenteritis may return to day care once they are asymptomatic. Approximately 50% of children younger than 5 years will continue to excrete *Salmonella* for 12 weeks after infection. Antimicrobial therapy is not indicated for uncomplicated *Salmonella* gastroenteritis because therapy does not shorten the disease course and may prolong duration of carriage.

11. **(C)** All symptomatic individuals in a child care facility with *Shigella* infection should receive antimicrobial therapy. In mild disease, the primary indication for treatment is to prevent spread of *Shigella* throughout the day care center. Child care attendees or staff members with symptomatic infection should be excluded until the diarrhea has resolved, and stool cultures are negative.

12. **(C)** The correct transmission based precautions in the hospital setting to prevent transmission of

respiratory syncytial virus infection is contact precautions.

13. **(C)** In the hospital setting, the correct transmission based precautions to prevent spread of *Mycobacterium tuberculosis* is airborne precautions. Children younger than 12 years of age with pulmonary tuberculosis are rarely contagious because cavitary disease is rare and cough is not productive so there is little or no expulsion of bacilli. If a patient is receiving adequate antituberculosis therapy with cough resolved and three sputum smears are negative for acid-fast bacilli, the person can be considered non-contagious.

14. **(C)** Child care or school providers need not be informed of the HIV status of a child who is attending a child care center or school. In the absence of blood exposure, HIV is not acquired through the types of contact that occurs in school settings, including contact with saliva or tears. The rate of transmission of HIV has continued to increase, and HIV transmission in adolescents is attributed primarily by sexual contact.

15. **(B)** There is no increased risk of transmission of hepatitis B infection in the school setting. An exception is that residents and staff of institutions for people with developmental disabilities represent a high-risk group for hepatitis B virus infection and should be immunized. In this clinical situation involving the school setting, the classmate of the 12-year-old who is the hepatitis B surface antigen positive should complete the three-dose series. It is not necessary to begin the

series again even though the last dose of vaccine was 1 year previously.

16. **(A)** The risk of transmission from a percutaneous needle accident is highest with hollow bore needles. Antiretroviral therapy is generally not recommended if the source of a needle-stick injury is not known in the non-occupational setting, such as injuries from discarded needles. Finally, needle-stick injuries can also result in hepatitis C virus transmission.

17. **(D)** Household contacts are in the high-risk category for contacts of individuals with meningococcal disease. Rifampin, ceftriaxone, and ciprofloxacin can be used for chemoprophylaxis for high-risk individuals with invasive meningococcal disease (see Table 93-1).

18. **(D)** Children living in residential institutions should receive all the routine childhood vaccines. In this setting children as well as staff are at increased risk of acquiring hepatitis B virus infection. Outbreaks of hepatitis A virus infection can occur in residential institutions. The routine vaccination of all children 1 year of age and older is now recommended. Hepatitis A vaccine, in addition to immunoglobulin, should be considered for staff and residents in an institutional setting where an outbreak of hepatitis A is occurring.

SUGGESTED READING
Pickering LK, Baker CJ, Overturf GD, et al: *Red Book: 2003 Report of the Committee on Infectious Diseases, 26th* ed. Elk Grove Village, IL: American Academy of Pediatrics, 2003.
Robinson J: Infectious diseases in schools and childcare facilities. *Pediatr Rev* 22:39, 2001.

CASE 94: A 3-YEAR-OLD CHILD WITH A FEBRILE SEIZURE

You are called during the middle of a busy day at the office on a Friday afternoon by the pediatric resident at the children's hospital emergency department. You have been very busy all week, seeing many children of all ages with fever associated with upper respiratory tract symptoms (especially cough, rhinorrhea, and sore throat). The pediatric resident tells you that one of your patients, a 3-year-old previously healthy child, was brought to the emergency department after being witnessed by parents at home to have a 5- to 10-minute episode of shaking of the arms and legs. The shaking of the arms and legs had stopped while en route to the emergency department with the parents.

At the emergency department the child was noted to be sleepy and non-responsive. The temperature was 103.1°F (39.5°C). There was minimal nasal congestion. The throat was erythematous. The neck was supple; bilateral anterior cervical adenopathy was present. The spleen tip was palpable. Examination of both lungs and heart were clear.

SELECT THE ONE BEST ANSWER TO THE FOLLOWING QUESTIONS

1. Since the month is December and you have been seeing many children with febrile respiratory illnesses in your office, you suspect influenza is the etiology. The most rapid and sensitive method to diagnose influenza A infection is:

   (A) viral culture of nasopharyngeal specimen
   (B) Influenza A EIA antigen detection on throat specimen
   (C) Influenza A DFA on nasopharyngeal specimen
   (D) Influenza A IgM serology on acute serum

2. The evaluation for influenza A in the child with the febrile seizure does not confirm that diagnosis. You next consider adenovirus in the differential diagnosis. The best method to diagnose adenovirus includes:

   (A) viral culture of nasopharyngeal specimen
   (B) PCR on nasopharyngeal specimen
   (C) adenovirus DFA on nasopharyngeal specimen
   (D) adenovirus complement fixation (IgG) antibody on convalescent serum

3. While hospitalized the child develops prominent respiratory symptoms, including cough, rhinorrhea, and wheezing, which is noted on physical exam. You now suspect that the child has RSV infection. The diagnostic test of choice for diagnosing RSV is:

   (A) enzyme immunoassay of nasal wash specimen
   (B) enzyme immunoassay of nasal swab specimen
   (C) virus isolation of nasopharyngeal aspirate specimen
   (D) immunofluorescent assay of throat specimen

4. You ask the clinical microbiologist about antimicrobial susceptibility testing of bacteria isolated from clinical specimens of children at the children's hospital where you admit children. You are told that there are difficulties in detecting which organism in the microbiology laboratory?

(A) penicillin-resistant *Streptococcus pneumoniae*
(B) vancomycin-resistant *Enterococcus faecium*
(C) ESBL producing *Escherichia coli*
(D) clindamycin-resistant methicillin susceptible *Staphylococcus aureus*

5. A 15-month-old boy presents with a 3-day history of fever to 103°F (39.4°C) followed by refusal to walk. On physical examination he is found to have swelling of the left knee. Arthrocentesis of the left knee joint reveals purulent fluid that grows *S. pneumoniae*. The MIC of the organism is 1.0 μg/mL. The organism is nonsusceptible to penicillin with intermediate resistance. The MIC for the *S. pneumoniae* isolate to be considered susceptible to ceftriaxone would be:

(A) less than or equal to 0.5 μg/mL
(B) less than or equal to 1.0 μg/mL
(C) 2.0 μg/mL
(D) greater than or equal to 4.0 μg/mL

6. A 2-year-old previously healthy boy develops orbital cellulitis with a positive blood culture for methicillin-resistant *S. aureus*. The child is treated with vancomycin at an initial dose of 40 mg/kg/day in four divided doses and serum concentrations of vancomycin are monitored. Adverse reactions to monitor for include all but:

(A) ototoxicity
(B) "red-man syndrome"
(C) hypotension
(D) dose-related anemia with reticulocytopenia

7. All but one of the following antibiotics are best monitored by both peak and trough measurements of serum concentrations:

(A) amikacin
(B) chloramphenicol
(C) linezolid
(D) vancomycin

8. An 18-month-old boy with recurrent otitis media develops fever, rhinorrhea, and fussiness. At your office he has purulent drainage from the left ear, which you send to the children's hospital microbiology laboratory for bacterial culture. The antibiotic amoxicillin is prescribed and 2 days later you receive a call from the microbiology laboratory that the culture is positive for *H. influenzae*. The method to determine whether or not the isolate is susceptible to amoxicillin is to ask the microbiology lab to:

(A) perform test for detection of β-lactamase production
(B) perform a disk diffusion (Bauer-Kirby) antibiotic susceptibility test
(C) perform the oxacillin disk diffusion test
(D) perform the antibiotic gradient method (E-test)

9. A 14-year-old adolescent boy who works on a dairy farm presents with a 4-day history of fever, headache, myalgias of the calf and abdominal pain. On physical exam he is febrile to 102°F (38.8°C) and also has conjunctival suffusion without purulent drainage. You suspect Leptospirosis. The most appropriate diagnostic test to perform to confirm the diagnosis is:

(A) blood culture
(B) serology for *Leptospira interrogans*
(C) anaerobic swab culture of conjunctiva
(D) PCR test of blood specimen

10. An 8-year-old girl develops monoarticular arthritis of the left knee 3 months after traveling with her family in Wisconsin. You suspect late disseminated disease manifesting as Lyme arthritis. Of the following, the most appropriate statement about the diagnosis of Lyme disease is:

(A) The EIA is usually positive in patients with erythema migrans.
(B) A positive EIA in a patient with chronic fatigue is indicative of late disseminated Lyme disease.
(C) Virtually all patients with late disseminated Lyme disease will have IgG antibodies to *Borrelia burgdorferi*.
(D) The EIA if positive should be confirmed by the PCR assay.

11. A 24-year-old woman has a pregnancy complicated by fever, headache, and lymphadenopathy during the first trimester. The mother reports that there are a number of stray cats in the neighborhood. The infant is born at 38 weeks' gestation and weighs 2.5 kg. On physical examination the infant has jaundice, hepatomegaly, chorioretinitis, and scattered punctate calcifications throughout the brain on CT scan. The diagnostic test to determine the etiology of this infant's infections is:

(A) herpes simplex virus serology on infant
(B) *Toxoplasma gondii* serology on maternal and infant sera
(C) culture of blood and cerebrospinal fluid for lymphocytic choriomeningitis virus
(D) cytomegalovirus serology on maternal and infant sera

12. A 3-month-old female infant is brought to your office by her mother for fever, nasal congestion, and poor feeding. On physical examination the infant has a temperature of 101°F, a maculopapular rash and hepatosplenomegaly. At the time of the visit the mother's obstetric record is not available. You suspect congenital syphilis. The following diagnostic test would be most useful in confirming infection with *Treponema pallidum*:

(A) a positive TP-PA test or positive FTA-ABS test
(B) a titer of 1:2 on a RPR test
(C) a hemoglobin concentration of 7.5 g/dL
(D) the presence of intracranial calcifications

12. A 4-year-old boy has a 3-day history of mild headache and decreased activity. This is followed by fever to 103°F (39.4°C), mild cough, and sore throat. On physical exam the child has anterior and posterior cervical lymphadenopathy and splenomegaly. The white blood cell count is 5000/mm³ with a normal differential. The alanine aminotransferase level is increased at 280 U/L. Of the following, the most appropriate diagnostic study to perform is:

(A) IgM for hepatitis A in serum
(B) IgM for the VCA of Epstein-Barr virus
(C) rapid heterophil slide test (monospot)
(D) isolation of HHV-6 from peripheral blood lymphocytes

14. A 14-day-old term infant develops fever to 100.8°F (38.2°C), poor feeding, and two vesicular-appearing skin lesions on the right arm. You suspect neonatal herpes simplex virus (HSV) infection. The most appropriate diagnostic test to perform is:

(A) DFA test of skin lesions
(B) Tzanck test of the skin lesions
(C) PCR of skin lesions
(D) serum for type-specific HSV-2 immunoglobulin IgG antibody

15. Of the following viruses, the one that can be identified by viral culture is:

(A) calicivirus
(B) measles
(C) parvovirus B19
(D) hepatitis E

16. An 8-year-old girl who has received bacilli Calmette-Guérin (BCG) vaccine at age 5 years and now has a positive tuberculin skin test measured using 5 tuberculin (TU) of purified protein derivative. Which of the factors would most support that the positive tuberculin skin test (TST) is caused by BCG?

(A) TST of 16 mm
(B) identification of the BCG immunization scar
(C) chest radiographic findings of hilar adenopathy
(D) child's mother known to have HIV infection

17. A 5-year-old healthy boy has been exposed to *Mycobacterium tuberculosis* by his aunt who is now hospitalized with cavitary pulmonary tuberculosis comes to your office for evaluation. You place a Mantoux test and order a chest radiograph. The Mantoux test is non-reactive but the chest radiograph is abnormal, showing mediastinal adenopathy with a left upper lobe segmental lesion. The most likely explanation for the negative Mantoux skin test is:

(A) receipt of measles vaccine 16 weeks earlier
(B) malnutrition
(C) selective anergy to PPD
(D) the child's young age

18. A 3-year-old girl has a large left, minimally tender, anterior cervical triangle lymph node that has

been present for approximately 5 weeks. All but one of the following factors would suggest a nontuberculosis mycobacterium (NTM) infection:

(A) bilateral location of lymphadenopathy
(B) Mantoux test <12 mm in duration
(C) normal chest radiograph
(D) age <6 years

Answers

1. **(C)** The rapid antigen tests commercially available for identification of influenza A or B have variable sensitivity and specificity compared to viral culture. The DFA is more sensitive than the rapid antigen tests and its sensitivity is high (90%) when compared with culture. Serologic testing with acute and convalescent serum can identify children with influenza not detected by other methods but is not helpful for rapid diagnosis.

2. **(A)** Viral culture is the preferred method of diagnosis of adenovirus infection. The DFA of nasopharyngeal secretions lacks sensitivity (only 60%) as does measurement of complement fixation antibodies. The one exception to viral culture is the detection of the enteric adenovirus types 40 and 41 that cannot be isolated in standard cell cultures. An enzyme immunoassay as well as PCR can be used to detect these enteric adenoviruses in fecal specimens.

3. **(A)** The enzyme immunoassay of nasal specimens has advantages including ease of performance, low cost compared with culture, technical simplicity, and short time to a result compared with immunofluorescence assays. The nasal wash is the preferred specimen for diagnostic testing with a higher yield than specimens obtained by swabs.

4. **(C)** Extended-spectrum β-lactamase producing *E. coli* may be difficult to detect in the laboratory. This is related to the difficulty in identifying those organisms that produce these β-lactamases. Currently, isolates of these species that have minimum inhibitory concentrations of greater than or equal to 2 μg/mL to cefpodoxime, ceftazidime, cefotaxime or ceftriaxone should be considered possible ESBL producers.

5. **(B)** For treatment of nonmeningeal infections caused by penicillin nonsusceptible *S. pneumoniae* isolates the organism is considered susceptible to ceftriaxone if the MIC is less than or equal to 1.0 μg/mL. For treatment of meningeal infections, the breakpoint for ceftriaxone susceptible is less than or equal to 0.5 μg/mL (see Table 94-1).

6. **(D)** Anemia is not an adverse reaction occurring with vancomycin. Dose-related anemia with reticulocytopenia is an adverse reaction reported commonly with chloramphenicol. This red-man syndrome results in flushing of the upper part of the body during rapid intravenous infusion of vancomycin.

7. **(C)** Linezolid does not require measurement of serum concentrations during therapy. Nonrenal pathways account for greater than 80% of total body clearance, and only minor age-related changes

Table 94-1. **INTERPRETATION OF SUSCEPTIBILITY TESTING FOR** *STREPTOCOCCUS PNEUMONIAE* **TO ANTIMICROBIAL AGENTS**

Drug	Susceptible (MIC, μg/ml)	Nonsusceptible (MIC, μg/ml)	
		Intermediate	Resistant
Penicillin	≤0.06	0.1–1.0	≥2.0
Amoxicillin	≤2.0	4.0	≥8.0
Cefotaxime/ceftriaxone			
Meningeal	≤0.5	1.0	≥2.0
Nonmeningeal	≤1.0	2.0	≥4.0

MIC, minimum inhibitory concentration.

in clearance have been observed in children of varying ages.

8. **(A)** β-lactamase production is the most frequent mechanism of ampicillin resistance with *Haemophilus* species and can be detected in the laboratory. The same test can be used to detect penicillin resistance in *Neisseria gonorrhoeae*.

9. **(B)** Isolation of *Leptospira* from blood or CSF specimen can be very difficult, requiring special media, techniques, and long incubation times. Serology is the method of choice for diagnosis, with the macroscopic slide agglutination test the most useful serologic test for screening. Antibodies usually develop during the second week of illness.

10. **(C)** Localized erythema migrans usually occurs 1 to 2 weeks after a tick bite so antibodies against *Borrelia burgdorferi* will not be detectable. IgM antibodies appear 3 to 4 weeks after infection begins and peak by 6 to 8 weeks. Specific IgG antibodies usually appear 4 to 8 weeks after onset of infection and peak 3 to 6 months later. The enzyme immunoassay (EIA) test should be corroborated with the Western immunoblot test. The practice of ordering serologic tests for patients with nonspecific symptoms such as fatigue or arthralgia is not recommended.

11. **(B)** The newborn infant most likely has toxoplasmosis. Serologic tests are the primary approach to the diagnosis of congenital toxoplasmosis. It is important to send blood specimens to a reference laboratory with expertise in performing toxoplasma neonatal serologic assays with appropriate interpretation. Herpes simplex virus and cytomegalovirus are best diagnosed by culture. The diagnosis of lymphocytic choriomeningitis virus is best diagnosed by serology, but virus isolation is possible.

12. **(A)** The nontreponemal tests for syphilis (RPR, VDRL) are sensitive but can produce false-positive results. The treponemal tests (TP-PA, FTA-ABS) are much more specific, and a positive TP-PA would provide the information to confirm the diagnosis of congenital syphilis.

13. **(B)** This child most likely has acute Epstein-Barr virus (EBV) infection. Young children under the age of 5 years with acute Epstein-Barr virus infection will often have results for heterophil antibody tests that are negative. With acute EBV infection VCA-IgM and VCA-IgG will be positive and serum antibody to the EBV nuclear antigen (EBNA) will be negative.

14. **(A)** Rapid diagnostic techniques such as the HSV DFA of skin lesions have the advantage of a rapid turn-around time. This technique is as specific but slightly less sensitive than viral culture. For the diagnosis of neonatal HSV infection, specimens for culture should also be obtained from skin vesicles, mouth or nasopharynx, eyes, urine, blood, stool or rectum, and CSF. The Tzanck test (examination for multinucleated giant cells and eosinophilic intranuclear inclusions) has lower sensitivity. The CSF should be tested for the presence of HSV DNA by PCR.

15. **(B)** Of the viruses listed, only measles can be diagnosed by culture although the simplest method of establishing the diagnosis of measles is by testing for the presence of measles immunoglobulin IgM antibody on a single serum specimen obtained during acute illness. Calicivirus and hepatitis E can be diagnosed with reverse-transcriptase-polymerase chain reaction (RT-PCR) assay for detection of viral RNA in stool as well as by serology. Parvovirus B19 can be diagnosed by serology or PCR assay.

16. **(B)** Vaccination with BCG vaccine can result in a positive TST. The interpretation of TST results in BCG recipients is the same for people who have not received BCG vaccine. The size of 16 mm induration, abnormal chest radiograph, and contact with an adult who has a risk factor (HIV) for tuberculosis, which makes it more likely the cause of the positive TST. The presence of a BCG scar decreases the likelihood that a positive TST is a result of LTBI (latent tuberculous infection).

17. **(C)** A negative Mantoux test does not exclude the diagnosis of tuberculosis disease such as pulmonary tuberculosis, or latent tuberculosis infection (LTBI). Approximately 10% of immunocompetent children with culture-proven tuberculosis do not react initially to a Mantoux test. Young age (younger than 1 year), malnutrition and re-

ceipt of measles vaccine can increase the likelihood for a negative Mantoux test. The effect of measles vaccine on tuberculin reactivity is temporary and should not last for more than 4 to 6 weeks after vaccination.

18. **(A)** All of the factors noted except bilateral location of lymphadenopathy are more likely associated with non-tuberculous mycobacterial species. Adenitis because of NTM is usually unilateral and most commonly involves the submandibular nodes or anterior superior cervical nodes.

SUGGESTED READING

Christenson JC, Kovgenski EK: Laboratory diagnosis of infection because of bacteria, fungi, parasites and rickettsiae. In: Long SS, Pickering LK, Prober CG (eds): *Principles and Practices of Infectious Diseases*, 2nd ed. Philadelphia: Churchill Livingstone, 2003, p 1380.

Miller MJ, Cherry JD: Use of the diagnostic virology laboratory. In: Feigin RD, Cherry JD, Demmler FJ, et al (eds): *Textbook of Pediatric Infectious Diseases*, 5th ed. Philadelphia: WB Saunders, 2004, p 3297.

CASE 95: A 9-MONTH-OLD INFANT WITH FEVER AND CEREBROSPINAL FLUID PLEOCYTOSIS

A 9-month-old male infant was seen by his pediatrician 7 days prior to admission to the hospital with fever to 101.3°F (38.5°C) and runny nose. He was diagnosed with an uncomplicated viral upper respiratory tract infection and sent home. Two days later the infant was brought to the children's hospital emergency department because of persistent fever. At that time he was diagnosed with bilateral otitis media, prescribed amoxicillin, and sent home. No laboratory work-up was done at the time. The infant was administered the amoxicillin as prescribed for the next 5 days but continued to be febrile. His appetite and activity level decreased. So the parents brought him back to the emergency department on day 6 because of these problems.

On physical examination the infant was noted to be irritable. Both tympanic membranes were dull grey with decreased mobility. Nuchal rigidity was present. Examinations of lungs, heart, and abdomen were normal. A spinal tap was performed with the results of: WBC 1200/mm^3 (S-65, L-30, M-5), RBC 10/mm^3, glucose 10 mg/dL and protein 100 mg/dL.

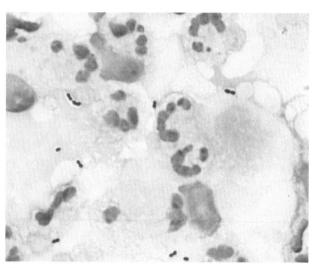

Figure 95-1. Gram stain of CSF that grew **S. pneumoniae** *revealing gram-positive diplococci. Note halo surrounding some of the organisms that represents the capsule. See color plates.*

SELECT THE ONE BEST ANSWER TO THE FOLLOWING QUESTIONS

1. The Gram stain of the CSF shows gram-positive diplococci and the culture of the CSF grows *S. pneumoniae* (see Figure 95-1). The minimum inhibitory concentration (MIC) of penicillin is 0.1 μg/mL and of cefotaxime is 0.25 μg/mL. The appropriate antibiotic therapy for treatment of this infection is:

   (A) ceftriaxone
   (B) chloramphenicol
   (C) penicillin G
   (D) rifampin

2. You are asked about the indications for treatment of different formulations of penicillin (pen) including Pen V, procaine pen G, and benzathine pen G. Procaine pen G is appropriate for treatment of the following infection:

   (A) congenital syphilis in neonates
   (B) group A streptococcal pharyngitis in a school-age child
   (C) actinomycosis in an adolescent
   (D) nosocomial urinary tract infection caused by *Enterococcus faecalis* in a hospitalized 3-year-old child

3. The penicillinase-resistant penicillin oxacillin is not inactivated by the action of the bacterial penicilli-

nase. Oxacillin would therefore be effective therapy for treatment of which of the following infections:

(A) *Enterococcus faecalis* bacteremia
(B) *Pasteurella multocida* wound infection caused by a cat bite
(C) *Streptococcus pyogenes* cellulitis of the lower leg
(D) methicillin-resistant coagulase-negative staphylococci causing a ventriculoperitoneal shunt infection

4. Ampicillin is the antibiotic of choice for which of the following infections:

(A) β-lactamase producing *Moraxella catarrhalis*
(B) *Listeria monocytogenes* causing meningitis in a 3-week-old infant
(C) MSSA causing pneumonia in a 12-month-old child
(D) *Clostridium difficile* causing diarrhea in a 4-year-old hospitalized child

5. A 3-year-old child recently diagnosed with acute myelogenous leukemia (AML) has received induction chemotherapy. The child is admitted to the children's hospital because of fever, neutropenia, and hypotension. The best initial empiric antimicrobial therapy would include:

(A) piperacillin-tazobactam and gentamicin
(B) ceftriaxone and tobramycin
(C) clindamycin and ceftriaxone
(D) vancomycin

6. A 6-week-old infant presents to your office with the insidious onset of cough and tachypnea. On examination the infant is afebrile with rales on pulmonary auscultation. You suspect *Chlamydia trachomatis* pneumonia that is supported by a chest radiograph demonstrating interstitial infiltrates. Erythromycin is prescribed and you tell the infant's mother that the most common adverse reaction of erythromycin is:

(A) cholestatic jaundice
(B) GI discomfort
(C) hearing loss
(D) maculopapular rash

7. Of the following situations, azithromycin would be most appropriate for treatment of the following infection:

(A) a 5-year-old boy with group A streptococcal pharyngitis
(B) a 2-year-old with impetigo caused by methicillin resistant *S. aureus*
(C) a 4-year-old child with lobar pneumonia caused by *S. pneumoniae* that is resistant (MIC = 2.0 μg/mL) to penicillin
(D) a 15-year-old adolescent girl with *C. trachomatis* cervicitis

8. An 18-month-old boy develops anterior cervical lymphadenitis requiring drainage of an abscess that has formed. The abscess culture grows methicillin-resistant *S. aureus* (MRSA) that is D-test negative. The most appropriate antibiotic for treatment would include:

(A) vancomycin
(B) imipenem
(C) cefepime
(D) clindamycin

9. A 5-year-old boy whom you follow for short bowel syndrome has a central venous catheter infection. He is admitted to the children's hospital with fever to 104°F (40°C). He is also known to be colonized with MRSA. A central line infection is strongly suspected and vancomycin is started. The blood culture grows vancomycin-resistant *E. faecalis*. Appropriate therapy would now include:

(A) linezolid
(B) meropenem
(C) clindamycin
(D) clofazimine

10. A 13-year-old adolescent male with HIV infection is being treated with trimethoprim-sulfamethoxazole (TMP-SMX) for *Pneumocystis jiroveci* pneumonia. Adverse reactions that can occur during TMP-SMX therapy include all but:

(A) Stevens-Johnson syndrome
(B) neutropenia
(C) renal dysfunction
(D) pancreatitis

11. Sulfonamides such as sulfadiazine, sulfamethoxazole, and sulfasoxazole all have indications for clinical use in children except:

(A) congenital toxoplasmosis

(B) prophylaxis of urinary tract infections

(C) secondary prophylaxis for rheumatic fever

(D) meningitis caused by *Neisseria meningitidis*

12. A 2½-year-old girl with ventriculoperitoneal shunt secondary to intraventricular hemorrhage (IVH) occurring as a premature neonate develops fever to 102.2°F (39°C), vomiting, and irritability. Examination of the CSF reveals pleocytosis and a Gram stain showing a few gram-positive cocci in clusters. You start empiric therapy with vancomycin. All of the following are appropriate uses of vancomycin except:

(A) treatment of serious infections attributable to β-lactam-resistant gram-positive organisms

(B) treatment of infections attributable to gram-positive microorganisms in patients with serious allergy to β-lactam agents

(C) empiric antimicrobial therapy for a febrile neutropenic patient

(D) prophylaxis for major surgical procedures involving implantation of prosthetic materials or devices at institutions with a high rate of infection caused by MRSA

13. A 5-year-old boy from New York comes to your office with a swollen, tender left knee and some limitation of motion. His mother remembers the child having been bitten by a tick a few months ago during the summer. You suspect Lyme disease, which is confirmed by serology. The mother was treated for Lyme disease 2 years ago with doxycycline and wonders if her child should also be treated with doxycycline. You tell her that:

(A) Doxycycline in only indicated for early Lyme disease with erythema migrans.

(B) Ceftriaxone is the antibiotic of choice for treatment of Lyme arthritis in children.

(C) Doxycycline can cause permanent dental discoloration in children younger than 8 years.

(D) Doxycycline is the antibiotic of choice if the arthritis does not initially respond to treatment with amoxicillin.

14. A 4-year-old child with *Streptococcus viridans* group endocarditis is being treated with penicillin and gentamicin. The following statement best describes the nephrotoxicity caused by the use of aminoglycosides.

(A) all aminoglycosides exert the same degree of risk for nephrotoxicity

(B) nephrotoxicity can be increased by the concomitant use with cyclosporine

(C) the dose of aminoglycosides is not correlated with development of nephrotoxicity

(D) gentamicin nephrotoxicity is usually irreversible

15. A 4-year-old girl returns from a trip to Pakistan with her family. On return she develops fever, headache and abdominal pain that persists for 1 week. She has mild intermittent diarrhea and a rash develops in the second week of the illness. *Salmonella typhi* is isolated from blood that is ampicillin resistant but chloramphenicol susceptible. The most common adverse effect occurring with chloramphenicol use includes:

(A) dose-dependent anemia with low reticulocyte count

(B) aplastic anemia

(C) ototoxicity

(D) myocardial toxicity

16. The use of fluoroquinolones in the pediatric age group has been limited since fluoroquinolones have been shown to cause cartilage damage in puppies and large joint arthropathy in other immature animals. Their use in children therefore has not been approved by the Food and Drug Administration (FDA) except for ciprofloxacin that has been recently FDA-approved for complicated urinary tract infections and pyelonephritis because of *E. coli*. Nevertheless, there has been an increasing experience in children with the use of fluoroquinolones in certain situations. Which of the following scenarios is a clinical situation in which the use of a fluoroquinolone is inappropriate:

(A) pulmonary exacerbation in cystic fibrosis patient

(B) cellulitis caused by methicillin-resistant *S. aureus*

(C) typhoid fever resistant to ampicillin, ceftriaxone, and TMP-SMX resistant *S. typhi*

(D) urinary tract infection caused by multidrug-resistant, gram-negative bacteria

17. A 4-year-old girl has had daily contact with her aunt for the past 2 months. The aunt has recently

been diagnosed with isoniazid-resistant pulmonary tuberculosis. A chest radiograph of the child is normal. Appropriate treatment of the child includes:

(A) azithromycin
(B) ethambutol
(C) rifampin
(D) clofazimine

18. A 6-year-old boy develops an intra-abdominal abscess following appendectomy for a ruptured appendix. Meropenem is being administered as part of empiric therapy. The organism that is susceptible to meropenem is:

(A) *Stenotrophomonas maltophilia*
(B) MRSA
(C) vancomycin-resistant *E. faecium*
(D) *Serratia marcescens*

Answers

1. **(A)** There is a difference in susceptibility break points for ceftriaxone or cefotaxime for meningeal versus nonmeningeal infections. For meningeal isolates, the MIC must be less than or equal to 0.5 µg/mL to be considered susceptible. For nonmeningeal isolates the susceptibility break point is doubled for less than or equal to 1.0 µg/mL.

2. **(A)** There are a number of difficult formulations for natural penicillins. Benzathine penicillin by intramuscular injection can be used for the treatment of group A streptococcal pharyngitis. Actinomycosis is best treated initially with intravenous penicillin G. *E. faecalis* causing a urinary tract infection is usually treated with oral amoxicillin or intravenous ampicillin.

3. **(C)** The penicillinase-resistant penicillin oxacillin is active against *S. pyogenes* (group A streptococcus). Enterococci and gram-negative bacilli (including *Pasteurella* species) cannot be treated with these semisynthetic penicillins.

4. **(B)** Ampicillin is considered the preferred antimicrobial agent for treatment of *Listeria* infections. Bacteria that produce the enzyme β-lactamase are resistant to ampicillin since the enzyme hydrolyzes the β-lactam antibiotic. Staphylococcal resis-

tance to ampicillin is also through production of a penicillinase. *C. difficile* pseudomembranous colitis can occur after treatment with ampicillin.

5. **(A)** In this clinical situation infection with *Pseudomonas aeruginosa* is of major concern. Piperacillin-tazobactam, an extended-spectrum penicillin, has the best activity of the antibiotic listed for treatment of *P. aeruginosa*. Piperacillin is a piperazine analogue of ampicillin and tazobactam is a synthetic penicillanic acid sulfone. Tazobactam irreversibly binds with a number of different plasmid encoded β-lactamases and also has activity against certain chromosomally mediated β-lactamases.

6. **(B)** The most common adverse effect of erythromycin is gastrointestinal discomfort and nausea. An association between oral erythromycin and infantile hypertrophic pyloric stenosis has been reported in infants younger than 6 weeks of age.

7. **(D)** Azithromycin can be used for treatment of uncomplicated Chlamydia cervicitis (single 1-g oral dose). Azithromycin is not active against methicillin resistant *S. aureus*. A high percent (>75%) of penicillin resistant *S. pneumoniae* are also resistant to azithromycin.

8. **(D)** The MRSA isolate is erythromycin resistant and clindamycin susceptible so the D-test was performed. The D-test is used to screen for the presence of the erythromycin ribosome methylase (erm) gene. If the D-test is positive, this suggests the presence of the erm gene in the *S. aureus* isolate. This mechanism of resistance to erythromycin is the production of the erythromycin ribosome methylase. Treatment of the *S. aureus* isolate with clindamycin can select for mutants during therapy that are also clindamycin resistant. Since the D-test is negative this risk does not exist.

9. **(A)** Linezolid represents a new class of antimicrobial agents called the oxazolidinones that bind to the 50S ribosomal subunit and inhibit protein synthesis. Linezolid is active against MRSA, VRE, and penicillin-resistant *S. pneumoniae*.

10. **(D)** The most common adverse events are GI and skin reactions. Adverse reactions to TMP-SMX

occur infrequently in non-AIDS patients (<5%) but frequently (15%) in children with AIDS. The most common adverse event is an erythematous maculopapular rash that is often transient and can clear without stopping the drug.

11. **(D)** TMP-SMX is not recommended for treatment of meningococcal meningitis but has been used to successfully treat meningitis caused by *Salmonella* and *Listeria*. TMP-SMX also is useful for the treatment of urinary tract infections and pyelonephritis, gastroenteritis because of susceptible strains of *Shigella* and is the treatment of choice for *P. jiroveci* pneumonia.

12. **(C)** The Centers for Disease Control and Prevention have established guidelines for situations in which the use of vancomycin is appropriate as well as situations in which the use of vancomycin is discouraged (see Table 95-1). Vancomycin is not recommended for empiric therapy of the patient with fever and neutropenia.

13. **(C)** Tetracyclines can combine with newly formed bone to produce a tetracycline-calcium orthophosphate complex that can inhibit bone growth in neonates and cause staining of the enamel of the teeth in children younger than 8

Table 95-1. SITUATIONS IN WHICH VANCOMYCIN USE SHOULD BE DISCOURAGED

Routine surgical prophylaxis (exception: life-threatening allergy to β-lactam antibiotics)

Empiric antimicrobial therapy for febrile neutropenic patients

Treatment of a single positive blood culture for coagulase negative staphylococcus, if other blood cultures around same time negative

Continued empiric use for presumed infections with no evidence β-lactam-resistant gram-positive bacteria

Selective decontamination of gastrointestinal tract

Attempted eradication of MRSA colonization

Primary treatment of antimicrobial associated colitis

Treatment of any infection caused by β-lactam-susceptible gram-positive bacteria

Topical application or irrigation

MRSA, methicillin-resistant *Staphylococcus aureus*.

years. For this 5-year-old child the treatment of choice for Lyme arthritis would be amoxicillin for a 28-day course (compared with amoxicillin for 14 to 21 days for early localized disease). For persistent or recurrent arthritis, the treatment of choice would be ceftriaxone.

14. **(B)** Gentamicin nephrotoxicity is characterized by proximal tubular necrosis in the kidneys. Risk factors for nephrotoxicity from aminoglycosides include high dose, prolonged course, liver disease, concomitant use of other nephrotoxic drugs such as cyclosporine and salt and water depletion (such as dehydration or sepsis).

15. **(A)** Bone marrow suppression can occur with chloramphenicol in two ways. The first is related to the duration of the dose and is reversible. It is usually seen after 7 days of therapy and manifests as anemia with a low reticulocyte count. It is associated with peak and trough serum chloramphenicol concentrations greater than 25 and 10 μg/mL, respectively. Chloramphenicol can also cause idiosyncratic aplastic anemia that is irreversible and occurs in about 1 in 40,000 patients treated with chloramphenicol. This is similar to the rate of fatal anaphylaxis with β-lactams such as penicillins and cephalosporins.

16. **(B)** Use of the fluoroquinolones is still generally contraindicated in children and adolescents younger than 18 years of age. There are certain situations in which fluoroquinolones may be useful including when no other oral agent is available or the infection is caused by a multidrug-resistant gram-negative enteric or other bacterium. MRSA are often fluoroquinolone resistant, resistance to them may develop rapidly, and for community-acquired MRSA infections in children, there are alternative antibiotics.

17. **(C)** Rifampin has been used alone for the treatment of latent tuberculosis infection (LTBI) infants, children and adolescents when INH could not be tolerated or the index case was infected with an INH resistant, rifampin susceptible organism. In this clinical situation rifampin should be given for at least 6 months. Patients should be informed that rifampin can cause orange urine, sweat and tears and discoloration of soft contact

lenses. Sexually active women on oral contraception should be informed that rifampin can make oral contraceptives ineffective.

18. **(D)** Meropenem is a carbapenem antibiotic that has a broad spectrum of activity against many gram-positive aerobic cocci, gram-negative enteric bacteria and anaerobes. In this example, meropenem would likely be active against *Serratia marcescens* but not active against MRSA or VRE. *Stenotrophomonas maltophilia* is commonly resistant to the carbapenems. Another carbapenem antibiotic imipenem-cilastin, has been associated with an increased risk of seizures. This risk appears to be related to high dose, age (elderly) and impaired renal function.

SUGGESTED READING

James LP, Abdel-Rahman, Farrar HC, et al: Antimicrobial agents. In: Long SS, Pickering LK, Prober CG (eds): *Principles and Practices of Infectious Diseases*, 2nd ed. Philadelphia: Churchill Livingstone, 2003, p 1458.

Jacob RF: Judicious use of antibiotics for common pediatric respiratory infections. *Pediatr Infect Dis J* 19:938, 2000.

CASE 96: AN 18-MONTH-OLD CHILD WITH FEVER AFTER RENAL TRANSPLANT

An 18-month-old boy whom you have followed in your practice since birth has been diagnosed with renal failure secondary to posterior urethral valves. As a result he has undergone a renal transplant with success. Renal function post-transplantation has been normal, and he is receiving a number of immunosuppressive medications to prevent rejection of the transplanted kidney. One month after the kidney transplant, he develops fever associated with cough and rhinorrhea.

On physical examination the child is sitting up in his mother's lap. He is alert and active. The temperature is 101.4°F (38.6°C). There is clear rhinorrhea but no abnormalities of the oropharynx. Lungs and heart examinations are normal. Examination of the abdomen reveals a palpable kidney in the right lower quadrant but no abdominal tenderness. The leukocyte count is 8900/mm³ (S-20, L-65, M-15), the hemoglobin concentration is 8.0 g/dL and the platelet count is 120,000/mm³. A chest radiograph reveals no evidence of pneumonia.

SELECT THE ONE BEST ANSWER TO THE FOLLOWING QUESTIONS

1. Prior to transplantation it was known that the child was seronegative for cytomegalovirus (CMV) and the donor of the kidney was seropositive. The antiviral agent of choice for prophylaxis of CMV infection is:

   (A) acyclovir
   (B) cidofovir
   (C) foscarnet
   (D) ganciclovir

2. The mother of the child asks you about adverse effects that can occur with the use of ganciclovir. You tell the mother that the most important toxic effect of ganciclovir is:

   (A) anemia
   (B) neutropenia
   (C) hallucinations
   (D) hepatitis

3. The mechanism of action of ganciclovir includes:

   (A) prevention of viral entry into the host cell
   (B) prevention of viral transcription by inhibiting viral DNA polymerase
   (C) interrupting viral protein assembly
   (D) modulation of host response to infection

4. An 1800-g infant is born at 35 weeks' gestation. Growth parameters are consistent with intrauterine growth retardation including microcephaly. The infant has scattered petechiae as well as hepatosplenomegaly. The diagnosis of congenital cytomegalovirus infection is confirmed by detection of virus in sequential urine specimens. Intravenous ganciclovir is discussed with the parents as a treatment option. The major benefit of IV ganciclovir in this clinical setting is:

   (A) prevention of sensorineural hearing loss
   (B) more rapid resolution of hepatosplenomegaly
   (C) more rapid resolution of CMV retinitis
   (D) improved weight gain and head circumference growth

5. A 3-year-old child is hospitalized for repair of congenital heart disease. Influenza A is known to be present in the community, and there has been

influenza A infection in several staff members. The child did not receive influenza vaccine. The best initial management is:

(A) initiation of rimantadine chemoprophylaxis
(B) vaccination with whole virus influenza vaccine
(C) vaccination with live attenuated influenza vaccine
(D) initiation of oseltamivir chemoprophylaxis

6. You are asked about the activity and treatment of antiviral agents against influenza. Which of the following antiviral agents are active against influenza A and influenza B and approved for treatment of infection caused by both viruses.

(A) amantadine
(B) rimantadine
(C) zanamivir
(D) interferon-α

7. A 15-year-old adolescent female develops a fever of 104°F (40°C), cough, rhinorrhea, headache, sore throat, and myalgias during the middle of an epidemic of influenza A. You are considering prescribing oseltamivir for treatment. Recommendations for use of oseltamivir include starting the medication within which of the following number of days of symptoms of influenza:

(A) 1 day
(B) 2 days
(C) 3 days
(D) 4 days

8. You are asked about the potential indications for acyclovir use. The infection for which your patient is most likely to benefit from the use of acyclovir is:

(A) a 14-year-old adolescent female with an initial genital herpes infection that began 2 days ago
(B) a 2-week-old female infant with microcephaly, hepatosplenomegaly, and shedding cytomegalovirus in the urine
(C) a 3-year-old with hepatitis associated with varicella zoster virus infection that began 2 days ago
(D) a 2-year-old boy with encephalitis caused by human herpes virus type 6

9. You are asked about the mechanism of action of acyclovir by a group of medical students. You reply that:

(A) Acyclovir in its triphosphate form inhibits the viral DNA polymerase of HSV.
(B) Acyclovir has metabolites that interfere with elongation of viral messenger RNA in HSV.
(C) Acyclovir results in the methylation of viral messenger RNA in HSV.
(D) Acyclovir interferes with viral protein synthesis in HSV.

10. The most serious side effect of acyclovir is:

(A) acute renal failure
(B) hematuria
(C) neurotoxicity
(D) neutropenia

11. You are asked about the appropriate indications for the use of foscarnet. Of the following indications listed, the one in which foscarnet would not be appropriate includes:

(A) cytomegalovirus retinitis in a 19-year-old male with AIDS
(B) cytomegalovirus infection that is unresponsive to ganciclovir in an 18-month-old child with a renal transplant
(C) primary acyclovir resistant varicella zoster virus infection in an 8-year-old girl with acute lymphoblastic leukemia
(D) Parainfluenza virus pneumonia in a 12-year-old boy with leukemia

12. The most common and serious adverse effect of foscarnet includes:

(A) hypocalcemia
(B) nephrotoxicity
(C) pancreatitis
(D) seizures

13. A 6-year-old Asian boy with perinatal hepatitis B infection has persistent hepatitis B surface antigen (HBsAg) in serum, no hepatitis B surface antibody (Anti-HBs) and a positive hepatitis B e antigen (HBeAg). These findings are consistent with chronic hepatitis B infection. An appropriate antiviral agent for treatment of this infection includes:

(A) cidofovir

(B) interferon-α

(C) trifluridine

(D) vidarabine

14. The most likely adverse reaction associated with the first week of therapy of the child with chronic hepatitis B infection in the previous question is:

(A) influenza-like illness with fever, chills, headache, myalgias, arthralgias

(B) seizures

(C) anemia

(D) renal insufficiency

15. An 8-year-old girl recently diagnosed with HIV infection has a CD4 count of 478/μL and percentage of 16%. The viral load measured is 10,500 copies/mL. All of the following are recommended regimens for initial therapy for HIV infection in children except:

(A) two NRTIs plus one PI

(B) two NRTIs plus one NNRTI

(C) two NRTIs

(D) one NRTI

16. Monotherapy with an antiretroviral agent is recommended in the following circumstances:

(A) a 14-year-old adolescent with a CD4 count of 300/μL and suspected poor compliance

(B) newborn infant born to an HIV positive mother

(C) 6-month old infant girl with viral load of 50,000 copies/mL and CD4 count of 750/μL

(D) a 10-year-old girl with a newly diagnosed HIV infection undetectable viral load, a CD4 count of 650 and percentage of 33%

17. The major toxicity associated with zidovudine in children is:

(A) anemia

(B) lactic acidosis

(C) pancreatitis

(D) peripheral neuropathy

18. You are considering using a protease inhibitor for use in a highly active antiretroviral combination regimen for treatment of HIV infection in a pediatric patient. Protease class disadvantages include all but:

(A) metabolic complications including dyslipidemia, fat maldistribution and insulin resistance

(B) higher pill burden than nucleoside or non-nucleoside analogue reverse transcriptase inhibitor based regimens

(C) poor palpability of liquid preparations

(D) a single mutation can confer resistance with cross resistance among other non-nucleoside reverse transcriptase inhibitors

Answers

1. **(D)** For renal transplant recipients, antiviral therapy is recommended when the recipient is seronegative for CMV and the donor is seropositive. If the donor or recipient is seropositive for CMV and antilymphocyte treatment is used, antiviral therapy is recommended. In one comparative trial of antiviral therapy for CMV prophylaxis in kidney transplant recipients, ganciclovir was superior to acyclovir.

2. **(B)** Myelosuppression is the most frequent toxic effect of ganciclovir. The incidence of neutropenia is 40%. Thrombocytopenia occurs in 20% of patients and anemia in 2% of ganciclovir recipients. Hallucinations and hepatitis are rare adverse events associated with ganciclovir.

3. **(B)** Ganciclovir is a nucleoside analogue that is phosphorylated first by virus encoded enzymes then by cellular enzymes. Ganciclovir triphosphate is a competitive inhibitor of herpes viral DNA polymerase but has some activity against cellular DNA polymerases.

4. **(A)** A randomized controlled trial of neonates with symptomatic CMV disease involving the central nervous system found that neonates treated with 6 weeks of intravenous ganciclovir prevented hearing deterioration at 6 months of age and may prevent hearing loss >12 months of age. Neutropenia is a significant side effect of the therapy.

5. **(A)** Chemoprophylaxis for prevention of influenza A is indicated to protect high-risk children, e.g. congenital heart disease during the 2 weeks after

immunization while an immune response is developing or if the child is immunized after influenza is circulating in the community. In addition to receiving rimantadine for chemoprophylaxis, influenza vaccine should also be administered for a 3 year-old child with congenital heart disease. Oseltamivir is licensed for prophylaxis against influenza for patients > 13 years of age.

6. **(C)** Amantadine and rimantadine are only active against influenza A. Interferon-α is not recommended for treatment of influenza.

7. **(B)** Based on placebo-controlled studies in both adults and children, patients who receive oseltamivir within 2 days of onset of symptoms of influenza had a shorter illness duration, more rapid return to normal health and activity and decreased frequency of secondary complications such as sinusitis and otitis media that required antibiotic prescriptions. Therapy should be considered for children at increased risk of severe or complicated influenza, healthy children with severe illness and for children in special environmental, family or social situations in which ongoing illness would be detrimental.

8. **(A)** Patients with the first episode of genital herpes may initially have mild symptoms but develop more severe or prolonged symptoms. Both acyclovir and valacyclovir decrease the duration of symptoms and viral shedding in genital herpes. If oral acyclovir is initiated within 6 days of the onset of disease, the duration of illness and viral shedding are shortened by 3–5 days.

9. **(A)** Acyclovir is a dioxygenase analogue that is monophosphorylated by virus-encoded thymidine kinase then diphosphorylated and triphosphorylated by host cell enzymes. Acyclovir triphosphate prevents viral DNA synthesis by inhibiting the viral DNA polymerase. Acyclovir also results in DNA chain termination.

10. **(C)** The most frequent neurologic manifestations are tremors, myoclonus, lethargy, agitation, and hallucinations. These side effects occur in patients with compromised renal function who achieve high concentrations of acyclovir. Neutropenia has been observed in neonates receiving high doses of intravenous acyclovir (60 mg/kg/day) for treatment as well as infants receiving oral acyclovir for suppressive therapy.

11. **(D)** Foscarnet is a non-competitive inhibitor of viral DNA polymerase. Foscarnet can be used for treatment of CMV retinitis in patients with AIDS. Foscarnet also is an option for a patient with severe CMV infection that is unresponsive to ganciclovir. Foscarnet also is the antiviral agent of choice for treatment of acyclovir resistant herpes simplex and varicella zoster infections. Parainfluenza virus is an RNA virus, and foscarnet is not active against RNA viruses.

12. **(B)** Azotemia, proteinuria, acute tubular necrosis, crystalluria, and interstitial nephritis can occur. Risk factors for renal dysfunction include pre-existing renal disease, use of other nephrotoxic drugs, dehydration, rapid injection of large doses, and continuous intravenous infusion. Hypocalcemia can occur and is because of chelation of ionized calcium by foscarnet. Seizures are one CNS complication that can occur. Seizures can also occur as a manifestation of hypocalcemia.

13. **(B)** Interferons are a family of nonspecific regulatory proteins associated with a variety of antiviral, antiproliferative and immunomodulatory activities. Interferon-α is approved for treatment of chronic hepatitis B and hepatitis C infection as well as papillomavirus-induced anogenital disease.

14. **(A)** The symptoms of an influenza-like illness usually remit with continued therapy. These symptoms rarely require discontinuing therapy or changing the dose. The two major therapy-limited toxicities of interferon are neuropsychiatric complications (somnolence, confusion, behavioral disturbances, depression, seizures) and bone marrow suppression. Neutropenia and thrombocytopenia are most commonly seen.

15. **(D)** Either choice A or B are strongly recommended for initial antiretroviral therapy and would be considered highly active antiretroviral therapy (HAART). Choice C, which is dual NRTI therapy, should only be used in special circumstances. The regimen should be considered when the healthcare provider or guardian/parent has

Table 96-1. RECOMMENDED ANTIVIRAL DRUGS FOR HUMAN IMMUNODEFICIENCY VIRUS INFECTION IN CHILDREN

Regimens	PI	NNRTI	NRTI
Strongly recommended	2 NRTIs plus lopinavir/ritonavir or nelfinavir or ritonavir	>3 yrs: 2 NRTIs plus efavirenz ≤3 yrs or can't swallow capsules: 2 NRTIs plus nevirapine	None
Alternative recommendation	2 NRTIs plus idinavir or amprenavir	2 NRTIs plus nevirapine	Zidovudine plus lamivudine plus abacavir

PI, protease inhibitor; NNRTI, nonnucleoside analogue reverse transcriptase inhibitor; NRTI, nucleoside analogue reverse transcriptase inhibitor.

concerns regarding the feasibility of adherence to more complex regimens. Choice D, which is monotherapy, should never be used as therapy for children with HIV infection (see Table 96-1).

16. **(B)** Monotherapy as initial therapy for HIV infection in children is only recommended for chemoprophylaxis administered to HIV-exposed infants during the first 6 weeks of life to prevent perinatal HIV transmission.

17. **(A)** The most common toxicities in children with zidovudine treatment are anemia and neutropenia, both of which will usually resolve with temporary cessation of drug or dose modification. The NRTI drugs didanosine (ddI) and stavudine (d4T) have peripheral neuropathy as their primary toxicity. Abacavir (ABC) has been associated with a hypersensitivity reaction consisting of fever, rash, nausea, vomiting, or abdominal pain. This reaction should result in permanent discontinuation of the drug.

18. **(D)** With the protease class inhibitors, resistance requires multiple mutations. The protease inhibitors target HIV at two steps of viral replication, the viral reverse transcriptase and protease enzymes.

SUGGESTED READING

Hayden FG: Antiviral drugs (other than antiretrovirals). In: Mandell GL, Bennett JE, Dolin R (eds): *Mandell, Douglas and Bennett's Principles and Practice of Infectious Diseases*, 5th ed. Philadelphia: Churchill Livingstone, 2000, p 460.

Centers for Disease Control and Prevention: Guidelines for using antiretroviral agents in pediatric HIV infection. *MMWR* 47(RR-4):1–38, 1998. Available at: http://AIDSinfo.nih.gov. Last accessed: November 3, 2005.

CASE 97: A 12-YEAR-OLD GIRL WITH LEUKEMIA AND PERSISTENT FEVER

A 12-year-old girl, whom you have followed in your practice since birth, was recently diagnosed with acute myelogenous leukemia after developing fever, fatigue, and epistaxis. Your patient had begun chemotherapy under the guidance of your pediatric oncology consultant. After induction chemotherapy was completed, you receive a phone call on a Saturday evening that your patient has developed fever at home. You direct your patient's parents to bring her to the children's hospital emergency department.

On physical examination at the emergency department, the adolescent girl is non-toxic in appearance. The temperature is 102.2°F (39°C). There is mild erythema of the posterior pharynx. Examination of both lungs and the heart are normal. A WBC count revealed an absolute neutrophil count of 200/mm^3, hemoglobin of 9.0 g/dL and platelet count of 130,000/mm^3. Ceftazidime empiric therapy was begun. However, fever persisted and after 4 days a repeat WBC count revealed an absolute neutrophil count of 0/mm^3.

SELECT THE ONE BEST ANSWER TO THE FOLLOWING QUESTIONS

1. The most appropriate course of action to follow with the persistence of fever includes:

   (A) addition of vancomycin to antibiotic regimen
   (B) change of ceftazidime to imipenem
   (C) addition of ketoconazole
   (D) addition of amphotericin B

2. One of the common adverse events to now monitor for in the 12-year-old patient after the above change in management is:

(A) hypocalcemia
(B) hypokalemia
(C) hypermagnesemia
(D) hyperuricemia

3. An 850-g very low birthweight infant now 24 days old has a central venous catheter and has completed a 10-day course of broad spectrum antibiotic therapy with cefotaxime and gentamicin for a bacteremia with *E. coli*. The infant develops apnea along with poor feeding and hypothermia. A blood culture sent to the microbiology laboratory is reported in 24 hours to be growing a yeast. Appropriate therapy would now include:

(A) amphotericin B
(B) fluconazole
(C) liposomal amphotericin B
(D) flucytosine

4. You prescribe ketoconazole for a 6-year-old child with tinea capitis who develops urticaria while receiving griseofulvin. The most severe adverse event associated with ketoconazole when administered alone includes:

(A) cardiac arrhythmia
(B) hemolytic anemia
(C) hepatic necrosis
(D) renal failure

5. You are asked about the appropriate indications for use of the triazole antifungal agent fluconazole. Which of the following infections would fluconazole be appropriate for first time therapy?

(A) Treatment of esophageal candidiasis caused by *Candida albicans* in a 6-year-old child with HIV infection.
(B) Treatment of hepatosplenic candidiasis in a 3-year-old child with acute myelogenous leukemia.
(C) A premature neonate with *Candida tropicalis* fungemia and a renal fungus ball.
(D) Catheter-associated fungemia with *Candida krusei*.

6. The most common adverse reactions reported with the triazoles include:

(A) hepatitis
(B) rash
(C) GI symptoms (nausea, vomiting, diarrhea)
(D) fatigue

7. A 12-year-old adolescent male has fever, cough, and productive sputum production for 4 weeks. A chest radiograph reveals a right lower lobe infiltrate. A sputum culture grows *Blastomyces dermatitis*. He is not vomiting and requires no supplemental oxygen. The antifungal agent of choice for treatment of this infection is:

(A) fluconazole
(B) itraconazole
(C) ketoconazole
(D) amphotericin B

8. Antifungal therapy is begun and the adolescent develops pedal edema. This finding is most likely an adverse effect associated with:

(A) fluconazole
(B) itraconazole
(C) ketoconazole
(D) amphotericin B

9. You are asked about the appropriate indications for the use of flucytosine (5-fluorocytosine). You indicate that flucytosine is the preferred treatment for the following infection in combination with amphotericin B:

(A) chronic mucocutaneous candidiasis
(B) cryptococcal meningitis
(C) pulmonary aspergillosis
(D) disseminated histoplasmosis

10. The antifungal agent of choice for treatment of invasive aspergillosis refractory to amphotericin B is:

(A) voriconazole
(B) fluconazole
(C) miconazole
(D) flucytosine

11. Itraconazole is the preferred antifungal therapy for moderate pulmonary infections caused by all but one of the following fungi:

(A) *Histoplasma capsulatum*
(B) *Cryptococcus neoformans*
(C) *Blastomyces dermatitidis*
(D) *Sporothrix schenckii*

12. A 13-year-old girl has developed soft disfigured nails with pits and grooves involving only the nails of her hands. A fungal culture grows *Tinea unguium*. The antifungal agent of choice for this infection is:

(A) fluconazole
(B) griseofulvin
(C) itraconazole
(D) terbinafine

13. The duration of therapy for the 13-year-old adolescent with *T. unguium* in the above example should be:

(A) 6 weeks
(B) 12 weeks
(C) 24 weeks
(D) 52 weeks

14. A 3-year-old child presents to your office because of persistent itching for the past 2 weeks. On physical examination the child is afebrile. The examination of the skin reveals scattered papules and burrows involving the arms, legs, palms, soles, and the trunk. You make the diagnosis of scabies examining the scrapings of a burrow to which mineral oil is first applied. The treatment of choice for this condition includes:

(A) Lindane 1% lotion
(B) Permethrin 5% cream
(C) Crotamiton 10% cream
(D) Single oral dose of ivermectin

15. A 3-year-old child develops abdominal pain, diarrhea about 4 weeks after returning with his family from a trip to South America. About 12 weeks later he is diagnosed with iron deficiency anemia and peripheral eosinophilia (20%). Intestinal hookworm infection is detected by identifying the hookworm eggs in feces. You recommend treatment with:

(A) Albendazole 400 mg in a single dose
(B) Mebendazole 100 mg in a single dose
(C) Pyrantel pamoate 11 mg/kg/dose (max 1.0 g) for 1 dose
(D) Niclosamide 1 g in a single dose

16. A 2-year-old child returns with parents from vacation in Southeast Asia. The child presents to your office with abdominal pain and bloody diarrhea with mucus. You diagnose infection with whipworm (*Trichuris trichiura*) by examination of stool for the characteristics *T. trichiura* eggs. Treatment of the infection should include:

(A) Albendazole 400 mg in a single dose
(B) Mebendazole 100 mg twice daily for 3 days
(C) Pyrantel pamoate 1 g in a single dose
(D) Ivermectin 200 μg/kg in a single dose

17. Metronidazole has both antibacterial and antiprotozoal properties. Major indications for the use of metronidazole include all but:

(A) actinomycosis
(B) brain abscess secondary to chronic sinusitis
(C) giardiasis
(D) *Trichomonas* vaginitis

18. A 4-year-old girl is going to travel with her family to West Africa where chloroquine resistant *Plasmodium falciparum* is reported. Appropriate chemoprophylaxis for the child would include:

(A) doxycycline
(B) atovaquone-proguanil
(C) sulfadoxine-pyrimethamine
(D) clindamycin

Answers

1. **(D)** Fungi are common causes of secondary infection among neutropenic patients who have received courses of broad spectrum antibiotic therapy. Fungi can also cause primary infections. Studies have indicated that up to one-third of febrile neutropenic patients who do not respond to a 1-week course of antibiotic therapy have systemic fungal infections.

2. **(B)** Nephrotoxicity and bone marrow suppression are the most frequent adverse events which can result in renal tubular acidosis, hypokalemia, hypomagnesemia from its effect on the kidneys as well as anemia. Amphotericin B inhibits erythropoietin production in the kidney resulting in anemia as the cumulative dose increases.

3. **(A)** The premature neonate likely has catheter-related fungemia caused by *Candida*. The infant could also have disseminated candidiasis. In both these instances a blood culture will yield *Candida*. Amphotericin B is the drug of choice for treatment of suspected fungal infections in premature infants.

4. **(C)** Common adverse reactions associated with ketoconazole include anorexia, nausea and vomiting. The most severe adverse event is fatal hepatic necrosis, a rare complication that occurs in about 1 in 10,000 treated patients. Administration of ketoconazole is contraindicated with the antihistamines astemizole and terfenadine because of potential prolongation of the cardiac QT interval.

5. **(A)** Fluconazole is also effective in preventing relapse of cryptococcal meningitis in patients with AIDS. *C. krusei* is resistant to fluconazole.

6. **(C)** Patients may also have transient asymptomatic elevations of liver enzymes. Rashes have been reported, and rare reports of an exfoliative dermatitis in AIDS patients receiving fluconazole have been described.

7. **(B)** Itraconazole is the preferred treatment for mild to moderate pulmonary disease caused by *B. dermatitidis*. Fluconazole and ketoconazole can be used as alternative treatment for pulmonary blastomycosis (see Table 97-1). For children who are immunocompromised or who have evidence of disseminated disease, amphotericin B is the treatment of choice.

8. **(B)** Itraconazole at high doses has been described to cause hypokalemia and pedal edema. Life-threatening ventricular tachycardias can occur when the antihistamines terfenadine or astemizole are administered with itraconazole.

9. **(B)** Flucytosine can be used in combination with amphotericin B for meningeal and other serious cryptococcal infections as well as for *C. albicans* infection involving the CNS. Drug levels in the CSF are up to 75% of those found in serum (see Table 97-1).

10. **(A)** Voriconazole is a triazole derivative of fluconazole that exhibits a wide spectrum of activity

Table 97-1. PREFERRED DRUGS FOR INITIAL TREATMENT OF SERIOUS FUNGAL INFECTIONS

Disease	Pulmonary, life-threatening or disseminated	Mild to moderate pulmonary
Aspergillosis	AmB[*]	Itr
Blastomycosis	AmB	Itr
Candidiasis	AmB[†]	Flu
Coccidioidomycosis	AmB	Itr or Flu
Cryptococcus	AmB[†]	Flu
Histoplasmosis	AmB	Itr
Sporotrichosis	AmB	Itr

[*]Alternative therapy for invasive aspergillosis is voriconazole.
[†]Flucytosine has been used in combination with AmB (particularly for meningitis).
AmB, amphotericin B; Flu, fluconazole; Itr, itraconazole.

against many important fungi including *Candida*, *Aspergillus*, *Cryptococcus*, and *Fusarium*. Voriconazole has been successful in the treatment of esophageal candidiasis in adults (see Table 97-1).

11. **(B)** For immunocompetent individuals with isolated symptomatic pulmonary infection, fluconazole is the drug of choice for pulmonary cryptococcosis.

12. **(D)** In the past griseofulvin has been the drug of choice for treatment of *T. unguium*. Topical antifungal agents are ineffective because of the inability to penetrate the nail bed. Oral terbinafine is well absorbed and penetrates the nail bed. Oral terbinafine is now the treatment of choice for onychomycosis because it has been used successfully to treat *T. unguium* in a much shorter period of time than previous antifungal medications.

13. **(A)** The duration of treatment recommended for onychomycosis of the fingernails is 6 weeks and 12 weeks for toenail onychomycosis.

14. **(B)** Permethrin 5% cream is a safe and effective therapy for scabies. The cure rate is greater than 90%. Side effects of permethrin 5% are minimal. In infants and young children the cream is applied to the entire head, neck, and body, then removed by bathing 8 to 14 hours later.

15. **(A)** The advantage of albendazole over mebendazole is its activity in a single oral dose of 400 mg for treatment of hookworm infection. Mebendazole (100 mg twice daily for 3 days) and pyrantel pamoate (11 mg/kg/day not to exceed 1 g/day for 3 days) are alternative treatments for hookworm infection.

16. **(B)** Either mebendazole or albendazole can be administered for the treatment of whipworm infection. Both should be given for a 3-day course. Albendazole (400 mg) and ivermectin (200 μg/kg) given together each in a single dose have been effective for treatment of whipworm infection.

17. **(A)** Metronidazole is an important drug as part of treatment for intra-abdominal anaerobic infections and brain abscess. It is also effective therapy for treatment of intestinal or extraintestinal (such as liver abscess) disease caused by *Entamoeba histolytica*.

18. **(B)** Travelers to areas where chloroquine-resistant *Plasmodium falciparum* can take one of three regimens which include mefloquine hydrochloride, doxycycline or atovaquone-proguanil. Chloroquine is still the drug of choice for malaria prophylaxis in areas in which *P. falciparum* is still susceptible or non-falciparum malaria (*P. vivax*, *P. ovale*, *P. malariae*) only exist.

SUGGESTED READING

Correa AG, Baker CG: Antifungal agents. In: Long SS, Pickering LK, Prober CG (eds): *Principles and Practices of Infectious Diseases*, 2nd ed. Philadelphia: Churchill Livingstone, 2003, p 1511.

John CC: Drug treatment of malaria. *Pediatr Infect Dis J* 22:649, 2003.

CASE 98: A 15-YEAR-OLD ADOLESCENT GIRL WITH FEVER, SHORTNESS OF BREATH, AND AN ABNORMAL CHEST RADIOGRAPH

A 15-year-old adolescent girl comes to your office on Friday morning with her 20-year-old sister. She indicates that she has not been feeling well for 1 to 2 months. She remembers fever and sore throat about 2 months ago that resolved after 1 to 2 weeks. Since then she has had fatigue and decreased appetite and thinks that she may have lost some weight. She has also been too tired to try out for the high school basketball team. Her older sister has noticed a change in her younger sister's activity level and insisted that she come to your office today because of her sister's complaint of shortness of breath.

On physical examination the adolescent girl was alert and cooperative but appeared tired. The temperature is 100.5°F (38.1°C). A fine, white exudate is present on the buccal mucosa, posterior pharynx, and tongue. Posterior cervical and axillary adenopathy are noted. The respiratory rate is 30 bpm and scattered rales are heard at both the right and left lung bases. The heart and abdominal examinations are normal.

SELECT THE ONE BEST ANSWER TO THE FOLLOWING QUESTIONS

1. You are concerned about the possibility of an immunodeficiency disorder in this adolescent girl. The first laboratory test to order for the evaluation for immunodeficiency should be:

    (A) complete blood count with differential
    (B) qualitative immunoglobulin levels
    (C) T-lymphocyte subsets
    (D) Total hemolytic complement activity

2. Human immunodeficiency virus infection is confirmed in this adolescent girl. In her case the major route of acquisition of HIV would likely be:

    (A) injecting drug use
    (B) heterosexual contact with an HIV-infected person
    (C) coagulation disorder
    (D) perinatal exposure

3. A chest radiograph reveals bilateral alveolar disease with involvement of perihilar regions. The most likely diagnosis for the pulmonary abnormalities is:

    (A) cytomegalovirus pneumonia
    (B) pulmonary candidiasis
    (C) *Mycobacterium avium* complex pneumonia
    (D) *Pneumocystis jiroveci* pneumonia

4. The major risk factor development of *P. jiroveci* infection in HIV-infected individuals is:

    (A) suppression of cell-mediated immunity measured by CD4+ lymphocytes

(B) impaired specific antibody production after immunization with T-cell independent antigens

(C) depressed neutrophil superoxide production

(D) diminished capability of NK lymphocytes to mediate antibody-dependent cell-mediated cytotoxicity of HIV infected cells

5. A 10-month-old male infant develops fever and shock, and a blood culture drawn before the start of antibiotic therapy grows *Pseudomonas aeruginosa*. The infant appears malnourished and has a weight that is less than two standard deviations below the mean for sex and age. The most likely underlying reason for the gram-negative septic shock is:

(A) X-linked agammaglobulinemia

(B) immunodeficiency with hyperimmunoglobulinemia M

(C) protein-calorie malnutrition

(D) leukocyte adhesion deficiency type I

6. Protein-caloried malnutrition is a clinical example of malnutrition that can result in a major category of immunodeficiencies. The immune deficit associated with malnutrition is primarily:

(A) T cell cellular immunity

(B) B cell humoral immunity

(C) neutrophil function

(D) complement system

7. A 4-year-old girl with a severe brain injury from intraventricular hemorrhage as a newborn does not develop fever in response to a documented infection with influenza virus. The most likely reason for this finding is:

(A) damage to the thermoregulatory center in the hypothalamus

(B) inability to generate production of tumor necrosis factor-α

(C) inability to generate production of interleukin-1-β

(D) deficiency of interferon-γ in the systemic circulation

8. A 3-year-old child presents to your office with fever of 103°F (39.4°C), cough, and rhinorrhea during the peak of an epidemic of influenza A. The child's mother is very concerned about the fever. You counsel her regarding the fever that:

(A) the high fever can increase the replication of influenza virus

(B) fever can enhance some immunologic responses such as movement and function of certain white blood cells

(C) fever is best treated with a cooling blanket

(D) antipyretic agents will shorten the duration and contagiousness of influenza

9. A 12-month-old boy develops septic arthritis of the left knee with a positive blood and joint fluid culture for *S. pneumoniae*. Protection against subsequent infection with the bacteria correlate best with:

(A) type specific IgG anticapsular antibody

(B) anti-C-polysaccharide antibody

(C) IgG 1 and IgG 3 subclass antibody

(D) maturation of the classical pathway of the complement system

10. A 16-year-old previously healthy adolescent male presents with a 2-week history of fever associated with malaise, anorexia, and weight loss. He is diagnosed with pneumonia but when three blood cultures are reported positive for *S. aureus*, an echocardiogram is performed. The results reveal tricuspid valve endocarditis. The major risk factor for development of endocarditis in this adolescent is:

(A) unrecognized congenital heart disease

(B) prior rheumatic heart disease

(C) intravenous drug use

(D) immunodeficiency with an underlying phagocyte function disorder

11. A 3-week-old female infant was born to a mother with a history of intravenous drug abuse. The mother had serologic testing for HIV, rapid plasma reagin (RPR) and hepatitis B surface antigen (HBsAg) during the second trimester of pregnancy. All results were negative. The infant now presents at 3 weeks of age with a diffuse vesiculobullous rash that involves the palms and soles. The diagnostic test that will most likely reveal the etiology of the rash is:

(A) culture of vesicle scrapings for herpes simplex virus

(B) direct fluorescent antibody staining of vesicle scraping for varicella-zoster-virus

(C) RPR and fluorescent treponemal antibody absorption (FTA-ABS) tests for syphilis

(D) Gram stain and bacterial culture of vesicle fluid

12. A 10-day-old term infant girl presents to your office with eyelid swelling, erythema, and mucopurulent drainage from the left eye. A culture of the conjunctiva does not grow *N. gonorrhoeae*. What important historical factor in the mother will help best in determining the etiology of the new newborn's conjunctivitis:

(A) sexual history

(B) medication history

(C) surgical history

(D) history of prior miscarriages

13. The mother of the 10-day-old infant with conjunctivitis should also have testing to determine possible infection with:

(A) herpes simplex virus

(B) HIV

(C) hepatitis B virus

(D) cytomegalovirus

14. The indigenous bacterial flora of the gut are important in the prevention of gastrointestinal tract infection caused by pathogenic bacteria. Antimicrobial therapy can result in diarrhea with alterations in the colonic microflora. Antimicrobial therapy can lead to diarrhea with the overgrowth of the following bacteria:

(A) *Campylobacter jejuni*

(B) enterotoxigenic *E. coli*

(C) *Aeromonas hydrophila*

(D) *Clostridium difficile*

15. A 7-year-old boy with newly diagnosed acute myelogenous leukemia (AML) has recently completed induction chemotherapy. He develops fever, neutropenia (absolute neutrophil count of 100 cells/mm³), and shock. All of the following bacteria are likely pathogens except:

(A) *S. pyogenes*

(B) *S. aureus*

(C) *S. epidermidis*

(D) *P. aeruginosa*

16. An 18-year-old girl with congenital asplenia associated with congenital heart disease develops fever to 104°F (40°C) associated with a faint maculopapular rash. The child is at high risk for fulminant infection with all of the following agents except:

(A) *H. influenzae* type b

(B) *N. meningitidis*

(C) *P. aeruginosa*

(D) *S. pneumoniae*

17. A 4-year-old boy with acute lymphoblastic leukemia develops fever to 103°F (39.4°C). He also has neutropenia with an absolute neutrophil count of 200 cells/mm³. An appropriate antimicrobial regimen for initial empiric therapy is:

(A) ceftazidime

(B) ceftriaxone

(C) cefazolin and gentamicin

(D) trimethoprim-sulfamethoxazole and vancomycin

18. Aspergillus can cause invasive pulmonary infection in children with underlying medical problems. Of the following patients, the one most likely to develop invasive pulmonary aspergillosis is:

(A) a 19-year-old adolescent boy with acute lymphoblastic leukemia in relapse with fever and neutropenia

(B) an 8-year-old girl with HIV infection and pneumonia and a CD4 percentage of 20%

(C) a 12-year-old girl with cystic fibrosis, new infiltrates on chest radiographs and hypoxia

(D) a 4-year-old boy with common variable immunodeficiency who develops pneumonia

Answers

1. **(A)** First obtaining a complete blood count, differential, and platelet count provides a great deal of information; the results give information regarding leukocytosis, leukopenia (lymphopenia, neutropenia), leukocyte morphology, the presence of Howell-Jolly bodies, anemia, and thrombocytopenia.

2. **(B)** Among adolescents in the 13- to 19-year age group, the proportion of cases of HIV infection in females is surpassing that in males (see Table

Table 98-1. DISTRIBUTION OF CASES OF HIV INFECTION CASES REPORTED AMONG ADOLESCENTS AND YOUNG ADULTS BY SEX AND AGE GROUPS*

Sex	Age in years		
	13–19	20–24	≥25
Female	51%	38%	30%
Male	49%	62%	70%

*From 39 areas with confidential HIV surveillance for adults and adolescents in 2002.
Source: US Centers for Disease Control.

98-1). The major route of transmission in adolescent females is heterosexual transmission. Most HIV-infected adolescents are asymptomatic and not aware they are infected.

3. **(D)** *P. jeroveci* most commonly occurs in HIV-infected children between 3 and 6 months of age. Nevertheless, in adolescents *Pneumocystis* pneumonia (PCP) is still a more common AIDS-defining diagnosis than *Candida*, cytomegalovirus, or *M. avium* complex (MAC) disease.

4. **(A)** Epidemics of PCP have occurred in malnourished infants and children, as well as premature infants. With HIV infection, the risk of PCP is related to the viral endured suppression of cell-mediated immunity. The decision to administer PCP prophylaxis is based on the total CD4 lymphocyte count and percentage.

5. **(C)** Protein calorie malnutrition is a condition that can predispose to recurrent infections. Cellular immunity is important for protection against enteric bacteria.

6. **(A)** With malnutrition such as protein/energy deficiencies, there are immune deficits involving cellular immunity and T cell function. Immunoglobulins (Ig)A and E may be decreased.

7. **(A)** The pathogenesis of fever involves cytokines stimulating the preoptic area of the hypothalamus (thermoregulatory center) which leads to the production of prostaglandin E2. This molecule is thought to activate thermoregulatory neu-

rons to raise the thermostat setpoint. Then peripheral mechanisms are activated that lead to vasoconstriction and muscle contraction, which result in the generation of fever. Also certain areas in the cerebral cortex are stimulated to promote behavioral changes designed to help control temperature.

8. **(B)** There is evidence that fever is more beneficial than harmful to the host. High temperatures also interfere with the replication and virulence of certain pathogens. Fever also represents a regulatory mechanism to reduce cytokine activation of the acute inflammatory response. Controversy exists about whether febrile episodes should be treated. A short course of an antipyretic drug has low risk for toxicity and most of the appropriate antipyretic drugs also have analgesic properties.

9. **(A)** Immunity to *S. pneumoniae* is related to the production of type specific humoral immunity. Development of type specific antibodies against the capsular polysaccharide correlates with immunity to that specific serotype. Children with deficiency of the classical pathway of complement such as C2 deficiency are at increased risk for invasive infections caused by *S. pneumoniae*. IgG subclass deficiencies are not associated with an increased risk for invasive pneumococcal infections.

10. **(C)** In this previously healthy adolescent intravenous drug use would be the most likely risk factor for development of right-sided endocarditis. Other risk factors for right-sided endocarditis include pacemakers, wires and long-term intravenous central venous catheterization.

11. **(C)** The description of the rash is most characteristic of congenital syphilis, even though the RPR drawn on the mother in the second trimester was non-reactive. A history of intravenous drug use should raise the suspicion of syphilis as well as HIV and hepatitis B infection. Another important risk factor for vertical transmission of syphilis is lack of prenatal care.

12. **(A)** The most likely pathogen in this case of mucopurulent conjunctivitis is *C. trachomatis*, which is an STD. Many men and women infected with *C. trachomatis* are either asymptomatic or mildly

symptomatic so a history of sexual activity is important to obtain.

13. **(B)** Individuals who have an STD such as *C. trachomatis* and *N. gonorrhoeae* should also be evaluated for infection with HIV.

14. **(D)** Diarrhea can occur during therapy with many different antimicrobial agents. Antimicrobial-associated diarrhea can result from either changes in small bowel peristalsis or from alteration in the normal flora found in the intestine. A good example of the latter is overgrowth in the colon of *C. difficile*.

15. **(C)** Patients with fever and neutropenia can develop infections caused by coagulase negative staphylococci such as *S. epidermidis*. However, this is a more indolent infection and a short delay in administration of specific antimicrobial therapy has not been shown to be detrimental to the patient's outcome. The other bacteria listed can all cause fulminant infection resulting in death.

16. **(C)** Patients with asplenia are at increased risk for overwhelming life-threatening infections. The most common organism involved is *S. pneumoniae* but other encapsulated bacteria can cause fulminant infections. Fulminant septicemia has also been reported in asplenic patients that is caused by *Capnocytophaga canimorsus*. This species is part of the normal mouth flora of dogs.

17. **(A)** A number of studies have shown no differences between monotherapy and multiple drug therapy for empirical treatment of uncomplicated episodes of fever in neutropenic patients. A third- or fourth-generation cephalosporin (ceftazidime or cefepime) or a carbapenem (imipenem-cilastin or meropenem) may also be used successfully. The other antibiotic regimens listed above except gentamicin do not have appreciable activity against *P. aeruginosa*.

18. **(A)** In children the most common presentation of invasive pulmonary aspergillosis occurs in the setting of fever and neutropenia without any initial respiratory tract symptoms, and there is a failure to respond to broad spectrum antibacterial therapy. Bacterial pathogens most commonly are the etiologic agents of pneumonia in patients with common variable immunodeficiency.

SUGGESTED READING

Goldman AS: Host responses to infection. *Pediatr Rev* 21: 342, 2000.

Maldanado YA, Shetty A: Epidemiology of HIV infection in children and adolescents. In: Long SS, Pickering LK, Prober CG (eds): *Principles and Practices of Infectious Diseases*, 2nd ed. Philadelphia: Churchill Livingstone, 2003, p 658.

CASE 99: A 2-WEEK-OLD INFANT WITH FEVER, RASH, AND A SEIZURE

A 3000-g infant was born at 40 weeks' gestation to a 24-year-old G1P1 white female by normal spontaneous vaginal delivery. The infant was discharged in 2 days, and mother was breast-feeding the infant without difficulty. An office visit in the first week of life revealed that the infant was afebrile, breast-feeding well and back to birth weight.

At 2 weeks of age the mother noticed that the infant was not breast-feeding as well. This continued for 24 hours when the mother then measured the infant's temperature at 101.1°F (38.4°C). The mother called you, and you advised her to bring the infant directly to the children's hospital emergency department.

On physical examination at the emergency department the infant is found to be sleepy but arousable. The temperature is 100.7°F (38.2°C). The infant has two papulovesicular lesions on the right arm. The oropharynx and eye exam is normal. Examination of the lungs and heart also is normal. There are no focal neurological deficits.

SELECT THE ONE BEST ANSWER TO THE FOLLOWING QUESTIONS

1. The most accurate statement regarding neonatal herpes simplex virus with disease localized to the skin, eyes, and mouth (SEM) is:

   (A) If untreated, 20% of neonates will progress to disseminated or CNS disease.
   (B) Most neonates infected at birth are born to women who are completely asymptomatic for genital HSV infection during pregnancy and at delivery.
   (C) Women who have recurrent HSV genital infection cannot transmit the virus by an ascending infection from the genital tract.

(D) Treatment includes acyclovir at a dose of 10 mg/kg every 8 hours by the intravenous route for 10 days.

2. The risk of herpes simplex virus (HSV) infection in a neonate varies based on type of HSV infection in the mother. The risk of neonatal infection in primary versus recurrent HSV infection in the mother is:

(A) 50% vs. 5%
(B) 50% vs. 10%
(C) 25% vs. 2%
(D) 25% vs. 20%

3. You suspect congenital cytomegalovirus (CMV) infection in a term newborn infant with bilateral sensorineural hearing loss. Vertical transmission of CMV to an infant occurs by all except one of the following methods:

(A) transplacental passage of blood-borne virus
(B) at delivery by exposure to virus in the maternal genital tract
(C) by ingestion of breast milk in postnatal period
(D) asymptomatic oral shedding of CMV in postnatal period

4. In healthy children and adolescents, infectious mononucleosis is a self-limited disease. However, some children can develop serious complications from EBV. The most likely disorder that is associated with complicated EBV infection is:

(A) primary immunodeficiency involving T lymphocytes
(B) primary immunodeficiency involving B lymphocytes
(C) primary immunodeficiency involving phagocytes
(D) primary immunodeficiency involving complement

5. A 5-year-old boy with acute lymphoblastic leukemia develops fever to 102.2°F (39°C) and a vesicular rash involving the face, trunk, extremities, palms, and soles. Some of the vesicular lesions are deepseated with surrounding erythema. You suspect varicella which is confirmed by direct fluorescent antibody staining of the skin lesions. The most common life-threatening complication of varicella in immunocompromised children is:

(A) encephalitis
(B) hepatitis
(C) pneumonia
(D) necrotizing fasciitis

6. An 8-month-old male infant who recently emigrated with his family from Mexico presents to your office with a 4-day history of fever associated cough, coryza, and conjunctivitis. On the third day of illness, a maculopapular rash then began along the hairline and spread to involve the face, neck, trunk, and extremities. You strongly suspect the diagnosis of measles. The complication that causes the most morbidity in young children with this disease is:

(A) encephalitis
(B) hemorrhagic shock
(C) pneumonia
(D) myocarditis

7. An 8-year-old girl develops fever to 102°F (38.8°C), bilateral swelling of the parotid glands and headache. You suspect the diagnosis of mumps. The most likely complication to occur with mumps is:

(A) pancreatitis
(B) meningitis
(C) sensorineural hearing loss
(D) myocarditis

8. A 17-year-old adolescent female in her junior year of high school develops a low-grade fever to 101°F (38.3°C), a maculopapular rash that first appears on the face, and suboccipital/postauricular lymphadenopathy. You suspect rubella and confirm the diagnosis by serology. Serologic surveys of young adults indicating the percentage that are susceptible to rubella are:

(A) 3%
(B) 5%
(C) 10%
(D) 15%

9. A 4-year-old boy with sickle cell disease (hemoglobulin SS disease) develops mild fever to 100.5°F (38°C) associated with fatigue for 2 days. On physical examination he is noted to have pallor. Laboratory results reveal a white blood cell

count of 6800/mm^3, hemoglobin 5.4 g/dL; reticulocyte count 0.7%; and platelet count 150,000/mm^3. The most likely etiology of the severe anemia in this child is:

(A) parvovirus B19
(B) human herpes virus type 6
(C) human herpes virus type 8
(D) Coxsackie virus A16

10. A 13-month-old infant boy has mild nasal congestion and eyelid edema associated with erythema of the palpebral conjunctiva for 1 day. He then develops fever to 104°F (30°C) that is associated on the same day with a 5- to 10-minute generalized tonic-clonic seizure. The child's parents bring him to the emergency department. After an observation period in the emergency department, the temperature has decreased to 101°F (38.3°C) and he is alert and consolable. The most likely etiology of the seizures is:

(A) adenovirus
(B) HHV-6
(C) influenza A
(D) *Shigella sonnei*

11. A 15-month-old infant boy is evaluated for recurrent bacterial infections (one episode of culture-proven pneumonia caused by *S. pneumoniae* and one episode of septic arthritis caused by *S. aureus*). On physical exam the infant is afebrile; the weight is at the 5th percentile for age and he has hepatosplenomegaly and generalized lymphadenopathy. The most likely etiology to explain these findings is:

(A) Epstein-Barr virus
(B) HIV
(C) cytomegalovirus
(D) *Histoplasma capsulatum* infection

12. Enteroviruses often cause a non-specific febrile illness in young children but can also cause exanthems. All of the following exanthems have been reported in the non-polio enteroviruses except:

(A) papular-purpuric rash in glove and stocking distribution
(B) papulovesicular rash
(C) papular urticaria
(D) petechial rash

13. In January you are seeing large numbers of children in your office with fever and respiratory symptoms. You suspect influenza as the likely etiology. Compared with children younger than 5 years old, children older than 5 years of age are more likely to have:

(A) flulike syndrome of fever, cough, headache, myalgia, malaise
(B) laryngotracheobronchitis
(C) an illness requiring hospitalization
(D) vomiting, diarrhea, abdominal pain

14. A 12-month-old boy develops fever, cough, rhinorrhea for 2 days followed by the onset of inspiratory stridor. The month is October, and you suspect laryngotracheobronchitis (croup) caused by parainfluenza virus. A true statement about the epidemiology of parainfluenza virus is:

(A) Parainfluenza virus type 4 causes epidemics of croup in the summer every year.
(B) Parainfluenza virus type 3 causes epidemics of croup in the spring of odd numbered years.
(C) Parainfluenza virus type 2 causes epidemics of croup in the fall of even numbered years.
(D) Parainfluenza virus type 1 causes epidemics of croup in the fall of odd numbered years.

15. During July a 6-year-old girl develops fever to 103°F (39.4°C) that persists for 5 days. Associated symptoms include sore throat. On physical examination the child has follicular injection of the tonsillar pillars, bilateral purulent conjunctivitis, cervical lymphadenopathy, and preauricular lymphadenopathy. The most likely etiologic agent is:

(A) enterovirus
(B) *C. trachomatis*
(C) adenovirus
(D) *H. influenzae*

16. A 4-month-old male infant is hospitalized in January with fever, cough, rhinorrhea, and bilateral wheezing associated with respiratory distress. Respiratory syncytial virus (RSV) infection is confirmed by enzyme immunoassay (EIA) of nasal secretions. All of the following strategies are important for reducing the risk of nosocomial transmission of RSV except:

(A) handwashing
(B) use of gowns, gloves, and goggles
(C) contact precautions for infected patients
(D) droplet precautions for infected patients

17. A 10-month-old infant girl is seen at the children's hospital emergency department in February with a 2-day history of fever to 103°F (39.4°C) associated with vomiting. The infant is admitted to the hospital with dehydration. After admission, she passes a large watery stool. The best diagnostic study to perform on the stool is:

(A) antigen testing for rotavirus
(B) culture for *Campylobacter jejuni*
(C) antigen testing for the Norwalk agent
(D) enzyme immunoassay for *C. difficile* toxin

18. A 12-year-old boy comes to your office with a sudden onset of vomiting associated with fever to 101°F (38.3°C) and myalgias, headache, and chills. The patient is not dehydrated, and you recommend symptomatic treatment. The next day you learn from the school nurse that more than one-half of the patient's classmates have similar symptoms and some also have diarrhea. The most likely etiology of your patient's illness is:

(A) astrovirus
(B) calicivirus
(C) hepatitis E
(D) pestivirus

Answers

1. **(B)** When SEM disease in neonates is not promptly treated, 75% of cases will progress to disseminated or central nervous system disease. Both primary and recurrent infections frequently are asymptomatic. The treatment of neonatal HSV infection includes acyclovir at a dose of 20 mg/kg every 8 hours by the intravenous route for 14 to 21 days.

2. **(A)** The risk of transmission to an infant born to a mother who has recurrent HSV infection is significantly less than a mother who has primary infection (3% to 5% versus 33% to 50%). This difference is largely related to the HSV antibody status of the mother.

3. **(D)** Approximately 10% of mothers seropositive for CMV shed the virus during delivery, and about 50% of infants exposed to the virus during birth are infected. Oral shedding is common in young children with rates as high as 70% in 1- to 3-year-old children in childcare centers. Spread of CMV in households and child care centers is well documented but oral shedding is not a method by which congenital CMV infections occur.

4. **(A)** EBV infection is controlled through the production of CD8 + cytotoxic T-lymphocytes, which limit primary infection and keep the pool of EBV-infected B lymphocytes in check. Natural killer (NK) cells also play a role in the lysis of EBV-infected lymphocytes. Examples of impairment of cell-mediated immunity by resulting in unchecked EBV infection include lymphoma, X-linked lymphoproliferative syndrome and post-transplant lymphoproliferative disorder.

5. **(C)** Hemorrhage into cutaneous lesions is also a sign of severe varicella in a pediatric patient who is immunocompromised. In contrast to the vesicles of varicella seen in healthy children, the vesicles in children who are immunocompromised are larger and often umbilicated. The lesions are widely distributed and also can occur on the palms and soles.

6. **(C)** Pneumonia is the most serious complication associated with measles, accounting for approximately 60% of the deaths in infants who have measles. The respiratory clinical manifestations of measles include bronchopneumonia, bronchiolitis, laryngotracheobronchitis, and lobar pneumonia. Mortality among children in the United States is 2 to 3 per 1000 with measles. Encephalitis occurs in 1 in 1000 cases of measles and is more common in older children and adolescents. Measles has not been endemic in the United States since 1997. Limited outbreaks of measles have occurred that are caused by imported cases.

7. **(B)** Although more than 50% of individuals with mumps parotitis will have CSF pleocytosis, only 1% to 10% have symptoms of CNS infection. Aseptic meningitis is the most frequent central nervous infection. Myocarditis is a rare complication of mumps. Orchitis can also be a compli-

cation that occurs in up to 35% of males with mumps. This complication is uncommon in pre-pubertal males and uncommonly bilateral.

8. **(C)** Rubella is a mild disease characterized by a generalized erythematous maculopapular rash, generalized lymphadenopathy and low-grade fever. The risk of acquiring rubella is low in all age groups. However, in the vaccine era, most cases have occurred in young, unimmunized adults in outbreaks on college campuses and in occupational settings. In March 2005, the Centers for Disease Control and Prevention declared that rubella is no longer endemic in the United States.

9. **(A)** Parvovirus B19 can cause a transient aplastic crisis that can be severe in individuals with hemolytic disorders, hemoglobinopathies, red cell enzyme deficiencies and autoimmune hemolytic anemias. Life-threatening anemia is common when aplastic crises develop, particularly in children who have homozygous sickle cell (SS) disease.

10. **(B)** CNS manifestations are common in infants with HHV-6 infection, with seizures being the most common CNS manifestation. Seizures occur during the febrile period in 10% to 15% of children with primary infection. The risk of seizures is greatest for children who develop primary HHV-6 infection during the second year of life.

11. **(B)** Children with HIV infection may present with multiple or recurrent serious bacterial infections. Combined with hepatosplenomegaly, lymphadenopathy and failure to thrive, HIV is by far the most likely diagnosis to consider. EBV, CMV, and *Histoplasma capsulatum* can cause hepatosplenomegaly and failure to thrive but are not associated with recurrent, serious bacterial infections.

12. **(A)** The rashes associated with enteroviruses include maculopapular, petechial, urticarial, and vesicular. The papular-purpuric glove and stocking distribution syndrome is caused by parvovirus B19.

13. **(A)** Older children and adults with influenza are more likely to have an abrupt onset of illness associated with fever and chills, headaches, sore throat, myalgia, and a dry cough. The rates of hospitalization in children younger than the age of 2 years are comparable with the rates of hospitalization in the elderly with underlying medical conditions.

14. **(D)** Since 1971 when surveillance for croup began in the United States, parainfluenza virus type 1 has caused epidemics of croup in the fall of odd-numbered years. Compared with the other parainfluenza viruses, infection with type 3 occurs more often in infants. Parainfluenza virus type 3 is second in frequency to respiratory syncytial virus as a cause of bronchiolitis.

15. **(C)** The child likely has pharyngoconjunctival fever. Outbreaks of pharyngoconjunctival fever have occurred at swimming pools and summer camps. The most common site of involvement of adenovirus is the upper respiratory tract. Infants and young children will often develop upper respiratory illness with serotypes 1 to 3, 5, and 7. Adenovirus infections occur year-round but can produce sporadic attacks, most commonly in the winter, spring, and early summer.

16. **(D)** Nosocomial transmission of RSV in the hospital setting is an annual problem, but studies have indicated that there are strategies that can by employed to decrease the risk of transmission. Outbreaks of RSV occur in temperate climates every year during winter and early spring. Most hospitalizations for RSV occur in 2- to 6-month-old children. Besides the most recognized clinical manifestations of bronchiolitis, RSV can also cause pneumonia, upper respiratory tract infection, croup, apnea, and otitis media.

17. **(A)** This young child most likely has rotavirus infection. Rotavirus has an annual peak of infection and illness in the winter. Children usually experience their first rotavirus infection between 3 and 24 months of age. Infections during the first 3 months of life and reinfections among older children are more likely to be asymptomatic. Rotavirus causes gastroenteritis and is more likely to cause dehydration than other viral agents that cause gastroenteritis. Vomiting and fever may precede the diarrhea in children ultimately requiring hospitalization.

Table 99-1. FACTORS CONTRIBUTING TO CALICIVIRUSES AS CAUSES OF OUTBREAKS

Factor	Observation
Low infectious dose	Less than 10^2 viral particles
Asymptomatic shedding	Up to 2 weeks
Stable in environment	Survives freezing, heating up to 60°C and 10 ppm chlorine
Strain diversity	Multiple genotypes
Immunity	Antibody not correlated with long-term protection
Multiple means of transmission	Fecal-oral, large droplets, environmental contamination

Source: Bresee JS, Widdowson M, Monroe SS, et al: Foodborne viral gastroenteritis: Challenges and opportunities. *Clin Infect Dis* 35:748, 2002.

18. **(B)** Caliciviruses have caused outbreaks of gastroenteritis in all age groups and are associated most commonly with contamination of seafood and water. There are a number of characteristics of caliciviruses that facilitate their causing outbreaks of gastroenteritis (see Table 99-1). Outbreaks have occurred on cruise ships, childcare centers, and nursing homes. Caliciviruses can also cause sporadic gastroenteritis in children and adults in community settings. Commercial assays to detect caliciviruses are not available but a reverse transcription polymerase chain reaction (RT-PCR) assay has been used to detect viral RNA in the stool. This assay is useful for identifying caliciviruses as the cause of an outbreak of gastroenteritis.

SUGGESTED READING

Pickering LK, Baker CJ, Overturf GD, et al: *Red Book: 2003 Report of the Committee on Infectious Diseases*, 26th ed. Elk Grove Village, IL: American Academy of Pediatrics, 2003.

Long SS, Pickering LK, Prober CG (eds): Principles and Practices of Infectious Diseases. Philadelphia: Churchill Livingstone, 2003.

CASE 100: A 15-MONTH-OLD INFANT WITH FEVER AND TACHYPNEA

A 15-month-old male infant has a 7-day history of cough and rhinorrhea. He had one previous episode of wheezing at age 4 months. His mother is concerned that he may be having difficulty breathing and is wheezing. There is also a strong family history of asthma in the paternal family. He is now brought to your office because of fever and some difficulty breathing. There is an older brother and uncle who live with the family who have been ill with cough and sore throat. The child has received three *H. influenzae* type b conjugate and three pneumococcal conjugate vaccines according to records.

On physical examination the child is sitting quietly in his mother's arms. The temperature is 102°F (38.9°C). There is nasal flaring along with clear rhinorrhea. The respiratory rate is 48 bpm and breath sounds are decreased under the right posterior chest. There is no hepatosplenomegaly. A pulse oximeter is available in your office. In room air the infant's oxygen saturation is found to be 92%.

SELECT THE ONE BEST ANSWER TO THE FOLLOWING QUESTIONS

1. You order a chest radiograph for the 15-month-old child that reveals right middle and right lower lobe infiltrates and a large pleural effusion. A thoracentesis is performed after the child is admitted to the hospital and purulent fluid with a leukocyte count of 55,000/mm³. The most likely etiology of the pneumonia and empyema is:

   (A) *S. aureus*
   (B) *Streptococcus pyogenes*
   (C) *Klebsiella pneumoniae*
   (D) *H. influenzae* type b

2. A 4-month-old infant girl develops fever to 102°F (38.8°C) with acute swelling of the left anterior neck. An abscess involving the anterior cervical triangle lymph node is drained and the culture grows methicillin-resistant *S. aureus* (MRSA). The isolate is susceptible to vancomycin, clindamycin, trimethoprim-sulfamethoxazole and rifampin but resistant to erythromycin. The D-test is negative. The antibiotic of choice for this infection is:

   (A) clindamycin
   (B) rifampin
   (C) azithromycin
   (D) vancomycin

3. A previously healthy 4-month-old infant boy presents with a history of decreased bowel move-

ments, poor feeding, and decreased activity. On physical examination the temperature is 100°F (37.8°C). The infant is alert, pupils are sluggishly reactive, and he exhibits poor head control and hypotonia. The most likely etiology to explain these findings is:

(A) hypothyroidism
(B) myasthenia gravis
(C) infant botulism
(D) Guillain-Barré syndrome

4. An 18-month-old girl develops a minor scalp wound and is well until 2 weeks later when she develops trismus and severe generalized muscular spasms. Her mother tells you that her daughter has received no immunizations. You suspect tetanus caused by *Clostridium tetani*. Initial treatment should first include:

(A) intravenous metronidazole
(B) intravenous penicillin
(C) IG
(D) TIG

5. A pregnant woman at 33 weeks' gestation develops fever, headache, diarrhea, and back pain. Labor ensues and a 2-kg premature infant girl is born with respiratory distress, apnea, and shock. Pneumonia is identified by chest radiograph. You obtain the history from the father that about 2 weeks prior to delivery, the mother ate some soft Mexican cheese. The most likely etiology for the findings in this neonate is:

(A) *Pseudomonas aeruginosa*
(B) *Listeria monocytogenes*
(C) *S. pyogenes*
(D) *S. aureus*

6. A 5-month-old infant boy with a 2-day history of rhinorrhea develops a persistent cough and an episode of apnea. *Bordetella pertussis* infection is confirmed by culture. The reservoir for *B. pertussis* in this case most likely is:

(A) 4-year-old sibling with cough and conjunctivitis
(B) 6-month-old cousin with rhinorrhea
(C) 13-year-old sibling with post-tussive emesis
(D) 65-year-old grandfather with a productive cough

7. An 8-month-old infant girl who has received three doses of *H. influenzae* type b conjugate vaccine develops fever, irritability, and vomiting. A Gram stain of CSF reveals small gram-negative coccobacilli. The most likely etiology of the meningitis is:

(A) *H. influenzae* type b
(B) *H. influenzae* type f
(C) *E. coli*
(D) *Salmonella choleraesuis*

8. A 2-year-old boy living in southeastern United States who attends day care develops acute otitis media. You suspect infection with penicillin non-susceptible *S. pneumoniae*. The drug of choice for treatment of this infection is:

(A) amoxicillin 80 mg/kg/day
(B) amoxicillin-clavulanate 80 mg/kg/day, amoxicillin component
(C) clindamycin 30 mg/kg/day
(D) azithromycin 10 mg/kg/day

9. A 12-month-old girl develops fever and a maculopapular rash that becomes petechial 6 hours later. The child has CSF pleocytosis, and both blood and CSF cultures grow *N. meningitidis* serogroup C. She initially receives a single dose of ceftriaxone followed by 4 more days of IV penicillin G. All of the following contacts should receive chemoprophylaxis except:

(A) 3-year-old sister
(B) 2-year-old nursery school contact
(C) pediatric resident who performed spinal tap
(D) 13-year-old cousin visiting from out of state for past week

10. An 8-year-old girl develops fever, and a blood culture drawn is positive for *Staphylococcus epidermidis*. In which setting is the blood culture most likely to be a contaminant:

(A) child with leukemia who develops fever and neutropenia
(B) child with a prosthetic mitral valve after mitral valve prolapse
(C) child with ventriculoperitoneal shunt secondary to hydrocephalus
(D) child with central venous catheter receiving total parenteral nutrition

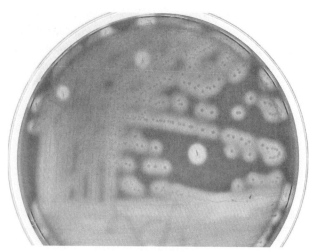

Figure 100-1. ***Blood agar plate that reveals characteristic β-hemolytic colonies characteristic of* S. pyogenes. *Note the areas of enhanced β-hemolysis where the agar was stabbed after the throat culture was plated.***

11. An 8-year-old girl develops fever to 103°F (39.4°C) for 2 days with cough, rhinorrhea, sore throat, and dyspnea. A chest radiograph reveals a small right lower lobe infiltrate. Antibiotic therapy with erythromycin is initiated, but 24 hours later the child is seen at the emergency department. Findings on physical examination reveal an ill-appearing child, temperature: 104°F (40°C), respiratory rate 30/min, blood pressure 80/45 mm Hg, hyperemic tonsils and posterior pharynx, and a generalized, erythematous, macular rash. A throat culture is obtained that reveals the finding in Figure 100-1. The most likely diagnosis is:

   (A) Stevens-Johnson syndrome
   (B) Kawasaki disease
   (C) Rocky mountain spotted fever
   (D) streptococcal toxic shock syndrome

12. A pregnant woman is screened for rectal and vaginal colonization with group B streptococcus (GBS) at 35 weeks' gestation. All of the following are indications for intrapartum prophylaxis to prevent early onset GBS disease except:

   (A) GBS bacteriuria during current pregnancy
   (B) delivery at 36 weeks' gestation with unknown GBS status
   (C) rupture of membranes for 18 hours during labor with unknown GBS status
   (D) previous pregnancy with a positive GBS screening culture

13. A 4-year-old girl develops fever and a blood culture drawn is positive for *E. faecalis*. In which clinical setting is enterococcal bacteremia most likely to occur with this young girl?

   (A) child hospitalized in the pediatric intensive care unit with a central venous catheter
   (B) child with first episode of a urinary tract infection
   (C) child with a seizure and a lumbar puncture revealing CSF pleocytosis
   (D) child with an isolated ventricular septal defect

14. A 15-year-old adolescent girl develops pain in the hands and wrists 4 days after the start of her menstrual period. She then develops scattered papules on both hands while the pain in the hands and wrists improves. She then develops swelling of her left knee, which prompts medical attention. You suspect disseminated gonococcal infection. The most reliable method to diagnose this infection is by:

   (A) culture of blood
   (B) culture of endocervix
   (C) culture of joint fluid
   (D) Gram stain smear of pharyngeal secretions

15. A 3-year-old boy is bitten on his right lower leg by a dog in the neighborhood. Twelve hours later he develops fever to 102°F (38.8°C) and chills. The bite wound has swelling, erythema, tenderness and a serosanguineous drainage. The most likely etiology of this wound infection is:

   (A) *Eikenella corrodens*
   (B) *Pasturella multocida*
   (C) *P. aeruginosa*
   (D) *S. pyogenes*

16. A 4-year-old girl develops fever, vomiting, and hematochezia. A stool culture grows *Salmonella marina*. The child recovers from the illness but a stool culture sent 12 weeks later is still positive for *S. marina*. The organism is ampicillin, ceftriaxone, trimethoprim-sulfamethoxazole, and gentamicin susceptible. At this point appropriate treatment would include:

   (A) trimethoprim-sulfamethoxazole
   (B) gentamicin

(C) high-dose amoxicillin combined with probenecid

(D) no antimicrobial therapy

17. A 3-year-old girl develops fever, abdominal cramps, and mucoid bloody stools. A stool culture grows *S. sonnei*, and the child is treated with trimethoprim-sulfamethoxazole based on susceptibility testing. Two days after the onset of the girl's symptoms, her 2-year-old brother also develops fever, vomiting, and profuse watery diarrhea. A stool culture is negative. Appropriate management of this sibling could include:

(A) antimicrobial therapy with trimethoprim-sulfamethoxazole

(B) diagnostic assay of stool for rotavirus antigen

(C) *C. difficile* toxin assay on stool

(D) complete blood count with differential

18. In December, a 6-month-old male infant develops fever, vomiting and diarrhea that contains mucus and blood. He is bottle-fed infant formula. A stool culture sent grows *Yersinia enterocolitica*. The most likely source of the *Y. enterocolitica* in this case is:

(A) contaminated well water

(B) pork intestines (chitterlings)

(C) pasteurized milk

(D) raspberry flavored baby food

Answers

1. **(A)** Although all of the bacterial pathogens listed can cause pneumonia with empyema, *S. aureus* is the most common cause worldwide. Some recent pediatric series in the United States have documented the emergence of *S. pneumoniae* as the most common cause of parapneumonic effusions in children. Overall, patients with staphylococcal disease are more likely to require chest tube drainage than those with pneumococcal disease.

2. **(A)** Clindamycin would be the most appropriate antibiotic choice in this case of community-acquired MRSA infection. There has been an increase in minor soft tissue as well as serious invasive infections because of *S. aureus* in many areas of the United States. Clindamycin therapy is effective and avoids the use of vancomycin.

3. **(C)** Botulism is caused by *Clostridium botulinum*, a gram-positive anaerobic bacillus that is found in soil and agricultural products. Ingestion of honey is a risk factor for infant botulism but in most infants, no source of the *C. botulinum* spores can be found. Decreased frequency of bowel movements is common as are the other symptoms and signs listed above. Diagnosis can be confirmed by culture of the organism or identification of *C. botulinum* toxin in the stool. The mainstay of management of infants with botulism is supportive care. Human botulism immune globulin intravenous (BIG-IV) is now also available for treatment.

4. **(D)** The goals of treatment of tetanus include neutralization of toxin, eradication of *C. tetani* and supportive care. Antimicrobial therapy to eradicate the organism can include: metronidazole, penicillin, or tetracycline. Immune globulin intravenous (IGIV) can be considered for treatment if TIG is not available.

5. **(B)** *Listeria* monocytogenes can manifest in a similar clinical pattern as *Streptococcus agalactiae* (group B streptococcus) with either early-onset sepsis or late-onset meningitis. Prematurity, pneumonia, and septicemia are common in early onset disease. Perinatal infection can result in stillbirth or neonatal death in approximately 20% of infections in pregnancy.

6. **(C)** There has been an increase in reported cases from 1997 to 2000 of pertussis in individuals 10 years and older with a peak in the 10- to 19-year age group. Up to a third of adolescents and adults with prolonged cough illness have been shown to have pertussis. Neonates with pertussis are likely to have been born to young mothers with a cough illness. These findings support the current concept that older individuals are the major reservoirs of *B. pertussis*.

7. **(B)** The Gram stain that reveals gram negative coccobacilli is consistent with *H. influenzae*. The incidence of *H. influenzae* type b meningitis has declined dramatically since routine immunization of young infants against *H. influenzae* type b. Invasive disease by non-type b encapsulated strains and nontypable strains still does occur, and in most states, the incidence of invasive disease because of non-type b strains is higher than with type b strains.

Table 100-1. FEATURES OF TOXIC SHOCK SYNDROME CAUSED BY *STAPHYLOCOCCUS AUREUS* AND *STREPTOCOCCUS PYOGENES* (GAS)

Feature	*Staphylococcus aureus*	*Streptococcus pyogenes*
Prodrome	Vomiting, diarrhea	Malaise, myalgia
Physical findings		
Rash	Diffuse macular erythroderma	Generalized erythematous macular rash
Conjunctivitis	Often present	Absent
Soft-tissue infection	Uncommon	Common
Foreign body at infection site	Common	Uncommon
Blood culture positive	<5%	>50%
Necrotizing fasciitis	No	Yes
Recurrent episodes	Yes	No
Toxin	TSST-1	SPE A, SPE B

TSST-1, toxic shock syndrome toxin–1; SPE, streptococcal pyrogenic exotoxin.

8. **(A)** Amoxicillin is the drug of choice for treatment of acute otitis media, including infection caused by penicillin nonsusceptible *S. pneumoniae*. With use of this dose of amoxicillin, the concentration of the antibiotic in middle ear fluid is believed to be high enough to eradicate penicillin nonsusceptible strains of *S. pneumoniae*.

9. **(C)** Chemoprophylaxis to prevent invasive meningococcal disease for health care professionals is not recommended unless there is intimate exposure to a patient with invasive meningococcal disease. This type of exposure would include: unprotected mouth-to-mouth resuscitation, intubation or suctioning of the patient before antimicrobial therapy was administered.

10. **(C)** Most of the coagulase negative staphylococci (CONS) associated with humans are common inhabitants of the skin and mucous membranes and procedural contaminants of blood culture techniques. Risk factors for actual CONS infection would include: catheter placement, medical device insertion or immunosuppression. CONS are common causes of ventriculoperitoneal shunt infections but secondary bacteremia or bacteremic seeding of the shunt does not occur. CONS may also cause urinary tract infections, particularly in adolescent girls and young adult women. The species involved is most commonly *S. saprophyticus*. Children with fever and neutropenia who develop CONS bacteremia most often have central venous catheters in place.

11. **(D)** Toxic shock syndrome (TSS) can be caused by toxin-producing *S. aureus* or *S. pyogenes*. The presence of a foreign body at the site of infection is common with *S. aureus* mediated by TSS but not with *S. pyogenes*. In children a major risk factor for streptococcal TSS is concomitant varicella. Both forms of TSS can occur without a clinically identifiable focus of infection (see Table 100-1).

12. **(D)** According to CDC recommendations, all pregnant women should be screened at 35 to 37 weeks' gestation for rectal and vaginal colonization for GBS. Intrapartum prophylaxis is also indicated if there was a previous infant with invasive GBS disease, if the GBS screening culture is positive during the current pregnancy or if the temperature is >100.4°F (38°C) with unknown GBS status. Colonization alone during a previous pregnancy is not an indication for intrapartum chemoprophylaxis unless screening results are positive in the current pregnancy.

13. **(A)** The enterococcus can cause neonatal infections as well as infections in older children. In older children nosocomially acquired infection is not rare. Risk factors include indwelling central venous catheters, GI disease, immunodeficiency, cardiovascular abnormalities, and hematologic

malignancy. Enterococcus spp. can occasionally cause meningitis, usually in neonates, and can occasionally cause urinary tract infections.

14. **(B)** In patients with disseminated gonococcal infection, isolation of *N. gonorrhoeae* from sterile sites such as blood or joint fluid occurs in less than half of the patients. However, the organism can be isolated from a mucosal site or from a sexual contact in approximately 80% of cases.

15. **(B)** A bite by a cat or a dog that results in cellulitis within 24 hours of the bite is most likely caused by *Pasteurella multocida*. Regional lymphadenopathy, fever, and chills are common. Tenosynovitis, septic arthritis, or osteomyelitis can also occur, associated with deeper bites by animals.

16. **(D)** Antimicrobial therapy is not indicated for uncomplicated *Salmonella* gastroenteritis in most cases since the therapy does not shorten the duration of disease and may prolong carriage. Antimicrobial therapy for *Salmonella* gastroenteritis is indicated for certain groups of patients, including infants younger than 3 months as well as patients with chronic gastrointestinal disease, malignancy, hemoglobinopathy, HIV infection or other immune deficiency, and severe colitis.

17. **(A)** Even though the stool culture is negative for bacterial pathogens, *Shigella* is still the most likely pathogen. The sensitivity of stool culture for diagnosing *Shigella* dysentery in approximately 70%. Treatment for patients with *Shigella* is recommended for patients with severe disease (such as bacteremia), dysentery or immunodeficiency.

18. **(B)** Infection caused by *Yersinia* is caused by ingestion of contaminated foods (pork intestine, milk, and other dairy products), by contaminated surface or well water and by direct or indirect contact with animals, and refrigerated stored blood. Infections in humans are more common in cooler climates during the winter months. *Y. enterocolitica* has also been reported to cause mesenteric adenitis, septicemia, meningitis, and postinfectious sequelae such as reactive arthritis, erythema nodosum, and uveitis.

SUGGESTED READING

Pickering LK, Baker CJ, Overturf GD, et al: *Red Book*: *2003 Report of the Committee on Infectious Diseases*, 26th ed. Elk Grove Village, IL: American Academy of Pediatrics, 2003.

Long SS, Pickering LK, Prober CG (eds): *Principles and Practices of Infectious Diseases*. Philadelphia: Churchill Livingstone, 2003.

CASE 101: A 13-YEAR-OLD ADOLESCENT MALE WITH A CHRONIC COUGH

A 13-year-old adolescent male, who has been previously healthy, is brought to your office, because he has had a persistent daytime and nighttime cough for the past 6 weeks. He had been diagnosed with pneumonia 4 weeks ago and treated with a 5-day course of azithromycin, then a 10-day course of amoxicillin-clavulanic acid but there was little improvement in his cough. In addition, he has developed intermittent chest pain and a sensation of fever. He now has blood-tinged sputum.

On physical examination he is alert and cooperative. He is non-toxic in appearance. The temperature is 100°F (37.8°C). There are no skin lesions present. There is mild anterior and posterior cervical lymphadenopathy. The respiratory rate is 30/minute. The lung examination revealed decreased breath sounds over the left anterior and posterior chest. The examination of the heart and abdomen is normal.

SELECT THE ONE BEST ANSWER TO THE FOLLOWING QUESTIONS

1. A chest radiograph is obtained, which reveals increased density in the inferior segment of the left lower lobe and marked interstitial disease in the left lower and right upper lobes. The left upper lobe is partially collapsed. A fungal culture of the sputum reveals no mycelia forms on smear but the culture grows a few *Blastomyces dermatitidis*. The most common extrapulmonary manifestation of blastomycosis involves the:

   (A) skin
   (B) bone and joints
   (C) genitourinary tract
   (D) spleen

2. An 8-year-old girl from Indiana develops fever, cough, malaise, and chest pain. A chest radiograph obtained reveals diffuse, reticulonodular infiltrates with hilar adenopathy. You obtain the history that she was playing in a barn 2 weeks be-

fore the illness started. The most likely etiology of the child's illness is:

(A) *B. dermatitidis*
(B) *Histoplasma capsulatum*
(C) *Mycobacterium tuberculosis*
(D) *Paracoccidioides brasiliensis*

3. A 15-year-old girl develops a papule on the dorsum of her left hand that in a 2-week period enlarges and becomes indurated. The skin lesion then develops into a painless ulcer with formation of subcutaneous nodules and erythema involving the forearm. There is no response to antibacterial therapy. The most likely diagnosis is:

(A) lymphocutaneous sporotrichosis
(B) lymphocutaneous blastomycosis
(C) lymphocutaneous aspergillosis
(D) lymphocutaneous tuberculosis

4. A 14-year-old girl develops fever to 102°F (38.8°C), chest pain, and rash 2 weeks after return from visiting relatives in Phoenix, Arizona. She took a few trips to desert areas outside Phoenix while visiting. On physical examination, she has fever of 102°F (38.8°C), and erythema nodosum is present on the lower extremities. A chest radiograph reveals a small right middle lobe infiltrate. Of the following, the pneumonia is most likely caused by:

(A) *Aspergillus fumigatus*
(B) *H. capsulatum*
(C) *Candida glabrata*
(D) *Coccidioides immitis*

5. Congenital candidiasis can occur both in term and premature infants. The clinical manifestations in these two age groups differ in all the following features except:

(A) Premature infants require treatment with amphotericin B.
(B) Premature infants are more likely to have pulmonary involvement.
(C) Premature infants with candidiasis more often have a positive blood culture.
(D) Premature infants more often have a leukemoid reaction.

6. A 7-year-old white girl has multiple hyperpigmented brown lesions with scaling that involve the upper trunk, proximal trunk, and neck. These are also a few scattered hypopigmented macular lesions on the face with fine scaling. You suspect *Pityriasis versicolor*. The etiologic agent of this skin disorder is:

(A) *Malassezia furfur*
(B) *Microsporum canis*
(C) *Trichophyton tonsurans*
(D) *Epidermophyton floccosum*

7. An 8-year-old boy develops fever, headache, cough, and dyspnea. A chest radiograph reveals diffuse interstitial infiltrates. He is treated with oral antibiotics (amoxicillin-clavulanate) for one week without improvement. Fever and headache persist. He then becomes somnolent and confused. A spinal tap is performed that shows a high protein concentration, low glucose concentration and pleocytosis, mostly lymphocytes. The diagnosis of cryptococcal meningitis is confirmed by cryptococcal antigen testing in the urine. The boy likely has an underlying disorder involving:

(A) humoral immunity
(B) cell-mediated immunity
(C) complement deficiency
(D) phagocytic function of neutrophils

8. A 6 month old infant boy develops progressive respiratory distress with tachypnea and intercostal retractions but no fever. Bilateral rales are heard on auscultation. The infant has hypoxia with an oxygen saturation of 89% and requires intubation. The diagnosis of *P. jiroveci* is confirmed by a fluorescein-conjugated monoclonal antibody stain of a tracheal aspirate specimen. All of the following drugs can be used alone for treatment of *P. jiroveci* except:

(A) atovaquone
(B) clindamycin
(C) pentamidine isethionate
(D) trimetrexate-leucovorin

9. A 3-year-old girl who lives in a large urban city develops fever to 102°F (38.8°C), irritability, and drowsiness in a 2-week period. The child then develops vomiting, lethargy, and nuchal rigidity. A CT scan of the brain shows hydrocephalus and a ventriculoperitoneal (VP) shunt is placed. The CSF shows a cell count of 500/mm^3 with a lym-

phocyte predominance. The protein concentration was 85 mg/dL and the glucose level was 40 mg/dL. A chest radiograph is normal, and the Mantoux test result is nonreactive. The child's mother reveals to you that she and her daughter have been living in a homeless shelter for the past 6 months. The most likely diagnosis is:

(A) cryptococcal meningitis
(B) neurocysticercosis
(C) tuberculous meningitis
(D) lymphocytic choriomeningitis

10. A full-term newborn infant boy is born to a 23-year-old mother who has a positive Mantoux test reaction, a result obtained 1 week before delivery. The infant should be evaluated for congenital tuberculosis in all of the following circumstances except when the:

(A) mother has miliary tuberculosis
(B) mother has tuberculous endometritis
(C) mother has tuberculous infection of the knee joint
(D) mother has apical scarring of the right upper lobe of lung with a negative sputum smear for acid-fast bacilli

11. A 4-year-old boy with HIV infection has a CD4 count of 80 cells/mm^3 (3%). He develops fever to 102°F (38.8°C) that persists for 1 week and is associated with weight loss, abdominal pain, fatigue, and diarrhea. Anemia is present with a hemoglobin of 9.0 g/dL. The most likely infectious etiology to explain these findings is:

(A) nontuberculous mycobacteria, disseminated
(B) histoplasmosis disseminated
(C) *M. tuberculosis*, disseminated
(D) brucellosis, disseminated

12. A 3-year-old girl has a one-month history of bilateral swelling of the submandibular lymph nodes. A chest radiograph is normal and a Mantoux test result is positive at 10 mm. All of the following are consistent with nontuberculous mycobacterial lymphadenitis except:

(A) age of the patient
(B) involvement of bilateral lymph nodes
(C) normal chest radiograph
(D) size of Mantoux test response

13. A 2-year-old boy who attends a child care center develops diarrhea that persists for 2 weeks and is associated with malaise, anorexia, abdominal distension, and abdominal cramps. You suspect giardiasis as the etiology. All of the following methods can be used to diagnose *Giardia lamblia* infection except:

(A) duodenal fluid specimen
(B) concentrated specimen of stool
(C) direct fluorescent antibody test of stool
(D) IgG-specific antibody to *Giardia* by enzyme immunoassay

14. Toxoplasmosis can cause both congenital infection as well as acquired infection in older children and adults. The most common physical finding in children with acquired toxoplasmosis is:

(A) lymphadenopathy
(B) pharyngitis
(C) conjunctivitis
(D) macular rash

15. A 16-year-old sexually active adolescent female presents to your office with a 1-week history of vaginal discharge and dysuria. She also reports a recent history of dyspareunia. A pelvic exam is performed that reveals vaginal and vulvar erythema with a frothy discharge. The cervix has a "strawberry appearance," related to friability and punctate hemorrhages. Based on these findings, you strongly suspect infection with:

(A) *Chlamydia trachomatis*
(B) *Gardnerella vaginalis*
(C) *Neisseria gonorrhoeae*
(D) *Trichomonas vaginalis*

16. A 3-year-old boy develops fever and malaise in a 10-day period. On physical examination he has a fever of 102°F (38.8°C) and hepatosplenomegaly. The leukocyte count is 9000/mm^3 with 50% eosinophils (4500/mm^3). An important epidemiologic finding to support the diagnosis of visceral larva migrans (VLM) caused by *Toxocara canis* is:

(A) recent visit to a cave
(B) recent play in a sandbox
(C) recent play in a barn
(D) family has two adult dogs as pets

17. The different *Plasmodium* species that cause malaria have unique geographic distribution and resistance patterns. The following statement regarding the epidemiology of malaria is correct:

    (A) *P. ovale* infections are common only in South Africa
    (B) *P. vivax* malaria is prevalent on the Indian subcontinent and in Central and South American
    (C) *P. malariae* has the same geographic distribution as *P. falciparum* and is more common in most areas they co-inhabit
    (D) Relapses can occur in *P. malariae* infection because of a persistent hepatic stage of infection

18. A 4-year-old girl returns from a trip to Bangladesh with her family where they traveled for the past 3 months. She develops diarrhea that persists for 2 weeks before being brought to your office by her parents. There is a history of bloody stools associated with abdominal pain and heme positive. You suspect intestinal amebiasis. An important extra-intestinal complication of *Entamoeba histolytica* to consider is:

    (A) ameboma
    (B) liver abscess
    (C) brain abscess
    (D) cutaneous amebiasis

Answers

1. **(A)** The skin lesions of blastomycosis usually begin as papules that usually evolve into verrucous, ulcerative lesions. Osteomyelitis is the second most common manifestation of disseminated blastomycosis. The CNS can also be involved with meningitis the most common complication.

2. **(B)** Areas of high incidence of histoplasmosis include the Mississippi and Ohio River Valleys. Some activities of children that can predispose to infection include playing in barns, hollow trees, caves, or bird roosts. Infection is usually self-limited in immunocompetent children but one form of infection called progressive disseminated histoplasmosis can occur. Prolonged fever, failure-to-thrive and hepatosplenomegaly can develop in

infants. A chest radiograph can show diffuse reticulonodular infiltrates. This form of the disease is often fatal if untreated.

3. **(A)** In children, sporotrichosis is localized to the skin and subcutaneous tissue. The disease most commonly affects the face and extremities, in particular hands and fingers. In most cases, infection will spread to regional lymph nodes that draw the primary site of infection. Skin lesions associated with tuberculosis include erythema nodosum, papulonecrotic tuberculids which are miliary lesions of the skin, verrucosa cutis which is a tuberculous wart-like lesion, and scrofuloderma which is an ulcer or sinus tract resulting from rupture of a lymph node.

4. **(D)** In this clinical situation, the travel history suggested that the patient has coccidioidomycosis. The infection is endemic to Southern California, Arizona, Western and Southern Texas, and New Mexico. In children with coccidioidomycosis, an acute diffuse erythematous rash and erythema multiforme are common. The primary infection involves the lungs, and in healthy children, symptoms improve without treatment within a few days to one month.

5. **(C)** In term infants, congenital cutaneous candidiasis is acquired from contaminated amniotic fluid. Skin findings include vesicles, pustules, or a widespread erythematous macular rash. In premature infants the skin findings may resemble a widespread erythematous dermatitis. The skin findings are associated with invasive pulmonary disease and early onset respiratory distress. Neither form has positive blood cultures for *Candida*.

6. **(A)** *Malassezia furfur* also can cause a chronic folliculitis in immunocompromised persons, such as with acquired immunodeficiency syndrome. In addition, systemic *Malassezia* infection can cause fungemia in infants receiving parenteral nutrition that contains intralipids. Fever, apnea, and bradycardia, interstitial pneumonia, and thrombocytopenia are common associated findings.

7. **(B)** Primary infection occurs through inhalation of airborne particles. After inhalation, the organism disseminates from the lungs to other organs,

the most important being the central nervous system. Dissemination of the fungus is rare in children without defects in cell-mediated immunity. CD4+ lymphocytes have been shown to play an important role in containing CNS infection caused by *Cryptococcus*.

8. **(B)** Trimethoprim-sulfamethoxazole is the drug of choice for treatment. Clindamycin plus primaquine has been used for treatment in adults. Prednisone is recommended as adjunctive therapy for moderate to severe *P. jiroveci* infection.

9. **(C)** Tuberculous meningitis is most common in children 6 months to 4 years old. Meningitis can occur within 2 to 6 months of initial infection. Chest radiographs are normal in 50% and the Mantoux test is nonreactive in 40% of children with tuberculosis meningitis. CT scan of brain can be useful for diagnosis with basilar enhancement, communicating hydrocephalus, and signs of cerebral edema (see Table 101-1). Hydrocephalus secondary to meningeal cysticercosis is rare, and cryptococcal meningitis also is not associated with hydrocephalus. Lymphocytic choriomeningitis virus can cause congenital infection characterized by chorioretinitis, hydrocephalus, and microcephaly. Intracranial calcifications are also present. Infection with lymphocytic choriomeningitis virus can also be acquired after contact with mice or hamsters.

10. **(D)** Congenital tuberculosis is rare. A pregnant woman with isolated pulmonary tuberculosis is unlikely to infect her infant until after birth. If congenital tuberculosis is suspected, a Mantoux test, chest radiograph, and lumbar puncture should be performed and antituberculous therapy started. The placenta should be sent to pathology and cultured for *M. tuberculosis*.

11. **(A)** All of the bacteria listed can cause disseminated infection in children with acquired immunodeficiency syndrome but infection with nontuberculous mycobacteria, particularly *M. avium* complex (MAC) is most common. The risk of developing disseminated MAC infection is inversely related to the CD4+ count. The incidence is as high as 24% in children with CD4+ counts less than 100 cells/mm^3. Manifestations

Table 101-1. CHARACTERISTIC FINDINGS WITH TUBERCULOUS MENINGITIS IN CHILDREN

Finding	Result
Exposure	Adult with tuberculosis
Age	Most common 6 months to 4 years
Cranial nerves	III, VI, VII
TST	Nonreactive in up to 40%
Chest radiograph	Normal in up to 50%
CSF	WBC 10–500/mm^3 (mononuclear)
	Glucose 20–40 mg/dl, protein >400 mg/dl
CT of brain	Basilar enhancement, communicating hydrocephalus

TST, tuberculin skin test; CSF, cerebrospinal fluid; CT, computed tomography.

of disseminated MAC infections include fever, weight loss, night sweats, abdominal pain, diarrhea, anemia, and neutropenia.

12. **(B)** Lymphadenitis or scrofula is the most common manifestation of nontuberculous mycobacterium (NTM) infection. Lymphadenitis because of NTM is usually unilateral and involves the submandibular or anterior cervical lymph nodes. For NTM lymphadenitis in healthy children, surgical excision is curative in most cases.

13. **(D)** Although enzyme immunoassay often provides rapid results, this method is not commercially available for *Giardia*. The other methods listed are more readily available, and a duodenal specimen should be considered when the organism is not found on repeated stool examination but clinical suspicion is high. Infection can occur either by hand to mouth transfer of cysts from feces of an infected person or ingestion of fecally contaminated food or water. Asymptomatic infection is common. Most community-wide epidemics have occurred from a contaminated water supply.

14. **(A)** Lymphadenopathy is frequently found in the cervical area of the neck. The classic triad of congenital toxoplasmosis is chorioretinitis, cerebral calcifications, and hydrocephalus. Humans develop infection with *T. gondii* by one of two

methods. These include consumption of raw or undercooked meat that contains cyst or accidental ingestion of oocysts from soil, contaminated food, or cat feces.

15. **(D)** *T. vaginalis* is a common, sexually transmitted organism. In addition to the signs and symptoms described above, abdominal pain can occur. This may indicate severe vaginitis but pelvic inflammatory disease should also be considered. In males, urethritis occurs with more than half of patients having urethral discharge. Neonates can develop infection after a vaginal delivery. Symptomatic infection in the female neonate involves a self-limited vaginal discharge.

16. **(B)** In children, infection with *T. canis* begins with ingestion of embryonated eggs. This occurs when children are playing in sandboxes and playgrounds contaminated with cat and dog feces. Other clinical manifestations of VLM include lower respiratory tract symptoms such as bronchospasm that mimics asthma. If the *T. canis* larvae invade the eye, the results is ocular larval migrans (OLM). The retina can be involved and cause loss of vision. The raccoon roundworm, *Baylisascaris procyonis*, rarely can also cause infection in children, and can result in severe encephalitis.

17. **(B)** Each *Plasmodium* species that causes malaria has a distinct geographic distribution. *P. ovale* occurs most often in West Africa. Malaria attributable to *P. vivax* and *P. falciparum* is common in Southeast Asia, Oceania, and South America. *P. falciparum* is prevalent in Africa, Haiti, and Papua New Guinea. *P. malariae* has the same distribution but is less common than *P. falciparum*.

18. **(B)** In approximately 10% of patients with invasive *Entamoeba histolytica* infection, a liver abscess develops. An ameboma is a mass of granulation tissue in the cecum or ascending colon. The clinical presentation usually includes a tender and palpable abdominal mass. Other organ system involvement is uncommon.

SUGGESTED READING

Pickering LK, Baker CJ, Overturf GD, et al: *Red Book: 2003 Report of the Committee on Infectious Diseases,* 26th ed. Elk Grove Village, IL: American Academy of Pediatrics, 2003.

Mandell FL, Bennett JE, Dolin R: *Mandell, Douglas and Bennett's Principles and Practice of Infectious Diseases.* Philadelphia: Churchill Livingstone, 2000.

CASE 102: A 4-YEAR-OLD BOY WITH FEVER AND A NECK MASS

A 4-year-old boy is brought to your office for evaluation of a right-sided neck mass. The child was well until about 10 days ago when he developed fever and a right-sided neck swelling. The swelling has increased in size over the past 1 week and is painful. There has been no cough, sore throat, or rhinorrhea. There has not been contact with anyone who has been ill. There also has not been any history of travel.

On physical examination the child is alert, active, and non-toxic in appearance. The temperature is 102.7°F (39.3°C). There are 3- × 4-cm and 1- × 2-cm right posterior cervical triangle lymph nodes palpable. The nodes are movable, firm, and tender to palpation. There are no skin lesions. Examination of the heart and lungs is normal. The leukocyte count is 8900/mm^3, the hemoglobin is 9.5 g/dL and the platelet count is 300,000/mm^3.

SELECT THE ONE BEST ANSWER TO THE FOLLOWING QUESTIONS

1. In obtaining further history you find out that there has been no contact with an adult who has a chronic cough or any exposure to ticks or rabbits. The mother does tell you that their family cat had kittens about 3 months ago. The most likely etiologic agent of this child's illness is:

    (A) *Bartonella henselae*
    (B) *Blastomyces dermatitidis*
    (C) *Francisella tularensis*
    (D) *Mycobacterium tuberculosis*

2. The diagnosis in this 4-year-old child can be confirmed most readily by:

    (A) culture of blood
    (B) culture of lymph node specimen
    (C) special stains of lymph node specimen
    (D) serology

3. Treatment of the infection in this 4-year-old should include:

(A) amphotericin B

(B) gentamicin

(C) doxycycline by oral route

(D) cefazolin

4. Endoscopy is performed on a 10-year-old girl with persistent epigastric abdominal pain and vomiting. A duodenal ulcer is found. Infection with *Helicobacter pylori* is confirmed by culture and histologic examination of duodenal biopsy samples. Treatment for this girl should include which of the following:

(A) omeprazole

(B) omeprazole and metronidazole

(C) amoxicillin, clarithromycin, and omeprazole

(D) amoxicillin, clarithromycin, omeprazole, and bismuth subsalicylate

5. A 5-year-old boy returns from Mexico with family after visiting with relatives that lived in a rural area. He develops fever to 103°F (39.4°C), anorexia, and decreased activity 2 weeks after returning home. His mother reports that he does not want to walk. On physical examination there is limitation of movement, swelling, and tenderness of the left knee joint. He also has splenomegaly. A definitive diagnosis can be made by:

(A) culture of blood

(B) enzyme immunoassay on acute serum

(C) PCR of serum

(D) urine for antigen detection

6. A 14-year-old boy develops severe conjunctivitis with pain followed by the development of enlarged painful preauricular lymph nodes. He reveals that 1 week ago he went hunting with his father and killed a number of squirrels. Which of the following should be considered in the differential diagnosis of the adolescent's illness?

(A) *Coccidioides immitis*

(B) *Francisella tularensis*

(C) *Bartonella quintana*

(D) *Mycobacterium tuberculosis*

7. *Kingella kingae* can be a normal inhabitant of the oropharynx of humans. The most common clinical infection caused by *K. kingae* in children is:

(A) endocarditis

(B) intervertebral diskitis

(C) occult bacteremia

(D) septic arthritis

8. *Legionella pneumophila* can rarely cause community acquired pneumonia in healthy children and infection usually resolves without treatment with effective antibiotics. *Legionella pneumophila* is likely to cause severe and fatal disease in children with:

(A) neoplasm receiving chemotherapy

(B) chronic persistent asthma

(C) X-linked agammaglobulinemia

(D) IgA deficiency

9. A 7-year-old girl from North Carolina develops fever to 102°F (38.8°C) in July associated with severe headache and myalgias. On the fifth day of fever the child develops a macular blanching rash that starts on the wrists, ankles, and forearms (see Figure 102-1). The rash then spreads centrally over the next 24 hours, and scattered petechiae are noted. Laboratory evaluation reveals a leukocyte count of 12,000/mm³, hemoglobin of 12.0 g/dL and platelet count of 100,000/mm³. The serum sodium is 130 meq/L. The etiologic agent of this child's illness is:

(A) Epstein-Barr virus

(B) *Neisseria meningitidis*

(C) *Rickettsia akari*

(D) *R. rickettsii*

10. The treatment of choice for this infection in this 7-year-old girl is:

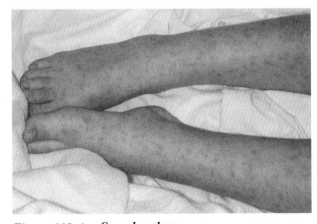

Figure 102-1. **See color plates.**

(A) azithromycin
(B) chloramphenicol
(C) doxycycline
(D) rifampin

11. An 8-year-old boy develops fever to 102°F (38.8°C) associated with headache, anorexia, and vomiting. He remembers being bitten by a tick 9 days prior to his illness. On physical exam he is alert. The temperature is 102°F (38.8°C) and a blanching macular rash involving the trunk is present. The leukocyte count is 3500/mm^3; the platelet count is 120,000/mm^3, the hemoglobin 12 g/dL and the aspartate aminotransferase (AST) is 110 U/L. The most likely diagnosis is:

(A) babesiosis
(B) ehrlichiosis
(C) rickettsialpox
(D) Rocky Mountain spotted fever

12. The treatment of choice for this infection in this 8-year-old boy is:

(A) azithromycin
(B) chloramphenicol
(C) doxycycline
(D) gentamicin

13. A 9-day-old male term infant develops a watery eye discharge that becomes purulent. The conjunctiva of the right eye becomes injected and the eyelid is swollen. A direct fluorescent antibody (DFA) test of a conjunctival specimen confirms the diagnosis of *C. trachomatis* infection. Treatment with systemic oral antibiotic therapy is recommended since:

(A) There is often co-infection with *N. gonorrhoeae*.
(B) The topical ophthalmic therapy does not eliminate nasopharyngeal carriage.
(C) There are no topical ophthalmic antibiotics active against *C. trachomatis*.
(D) Resistance develops rapidly when ophthalmic antibiotics are used.

14. A 5-year-old boy has an illness that includes a 2-week history of cough, sore throat, and fever. The coughing persists, and bilateral rales are

heard on auscultation of the lungs. A chest radiograph reveals bilateral infiltrates. The most likely etiology of the following choices for this pneumonia is:

(A) *Chlamydophila pneumoniae*
(B) *Chlamydia trachomatis*
(C) influenza A
(D) Epstein-Barr virus

15. *Mycoplasma pneumoniae* is well known to cause lower respiratory tract disease, primarily in school-age children and young adults. Severe and fatal pneumonia caused by *M. pneumoniae* has been described in children with the following disorder:

(A) hypogammaglobulinemia
(B) asthma
(C) cystic fibrosis
(D) prematurity

16. Appropriate antimicrobial therapy for a 5-year-old child with pneumonia caused by *M. pneumoniae* or *C. pneumoniae* is:

(A) azithromycin
(B) ciprofloxacin
(C) doxycycline
(D) ceftriaxone

17. A 6-year-old boy develops fever, headache, vomiting, and muscle pain. You obtain a history from his mother that he handled a dead rat in the alley of the family's apartment 2 weeks ago. On physical examination the child has a fever of 102°F (38.8°C) and a maculopapular rash involving the extremities, including the palms and soles. There is no evidence of any bite wound. The causative agent of this child's illness is likely:

(A) *Ehrlichia chaffeensis*
(B) *R. rickettsia*
(C) *Spirillum minus*
(D) *Streptobacillus moniliformis*

18. The treatment of choice for the infection in the 6-year-old boy noted above should include:

(A) doxycycline
(B) erythromycin
(C) penicillin
(D) vancomycin

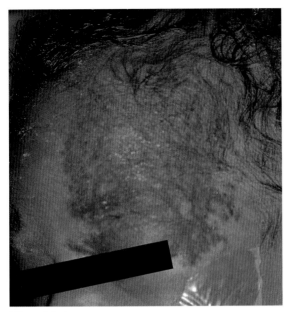

Plate 16-1.

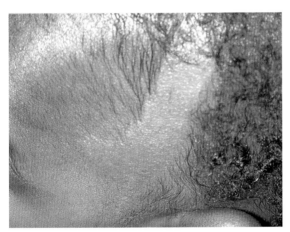

Plate 16-2.

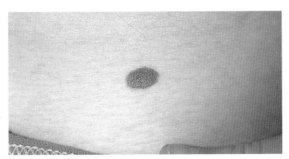

Plate 16-3.

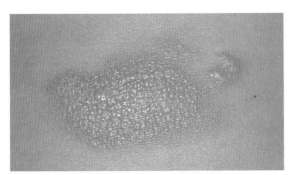

Plate 16-4.

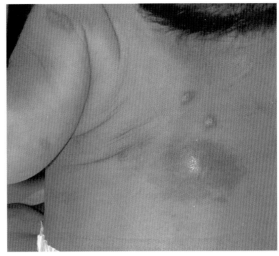

Plate 16-5.

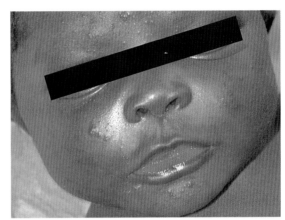

Plate 17-1.

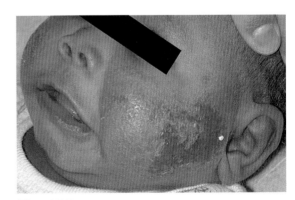

Plate 17-2.

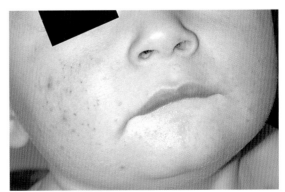

Plate 17-3.

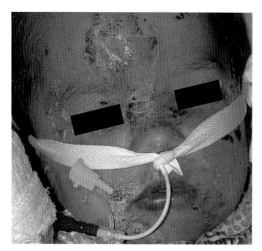

Plate 17-4.

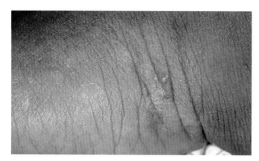

Plate 18-1A.

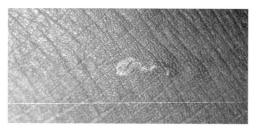

Plate 18-1B.

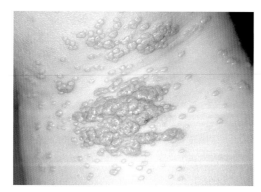

Plate 18-2.

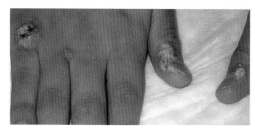

Plate 18-3.

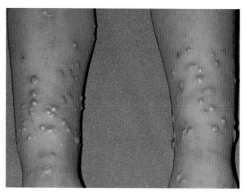

Plate 18-4B.

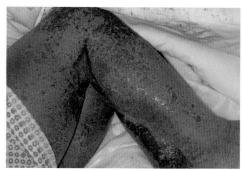

Plate 19-1.

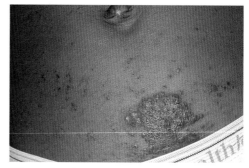

Plate 19-2A.

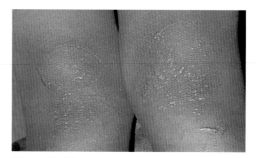

Plate 19-2B.

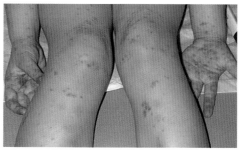

Plate 19-3.

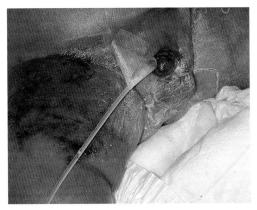

Plate 19-4.

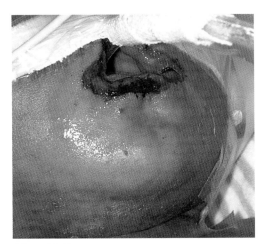

Plate 19-5.

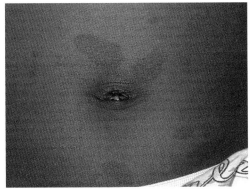

Plate 21-1.

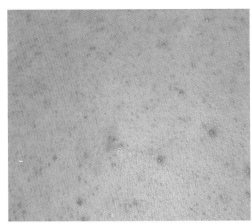

Plate 21-2.

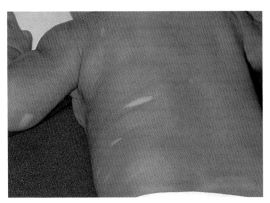

Plate 21-3.

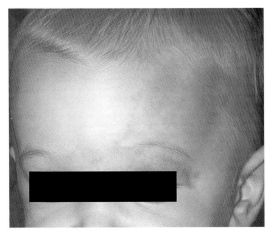

Plate 21-4.

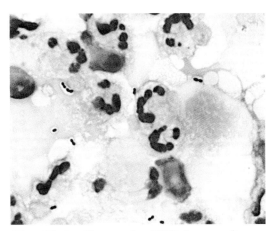

Plate 95-1.   *Gram stain of CSF that grew* S. pneumoniae *revealing gram-positive diplococci. Note halo surrounding some of the organisms that represents the capsule.*

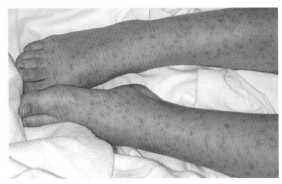

Plate 102-1.

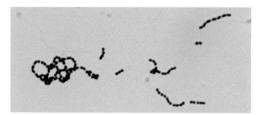

Plate 103-1.

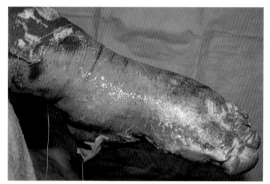

Plate 105-1. **Scald burn to the lower extremity of a 2-year-old.**

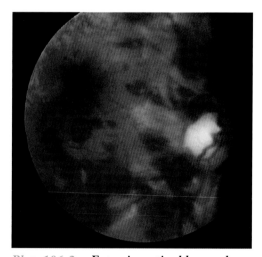

Plate 106-2. **Extensive retinal hemorrhages.**

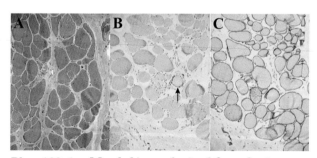

Plate 132-1. **Muscle biopsy obtained from the 4-year-old patient described in question 8. (A) Muscle stained with hematoxylin and eosin. (B) Immunohistochemical staining for the C-terminus of dystrophin. The arrow indicates a "revertant fiber." (C) Immunohistochemical staining of the same region of muscle for merosin. (Photographs courtesy of Dr. Manuel Utset, The University of Chicago.)**

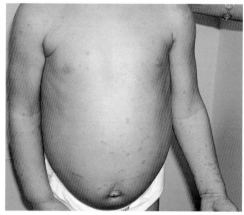

Plate 138-1. **Evanescent salmon-colored, macular or maculopapular rash of systemic-onset arthritis.**

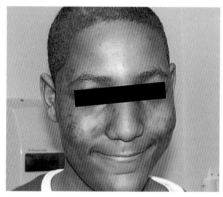

Plate 139-1. **Malar rash in a teenage boy with systemic lupus erythematosus.**

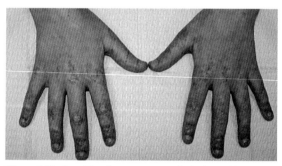

Plate 139-2. **Erythematous, scaly lesions (Gottron's papules) over the dorsal aspects of the metacarpophalangeal and interphalangeal joints in a 10-year-old girl with dermatomyositis. Nailfold telangiectasias can also be seen.**

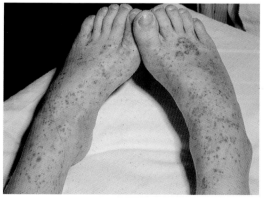

Plate 139-3. **Palpable, purpuric lesions on the legs of a child with Henoch-Schönlein purpura.**

Answers

1. **(A)** The most common clinical presentation with cat scratch disease is unilateral regional lymphadenitis. The lymphadenitis usually involves nodes that drain the site of inoculation but in up to 20% of cases additional lymph node groups are involved. At a particular site of lymphadenitis, multiple nodes are involved about half the time. The most common site is axilla, followed by cervical, submandibular and inguinal nodes. Most patients with cat scratch disease are afebrile. However, systemic cat scratch disease can occur in which the presentation includes prolonged fever of 1 to 3 weeks, malaise, myalgias, and arthralgias. Weight loss, abdominal pain, generalized lymphadenopathy, hepatomegaly, and splenomegaly can occur. Ultrasound of the liver or spleen can identify multiple microabscesses. Encephalopathy is the most serious complication of cat scratch disease, occurring in up to 5% of patients.

2. **(D)** Serology is the method of choice for diagnosis. Both IgG and IgM antibodies to *B. henselae* can be measured. Most patients with cat scratch disease have high IgG antibodies at presentation. The IgM test lacks sensitivity. If lymph node tissue is available, the organism may be seen with the Warthin-Starry silver impregnation stain, but this stain is not specific for *B. henselae*.

3. **(B)** Surgical excision of lymph nodes is unnecessary. Antimicrobial therapy may be beneficial for severely ill patients with systemic cat scratch disease and is recommended for immunocompromised patients. There are two other manifestations of *B. henselae* or *B. quintana* infections reported in immunocompromised patients. With *B. henselae* infection there often is a history of cat exposure. Bacillary angiomatosis is a vascular proliferative disorder that involves the skin and subcutaneous tissues which occurs in immunocompromised individuals. Bacillary peliosis occurs primarily in patients with AIDS and is characterized by reticuloendothelial lesions on the liver primarily but can also involve the spleen, abdominal lymph nodes and bone marrow. The lesions of these two diseases respond rapidly to erythromycin or doxycycline.

4. **(C)** Treatment is recommended only for patients who have a history of or active peptic ulcer disease, gastric mucosa-associated lymphoid tissue-type lymphoma (MALToma) or early gastric cancer. The most effective regimen in children includes a 2-week, three-agent therapy that consists of a protein pump inhibitor (omeprazole or lansoprazole), amoxicillin, and clarithromycin.

5. **(A)** The child likely has brucellosis with osteoarticular involvement. Childhood brucellosis most often affects the large peripheral joints, including the knees, hips, and ankles. A definitive diagnosis is established by recovery of *Brucella* species from blood, bone marrow, or other tissues. If brucellosis is suspected, the clinical microbiology laboratory personnel should be informed so blood cultures can be incubated for 4 weeks. A serum agglutination test (SAT) and enzyme immunoassay (EIA) are also available for diagnosis. It is recommended to send the SAT first and measure antibody titers in serum specimens collected at least 2 weeks apart.

6. **(B)** The adolescent has a clinical form of tularemia called oculoglandular syndrome that results from conjunctival infection and is acquired from contaminated fingers. *F. tularensis* can be transmitted by direct contact with infected animals, through tick bites and also by contaminated food or water. The most common clinical manifestation is the ulceroglandular syndrome. This disease manifests as swollen, tender lymph nodes in the inguinal, cervical or axillary regions that are preceded by painful maculopapular lesions at the portal of entry that develop into an ulcerated lesion (see Table 102-1).

7. **(D)** Osteoarticular infection is the most common clinical infection of *K. kingae* in children. Studies have shown that inoculating of joint fluid directly into BACTEC aerobic blood culture bottles increases the likelihood of isolating the bacteria. Most infections occur in children younger than 5 years of age. *K. kingae* is a common cause of septic arthritis in young children in Israel but less frequently has been reported in the United States.

8. **(A)** The most important clinical infection caused by *L. pneumophila* in both children and adults is

Table 102-1. CLINICAL MANIFESTATIONS OF TULAREMIA

Clinical Syndrome	Comment
Glandular	Most common form; adenitis ± ulcer
Oculoglandular	Nodular conjunctivitis; enlarged painful preauricular nodes
Oropharyngeal	Pseudomembrane simulating diphtheria; fever; associated with ingestion of contaminated meat, milk, or water
Typhoidal tularemia	High fever; signs of sepsis; hepato-splenomegaly common; ingestion of contaminated food; can have ne-crotic lesions in bowel
Gastrointestinal	Ingestion of contaminated food; persistent diarrhea and abdominal or back pain

pneumonia. Infections in immunocompromised children such as receipt of anticancer therapy represent the most severe form of the disease in pediatrics. At the other end of the spectrum, *Legionella* is responsible for 1% to 5% of commu-nity-acquired pneumonia in healthy children and the infection is self-limited. Severe disease with pneumonia and septicemia can also occur in neonates.

9. **(D)** The child's clinical presentation is most con-sistent with Rocky Mountain spotted fever. One must have a high index of suspicion since the signs and symptoms during the prodrome are nonspecific. Other findings in children include irritability, severe abdominal pain, conjunctivitis, preseptal edema and splenomegaly. The rash of Rocky Mountain spotted fever is absent until the third to fifth day of illness. The rash also typi-cally involves the palms and soles. The rash is the hallmark feature of the disease but may not occur in up to 20% of cases.

10. **(C)** Doxycycline is the drug of choice, even in children younger than 8 years. The reasons for this choice include tetracycline staining of teeth is dose-related; doxycycline is less likely than other tetracyclines to stain teeth and use of the alternative antibiotic chloramphenicol has signif-

icant potential toxicity. In addition a retrospec-tive study indicates that chloramphenicol may be less effective than doxycycline for treatment of Rocky Mountain spotted fever.

11. **(B)** In children most cases of ehrlichiosis have been associated with *E. chaffeensis*, which causes human monocytic ehrlichiosis. Most human monocytic ehrlichiosis infections occur in people from southeastern and south central United States but cases of ehrlichiosis have been re-ported in 48 states. Pediatric cases have a male predominance and the peak incidence occurs from May to August. The most common symp-toms reported in children include fever, myalgia, and rash. Lymphopenia, thrombocytopenia, and increased serum AST are common.

12. **(C)** Treatment with doxycycline should continue until at least 3 days after defervescence for a min-imum of 5 to 10 days.

13. **(B)** The risk that a neonate will acquire *C. tra-chomatis* is 50% if the mother has chlamydial in-fection. The risk for neonatal conjunctivitis is 25% to 50% and pneumonia is 5% to 20%. Pneumonia caused by *C. trachomatis* occurs be-tween 2 to 10 weeks of age. A staccato cough, tachypnea, and rales is characteristic. Wheezing is typically absent. A chest radiograph reveals bi-lateral interstitial infiltrates and hyperinflation. A diagnostic clue may be the presence of eosin-ophilia (>400 cells/mm^3).

14. **(A)** *Chlamydophila pneumoniae* causes community-acquired pneumonia, prolonged cough illness, and acute bronchitis in children. The organism has been implicated as the course in 5% to 10% of commonly acquired pneumonias in children. The illness tends to have subacute presentation that is indistinguishable from *Mycoplasma pneumoniae*. Cough often is prolonged with persistence for 2 to 6 weeks, and the illness can have a biphasic course.

15. **(A)** In patients with an underlying immunodefi-ciency (particularly hypogammaglobulinemia), sickle cell disease, Down syndrome, and chronic pulmonary and cardiac disorders, severe pneu-monia with pleural effusion can develop. Infec-tion with *M. pneumoniae* has been best described

as an influenza-like illness with gradual onset. Many extrapulmonary manifestations have been ascribed to *M. pneumoniae*. The detection of *M. pneumoniae* DNA by PCR has suggested a role for it in extrapulmonary manifestations such as encephalitis, transverse myelitis, pleural effusion, and bacteremia.

16. **(A)** The newer macrolide and azalide antibiotics are as effective as erythromycin in achieving clinical and microbiological cure in children with community-acquired pneumonia caused by *M. pneumoniae*. Doxycycline is also effective and can be used for children 8 years and older.

17. **(D)** Rat bite fever in the United States is mainly caused by *S. moniliformis*. Non-suppurative migratory polyarthritis or arthralgias occurs in 50% of patients. Generalized adenopathy also occurs. Rat bite fever caused by the spirochete *S. minus* manifests with fever and ulceration at the site of the bite. Regional lymphadenitis and lymphadenopathy are associated with the illness. *S. minus* infection occurs primarily in Asia.

18. **(C)** Penicillin is the drug of choice for rat bite fever caused by either organism. Alternative drugs include ampicillin, cefuroxime and cefotaxime. Doxycycline can be used in penicillin allergic patients who are 8 years of age or older.

SUGGESTED READING
Pickering LK, Baker CJ, Overturf GD, et al: *Red Book: 2003 Report of the Committee on Infectious Diseases*, 26th ed. Elk Grove Village, IL: American Academy of Pediatrics, 2003.
Feigin RD, Cherry JD, Demmler GJ, et al: *Textbook of Pediatric Infectious Diseases*. Philadelphia: WB Saunders, 2004.

CASE 103: A 2-YEAR-OLD GIRL WITH ABDOMINAL PAIN AND FEVER

A 2-year-old girl presents to the children's hospital emergency department with abdominal pain and fever. The child was well until 5 days ago when she developed fever. The next day abdominal pain began. The abdominal pain persisted and was then associated with intermittent vomiting. The child was healthy with no previous hospitalizations, operations or serious medical illnesses. One month previously, she received a 10-day course of amoxicillin for otitis media.

On physical examination the child is ill-appearing and seems to be in pain. The temperature is 104°F (40°C). There are no skin lesions. Examination of the lungs and heart is normal. There is mild abdominal distention and diffuse abdominal tenderness. A leukocyte count is 28,000/mm³ with 60% PMNS, 15% basophils, and 25% lymphocytes. The hemoglobin is 9.8g/dL and the platelet count was 18,000/mm³.

SELECT THE ONE BEST ANSWER TO THE FOLLOWING QUESTIONS

1. In this 2-year-old previously healthy child, an abdominal ultrasound is performed that demonstrates free fluid in the abdomen. You suspect primary peritonitis. The most likely etiologic agent in this setting is:

   (A) *Escherichia coli*
   (B) *Neisseria meningitidis*
   (C) *Staphylococcus aureus*
   (D) *Streptococcus pneumoniae*

2. The most common underlying condition associated with primary peritonitis caused by *S. pneumoniae* is:

   (A) B-cell immunodeficiency
   (B) HIV infection
   (C) complement deficiency
   (D) nephrotic syndrome

3. A 3-year-old girl presents with a one week history of a mucopurulent vaginal discharge. She has a fever to 103°F (39.4°C) and diffuse abdominal pain. An abdominal ultrasound reveals ascites. The most likely cause of these symptoms is primary peritonitis. The most likely pathogen is this setting is:

   (A) *Chlamydia trachomatis*
   (B) *Haemophilus influenzae*
   (C) *Neisseria gonorrhoeae*
   (D) *Staphylococcus aureus*

4. The most common complication of continuous ambulatory peritoneal dialysis (CAPD) is peritonitis. The most common organism responsible for peritonitis in this setting is:

(A) *Candida albicans*
(B) *Mycobacterium tuberculosis*
(C) *Pseudomonas aeruginosa*
(D) *Staphylococcus epidermidis*

5. During January, a 12-month-old male infant develops a fever to 104°F (40°C). The physical examination is normal and a leukocyte count is 20,000/mm³. All of the following are risk factors for occult bacteremia caused by *S. pneumoniae* except:

(A) age
(B) height of fever
(C) leukocytosis
(D) season of the year

6. In a 2-month-old infant the most likely cause of occult bacteremia is:

(A) *Neisseria meningitidis*
(B) *Streptococcus agalactiae* (group B streptococcus)
(C) *Streptococcus pyogenes*
(D) *Staphylococcus aureus*

7. An important reason that sepsis can progress to septic shock and multiorgan dysfunction syndrome (MODS) in spite of appropriate antimicrobial therapy is the systemic inflammatory response syndrome (SIRS). The stages of SIRS include all but:

(A) ARDS
(B) severe sepsis
(C) septic shock
(D) MODS

8. A 2½-year-old boy develops fever to 103°F (39.4°C) that persists for 6 days. His mother reports that he has become increasingly cranky. He then develops red eyes and a rash. On physical exam there is fever of 102°F (38.8°C), the child appears fussy and has a generalized erythematous maculopapular rash. His blood pressure is normal. He also has bilateral bulbar conjunctivitis with red, cracked lips. There is also mild swelling of the hands and feet. The correct therapy for this child would include:

(A) immune globulin intravenous (IGIV)
(B) intravenous penicillin and clindamycin
(C) intravenous corticosteroid therapy
(D) oral nonsteroidal anti-inflammatory drug

9. A 4-year-old girl develops bullous erythema multiforme over the extensor surface of the extremities which then spreads over the trunk. There is bilateral bulbar conjunctivitis, and the lips are swollen, denuded and bleeding. You suspect Stevens-Johnson syndrome. The infectious agent most clearly established as a cause of this disorder:

(A) herpes simplex virus
(B) *M. pneumoniae*
(C) adenovirus
(D) *S. pyogenes*

10. A 10-year-old boy develops fever documented daily of ≥100.4°F (38.0°C) for 14 days. All of the following infectious causes should be considered if there is history of travel outside of the United States except:

(A) cat scratch disease
(B) brucellosis
(C) malaria
(D) salmonellosis

11. Children with fever of unknown origin (FUO) will have infection as the etiology in more than one-third of the cases. The etiology of an FUO in children may be an uncommon presentation of a common infection. This would include all but:

(A) endocarditis
(B) pneumonia
(C) sinusitis
(D) urinary tract infection

12. In children with FUO the likelihood of establishing a diagnosis is low in patients with a normal laboratory value for:

(A) amylase
(B) erythrocyte sedimentation rate
(C) ferritin
(D) platelet count

13. In some children there is a syndrome of FUO that is associated with episodic fevers with fever-free intervals. All of the following disorders are examples of this pattern of recurrent fevers except:

(A) cyclic neutropenia
(B) hyper-IgD syndrome

(C) tumor necrosis receptor-associated periodic fever syndrome

(D) Kikuchi-Fujimoto disease

14. Systemic infections are the most common causes of generalized lymphadenopathy. All of the following organisms have a characteristic association with generalized lymphadenopathy except:

(A) *Ehrlichia chaffeensis*

(B) Epstein-Barr virus

(C) human herpes virus type 6

(D) *Yersinia enterocolitica*

15. A 7-year-old girl develops migratory arthritis that first involved the left knee and then the right elbow. There is no history of antecedent illness. On physical examination the child is febrile with temperature of 102°F (38.8°C). The right elbow is red, swollen, and tender with movement. The lung and cardiovascular examinations are normal. The erythrocyte sedimentation rate is 60 mm/hr. A throat culture reveals the organism depicted in Figure 103-1. The most likely diagnosis of the following choices is:

(A) acute rheumatic fever

(B) reactive arthritis

(C) serum sickness

(D) systemic lupus erythematosus

16. A 33-week-gestation newborn infant boy is born to a 19-year-old mother who has not received

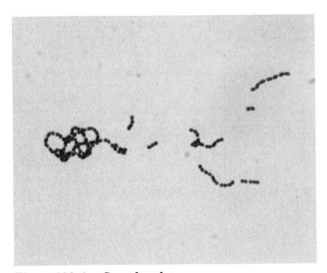

Figure 103-1. **See color plates.**

prenatal care. The mother admits that she used cocaine during the pregnancy. At birth, the infant has a generalized maculopapular rash, splenomegaly, and a slightly distended abdomen. The infant has anemia (hemoglobin of 11.0 g/dL) and urinalysis reveals 3+ protein. The CSF is normal, as is an eye examination. An HIV enzyme immunoassay and nontreponemal test for syphilis (RPR) are negative on the infant. The most likely diagnosis is:

(A) HIV infection

(B) congenital cytomegalovirus

(C) congenital syphilis

(D) congenital toxoplasmosis

17. A 10-year-old girl develops fever to 102°F (38.8°C) and a swollen, tender left knee joint 4 weeks after returning to school in the fall. There is also pain and limitation of movement of the joint. She had visited relatives in Northern California in July about 3 months ago. Neither she nor her parents recall an illness when visiting in California. You suspect arthritis, a manifestation of late, disseminated Lyme disease. The diagnostic test of choice to confirm the diagnosis is:

(A) culture of joint fluid for *Borrelia burgdorferi*

(B) EIA on serum for *B. burgdorferi* antibody

(C) polymerase chain reaction on serum to detect *B. burgdorferi* DNA

(D) urine antigen detection for *B. burgdorferi*

18. Of the following, the most appropriate antibiotic for treatment of Lyme arthritis in the 10-year-old girl is:

(A) azithromycin

(B) ceftriaxone

(C) doxycycline

(D) trimethoprim-sulfamethoxazole

Answers

1. **(D)** *S. pneumoniae* is the most common cause of primary peritonitis in children with no underlying immune or anatomic defect. Less common causes include other gram-positive organisms (*S. aureus*, group B streptococcus) and a variety of gram-negative organisms such as *E. coli* and *Klebsiella* species.

Table 103-1   CLASSIFICATION AND ETIOLOGY OF PERITONITIS IN CHILDREN

Classification	Setting	Etiologic agents
Primary	Intact gastrointestinal tract	
	1. Bacteremia	1. Spn, *S. aureus*, GBS
	2. Nephrotic syndrome/cirrhosis	2. Spn, enteric GNB
	3. VP shunt/CAPD	3. *S. aureus*, CONS
	4. Vaginitis	4. *N. gonorrhoeae*
	5. Tuberculosis	5. *M. tuberculosis*
Secondary	Defect or rupture of gastrointestinal tract	
	1. Ruptured appendix, perforation of small or large bowel	1. Enteric GNB, enterococcus, and anaerobes
	2. Perforation of stomach	2. Upper respiratory tract and aerobic bowel flora, *Candida* spp.

VP, ventriculoperitoneal; CAPD, continuous ambulatory peritoneal dialysis; Spn, *Streptococcus pneumoniae*; GBS, Group B streptococcus; GNB, gram-negative bacilli; CONS, coagulase negative staphylococci.

N. meningitidis and *N. gonorrhoeae* primary peritonitis has also been reported (see Table 103-1).

2. **(D)** The serum opsonizing activity of children with nephrotic syndrome is decreased. Children with nephrotic syndrome are at greatest risk for pneumococcal sepsis and peritonitis when in relapse and spilling large amounts of protein, which includes factor B of the alternative complement pathway. Children with nephrotic syndrome can also have low serum IgG levels.

3. **(C)** Prepubertal children with gonococcal vaginitis can develop peritonitis. The diagnosis can be confirmed by culture of the vagina for *N. gonorrhoeae*. In this circumstance an evaluation for sexual abuse must be undertaken.

4. **(D)** Gram-positive organisms including *S. epidermidis* and *S. aureus* account for 50% of episodes. Gram-negative organisms account for 20% and fungal peritonitis occurs in 2% (see Table 103-1). The classic triad of peritonitis in CAPD is fever, abdominal pain, and pleocytosis of the peritoneal fluid.

5. **(D)** There is no one historical item or diagnostic test that will identify all children with occult bacteremia. Fever greater than 103.1°F (39.5°C) age 3 to 36 months and a leukocyte count >15,000/ mm^3 increase the risk of occult bacteremia. The most common etiology of occult bacteremia is *S. pneumoniae*. *H. influenzae* type b was the second most common cause but has been virtually eliminated with the routine immunization of infants with *H. influenzae* type b conjugate vaccine.

6. **(B)** Late onset disease with *S. agalactiae* should be considered as a cause of occult bacteremia in infants younger than 3 months of age. Meningitis is the most serious complication that can occur as a result of occult bacteremia but osteomyelitis, arthritis, cellulitis, or adenitis can occur. GBS has also been reported to cause bacteremia without a focus. Some of these occult infections have occurred in very low birth weight infants with prolonged hospitalization. This clinical manifestation of group B streptococcus has been termed very late-onset infection.

7. **(A)** SIRS comprises several stages including sepsis, septic shock, multiorgan dysfunction and death. Severe sepsis includes sepsis but evidence of altered organ perfusion (e.g., altered consciousness, oliguria, elevated lactate, hypoxemia, hypotension responding rapidly to parenteral fluids). ARDS is one category of the multiorgan dysfunction syndrome.

8. **(A)** The child fulfills the "classic" diagnostic criteria for Kawasaki disease with fever persisting at

least 5 days plus the presence of at least four of five designated clinical criteria. These include bilateral bulbar conjunctival injection, changes of the lips and oral cavity, erythema and swelling of the hands and feet, and an erythematous rash. One feature the child did not have was one or more enlarged lymph nodes >1.5 cm in diameter. In the presence of more than or equal to four principal features, the diagnosis of Kawasaki disease can be made on day 4 of illness. The diagnosis should be considered in a young child with fever ≥5 days and any of the principal clinical features of the disease. An algorithm has been developed by the AHA and AAP to aid clinicians in deciding which patients with fever and less than four classic criteria should also undergo echocardiography or receive IVIG treatment or both for Kawasaki disease. This includes a combination of assessing whether the patient's characteristics are consistent with Kawasaki disease and assessing a number of laboratory tests including CRP and ESR.

Treatment of Kawasaki disease includes IGIV 2 g/kg given as a single infusion plus an antiinflammatory dose of aspirin, 80 to 100 mg/kg/day in four divided doses. Retreatment with IGIV is recommended for patients with persistent fever for 48 hours after the initial infusion or recurrence of fever after an initial period of being afebrile for 48 hours or less.

9. **(B)** Many infectious agents have been associated with the development of erythema multiforme minor (involvement of no more than one mucosal surface). However, *M. pneumoniae* is the most convincingly demonstrated cause of erythema multiforme and Stevens-Johnson syndrome.

10. **(A)** Brucellosis is prevalent in the Mediterranean basin, India subcontinent as well as Mexico and Central and South America. Malaria occurs in tropical climates and Salmonellosis in the form of typhoid fever usually is related to travel in a developing country in the 6 weeks prior to illness onset. *Bartonella henselae* causing cat scratch disease occurs sporadically throughout the United States. *B. bacilliformis* occurs in a restricted geographic region in the Andes Mountains in Western South America. The acute form is a febrile illness with high mortality and is called Oroya fever. This is a

bacteremic illness resulting in severe hemolytic anemia and transient immune suppression.

11. **(A)** The definition of FUO includes a minimum of 14 days of daily temperature of 100.9°F (38.3°C) or greater with no cause, after performance of repeated physical examination and screening laboratory tests. Infections account for more than one-third of cases of FUO, and in general are common infections with an uncommon presentation. In a recent series of children with FUO, Epstein-Barr virus infection, vertebral and pelvic osteomyelitis, cat scratch disease and urinary tract infection were the most common infections described.

12. **(B)** The likelihood of establishing a diagnosis in a child with FUO is low in patients with a normal erythrocyte sedimentation rate and hemoglobin value.

13. **(D)** Other disorders causing periodic, recurrent, or episodic fevers include periodic fever, aphthous stomatitis, pharyngitis, and adenitis (PFAPA syndrome), relapsing fever caused by *Borrelia recurrentis*, and Familial Mediterranean fever. Kikuchi-Fujimoto disease is a histiocytic necrotizing lymphadenitis and is in the differential diagnosis of regional or generalized lymphadenopathy that may present as an FUO but not as a periodic fever syndrome.

14. **(D)** There are many infectious and noninfectious diseases that cause generalized lymphadenopathy. Both *Salmonella typhi* and *Y. enterocolitica* can cause mesenteric lymphadenitis. *S. typhi* can cause hepatosplenomegaly and generalized lymphadenopathy although the lymphadenopathy of *Y. enterocolitica* is seldom generalized. Generalized lymphadenopathy can occur in association with *E. chaffeensis* which causes human monocytic ehrlichiosis, a tick-borne disease.

15. **(A)** The 7-year-old fulfills the Jones criteria for the diagnosis of acute rheumatic fever with one major criterion (polyarthritis) found in approximately 75% of cases and two minor criteria (fever and accelerated ESR) along with supporting evidence of antecedent group A streptococcus infection. Figure 103-1 shows a Gram stain of a

broth culture obtained from a β-hemolytic colony from a blood agar plate revealing gram-positive cocci in chains identified as *S. pyogenes* (group A streptococcus). Other major criteria include carditis (50% to 60% of cases), chorea (10% to 15% of cases), erythema marginatum (<3% of cases) and subcutaneous nodules (1% or less of cases).

16. **(C)** The neonate described above with rash and splenomegaly also has nephrotic syndrome and anemia. Nephrotic syndrome occurs in infants with congenital syphilis and is caused by immune complex disease. The negative RPR may be secondary to the prozone phenomenon. This results from excess antibody concentration that inhibits the formation of the antigen-antibody complex that is needed for flocculation. Diluting the same serum and retesting will result is a positive test. The clinical laboratory should be alerted to this possibility. A specific treponemal test such as the FTA-ABS or TP-PA tests should also be positive. Toxoplasmosis is less likely with the normal eye and CSF examinations, and HIV is less likely with the negative HIV ELISA. Infants with symptomatic congenital CMV infection will often have neurologic sequelae, including microcephaly, hypotonia, hearing loss, and seizures.

17. **(B)** The EIA used to detect antibodies against *B. burgdorferi* is usually negative in patients with early localized disease, such as a single erythema migrans lesion. Some patients who are treated early with an antimicrobial agent never develop antibodies against *B. burgdorferi*. Most patients with early disseminated Lyme disease, and all patients with late disseminated disease (arthritis is the most common manifestations) have a strong IgG antibody response to *B. burgdorferi*.

18. **(C)** The antibiotic of choice for late, disseminated disease manifesting as Lyme arthritis is doxycycline for children 8 years and older or amoxicillin for children younger than 8 years of age. The recommended duration of therapy is 28 days, compared with 14 to 21 days for early localized disease. Meningitis, or other CNS disease and carditis, with third-degree heart block should be treated with ceftriaxone for 14 to 28 days.

SUGGESTED READING

Long SS, Edwards KM: Fever of unknown origin and periodic fever syndromes. In: Long SS, Pickering LK, Prober CG (eds): *Principles and Practices of Infectious Disease*, 2nd ed. Philadelphia: Churchill Livingstone, 2003, p 114.

Shapiro ED: Lyme disease. *Pediatr Rev* 19:147, 1998.

Neglect and Abuse

13

CASE 104: A 4-MONTH-OLD INFANT WITH WEIGHT LOSS

A 4-month-old male is brought to the emergency department for evaluation of a cough and a tactile fever. On examination the patient is afebrile and has upper airway congestion, but you immediately note that this child appears small for his age, malnourished with loss of subcutaneous fat, and has an erythematous candidal-appearing diaper rash. The baby is alert, follows well, and appears to have appropriate tone.

The mother states that she has been concerned about her infant's small size and has brought her baby to the doctor requesting advice to help her baby grow, but she has not seen a physician in 4 weeks. The child has been fed standard formula mixed appropriately by the mother since birth and according to mother is a good eater.

The mother is 34 years old and has two other children at home who are well; both are in school and according to mother have no growth problems. You measure the child's weight, head circumference and height, and you plot the values on a growth curve (Figure 104-1 and Figure 104-2).

SELECT THE ONE BEST ANSWER

1. You are concerned about this baby's current state of malnutrition. Your immediate plan is to:

   (A) review the past medical history, inquire about risk factors for immune system disorders, and perform screening tests. You also ask the mother to keep a calorie calendar of daily input and plan to see her and her infant next week

   (B) order screening CBC, metabolic panel, pre-albumin, albumin, ferritin, thyroid-stimu-lating hormone (TSH), and a home visiting health nurse for dietary education and weight assessment

   (C) admit your patient to the hospital for evaluation

   (D) send the child home since your presumptive diagnosis is intrauterine growth retardation because of the symmetry of the growth failure, and change the child's formula to an increased calorie per ounce formula

   (E) send the child for a genetics consultation

2. In order to assess this child's growth, what would be the next important step?

   (A) obtain consent from the mother to review the patient's medical record and growth chart from her pediatrician

   (B) measure the pre-albumin, ferritin, and place a Mantoux test

   (C) obtain a bone age by radiograph

   (D) obtain the sibling's growth charts

   (E) obtain electrolytes with a complete metabolic panel to assess for hydration

3. You are able to obtain your patient's prior growth measurements from his pediatrician and you find the following: birth weight, length, and head circumference were all at the 50th percentile. Only one subsequent visit occurred at 2 months of age when the child was found to be between the 10th to 25th percentiles on the growth chart. True statements regarding growth parameters include the following except:

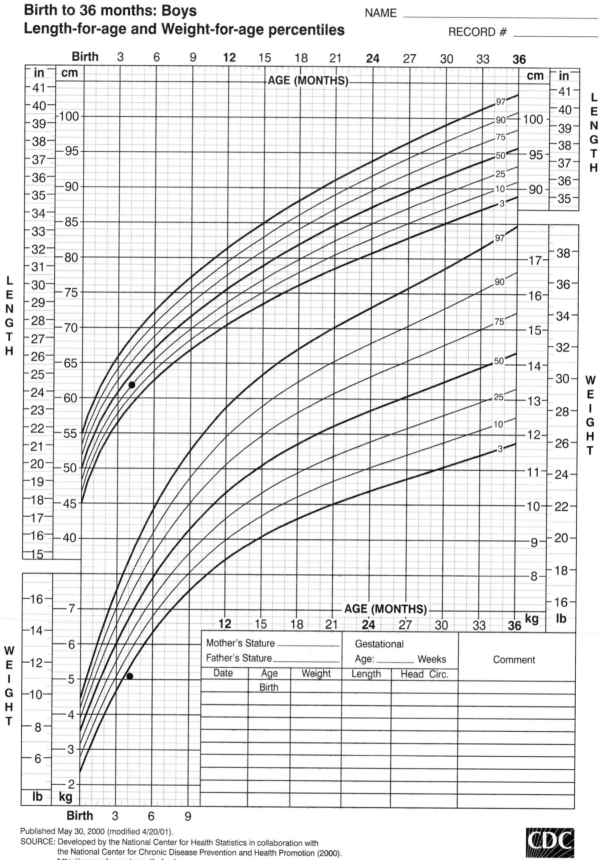

Birth to 36 months: Boys
Length-for-age and Weight-for-age percentiles

NAME _____

RECORD # _____

Published May 30, 2000 (modified 4/20/01).
SOURCE: Developed by the National Center for Health Statistics in collaboration with
the National Center for Chronic Disease Prevention and Health Promotion (2000).
http://www.cdc.gov/growthcharts

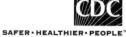

SAFER·HEALTHIER·PEOPLE™

Figure 104-1. Growth charts of 4-month-old infant with weight loss.

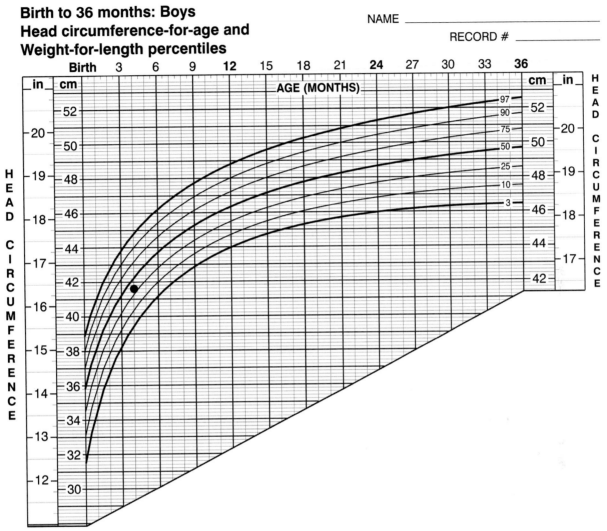

Birth to 36 months: Boys
Head circumference-for-age and
Weight-for-length percentiles

Figure 104-2. *Growth charts of 4-month-old infant with weight loss.*

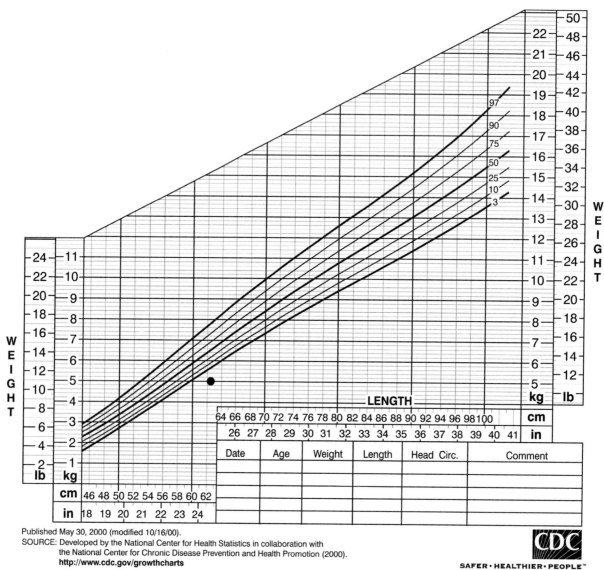

Published May 30, 2000 (modified 10/16/00).
SOURCE: Developed by the National Center for Health Statistics in collaboration with
the National Center for Chronic Disease Prevention and Health Promotion (2000).
http://www.cdc.gov/growthcharts

Figure 104-2. **Growth charts of 4-month-old infant with weight loss.** **(Continued)**

(A) weight for age reflects multiple factors including current and past growth problems

(B) depressed weight for height reflects more acute nutritional deprivation

(C) a depressed height reflects chronic malnutrition

(D) adjustments for prematurity are unnecessary past 1 year of age

(E) assessing the grade of nutrition guides both management and intervention

4. True statements regarding examination and laboratory evaluation for children with failure to thrive (FTT) include all of the following except:

(A) all children with FTT should have baseline metabolic evaluation, HIV, sweat test, thyroid studies, screening EKG, and stool for parasites

(B) short children should have a bone age performed

(C) the physical examination aids in identifying findings suggestive of chronic illnesses and potentially growth-retarding syndromes

(D) laboratory testing is guided by history and physical examination

(E) evaluation for gastrointestinal (GI) abnormalities should be considered in children with unexplained vomiting

5. True statements regarding FTT management include all but the following:

(A) ensuring appropriate nutrition for a child with FTT incorporates both catch-up and maintenance nutrition

(B) the amount of expected growth of a normal child varies with age

(C) heavy prenatal exposure to alcohol is associated with microcephaly and short stature

(D) demonstrating growth with provision of adequate nutrition in the hospital suggests a diagnosis of "nonorganic" FTT

(E) optimizing management includes an interdisciplinary approach, daily intake evaluation, and integration of the family in understanding the goal of a hospital admission for FTT evaluation

6. Parental competency is affected by all of the family characteristics except:

(A) parental resources

(B) maternal mental health

(C) lack of college education

(D) child characteristics

(E) family social context

7. The most common form of child maltreatment is:

(A) physical abuse

(B) sexual abuse

(C) infanticide

(D) neglect

(E) lack of supervision

8. The number of annual reports made nationally to a child abuse hotline is:

(A) 3 million

(B) 60,000

(C) 1 million

(D) 2 million

(E) 5 million

9. During your evaluation of the child with FTT, you find out that the mother has just moved into a domestic violence shelter and discloses that up until this recent move, her partner had been limiting her ability to purchase food and access medical care for her baby. During the hospitalization the mother is engaging with the child and the child takes nutrition well from the mother. She has just obtained a protective order from the courts with regard to her partner. All of the following are true except:

(A) in some jurisdictions the only access to necessary services for this mother is through a child welfare referral

(B) all children with FTT are required by law to be reported to child welfare services

(C) protective service intervention with placement out of the home of the child may be necessary in noncompliant family situations to enhance parental compliance

(D) referral to a child protection agency is warranted when safety cannot be ensured in the current environment

(E) foster care placement has a potential for suboptimal placement

10. The most common risk factor for FTT in a child is:

(A) maternal depression
(B) poverty
(C) prematurity
(D) poor oral motor skills
(E) maternal drug use

11. A skeletal survey is performed and a healing clavicle fracture is found. The following is a true statement:

(A) the finding of a fracture on the skeletal survey is diagnostic of child abuse
(B) clavicular fractures in toddlers are rare and should raise suspicion of child abuse
(C) because of the finding of a clavicular fracture, a head CT and ophthalmologic exam should be ordered
(D) a thorough history of the caretakers is warranted to assess whether there is an adequate explanation for this injury
(E) sternal fractures are the most common abusive injury in infants

12. On examination you note two healing lesions. They are dime-sized, scabbed over "mirror images" on each buttock. You are worried that these are because of cigarette burns. The mother denies smoking or hurting her child. Which of the following statements is false?

(A) Skin conditions such as impetigo can mimic abusive lesions.
(B) "Accidental" contact burns are often brushed burns and not ovoid.
(C) Intentional cigarette burns are ovoid and first-degree burns.
(D) The healing patterns of intentional cigarette burns differ from the scars that result from skin infection.
(E) Abusive burns are found more often in younger children; they are more serious and require longer hospital stays.

13. Four months after you evaluated and reported a child for suspected child abuse, you receive a subpoena to appear in juvenile court. Which of the following is true?

(A) The standard of proof is equal to criminal proceedings.
(B) The standard of proof is preponderance of evidence.

(C) Subpoena duces tecum is a subpoena that requires you to testify only.
(D) You should prepare an opinion for the court as to what your findings were.
(E) You are obligated to contact the family and inform them of your testimony.

14. The 4-month-old gains weight in the hospital. His siblings, who are 2 and 4 years of age, are evaluated and found to have mild malnutrition but have not seen a physician in more than a year. With regard to neglect, all of the following are true except:

(A) neglect is a failure to meet a child's needs with regard to food, shelter, or clothing, and medical, emotional, and educational needs
(B) neglect has variable manifestations
(C) often neglect is defined in terms of acts of omission by the caretaker
(D) harm or potential injury as a result of omission is often the basis for laws defining neglect
(E) lack of supervision is not a category of neglect

15. Medical conditions that will interfere with caloric intake and retention include all of the following except:

(A) GI conditions
(B) infections—e.g., parasitic GI tract infestation or urinary tract infection (UTI)
(C) renal tubular acidosis
(D) HIV
(E) prenatal exposure to marijuana and cocaine

16. Effective management of child neglect must rely on a systematic and thorough approach by the clinician. Which of the following is not a true statement regarding the management of child neglect?

(A) In order to initiate intervention, the clinician must convey to the family his or her specific concerns and show an interest in assisting the family.
(B) Early engagement of the child welfare system will ensure intervention.
(C) The clinician must recognize that intervention often requires long-term investment, support, and case tracking.

(D) Early efforts by the clinician should assess family and community supports and assessment of the available services.

(E) Development of a care plan with the family outlining efforts needed by the family and concrete plans for follow-up involving the family's input and agreement is a fundamental management step.

17. Your patient required a short admission and your final diagnosis was FTT. Your understanding of the etiology of this case had to do with social factors affecting safety and access to appropriate food and medical care. The mother now has a protective order, has moved to a shelter, and the children have all been assessed as well. Which of the following is a true statement about disposition of children with FTT?

(A) Most infants with FTT require transitional placement in foster care until the caretaker can demonstrate ability to care for the child.

(B) Assessment of the family's willingness, ability, and insight determine the disposition of the child with regard to child welfare contact and home disposition.

(C) Child welfare systems have well-developed interdisciplinary interventional models that include medical expertise, case management, and legal and mental health services to provide longitudinal interventional services for children with FTT.

(D) Children with FTT do not benefit from early interventional services as a result of the brain development insults from starvation.

(E) Catch-up growth often requires nasogastric or gastrostomy tube placement and feedings.

18. Which of the following require an immediate report to child welfare?

(A) a 15-month-old who has missed his last two immunization visits

(B) a 9-month-old who rolled off the bed and sustained a bruise to his forehead when his mother fell asleep

(C) a 12-year-old with Ewing's sarcoma who has failed two rounds of chemotherapy. His prognosis for recovery with an experimental regimen is poor and the parents refuse treatment

(D) a 10-year-old with sickle cell disease presents in aplastic crisis with a hemoglobin of 3 g/dL. The parents refuse transfusion because they are Jehovah's Witnesses

(E) a 2-year-old admitted for ingestion of his grandmother's cardiac medication

Answers

1. **(C)** This baby has "failure to thrive" that warrants immediate evaluation, which includes a review of family history, including assessment for potentially growth-retarding family illnesses such as cystic fibrosis (CF), celiac, inflammatory bowel disease or lactose intolerance, and HIV risk. The parent's height and weight and any family history of growth delay should be elucidated. A psychosocial assessment should also be obtained looking for stressors, domestic violence, or mental illness and a review of access resources. Prenatal and perinatal issues, e.g., low birth weight or drug exposures, are known to be predictors of FTT.

2. **(A)** To assess the child's current growth status it is important to obtain all prior growth measurements. Measurements are used to identify children with growth failure, guide treatment, and also aid prognostically. It is very important that measurements are performed appropriately, e.g., the same scale for weights. Infants and toddlers should be weighed without clothing and older children weighed in underwear. Growth measurements at one time point are difficult to interpret; what is most important is to assess growth over time or lack of it. The rest of the diagnostic evaluation must be guided by history and physical examination once FTT has been established. The most important guides to evaluation are the history and physical findings. The other answer choices in the question are potentially correct based on the initial findings, e.g., a pre-albumin would be helpful in assessment of a severely malnourished infant, the ferritin level may be indicated in an iron-deficient child, a bone age is appropriate in a child with short stature, and electrolytes are most often useful when a child is clinically dehydrated. In severe malnourishment, hypokalemia can be seen.

3. **(D)** Weight for age reflects multiple factors including current and past growth problems and is the single most powerful predictor of mortality compared with other measurements. Depressed weight for height reflects more acute nutritional deprivation, and a depressed height reflects chronic malnutrition. Growth chart adjustment for prematurity depends on both the severity of the prematurity and which growth index is being adjusted. Correction for prematurity may take up to 3 years of age. Adjustment for weight often takes 2 years postnatally; head circumference 18 months and length can take up to 40 months.

4. **(A)** An FTT evaluation must be directed by history and physical examination findings. There is no standard screening protocol. It is important to focus the workup to diagnose occult diseases and to assess any metabolic derangements causing FTT. All children should have a CBC, consideration for lead exposure, and a urinalysis to assess possible renal tubular acidosis. Metabolic testing, e.g., electrolytes, glucose, BUN, and creatinine should be considered in children with vomiting and diarrhea. Children who are severely malnourished should have a total protein, albumin, calcium, alkaline phosphatase (low in zinc deficiency), and a phosphorus level if rickets is of concern. Consideration of HIV, cystic fibrosis, or GI tract infection should be considered in "at-risk" populations, and food allergies should be considered in children with skin manifestations, e.g., urticaria or other rashes. If a child has unexplained respiratory symptoms, a GI evaluation for reflux should be considered. Children with medical diagnoses associated with FTT or children who have swallowing dysfunction warrant an oral motor evaluation.

5. **(D)** Unfortunately, there are current beliefs that demonstration of growth in the hospital is diagnostic of "nonorganic" FTT, that children with chronic and serious medical diseases do not grow and that those with "environmental FTT" will grow in the hospital. In reality, those inferences are too simplistic and imprecise. Growth is expected for most children with FTT if given appropriate nutrition and administration. Therefore growth in the hospital is not a definitive test to distinguish between nonorganic versus organic FTT. It is important for the medical community to self-educate and to train the child welfare community that the diagnosis of FTT is more complex than demonstrating growth, and that demonstrating growth is a poor discriminator of major organic disease from purely "environmental" causes of FTT. FTT is usually defined as a child whose growth is less than expected, with the weight falling below the fifth percentile, weight for height falling below the 10th percentile, or the weight falling across two major percentiles over time. The proximate issue with children with FTT is that they are malnourished. The etiology of this growth failure must be considered from a nutritional, medical, developmental, and social perspective. It is imperative that catch-up growth is considered along with required daily intake. Expected growth is based on age. An infant is expected to grow 25 to 30 g daily, a 3- to 6-month-old 17 to 18 g daily, a 6- to 9-month-old, 12 to 13 g daily, a 9- to 12-month-old 9 g daily, and a 12+-month-old 7 to 9 g daily. In most circumstances children will need 1.5 to 2 times their expected oral intake to catch up. It is known that heavy prenatal exposure to alcohol is associated with microcephaly and short stature.

6. **(C)** All of the family characteristics are important to assess in children with a FTT diagnosis. Effective treatment will need to incorporate this information by addressing the stressor that incites or hinders growth. A psychosocial perspective should be a core component of an FTT evaluation.

7. **(D)** The most common form of child maltreatment is neglect, based on national reporting data collected by the National Child Abuse And Neglect Data System (NCANDS 2001).

8. **(A)** Based on national data, 3 million children are reported to the child welfare system annually and about one-third of these reports are substantiated. Nearly 56% of the reports were made by a mandated reporter.

9. **(B)** It is an incorrect statement to state that *all* children with FTT must be reported to child welfare. There are many children who have growth-limiting illnesses and by definition fit the

diagnosis of FTT. It is very important to assess the family's strengths and ability to provide a child with the necessary environment to improve growth; if, in the judgment of the clinical team, a child requires out-of-home placement because the child is in jeopardy or if monitoring by child welfare and obtaining services and support would enhance compliance and therefore growth, child welfare referral and reporting are indicated.

10. **(B)** Poverty is the single most common risk factor associated with neglect and therefore FTT. The other factors listed are associated as well, but less strongly.

11. **(D)** Assessing findings on a skeletal survey must include a review of past medical history to elucidate if this was a documented and evaluated injury with treatment in the past. The relative suspicion for an injury to be associated with abuse is based on the child's age and the injury, e.g., a clavicular fracture in a toddler with a history of a fall is low suspicion unless there are mitigating issues. Conversely, a sternal fracture is rare and would absolutely warrant a meticulous evaluation.

12. **(C)** Healed round or ovoid lesions are often cigarette burns. Cigarette burns that are inflicted are usually ovoid and deep, partial-thickness burns that leave a scar. They are about 1 cm in diameter. Round, nonspecific lesions that are hypopigmented are often indeterminate in terms of etiology. In this case, the location of the lesions that are mirror images or kissing lesions on the buttocks raises the question of an infectious etiology, e.g., bullous impetigo. Key to making a diagnosis is eliciting a good history from the caretakers as to the presentation, age, and timing of the lesions' appearance, as well as healing and associated symptoms at the time of presentation.

13. **(B)** When a physician receives a subpoena, he or she must recognize that the subpoena is a court order and cannot be ignored. The subpoena may ask for the physician to testify, which is a subpoena ad testificandum, or it may ask for the doctor to appear and bring records or documents. A subpoena that requests documents is called a subpoena duces tecum. The judgment

standard required in civil or family court is "preponderance of evidence," i.e., more likely than not. In criminal court, the judgment standard is "beyond reasonable doubt." An expert witness provides testimony that is either an opinion, an answer to a hypothetical question, or an educational process, e.g., lectures on a given subject. The doctor who receives a subpoena as a treating physician will be asked questions with regard to his or her evaluation, e.g., historical findings, medical tests, and diagnosis. The judge must be convinced that the expert possesses sufficient knowledge, skill, and experience to qualify.

14. **(E)** Lack of supervision is an identifiable form of neglect. Child neglect is the failure to meet a child's medical, emotional, environmental, and education needs. Broadly defined it does not discuss resource or intent of the parent. Neglect should be viewed within a societal and cultural context. The potential of a lack of supervision must be recognized as potentially fatal. It is important for the pediatrician to be familiar with his or her jurisdiction's legal definitions and recognize that not all catastrophic outcomes are because of negligence. On the other hand, pediatricians have a unique opportunity to help screen preschool age children who are at risk for neglect and abuse.

15. **(E)** Although prenatal exposure to alcohol and opiates can lead to microcephaly and alcohol is associated with short stature (in addition to other characteristics of fetal alcohol syndrome [FAS]), cocaine and marijuana are not currently accepted explanations for postnatal growth failure. The medical evaluation should be based on family history, medical history, and physical examination.

16. **(B)** Effective management of child neglect must employ a systematic and thorough approach by the clinician. Intervention often requires a long-term investment. Assessment using social services is often a successful strategy to engage the family and develop a care plan. Depending on the circumstances that lead to a neglect concern, child welfare referrals for services without a report are possible in some states. Timely reporting of children who are at risk for harm where

the physician either feels he or she cannot assess the level of risk, or where the initial assessment is that the family is not invested in a care plan does push the response toward a consideration of formal reporting to child welfare authorities.

17. **(B)** Unfortunately, child welfare systems vary in their expertise with regard to interventional services for FTT and physicians should not assume that child welfare systems have integrated programs replete with medical expertise to provide a long-term care plan for children with FTT. Children with FTT do benefit from early interventional services, another system for monitoring and engagement with the family. Enteral feedings may be necessary for catch-up growth, but the need for this intervention depends on many factors.

18. **(D)** A 10-year-old with sickle cell disease who presents with life-threatening anemia warrants life-sustaining intervention and will require the treating team to take protective custody to treat this child in crisis. The process for this should be known by the physician in advance as it will vary by geographic locale.

SUGGESTED READING
Dubowitz H, Giardino A, Gustavson E: Child neglect: Guidance for pediatricians. *Pediatr Rev* 21:111–116, 2002.

Reece RM, Ludwig S, et al: *Child Abuse: Medical Diagnosis and Management*. Philadelphia: Lippincott, Williams & Wilkins, 2001.

CASE 105: A 2-YEAR-OLD WITH A BURN

A 2-year-old African-American female presents with her aunt for evaluation of a sharply demarcated burn to her right lower leg. The patient is in pain but consoled when sitting in her aunt's lap. On examination, the child has sustained a burn to the left lower extremity in a stocking distribution (Figure 105-1). The child is alert and appears to be in good health.

1. Which of the following descriptions is most consistent with your exam?

   (A) 5% to 10% first-degree scald burn
   (B) 3% to 5% partial-thickness scald burn

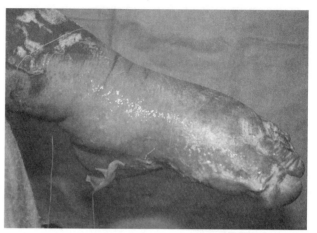

Figure 105-1. Scald burn to the lower extremity of a 2-year-old. See color plates.

   (C) 5% partial-thickness flame burn
   (D) 9% second-degree contact burn
   (E) 5% to 10% chemical burn

2. Which of the following statements about the depth of a burn is not true?

   (A) The depth of a burn is an important determinant of severity, management, and potential complications.
   (B) A first-degree burn or superficial partial-thickness burn is painful. They are confined to the epidermis and are red because of an inflammatory response in the skin. Healing occurs in 3–5 days without scar formation.
   (C) A second-degree burn is a partial-thickness burn that involves the epidermis and the dermis. The involvement of the dermis distinguishes between a superficial partial-thickness versus a deep partial-thickness burn where the superficial burn involves less than half of the dermis, has blisters, redness, and swelling; it takes about 2 weeks to heal with minimal scar formation.
   (D) Fourth-degree burns are third-degree burns with secondary infection.
   (E) Full-thickness burns involve destruction of the epidermis and dermis. They are pale, nontender, and cannot heal because they cannot re-epithelialize. Grafting is required in most of these burns.

3. Appropriate immediate management of this patient would include:

(A) debridement, application of silver sulfadiazine cream, and discharge to follow up with a plastic surgeon

(B) debridement, application of 1% silver sulfadiazine cream, admission, and oral hydration

(C) IV hydration, hospitalization, prophylactic oral antibiotics, and pain management

(D) IV hydration and pain control, wound management, and surgical consultation

(E) IV hydration, wound management, IV antibiotics, and consultation with child welfare

4. Which is a true statement regarding burn injuries and children?

(A) Children make up one-half to two-thirds of all burn admissions annually.

(B) The most frequent type of burn in children younger than 4 are electrical burns.

(C) Nearly 25% of burns in children are life threatening.

(D) Flame burns related to cooking injuries are responsible for the majority of thermal injuries in children younger than 4 years of age.

(E) The risk of thermal injury in children may be reduced by lowering the water heater temperature to 120°F (48.8°C).

5. The aunt does not know the child's immunization status; the mother is currently unavailable by phone. Because of the seriousness of this burn you elect to do which of the following?

(A) Initiate antibiotic prophylaxis to protect against streptococcal infection.

(B) Administer tetanus toxoid.

(C) Administer tetanus immune globulin.

(D) Administer tetanus toxoid and immune globulin.

(E) Provide local wound care at this point.

6. Once the child is stabilized, you start to obtain a more extensive history of the injury. According to the aunt, who was the caretaker of this child when the injury occurred, she had just boiled water to use to wash the floor because her hot water heater is broken. She had the hot water in a bucket on the floor in the kitchen. She thought the child was napping and went to get the mop from the closet when she heard the child crying and found her lying on the floor. She examined

the child, took her sock off, and found that her foot was red. She ran the child's foot under cold water. Blisters started to appear and she called 911. No one else was home at the time of the injury, but the aunt did run to the next apartment to ask her neighbor to help as they waited for the ambulance. The next appropriate management steps would include the following:

(A) call the neighbor to corroborate the history

(B) inform the caretaker that you are a mandated reporter and you are obligated to contact the regional child welfare agency

(C) call the regional child welfare agency and not inform the aunt about the report so that she does not have time to contact her neighbor

(D) admit the child and have the hospital social worker continue the investigation

(E) perform a skeletal survey; if the skeletal survey is negative, the suspicion of abuse is ruled out

7. You elect to admit this child and have a consultation with a burn specialist. On your examination, the child is well nourished and developmentally appropriate and there are no other cutaneous lesions of concern. The specialist concurs that the burn is a superficial partial-thickness burn that involves all surfaces of the skin, with the bottom of the foot minimally involved. Treatment will include hydrotherapy and wound management. What tests with respect to the child abuse investigation are warranted at this point?

(A) skeletal survey, head CT, and ophthalmologic eye examination

(B) a complete trauma evaluation, including a complete blood count, coagulation studies and sickle cell screen, liver function, pancreatic enzymes, and urinalysis

(C) vaginal cultures

(D) skeletal survey and MRI

(E) skeletal survey

8. The mother comes to the hospital and is appropriately upset about her child's injury. Her interaction with the child appears appropriate. Upon obtaining more information from the mother, you learn that an aunt has been caring for this child for more than 2 years and they are well bonded. The child is in the midst of toilet train-

ing and doing very well under the aunt's guidance. You also learn that the aunt cares for three other children during the week, all in the preschool age group. Which of the following statements about risk factors for child physical abuse is false?

(A) Children with child-related stressors including developmental disability or behavior problems are at increased risk for child abuse.
(B) Developmentally related stressors, e.g., colic and toilet training, appear to be stressors related to child abuse.
(C) Unrelated caretakers are more likely to abuse children than relatives.
(D) Social or situational stressors that are risk factors for physical abuse of children include social isolation, poverty, family discord, and violence.
(E) Parental stressors include prior abuse, depression, and substance abuse.

9. All are true statements about inflicted burns except:

(A) inflicted cigarette burns are round, vary in depth, and are often seen on the distal extremities; once healed, one can often appreciate a crater effect
(B) a burn with a symmetric stocking or glove distribution without splash marks is highly suspicious of being inflicted
(C) non-inflicted spill or splash burns often show an inverted tree–like pattern, with the depth of the burn worse at the initial site of contact
(D) the classic inflicted burn lesion is the immersion burn where the buttocks and/or extremities are held and restrained from moving in hot water
(E) patterned contact burns are the most common forms of inflicted burn injury

10. Which of the following statements regarding electrical burns in children is correct?

(A) The most serious form of electrical burn in children is exposure to high-voltage electric shock (>1000 V).
(B) Electrical burns in the home are from contact with low-voltage alternating household current (120 V).

(C) Current preferentially flows through tissues with less resistance, e.g., blood vessels, nerves, and muscles, and moisture decreases the resistance.
(D) A common injury to toddlers is when they suck on extension cords and sustain an electrical burn to the lip and mouth.
(E) Management of electrical burns is different than management of scald or contact burns because less skin surface area is involved.

11. The skeletal survey is negative and your review of the prior medical history reveals no prior injuries and normal development along the 75th percentile. The police and child welfare system interview the neighbor and the 911 emergency responders and investigate the scene. They corroborate that the water heater was not working at the time of the injury. When determining whether an injury is accidental versus inflicted, the following directly impact your determination except:

(A) type of injury
(B) age and developmental ability of the child
(C) physician's experience and training in the treatment of children with suspected child abuse
(D) mechanism provided by the caretaker to explain the injury
(E) prior involvement of the caretaker with child welfare system

12. Which characteristic should not be taken into consideration when differentiating between inflicted and non-inflicted bruises?

(A) age of the child
(B) pattern of the lesion
(C) location of the bruise on the child's body
(D) depth of the bruise
(E) skin disorder or condition

13. Doctors are often asked to date bruising. Which is the most accurate statement regarding this issue?

(A) Bruises of the same age in the same individual will be the same color at the same time.
(B) Skin color, location, amount of force, and local healing effects all impact the color changes as a bruise heals.
(C) There is a predictable order of color change progression as bruises heal.

(D) A bruise with yellow coloration must be at least 6 hours old.

(E) Mongolian spots are a form of healed bruise.

14. A new patient has blue to gray discoloration over the lower sacral area and the side of the head. You note no pattern to these lesions and the mother states they have been there since birth. You are concerned that they are bruises. To aid in your diagnosis, you:

(A) send the child to see a dermatologist for an assessment

(B) order a CBC and bleeding studies

(C) re-examine your patient in 2 weeks

(D) apply topical steroid cream

(E) order a skeletal survey

15. Which is an incorrect statement regarding human bites?

(A) Human bites may be a manifestation of child abuse.

(B) Dental impressions are an important tool to aid in the identification of the person who caused the bite in suspected cases of abuse.

(C) Adult bite marks look different than those of a child.

(D) Swabs of the bite marks should be obtained to assess the flora of the perpetrator's mouth.

(E) The physician is advised to obtain photo documentation of the bite mark in suspected child abuse cases.

16. One form of child abuse is Munchausen syndrome by proxy (MSBP), where the child is a victim of abuse as a result of the fabrication of illness in the child. All of the following define MSBP except:

(A) the mother, in the majority of the cases, is the perpetrator

(B) in most cases the child has a history of prematurity or a chronic disease

(C) the illness is produced or simulated (symptoms are fabricated) by a parent or someone who is *in loco parentis*

(D) the child repeatedly presents for medical care, inevitably resulting in multiple medical procedures that are unnecessary

(E) the parent denies knowledge of the cause of the illness

17. True statements regarding the diagnosis and outcome of MSBP include all of the following except:

(A) separation of the child from the parent-perpetrator will result in the symptoms disappearing

(B) covert video is a strategy to diagnose MSBP when the method of production of the symptoms is a result of an overt act by the parent, e.g., smothering, contaminating IV lines

(C) in the majority of cases the mother will confess to simulating the illness

(D) siblings are often at risk

(E) most cases go undiagnosed

18. The intention of foster care is to be a temporary situation that provides respite to a family in crisis. Which of the following is true regarding foster care?

(A) Parents must terminate their guardianship or custodial rights at the time a child is placed in foster care.

(B) The goal of foster care includes family reunification.

(C) The length of stay a child has in foster care does not impact the likelihood of family reunification.

(D) Children who have been abused by their parents feel safer in foster care.

(E) Reimbursement for foster care parents is based on the care difficulty and mental health demands of the child.

Answers

1. **(B)** The most consistent description of this burn is a 3% to 5% partial-thickness (second-degree) scald burn involving the lower left extremity in a stocking distribution. The percent surface area involved is based on age. At 16 years of age the rule of 9s can be used to estimate involved surface area. The rule of 9s at 16 years old is that surface area is 9% for the head and neck, anterior trunk 18%, and the posterior trunk 18%. Each leg is 18%, each arm is 9%, and the anorectal region is 1%.

Use of a body reference chart to estimate surface area is important to guide subsequent management for patients younger than 18 years.

2. **(D)** Fourth-degree burns are burns that are third-degree but also involve the fascia, muscle, or bone. Deep partial-thickness burns involve the epidermis and the majority of the dermis. These burns can be paler, less tender, and speckled because of edema, sensory receptors, and thrombosed vessels. They are difficult to distinguish from full-thickness burns and can evolve into full-thickness burns if they are hypoperfused or become infected. Scarring often occurs and these burns can take weeks to heal. Evolution into a full-thickness burn can occur because of infection or hypoperfusion.

3. **(D)** Burns involving the hands, face, eye, ears, feet, or perineum are considered major burns and warrant a surgical evaluation. IV hydration requirement is based on the burn's percent surface area and depth as well as other factors, e.g., pain control. In general, IV fluid resuscitation is warranted for children with either a 15% partial-thickness or 10% full-thickness burn. In this particular case, the combination of pain management and burn location justifies placement of an IV. Patients with burns that are minor or moderate, e.g., less than 10% body surface area, or full-thickness less than 2% where there are no concerns for child abuse, compliance, or other health risks, may be discharged home with follow-up.

4. **(E)** Decreasing the temperature of water heaters to 120°F (48.8°C) is a preventive strategy that decreases the risk of thermal injury. At 130°F (54.4°C) it takes 10 to 30 seconds of exposure to cause a partial- to full-thickness burn. Reduction to 120°F (48.8°C) increases the exposure time to several minutes in order to cause a thermal burn. Children make up one-third to one-half of hospitalizations for burn injury annually, and the most common burn type in children younger than 4 are scald burns. Three to five percent of all burn injuries in children are life threatening.

5. **(E)** Because this child is only 2 years old, and because tetanus immunization is required if there has not been immunization in the last 5 years, providing local wound care until the immunization status can be ascertained is the correct answer. An unimmunized child requires tetanus immune globulin. Empiric treatment for streptococcal infection is no longer warranted because of the routine use of topical antibiotics in burn care.

6. **(B)** The history the caretaker gives appears to be consistent with the injury sustained. The burn is in a stocking distribution but there are no splash burns noted. The burn is also consistent with a possible dunk or immersion that could have been intentional. By contacting the child welfare system and providing them your opinion that this could be consistent, you allow investigational agencies to corroborate many of the historical details you obtained, e.g., that the heater was broken, the neighbor was contacted, and the caretaker had called 911 within the time frame she provided.

7. **(E)** At this point a skeletal survey would be the best choice. With regard to the evaluation for suspected child abuse, your examination can guide you to necessary tests. On examination this child is alert and well nourished. Her mental status is normal so you can assess for other traumatic injuries clinically, e.g., evidence for acute brain injury or acute abdominal trauma. If, while obtaining prior medical information, there is concern for an old intracranial injury (e.g., a change in head circumference), one can obtain a head CT. If the child starts to show symptoms such as vomiting, a workup for an occult CNS or GI injury can be ordered. At this point a skeletal survey alone would be the best choice.

8. **(C)** Epidemiologically speaking, related caretakers are more likely to abuse children than unrelated caretakers.

9. **(E)** The most common inflicted injury will be a scald injury.

10. **(E)** Although they may not affect as much surface area, electrical burn injuries are more extensive than what can be visualized. The injuries are often internal and depend on the voltage and pathway of the electrical current. Myoglobinuria and renal failure can be anticipated with major elec-

trical injuries and management should include monitoring for cardiac arrhythmias.

11. **(E)** Prior involvement of the caretaker with the child welfare system may impact the disposition of the case, but it does not prove or disprove if a specific injury was inflicted. Distinguishing between an inflicted and non-inflicted injury should be based on the consistency of the history provided with the sustained injury. A collaborative and comprehensive multidisciplinary approach among child welfare, police, and medical staff with training and expertise in child abuse assessment is necessary to increase the likelihood of a correct decision.

12. **(D)** All of the characteristics are important to consider; depth of the bruise is not a characteristic that can be assessed on exam. The age of the patient is important as young infants with bruises should lead the doctor to inquire and ensure that the bruises are adequately explained since truly accidental bruising is rarely found in infants.

13. **(B)** Assessing the age of a bruise is a very imprecise process. Many factors affect the rate of healing and resulting color changes, and bruises in the same person that are of identical age and mechanism may not appear the same on examination. One study indicated that yellow discoloration implies at least 18 hours of healing, but it must be emphasized that aging of bruising is very imprecise. A physician can, however, comment on patterns, location, and, in some circumstances, varying ages between healed bruises or between old lesions and new ones.

14. **(C)** These lesions are most likely Mongolian spots or birth marks because the mother states that the child has had them since birth. Bruising is transient and will heal so re-examination at a later time will elucidate the diagnosis. Mongolian birth marks are most often seen in Asian and African-American children and disappear by 4 years of age.

15. **(D)** Saline swabs should be obtained from a fresh bite in order to perform forensic analysis, not to ascertain the flora of the perpetrator's mouth. The adult bite pattern is different than that of a child's in that the adult bite will usually only show one arch and it will only contain dentition marks between the canine teeth. Children's bite marks often will exhibit both arches and include the molars. Photo documentation including a ruler for measurement is invaluable for forensic investigation.

16. **(B)** All of the other answers define Munchausen syndrome by proxy, first described by Sir Roy Meadow in 1977.

17. **(C)** The perpetrators in Munchausen syndrome by proxy rarely confess on their own volition.

18. **(B)** The ultimate goal of foster care is family reunification.

SUGGESTED READING

Fleisher GR, Ludwig S, et al: *Pediatric Emergency Medicine*. Philadelphia: Lippincott, Williams & Wilkins, 2000.

Hansbrough JF, Hansbrough W: Pediatric burns. *Pediatr Rev* 20:117–123, 1999.

Reece RM, Ludwig S, et al: *Child Abuse: Medical Diagnosis and Management*. Philadelphia: Lippincott, Williams & Wilkins, 2001.

CASE 106: AN 8-MONTH-OLD INFANT WITH IRRITABILITY

A colleague contacts you requesting advice regarding her 8-month-old girl who has been very fussy for 2 days. The child has been sleepier, irritable, intermittently vomiting, and less consolable than usual. She has had no fever although frequently has felt warm to touch. Your colleague also thought she saw some tremors on one occasion. The pediatrician diagnosed a viral infection and instructed her to encourage fluids and use an antipyretic as necessary. You ultimately agree to evaluate your colleague's child.

During your assessment you find out that the girl is a first-born child, a product of a 36-week gestation, born by vaginal delivery without complications. The child is breast-fed; mother does pump breast milk so that her daytime caretaker can provide breast milk exclusively. The child has grown well and developmentally there have been no concerns to date.

On examination, her vital signs are stable; she appears mildly dehydrated and has no fever. She is sleepy but arousable; her eyes remain closed. She seems to be more irritable with holding, and her fontanel appears full but not tense. Her pupils are equal and reactive, tone appears symmetric, no murmurs are appreciated, lung fields are clear, abdomen is soft without any masses, and her skin shows no lesions. You advise your colleague that a sepsis evaluation is warranted. The spinal tap yields bloody fluid on two attempts. The white count is 7600/mm³, the hemoglobin is 9.5 g/dL, and the hematocrit is 29.6%. A urinalysis, blood electrolytes, and glucose measurements are normal. You elect to admit the patient for observation and empirically treat for sepsis.

SELECT THE ONE BEST ANSWER

1. Based on this child's history and examination, all of the following tests are indicated except:

   (A) head CT
   (B) abdominal ultrasound
   (C) skeletal survey
   (D) toxicologic screen
   (E) EEG

2. You are concerned that this child may have been abused; you attempt a funduscopic exam but the child is uncooperative. Which of the following statements is true?

   (A) The lack of retinal hemorrhages on examination rules out the diagnosis of inflicted head trauma.
   (B) Retinal hemorrhaging because of abuse is most often bilateral.
   (C) Examination by an ophthalmologist is indicated.
   (D) A neurologically intact child will not have retinal hemorrhages.
   (E) Cardiopulmonary resuscitation is known to cause retinal hemorrhage.

3. A head CT is performed and the results show an acute (high-intensity signal) subdural hemorrhage along the right cerebral convexity (Figure 106-1). You provide this information to your colleague. In the process of obtaining more history, your colleague shares with you that the child fell off the bed 3 days ago. Which of the following is true?

   (A) Subdural hematomas are pathognomonic for inflicted head trauma.
   (B) Household falls from furniture most commonly result in subarachnoid and parenchymal bleeding.

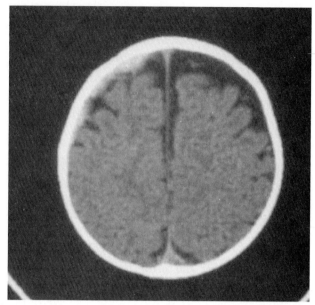

Figure 106-1. **Head CT of 8-month-old with irritability.**

   (C) A CT scan is superior to MRI to detect subarachnoid bleeding.
   (D) MRI is the study of choice to detect a skull fracture.
   (E) Epidural hematomas occur because of rotational forces on the skull, most prominently in the occipital region.

4. A skeletal survey has been performed. Which statement is incorrect?

   (A) A skeletal survey includes 14 to 19 views of the skeletal system.
   (B) A babygram is sufficient to perform as a screening tool for abuse.
   (C) A skeletal survey is indicated for children who are younger than 2 years of age with suspicion of child maltreatment.
   (D) A bone scan is inferior to a skeletal survey to age skeletal trauma.
   (E) Radiograph images of the hands and feet are not warranted in children younger than 1 year of age.

5. Which statement about inflicted traumatic brain injury is false?

   (A) Inflicted head trauma is the most common cause of death in traumatically injured infants.
   (B) About 2000 cases of traumatic brain injury annually are because of inflicted injury.

(C) The peak incidence of inflicted traumatic brain injury coincides with the peak incidences of colic, from 6 weeks to 4 months.

(D) Female babysitters are the most common perpetrators of inflicted head trauma.

(E) Physicians can "miss" a diagnosis of traumatic brain injury because of the lack of external evidence of trauma.

6. Which is not a predisposing factor for inflicted head trauma?

(A) the relatively large head size of an infant in proportion to the rest of the body

(B) open anterior fontanel

(C) high water content of the brain

(D) disparity of size between caretaker and child

(E) helplessness of the baby

7. A skeletal survey is performed on the patient and callous formation is seen on three ribs. Which of the following is true?

(A) The time to form callus observable on radiograph is 7 to 10 days.

(B) Acute rib fractures are easily visualized by radiograph.

(C) Bone scan can assist in aging the fractures.

(D) Rib fractures are a common form of birth trauma seen in children delivered by cesarean section.

(E) The rib injuries and head trauma occurred at the same time.

8. Which is a true statement about classic metaphyseal fractures?

(A) Treatment includes provision of a posterior mold and rest.

(B) They are initially painful with movement.

(C) They occur in soccer and hockey players.

(D) They result from a planar fracture through the region of the metaphysis where it is contiguous to the physis.

(E) High-risk locations for metaphyseal lesions are the wrist and hand joints.

9. Of the injuries listed below, which bone fracture is the most suspicious bone fracture for abuse and always warrants an investigation?

(A) a healing rib fracture found on radiograph of a premature baby in the NICU

(B) a spiral femur fracture in a 5-year-old

(C) a skull fracture in an 8-month-old after a witnessed fall

(D) an unwitnessed buckle or torus fracture of the distal radius of a 7-year-old

(E) a 6-month-old with a humeral fracture that occurred after being dropped by a sibling

10. Select the factor that would not raise concern that an injury is more likely inflicted.

(A) delay in seeking care

(B) discrepancies in the history provided by caretakers

(C) inconsistency between the history and the child's developmental abilities

(D) parent smells of alcohol or appears intoxicated

(E) injury was said to be caused by a sibling or self-inflicted

11. You inform your colleague that your diagnosis is inflicted head trauma and skeletal injuries. Which of the following steps is not necessary?

(A) Contact the regional child welfare system and report this as a case of suspected child abuse.

(B) Document in the medical record your history, physical, results of studies, and your impression.

(C) Restrict all visitation to the child until the investigation is completed in order to protect the child from further potential harm.

(D) Provide materials to investigational authorities according to your hospital protocols and state law.

(E) Offer the child welfare system and police investigators assistance in assessing other children in the current caretaker's environment.

12. On further investigation you find out that the baby had an admission for a gastroenteritis 1 month prior to this presentation. Choose the most appropriate statement below.

(A) Children diagnosed with abusive head trauma rarely have episodes of prior traumatic brain injury.

(B) Further evaluation of this child would include an MRI and imaging of the GI system.

(C) An evaluation for glutaric aciduria is warranted.

(D) The most common presentation of inflicted head trauma is cardiopulmonary arrest.

(E) The treating physician should obtain consent to review these prior medical records to re-evaluate the given diagnosis and findings.

13. Which statement accurately reflects the mechanism of inflicted head trauma?

(A) Impact from a fall less than 3 feet can cause serious life-threatening traumatic brain injury.

(B) Shearing injury because of acceleration-deceleration forces leads to the disruption of bridging veins and development of subdural bleeding; shearing of other tissue interfaces can cause brain damage.

(C) Lack of impact findings, e.g., bruising on examination, rules out an impact injury.

(D) Tin ear syndrome is caused by an isolated linear impact injury.

(E) The force required to cause shaking injuries is mild and within the realm of normal caretaking behavior.

14. Identify the abusive injury *not* associated with violent shaking.

(A) retinal hemorrhages
(B) rib fractures
(C) axonal brain injury
(D) diaphyseal fractures of the long bones
(E) subdural hematomas

15. Which is a true statement about the outcomes for children with inflicted traumatic brain injuries?

(A) Mortality is low from abusive head trauma.

(B) Neurodevelopmental delays are expected and careful follow-up is required.

(C) The infant brain is pliable and will regenerate after insult.

(D) Brain injuries are mostly motor-based impairments.

(E) Cognitive and behavioral delays are rarely seen in children with significant traumatic brain injury.

16. Which is a true statement regarding the Glasgow Coma Scale (GCS) system and the assessment of the severity of head trauma in children?

(A) There are three categories of head trauma (minor, moderate, and severe), which are based on CT findings.

(B) Three clinical examination categories are the basis for the GCS.

(C) The GCS scoring system ranges from 0 to 15.

(D) The GCS system uses clinical findings and assigns the same points for adults and children.

(E) The GCS system is not widely used for assessment of head trauma in children.

17. Which is an erroneous statement regarding the treatment of serious head trauma?

(A) Initial focus on adequate hemodynamics and oxygenation is imperative.

(B) Intubation and ventilation are indicated for children with a GCS <8.

(C) Cervical spine immobilization should be considered in the initial assessment and ensured in children with a mental status change.

(D) Immediate imaging of the head should include an MRI to delineate the extent of gray matter injury.

(E) Maintenance of cerebral perfusion pressure and lowering of high intracranial pressure are the main goals of treatment of a severe head injury.

18. Your colleague, her domestic partner, and the babysitter are being investigated because of your diagnosis of abusive head trauma and skeletal injuries. Which is the best statement regarding outcome from traumatic brain injury?

(A) Based on the initial GCS, which was >10, her child should have no long-term sequelae from the brain injury.

(B) Infants and children with brain injury have better outcomes because of the plasticity and myelination of the brain compared to older children with the same injury.

(C) Long-term cognitive, behavioral, and/or neurological deficits are common in children who have sustained inflicted head trauma and warrant close follow-up care.

(D) Children who show a normal neurological examination after serious brain trauma will have no long-term effects.

(E) Prophylactic administration of anticonvulsants seems to correlate with better behavioral outcome in children with serious head trauma.

Answers

1. **(B)** This patient's clinical examination and history lead to a differential diagnosis that includes entities that would cause mental status change in a child. CNS infection, central trauma, ingestion, and dehydration are the most likely causes of her clinical state. On exam she is not significantly dehydrated and her electrolytes are normal. Therefore, there seems to be no metabolic derangement. Because the lumbar taps yielded grossly bloody fluid, and because of the history of tremors, a head CT is warranted. Although the child does not have a classic toxicologic syndrome, a standard toxicology screen is appropriate as is a review of medications in the home. The depressed mental status, irritability, anemia, and grossly bloody lumbar tap put head trauma high on the differential, and a skeletal survey would be indicated even if the initial head CT was negative. The child also seems to be uncomfortable with movement; this paradoxical finding could indicate central infection or be because of an acute injury, e.g., an acute skeletal injury. An abdominal ultrasound does not aid in the evaluation of this child; if abdominal trauma was being considered, ordering liver enzymes, an amylase and lipase, as well as an abdominal CT to rule out a duodenal hematoma or a solid organ injury would be appropriate.

2. **(C)** Examination of a child for retinal hemorrhages requires the expertise of an ophthalmologist who can dilate the child's eyes and perform a thorough exam of the retina. Ophthalmologic exam in this case reveals bilateral retinal hemorrhages (Figure 106-2). The ophthalmologist will be able to document the number of hemorrhages, the layers they are contained in, and their extent. The ophthalmologist will also look for retinoschisis (a tear of the retina). Retinal hemorrhages are not necessary to diagnose traumatic brain injury and they can be bilateral or unilateral. Classic findings for inflicted brain injury are retinal hemorrhages that involve multiple layers and extend out to the periphery. Retinal hemorrhages can last for weeks after an injury. After a

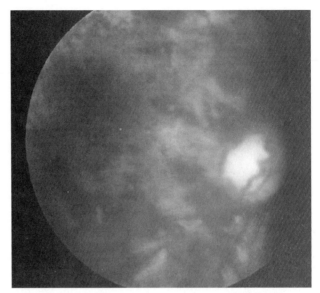

Figure 106-2. **Extensive retinal hemorrhages. See color plates.**

period of healing, a child can appear well on clinical exam. An evaluation for retinal hemorrhages would be warranted if head trauma was suspected. Current data support the notion that CPR does not cause retinal hemorrhaging.

3. **(C)** A head CT scan is more likely than an MRI to demonstrate an acute subarachnoid bleed. The preferred neuroimaging in a child with suspected head trauma should be a CT scan because of its availability and the ease with which it can be obtained. It will also be valuable as serial CT scans are often used to assess progression of a central finding. An MRI is indicated after the initial head CT in children with central injury because it is able to detect intracranial hemorrhages in various stages and also to delineate the location of extraaxial hemorrhages (e.g., subdural vs. subarachnoid bleeding). The significance of a subdural hemorrhage must be analyzed within the context of the child's examination, patient's clinical status, and the history of the injury. It is important not to label a subdural bleed as pathognomonic for inflicted trauma. Epidural hemorrhages are because of impact injuries. A skull radiograph is the best study to visualize a skull fracture; skull fractures may also be seen on CT depending on the direction of the fracture in relation to the CT slices. If the fracture is parallel to the cuts of the CT it may be missed. Most household falls do not

cause any injury more than a skin contusion or subgaleal bleed. A skull fracture in the temporo-parietal area can result from an impact injury; it is also possible, but rare, to see an impact-induced subdural hemorrhage.

4. **(B)** A babygram is not sufficient to evaluate a child for occult skeletal injury; clinically relevant injuries such as metaphyseal injuries will be missed. A complete skeletal survey includes 19 views: AP views of the skull, thorax, pelvis, humeri, forearms, femurs, tibias, and feet, lateral views of the skull, cervical spine, thorax, lumbar spine, and oblique views of the hands. A bone scan augments a skeletal survey in that it can visualize injuries that are too acute to be seen on a skeletal survey and can aid in elucidating the difference between a normal variant and a traumatic injury. However, a bone scan is limited in its ability to age injuries and it requires injection of a radionuclide. The child must be still or sedated and the scan must be directed by a radiologist to ensure that the correct images are obtained. Improper views or images result in an inability to visualize injuries related to abuse in children.

5. **(D)** Male caretakers are at greater risk to inflict traumatic brain injury in an infant.

6. **(B)** All the choices except B are thought to increase the susceptibility of the infant brain to inflicted brain trauma.

7. **(A)** Depending on many factors, rib fractures will be visualized by radiograph in 7 to 10 days. Acute rib fractures will not be visible by radiography until there is healing and new bone formation. As this continues with callus formation, rib fractures become visible. A technetium bone scan can visualize acute rib fractures within a few days of the injury but there are limitations of this study as well, i.e., it is more labor intensive, involves an injection, and cannot assist in aging the injury. Rib fractures are not known to result from cesarean section delivery. Because the rib fractures are calloused and the mental status changes appear to be more acute, the head and rib trauma appear to have been inflicted at different times. It is important to acknowledge that our ability to age bleeding in the extra-axial space is limited.

8. **(D)** Classic metaphyseal fractures of the long bones, e.g., bucket handle fractures or chip fractures, are injuries that are highly specific for child abuse. The mechanism for these injuries in infants is the application of rotational forces generated as an infant is shaken by the trunk or when the child's extremity is used as a handle for shaking the child. Classic metaphyseal injuries are not painful and do not require treatment. They occur near the joints of the long bones.

9. **(E)** The age of the patient and the belief that a sibling was allegedly responsible for the injury make "E" the best choice. Fractures in nonambulatory children should raise concern. A thorough investigation should be initiated to ensure the injury is well explained.

10. **(D)** Delay in seeking care, discrepancies in the history of the injury, injuries caused by a sibling, and inconsistencies between the child's developmental abilities and the sustained injury focus investigational efforts toward evaluating the consistency of the injury and the history. If a parent is disheveled or smells of alcohol, this has implications with regard to child welfare issues, but this does not diagnose an inflicted injury.

11. **(C)** Protection of a child who is hospitalized and being investigated for child maltreatment from further injury is a priority for the hospital and medical staff. Restriction of the parents is generally not necessary.

12. **(E)** Because this child has healing rib fractures, one would want to review the medical presentation and evaluation of the prior gastroenteritis. The diagnosis of inflicted head trauma can be missed by the treating physician because of the lack of external findings of trauma; the symptoms of central nervous system injury can often masquerade as a viral syndrome or gastroenteritis. A study by Jenny et al. indicates that 30% of children with abusive head trauma had a prior head injury that was not diagnosed.

13. **(B)** Many studies show that minor falls from less than 3 feet do not cause significant intracranial injury. The lack of a cutaneous finding of an im-

pact does not rule out an impact injury. Tin ear syndrome involves rotational injuries and includes unilateral internal ear injury and intracranial bleeding. The force necessary to cause traumatic brain injury, e.g., shaken baby syndrome, is out of the realm of normal caretaking behavior and resuscitation efforts.

14. **(D)** Diaphyseal fractures are not typical of the shearing injuries associated with violent shaking of an infant, although classic metaphyseal fractures are.

15. **(B)** Abusive head trauma is the leading cause of death because of trauma in infancy. All children with brain trauma need to have high-risk developmental follow-up because of irreversible brain injury, which may be manifested as cognitive delays or behavioral problems.

16. **(B)** The Glasgow Coma Scale is a universally used assessment tool to aid in assessing the severity of a central injury. The scale has three examination categories: eye, motor, and verbal response. Scores range from 3 to 15. Rules for use of the GCS system differ based on age of the patient.

17. **(D)** A head CT scan should be the first line of imaging, not an MRI.

18. **(C)** Cognitive impairment is difficult to assess in this child because the diagnosis of traumatic brain injury was occult. This differs from the situation with witnessed or "accidental" brain injury where the mechanism of injury is clear. In this circumstance the amount of time before medical intervention is sought decreases the likelihood and extent of secondary brain injury (e.g., development of cerebral edema and injury from untreated hypoxia).

SUGGESTED READING

Jenny C, Hymel KP, Ritzen A, et al: Analysis of missed cases of abusive head trauma. *JAMA* 282(7):621–626, 1999.

Rainer G: Head trauma. *Pediatr Rev* 22:118, 2001.

Reece RM, Ludwig S, et al: *Child Abuse: Medical Diagnosis and Management*. Philadelphia: Lippincott, Williams & Wilkins, 2001.

CASE 107: A 6-YEAR-OLD WITH VAGINAL DISCHARGE

A 6-year-old female is brought to your office for evaluation of malodorous blood-tinged vaginal discharge. The mother noted scant discharge on her daughter's underwear for 1 week. The child has not had any fever, although she did have a stomachache 1 week ago. There was no history of vomiting, diarrhea, constipation, or dysuria. The child has taken more frequent baths for the last 3 weeks because she is now participating in sports. She lives with her mother and sister; her parents are divorced but she does have weekend visits with her biological father. She has been a good student, although after the divorce her school performance declined. The mother feels her daughter is currently doing well at school.

On physical examination the child is well nourished with stable vital signs. She is quiet, yet willing to answer questions. The head and neck, respiratory, and cardiovascular examinations are normal. Her abdomen is soft and nontender. You order a urinalysis and urine culture; the urinalysis shows 10 to 15 white blood cells/HPF and 5 to 10 red blood cells/HPF. You culture the urine.

SELECT THE ONE BEST ANSWER

1. Which is an appropriate next step toward evaluating this patient?

   (A) Presumptive treatments with oral antibiotics until the culture results are confirmed.
   (B) Advise baths without bubble bath and reassure that the discharge is nothing more than a response to irritation from harsh soap.
   (C) Provide the child with a topical steroid and instruct application to any areas of vaginal redness.
   (D) Interview the mother and child with regard to concerns for sexual abuse.
   (E) Refer the child to an advocacy center or contact the child welfare system to evaluate for suspected abuse.

2. The differential diagnosis for vaginal bleeding in this age group includes all but the following:

   (A) vulvovaginitis
   (B) precocious puberty
   (C) foreign body
   (D) trauma
   (E) labial adhesions

3. Which is a true statement regarding genital examinations in prepubertal females?

   (A) Insufficient labial traction to adequately visualize the hymenal margins and vestibule is a common examination error.
   (B) Examination in the frog leg position with feet together is optimal to visualize the posterior hymenal area.
   (C) Sedation is often required to examine prepubertal girls.
   (D) Examination should be performed without a caretaker, allowing the child an opportunity to make a disclosure or reduce embarrassment.
   (E) Speculum examination is indicated if there is concern for a foreign body.

4. You interview the child and mother separately. The mother has noticed that the child has been quieter lately and not complaining of any vaginal or abdominal pain; she has no concerns about the father sexually abusing her child. You interview the child and she makes no disclosure regarding sexual abuse. A true statement regarding the presentation of child sexual abuse is:

   (A) specific signs and symptoms for sexual abuse include rectal or genital bleeding, developmentally unusual sexual behavior, and the presence of an STD
   (B) an STD in this child is diagnostic of child sexual abuse
   (C) sexual abuse represents 25% of all confirmed cases of child maltreatment
   (D) penetration defines child sexual abuse
   (E) sexual play is determined by the parents' standards of behavior

5. Which is a correct statement regarding findings indicative of child sexual abuse on examination?

   (A) A fimbriated hymen is suspicious for child abuse.
   (B) Children who have experienced penetration will not have a finding on genital examination in the majority of cases.
   (C) Hymenal diameter is a sensitive measure for child sexual abuse.
   (D) Hymenal tears are frequently seen in straddle injuries.
   (E) An intact hymen rules out child abuse.

6. The normal patterns of the prepubertal hymen include all of the following except:

   (A) crescentic
   (B) fimbriated
   (C) annular
   (D) septate
   (E) congenital absence of the hymen

7. On examination of your 6-year-old patient you find that she is not cooperative to perform a thorough genital examination. You note that she has a malodorous discharge and some dried blood on her labia. At this point what would be the best management?

   (A) The examination is consistent with a straddle injury; reassure the mother that this is a normal injury for her child's age.
   (B) Obtain vaginal cultures for gonorrhea and chlamydia. Presumptively treat for an STD and contact the regional child welfare system.
   (C) Arrange for an exam under anesthesia.
   (D) Reassure mother this is a hygiene issue and schedule an appointment in 2 weeks.
   (E) Attempt re-examination with support staff who can hold the child in place.

8. You are now examining a different 6-year-old with a chief complaint of finding drops of blood on her underwear. There have been no complains of dysuria, history of trauma, fevers, or discharge. On genital examination you note a purplish doughnut-shaped mass that obscures the vaginal opening. Which of the following is true?

   (A) This condition is mostly seen in Caucasian children.
   (B) Sudden or recurrent increases of intra-abdominal pressure are felt to be precursors for this condition.
   (C) The child should immediately be referred to an oncologist.
   (D) This is a prolapsed hymen and warrants immediate treatment by a gynecologist.
   (E) Surgery is required to correct this problem.

9. A 9-year-old is seen in your clinic for recurring abdominal pain. This pain is described as lasting for 4 months, intermittent, and periumbilical.

She has had no history of fever, vomiting, mouth sores, weight loss, joint pain, or rashes, although she has intermittent diarrhea. The pain does not interfere with her activity. Examination reveals a normally developing 6-year-old. The most correct choice is:

(A) obtaining ESR, CBC, stool for occult blood, culture, ova and parasites, and urinalysis
(B) referral to a regional child abuse advocacy center because of suspicions of child sexual abuse
(C) empiric administration of an anti-reflux medication
(D) order an upper GI to rule out juvenile peptic ulcer disease
(E) referral to a psychiatrist for antidepressants

10. In your clinic you have a 15-year-old female who presents with a 4-day history of nausea, vomiting, and diffuse lower abdominal pain. She has had fever, no diarrhea, and denies dysuria. She has a history of irritable bowel syndrome, which has been under control per her mother. She denies sexual activity when her mother is in the room. Her menstrual cycles have been regular and she just started her menses about 1 week prior to this visit. On exam her neck is supple, she has no oral lesions, but she does have right upper quadrant pain and lower abdominal tenderness. You interview the patient alone and she admits to sexual activity. You perform a pelvic examination and she is tender on cervical and adnexal examination. You obtain cultures. The most likely diagnosis is:

(A) chronic pelvic inflammatory disease (PID) because of chlamydia infection
(B) gonococcal cervicitis
(C) appendicitis
(D) mesenteric adenitis
(E) Fitz-Hugh Curtis syndrome

11. Which of the following is false statement regarding the Fitz-Hugh Curtis syndrome?

(A) Perihepatitis or Fitz-Hugh Curtis syndrome develops in 5% to 20% of women with acute salpingitis.
(B) Liver function tests are usually abnormal in Fitz-Hugh Curtis syndrome.

(C) Causative agents include chlamydia trachomatis, *Neisseria gonorrhoeae*, anaerobes, and mycoplasma.
(D) Complaints of upper right quadrant pain because of Fitz-Hugh Curtis may continue weeks after the lower abdominal pain has resolved.
(E) The risk of ectopic pregnancy because of tubal closure is a sequela of PID.

12. A 5-year-old is brought to your office with a complaint of vaginal discharge that can be seen on her underwear for 1 week. She has no fever, has had no rashes, but does complain that it hurts when she urinates, although she has no frequency or urgency. A true statement about vulvovaginitis in prepubertal girls is:

(A) nonspecific vulvovaginitis accounts for the majority of vulvovaginitis in prepubertal girls and often is related to poor hygiene
(B) candida is a common cause of prepubertal vulvovaginitis
(C) specific pathogens for complaints of vulvovaginitis are mostly a result of STDs
(D) estrogenization produces vaginal discharge seen in infants and prepubertal girls
(E) immune evaluation should be considered in prepubertal girls who have a specific respiratory and enteric pathogen causing vulvovaginitis

13. All of the following are diagnostic of child sexual abuse except:

(A) culture-positive gonorrhea infection
(B) non-perinatally transmitted (or transfusion acquired) HIV or syphilis
(C) disclosure by child of sexual abuse
(D) *Condyloma acuminata* (anogenital warts)
(E) documented presence of semen or sperm

14. Which is a true statement about straddle injuries to children?

(A) Straddle injuries are seen in nonambulatory children.
(B) Penetration in the majority of cases will exhibit hymenal injuries.
(C) Bruising or laceration near or between the labia majora and minora can occur.

(D) Straddle injuries often involve the posterior hymenal area.

(E) Boys with straddle injuries often have anal tears.

15. A mother brings her 8-month-old female infant in to see you because she noted on examination of her daughter's vagina that she "does not look right down there." She is worried the baby was possibly sexually abused. You examine the child's genital area and note that she has labial adhesions. A true statement regarding labial adhesions is:

(A) the urethral opening is always obscured in labial adhesion

(B) if there is no urinary obstruction, topical estrogen is an optional treatment

(C) the child needs immediate referral to a urologist due to the relationship of labial adhesions and urinary tract anomalies

(D) labial adhesions in this age group are most often a result of sexual abuse

(E) the first line of treatment for labial adhesion is surgical

16. A 9-year-old boy presents with a history of anal pain for 3 days. He has complained of a painful perianal rash, pain with defecation, and his mother noted blood on his stool last night. Your history reveals that his 6-year-old sister just recovered from a sore throat and your interview with mother reveals no concerns for a traumatic injury or sexual abuse. On examination, the child is cooperative. The eyes, ears, throat, lung, and skin examination are all normal. Examination of his anal region reveals a very erythematous perianal rash without ulcers. You also note one or two superficial rectal fissures. Which of the following is true?

(A) Streptococcal infection in the anogenital region is very suspicious of child sexual abuse and a report to child welfare is indicated.

(B) Topical treatment with a steroid cream is indicated.

(C) A rectal swab used for enteric pathogens will detect streptococcal infection.

(D) Streptococcal skin infections are not painful.

(E) Group A β-hemolytic streptococci can cause balanitis and vulvovaginitis.

17. Anal dilatation is a concerning finding for suspected child sexual abuse. Which of the following is not true?

(A) Stool in the vault can cause anal dilatation.

(B) A history of encopresis can be associated with anal dilatation.

(C) A child who has been in the knee-chest position for more than 30 seconds may have a dilated anal opening.

(D) Digital examination of the anus most often is the method that can elucidate if there has been acute trauma.

(E) Venous congestion is a normal finding on anal examination.

18. Which is a true statement regarding the role of the pediatrician in child sexual abuse evaluations?

(A) Each state has it own standards with regard to when a pediatrician must report a suspected case.

(B) Pediatricians are advised to keep minimally detailed documentation in reported cases because, in court, information may be used to discount the doctor's findings.

(C) The more explicit the record keeping the less likely a physician may have to testify in civil court where the legal standard for evidence is "preponderance of evidence."

(D) If a pediatrician is concerned that a child is sexually abused based on a behavioral change, e.g., new-onset enuresis in a 6-year-old, or a nonspecific physical finding, e.g., labial adhesion or vaginal rash, he or she is mandated to report their concern to regional authorities.

(E) Referral to a child advocacy center or regional multidisciplinary teams should only occur when there is sufficient physical evidence to support child sexual abuse.

Answers

1. **(D)** The next appropriate step would be to interview the caretaker and child separately to elucidate if there are any concerns for sexual abuse. Although at this point there are multiple etiologies to consider that can cause a vaginal discharge in this age group, the topic of sexual

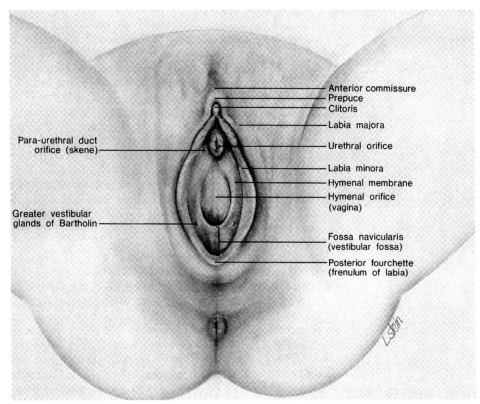

Figure 107-1. **External structures of the female genitalia. (Reproduced with permission from Finkle M, Giardino A: Medical Evaluation of Child Sexual Abuse, A Practical Guide, 2nd ed. California: Sage, 2002, p 46.)**

abuse must be explored with both the child and parent. It is in the purview of the pediatrician to do an initial screening with regard to the possibility of child sexual abuse before referral to a child advocacy center or specialists in the area of child sexual abuse. Vulvovaginitis is not usually blood-tinged or malodorous, and topical treatment without examination is inappropriate.

2. (**E**) In most of the cases of labial adhesions vaginal bleeding is not primary presentation.

3. (**A**) Genital examination of the prepubertal child should have the caretaker in the room in most circumstances to provide support for the patient. Examination rarely should require sedation, and all attempts prior to the examination to explain the examination will often help the child to be cooperative. The physician should ensure that he or she can visualize the inner thighs, the labia majora and minora, clitoris, urethra and periurethral tissues, the hymen and the hymenal opening, the fossa navicularis,

and the posterior fourchette (Figure 107-1). Often it is advised that two positions be used to visualize all of the structures mentioned; both the supine frog leg position and the knee-chest prone position work well. Examining the child prone in the knee-chest position greatly enhances the examiner's ability to visualize the posterior hymenal rim. A speculum exam is not indicated on a prepubertal child even if a foreign body is suspected.

4. (**A**) Ten percent of confirmed cases of maltreatment in children are a result of sexual abuse. Perinatal transmission of chlamydia and HPV, if detected in the newborn period, are not indicative of sexual abuse. The definition of child sexual abuse is not based on penetration; it is operationally and developmentally defined. When children are engaged in sexual activities they don't understand, they are developmentally not prepared and they cannot give consent. These acts violate social taboos and are proscribed by society's, not parental, standards.

5. **(B)** A fimbriated hymen is a normal variant. The majority of children who are sexually abused have a normal examination without sign of trauma, scarring or obvious bleeding, and/or discharge. Our current examination standards do not focus on the diameter of the hymenal opening but on findings specific to the hymenal ring and surrounding structures. Straddle injuries rarely involve the hymen but usually affect more lateral anatomic structures.

6. **(E)** All girls are born with a hymen; congenital absence of the hymen has not been described.

7. **(C)** Any child with a malodorous or blood-tinged discharge deserves a thorough examination. One approach could be to culture this child and if the cultures are negative to perform an exam under anesthesia. Another approach is a direct referral for performance of this procedure depending on your clinical suspicion.

8. **(B)** Urethral prolapse most often occurs in African-American females. A common presentation is vaginal bleeding or spotting. Most of the time urethral prolapse is not associated with tenderness on examination and can be conservatively managed with sitz baths and estrogen cream if the prolapsed area is non-necrotic.

9. **(A)** This child most likely has the syndrome of recurrent abdominal pain. The pain is very real to the patient. Criteria for diagnosis include recurrent pain for more than 3 months, usually female gender, age from 4 to 8 years, normal physical examination, growth, and laboratory testing. The physician should explore with the family detection of stressors that could underlie this entity. Treatment is supportive and, obviously, aimed at trying to modify any perceived stressors.

10. **(E)** The patient described in the vignette presents with a clinical picture for acute PID and, possibly, perihepatitis, the Fitz-Hugh Curtis syndrome. Bilateral lower abdominal pain and tenderness on examination, cervical motion tenderness, and adnexal tenderness may be present. There is usually a history of fever and continuous abdominal pain. Very few patients with PID have unilateral tenderness. Such a finding would warrant consideration of other etiologies such as appendicitis, ectopic pregnancy or urinary tract disease. In general, symptomatic *N. gonorrhoeae* infection is more acute and severe and is usually associated with menses.

11. **(B)** Liver function tests in Fitz-Hugh Curtis syndrome, a complication of acute PID, are usually normal. The risk of tubal closure and, therefore, ectopic pregnancy is significant. With repeated episodes of PID, the risk of infertility increases.

12. **(A)** Nonspecific vulvovaginitis accounts for the majority of vulvovaginitis seen in prepubertal girls. It is related to poor hygiene but also occurs because of the decreased estrogen level. The process is more atrophic in nature and the vulvar skin is more easily traumatized. Normal flora such as *Staphylococcus epidermitis*, α-hemolytic streptococci, diphtheroids, lactobacilli, and gram-negative bacteria may be isolated. Nonspecific treatment involving good hygiene, protective ointments, no harsh soaps, and sitz baths is initially tried to eradicate symptoms. Specific respiratory and enteric pathogens can cause vulvovaginitis (e.g., *Streptococcus pyogenes*, *S. pneumoniae*, *S. aureus*, and Shigella species). Candida species are unusual unless there has been some predisposing condition, e.g., recent antibiotic therapy.

13. **(D)** The presence of condyloma acuminata, anogenital warts, is suspicious for child sexual abuse if they were not perinatally transmitted. The classic lesions are irregular multidigitated wart-like growths. Perinatal maternal-infant transmission has been documented but the time to presentation is variable, with reports up to around 20 months of age. The mode of transmission of HPV, the wart virus, is also unclear and the variable incubation period and subclinical presentation make it difficult to identify the contact source. Any child with the presentation of HPV infection warrants an in-depth family history and assessment for any risk of child sexual abuse. A higher suspicion for child sexual abuse is warranted in children who present with new warts when older than 2 years of age.

14. **(C)** Straddle injuries to the genital region of children are common and rarely involve penetration.

In accidental straddle injuries there is often a history of a fall onto an object to cause a crush injury. Characteristically the injuries are localized to the labia minor and majora and rarely involve the hymenal area or posterior aspect of the fourchette. Ecchymoses on the scrotum or a minor laceration to the penis or scrotum are associated injuries in boys. Straddle injuries are rare in nonambulatory children, rarely involve major trauma, and are rarely associated with coexisting anal trauma.

15. **(B)** If there is no urinary obstruction, in addition to ongoing monitoring by the physician, topical estrogen treatment is an option.

16. **(E)** Group A β-hemolytic streptococci can cause perianal disease, vaginitis, and balanitis. The diagnosis is made by history and culture of the throat and rectum. The culture request must indicate that GAS is suspected so that appropriate culture techniques are used. The pain, itching, and blood-tinged stool are typical; there may also be a family history of recent streptococcal illness that could be the source of the infective organism. Nasopharyngeal carriers and autoinoculation are postulated as the mechanism by which the disease occurs. A throat culture in one study was positive 60% of the time in this type of scenario.

17. **(D)** Venous congestion is a normal finding on anal examination. Stool in the anal vault, a history of encopresis, and a child who sits in the knee-chest position for a period of time will all have normal anal dilatation. A digital examination in a child who has been anally sexually abused often does not reveal any abnormal findings.

18. **(C)** In the United States all pediatricians are required by law to report suspected cases of child sexual abuse. It is highly advised that pediatricians keep detailed records of their evaluation to assist the investigational agencies and for purposes of recreating findings. The more detailed the report, the more likely that a doctor may not have to testify in civil court. Pediatricians should report cases where they have an intermediate or high index of suspicion for child sexual abuse; consultation with regional experts is always encouraged.

SUGGESTED READING

American Academy of Pediatrics, Committee on Child Abuse and Neglect: Guidelines for the evaluation of sexual abuse of children: subject review. *Pediatrics* 103(1):186–191, 1999.

Reece RM, Ludwig S, et al: *Child Abuse: Medical Diagnosis and Management*. Philadelphia: Lippincott, Williams & Wilkins, 2001.

Vandeven AM, Emans SJ: Vulvovaginitis in the child and adolescent. *Pediatr Rev* 14:141–147, 1993.

14

Neonatology

CASE 108: A TERM BABY WITH RESPIRATORY DISTRESS

A baby weighing 3500 g is born at 40 weeks' gestation to a 35-year-old G2P1 mother by emergency C-section for fetal distress and late decelerations. Rupture of maternal membranes occurred 28 hours prior to delivery. Thick meconium stained amniotic fluid was noted at that time. The mother received four doses of ampicillin prior to delivery.

The baby is vigorous at birth. The APGAR scores are 8 and 9 at 1 and 5 minutes, respectively.

SELECT THE ONE BEST ANSWER TO THE FOLLOWING QUESTIONS

1. What is the delivery room management of this patient?

   (A) suction of the oropharynx and nasopharynx by the obstetrician before delivery of the shoulders
   (B) suction of the oropharynx and nasopharynx after delivery
   (C) intubation and suctioning
   (D) A, B, and C
   (E) A and B

2. Shortly after birth, the baby has subcostal and intercostal retractions. The O_2 saturation of room air is 72%. The baby is placed under a 60% O_2 hood with improvement in O_2 saturation to 88% to 92%. What is your differential diagnosis?

   (A) sepsis and/or meconium aspiration
   (B) transient tachypnea of the newborn
   (C) cyanotic congenital heart disease
   (D) A and B
   (E) all of the above

3. What further work-up is indicated?

   (A) chest radiograph and complete blood count with differential leukocyte count
   (B) blood culture and arterial blood gas determination
   (C) glucose measured by Dextrostix
   (D) A and B
   (E) all of the above

4. What is the management of the patient at this time?

   (A) intravenous maintenance fluids
   (B) antibiotics
   (C) monitoring O_2 saturation
   (D) monitoring blood glucose concentration
   (E) all of the above

5. The arterial blood gas (ABG) determination on 60% O_2 delivered by hood reveal: pH 7.35, PCO_2 45, PO_2 52. What are the likely diagnosis/ diagnoses based on those ABG data and the chest radiograph seen in Figure 108-1?

   (A) pneumonia, probably bacterial
   (B) meconium aspiration pneumonitis
   (C) transient tachypnea of the newborn

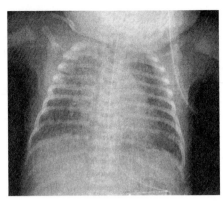

Figure 108-1.

(D) heart disease
(E) A or B

6. After the blood gas result was obtained, the FiO_2 was increased to 1.0; the O_2 saturation was still in the 88% to 92% range. The baby was intubated and mechanically ventilated with an FiO_2 1.0, PIP 25, PEEP 5 rate 60, I-time 0.4. The ABG values were: pH 7.37, PCO_2 40, PO_2 50, MAP 13.

   What other treatment(s) do you want to initiate at this time?

   (A) surfactant
   (B) inhaled NO, 20 ppm
   (C) prostaglandin
   (D) A and B
   (E) B and C

7. What is the next most important diagnostic test?

   (A) echocardiography
   (B) cardiac catheterization
   (C) head ultrasound
   (D) A and B
   (E) no additional diagnostic test is needed

8. The echocardiogram shows a bidirectional shunt at the atrial level, a tricuspid jet of 4.0, bulging of the interatrial septum toward the left side, normal valves, pulmonary veins and aorta, and good myocardial function. These echocardiographic findings are diagnostic of:

   (A) pulmonary hypertension
   (B) cyanotic heart disease
   (C) idiopathic hypertrophic subaortic stenosis (IHSS)

(D) congenital cardiomyopathy
(E) none of the above

9. What is the closest approximation to the pulmonary pressure in mm Hg based on the echo result?

   (A) 8
   (B) 16
   (C) 32
   (D) 64
   (E) 96

10. What factors at birth decrease the pulmonary vascular resistance?

   (A) cold stimulus
   (B) increase in PaO_2
   (C) hypercarbia
   (D) leukotrienes
   (E) all of the above

11. The patient's pre- and postductal O_2 saturation is 90% to 92%. The mean blood pressure is 45 and is very labile. Any intervention makes the O_2 saturation go down to the 70% range. What other treatments do you want to start?

   (A) inotropes and increased ventilatory settings
   (B) more surfactant and increased NO from 20 to 40 ppm
   (C) sodium bicarbonate
   (D) A and C
   (E) all of the above

12. What are the causes of pulmonary hypertension?

   (A) sepsis
   (B) asphyxia or meconium aspiration
   (C) respiratory distress syndrome
   (D) diaphragmatic hernia
   (E) all of the above

13. The ventilatory settings are increased to PIP 35, PEEP 5, rate 60, and I-time 0.4. The mean airway pressure is 15. The ABGs on these settings are pH 7.40, PCO_2 38, and PaO_2 50. What is the oxygenation index of this patient?

   (A) 3%
   (B) 30%
   (C) 33%
   (D) 53%
   (E) 60%

14. Since the PIP is 35 and the PaO_2 is still 50, you are worried about barotrauma and change the ventilator to a high frequency oscillator (HFOV). The ABGs on the HFOV at an FiO_2 1.0, MAP 17, ΔP 35 Hz10, and 20 ppm NO are pH 7.41, PCO_2 35 and PO_2 200. Pre- and postductal O_2 saturation is 100%. The baby does well for a few hours and then desaturates to the 60% range. The heart rate drops to 80 and the mean blood pressure is 28. Immediate management includes all but which of the following?

    (A) check ET placement
    (B) check for pneumothorax
    (C) give intravascular volume expansion
    (D) give surfactant
    (E) all of the above

15. The patient stabilizes after intravenous fluid bolus and an increase in ventilatory settings. In the next few hours, the baby is very labile and requires frequent volume pushes to keep the mean blood pressure in the 60 mm Hg range. Dopamine is being administered at 20 µg/kg/min. The baby desaturates when the mean blood pressure is <50 mm Hg. ABG values on HFOV FiO_2 1.0, MAP 20, ΔP 40, Hz 10 are: pH 7.45, PCO_2 32 and PO_2 48. A chest radiograph shows a ten-rib expansion and no air leak. The cardiothymic shadow is normal. What is the next step in management?

    (A) increase ventilatory settings
    (B) ↑ NO to 40 ppm
    (C) prepare for extracorporeal membrane oxygenation (ECMO)
    (D) all of the above
    (E) none of the above

16. Indications for ECMO are:

    (A) severe meconium aspiration
    (B) cyanotic heart disease
    (C) fulminant sepsis
    (D) A, B, and C
    (E) B and C only

Answers:

1. **(E)** Meconium staining of amniotic fluid occurs in 10% to 15% of deliveries. Meconium aspiration occurs in 1% of these cases. Whenever meconium is noted in amniotic fluid, whether it is thin or thick, obstetricians should suction the infant's oropharynx and nasopharynx before delivery of the shoulders. Babies that are vigorous at birth will not benefit from intubation and suctioning.

2. **(E)** Any of these can cause respiratory distress in a newborn. Babies with transient tachypnea generally do not have retractions. Cyanotic heart disease obviously presents with cyanosis but without the retractions present in this case.

3. **(E)**.

4. **(E)** Any newborn baby with respiratory distress should have a chest radiograph. A sepsis work-up should also be done and the patient should be started on antibiotics. This is especially so in this patient since there is a history of prolonged rupture of membranes that places this child at high risk for infection. Hypoglycemia can present with a wide range of non-specific symptoms. In a term baby with respiratory distress, the aim is to maintain the O_2 saturation at 96% to 100%.

5. **(E)** The chest radiograph shows bilateral scattered infiltrates. The cardiothymic shadow is normal. This fits best with a picture of pneumonitis, etiology uncertain.

6. **(D)** Surfactant administration is recommended for meconium aspiration. Meconium inactivates native surfactant and there is decreased surfactant production following alveolar injury. Inhaled NO is a pulmonary vasodilator. Meconium aspiration syndrome is associated with persistent pulmonary hypertension in many cases. If you are in a hospital where echocardiography cannot be done to rule out cyanotic heart disease, and despite high vent settings and other supportive measures the PaO_2 is low, it is appropriate to start a prostaglandin drip.

7. **(A)** Before making the diagnosis of persistent pulmonary hypertension as the cause of hypoxemia/low PaO_2 in a term baby with respiratory distress, an echocardiogram should be done to rule out cyanotic congenital heart disease.

8. **(A)** In persistent pulmonary hypertension (PPHN), pulmonary pressures remain higher than systemic

pressures, resulting in right-to-left shunting at the ductal or atrial level. In this patient, bidirectional shunting at the atrial level and bulging of the interatrial septum to the left indicates high pulmonary pressure compared with systemic pressure.

PPHN generally occurs in a full-term or post-term infant on day of life 1 with hypoxia and cyanosis. The patient can be very labile. The PaO_2 can increase from 45 to 200 without any change in therapy. If the shunt is at the ductal level, there will be a difference in the pre- and postductal O_2 saturation. This difference in pre- and postductal O_2 blood saturation is not seen if the shunt is at the atrial level or intrapulmonary.

9. **(D)** The pulmonary artery pressure (PAP) is measured by knowing the tricuspid jet pressure. The PAP = $4v^2$ + CVP where v is the tricuspid jet pressure and CVP is the central venous pressure. So PAP = 4×4^2 = 64/mm Hg (approx.).

10. **(B)** Pulmonary vascular resistance is high in the normal fetus because of mechanical factors, low fetal PaO_2 (normal PaO_2 of fetus is 30/mm Hg), increased constrictor stimuli like leukotrienes and endothelin and lack of dilator stimuli like NO. At birth, mechanical distention of the lung, an increase in PaO_2, a decrease in $PaCO_2$ and an increase in pH causes decreased pulmonary vascular resistance. Mechanical distention of the lung helps pulmonary vasodilatation both mechanically and by the production of endogenous vasodilators.

11. **(D)** Inotropes are used in PPHN to increase the systemic blood pressure so that right-to-left shunting will reverse. Increasing ventilator settings and the mean airway pressure will improve oxygenation. Studies in animals have shown that respiratory and metabolic alkalosis lowers pulmonary vascular resistance. There is no consensus about the effectiveness of surfactant use in patients with meconium aspiration. The FDA-approved dose of NO for term babies with respiratory distress is 20 ppm.

12. **(E)** The normal transition from intrauterine to extrauterine life requires a precipitous drop in pulmonary vascular resistance. Any factor that impairs this normal transition can cause persis-

tent pulmonary hypertension. The pulmonary vasculature is very labile in the first few days of life. Active contraction of pulmonary vessels can occur in sepsis, pneumonia, and meconium aspiration. A ventilation-perfusion mismatch may contribute to intraparenchymal right-to-left shunting. In congenital diaphragmatic hernia, pulmonary hypertension is secondary to the associated small cross-sectional area of pulmonary vessels.

13. **(B)** Oxygenation Index (OI) = [Mean Airway Pressure $\times$ FiO$_2$ $\times$ 100]/ PaO$_2$.
    In this patient, OI = [15 $\times$ 1.0 $\times$ 100]/50 = 30%.

14. **(D)** When a patient acutely decompensates, mechanical causes like ET tube placement, the presence or absence of pneumothorax or mechanical factors related to the ventilator should be checked. If mechanical factors are noncontributory, the patient likely has high pulmonary pressure. Any time systemic pressures decreases, there will be right-to-left shunting. Administration of intravascular volume expansion is appropriate to increase the systemic pressure. Surfactant will not help.

15. **(D)** The FDA-approved dose for inhaled NO is 20 ppm. There is a very small subset of patients that do not respond to 20 ppm but respond to 40 ppm. The oxygen intake (OI) of the patient at this time is 41%. An OI >40% is predictive of 80% mortality. If the OI for the next couple of hours remains high then this patient will be a candidate for ECMO.

16. **(D)** ECMO provides cardiopulmonary bypass and is used in babies >34 weeks' gestation that have reversible respiratory or cardiac failure. Since a patient on ECMO needs to be heparinized, babies with IVH or bleeding disorders are not candidates for ECMO. Sometimes ECMO is used for cyanotic heart disease as a bridge to corrective surgery.

SUGGESTED READING:

Hany A: Respiratory disorders in the newborn: Identification and diagnosis. *Pediatr Rev* 25;201–207, 2004.

Konduri GG: New approaches for persistent pulmonary hypertension of newborn. *Clin Perinatol* 31;591–611, 2004.

CASE 109: A PREMATURE BABY WITH RDS AND NEC

A 650-g baby at 26 weeks' gestation is born to a 20-year-old G2P1 mother by vaginal delivery. Mom presented in preterm labor 6 hours prior to delivery. The maternal membranes were intact; mom had no fever. The mother received one dose of betamethasone and one dose of penicillin 4 hours prior to delivery. Serologic tests for syphilis, hepatitis B surface antigen, and HIV were all negative. The baby is depressed at birth with a heart rate of 100 beats/min, and is dusky. The respiratory effort is poor. The patient is suctioned and positive pressure ventilation is given for about 1 minute with improvement in heart rate and color. However, the respiratory effort remains poor. The baby becomes dusky each time bagging is stopped at which time you decide to intubate with a size 2.5 ET tube. The endotracheal tube is secured with tape and bagging is continued with the endotracheal tube in place. The color and heart rate improve. The baby now has some spontaneous respiratory effort and begins to move. The baby is taken to the special care nursery. The APGAR scores are 3 and 7 at 1 and 5 minutes, respectively.

SELECT THE ONE BEST ANSWER TO THE FOLLOWING QUESTIONS

1. Administration of steroids to the mother probably helped the baby.

    (A) Yes
    (B) No

2. What are the problems that you anticipate in the first 24 hours in this premature baby?

    (A) fluid/electrolyte imbalance
    (B) respiratory distress syndrome
    (C) sepsis
    (D) hypoglycemia
    (E) all of the above

3. After admission to the NICU, the baby is put on a ventilator with settings as follows: FiO_2 of 1.0, PIP of 20, PEEP of 5, rate of 40 and I-time of 0.3. The O_2 saturation is in the mid-90% range. The perfusion is good, the mean BP is 28, the heart rate is 140/min and the respiratory rate is 40 to 50/min. The baby has mild to moderate subcostal retractions. What is the differential diagnosis of the respiratory distress?

    (A) respiratory distress syndrome (RDS)
    (B) sepsis
    (C) hypoglycemia
    (D) A and B
    (E) all of the above

4. What is the initial management?

    (A) surfactant administration
    (B) insertion of umbilical lines
    (C) sepsis work-up and antibiotic administration
    (D) IV maintenance fluids and a chest radiograph
    (E) all of the above would be included in the initial management

5. All of the following monitoring is required *except:*

    (A) ABGs and O_2 saturation
    (B) electrolytes, calcium, and glucose
    (C) blood pressure
    (D) bilirubin
    (E) all of the above are required (no exceptions)

6. The baby is under a radiant warmer and receiving 100 mL/kg of IV fluids. The first set of serum electrolytes at 12 hours of age includes an Na 150 mEq/mL, K 5.8 mEq/mL, Cl 108 mEq/mL, and a CO_2 18. What do you want to do?

    (A) Increase fluid administration
    (B) Decrease fluid administration
    (C) Increase Na concentration in the administered fluids
    (D) A and C
    (E) Make no change and repeat electrolytes in 12 hours

7. On day 2 of life the patient's weight is 550 g and the urine output is 1 mL/kg/hr. The ventilatory settings are: FiO_2 40%, PIP 18, PEEP 5, I-time 0.3 and a rate of 40/min. An ABG shows a pH of 7.38, $PaCO_2$ of 38, and a PaO_2 of 95. Serum electrolytes revealed Na 152 mEq/mL, K 5.6 mEq/mL, Cl 110 mEq/mL, CO_2 18, calcium of 6.5 mEq/mL and bilirubin of 4.0 mg/dL. What is the next step?

    (A) Increase fluid administration rate and add calcium to fluids.
    (B) Increase fluid administration rate and add calcium and potassium to fluids.
    (C) Make ventilatory setting changes.

(D) Start hyperalimentation.

(E) A, C, and D

8. On day 3 of life the patient's weight is 570 g and the urine output is 3 mL/kg/hr. The ventilatory settings are: FiO_2 0.3, PIP 16, PEEP 5, I-time 0.3 and a rate of 30/min. IV fluids are being given at 140 mL/kg. Determination of serum electrolytes reveals an Na 148 mEq/mL, K 3.5 mEq/mL, Cl 108 mEq/mL, CO_2 18 and Ca 7.5 mEq/mL. What is the next step?

(A) Increase IV fluids and add potassium.

(B) Administer IV fluids at the same rate and add potassium.

(C) Increase IV fluids and do not add potassium.

(D) No change.

(E) Decrease total fluids.

9. On day 4 of life, the ventilatory settings have increased to FiO_2 0.5, PIP 20, PEEP 6 and a rate of 50/min. On examination, there is an active precordium. The peripheral pulses are full; the blood pressure is 35/16 and, on auscultation, there is a grade II/VI systolic murmur. The hematocrit is 32%. What is the likely diagnosis that explains these changes?

(A) patent ductus arteriosus

(B) systolic murmur secondary to anemia

(C) pulmonary artery hypertension

(D) dehydration

(E) physiologic anemia

10. If an echocardiogram shows a ductus arteriosus of moderate size with left-to-right shunting and a chest radiograph shows bilateral haziness and an increase in the size of the cardiothymic shadow, what would you do?

(A) Restrict fluids.

(B) Give packed RBC to make the hematocrit >40%.

(C) Administer IV indomethacin.

(D) All of the above.

(E) Continue to monitor with no action at this time.

11. IV indomethacin could adversely affect which of the following?

(A) urine output

(B) serum sodium

(C) serum creatinine

(D) all of the above

(E) none of the above

12. After three doses of IV indomethacin, the patient improves. The ventilatory settings are down to FiO_2 30%, PIP 16, PEEP 5, and a rate of 30/min. No murmur is heard. You start nasogastric feedings. After 3 to 4 days, the patient develops abdominal distention and has increased residual feeds. On abdominal examination the baby has some guarding. All would be appropriate actions except:

(A) Make the patient NPO (nothing by mouth) and institute gastric suction.

(B) Order an abdominal radiograph.

(C) Order sepsis work-up.

(D) Start antibiotics.

(E) Order an abdominal CT.

13. The patient's abdominal radiographs can be seen in Figure 109-1. What is the next step?

(A) Order serial abdominal radiographs.

(B) Monitor platelet count.

(C) Monitor urine output closely.

(D) Monitor ABGs.

(E) All of the above.

14. The patient in Figure 109-2 requires surgery. What is an absolute indication for surgery in a patient with necrotizing enterocolitis (NEC)?

(A) free air

(B) fixed loop sign

(C) intractable thrombocytopenia

(D) intractable acidosis

(E) signs of peritonitis

15. The patient's abdominal radiograph improves during the next few days. The platelet count is stable. What complications might you expect?

(A) stricture

(B) sepsis

(C) neurodevelopmental problems

(D) A and B

(E) A and C

16. What routine monitoring is done in the first week of life in all premature babies?

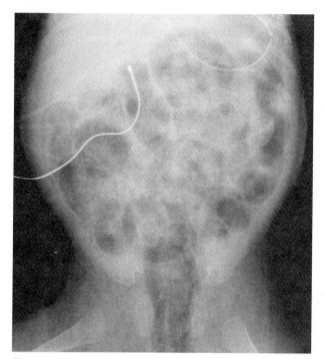

Figure 109-1.

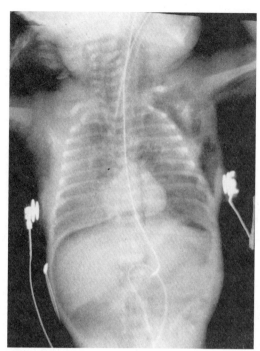

Figure 109-2.

(A) head ultrasound
(B) echocardiogram
(C) cardiac catheterization
(D) ophthalmology examination
(E) A, B, and D

Answers

1. **(B)** Antenatal corticosteroids, betamethasone or dexamethasone decrease morbidity from respiratory distress, necrotizing enterocolitis and intraventricular hemorrhage. Steroids are most effective if delivery occurs 48 hours to 7 days after administration but some beneficial effect has been seen as early as 12 hours after the first dose of steroids.

2. **(E)** Premature babies lighter than 750 g and less than 28 weeks' gestation have very high insensible water loss. The insensible water loss is increased under a radiant warmer, in low ambient humidity and under phototherapy. Respiratory distress syndrome is caused by surfactant deficiency. Surfactant is produced by type II alveolar cells. Surfactant decreases surface tension and so decreases the pressure required to stabilize the alveolus. Sepsis should always be considered in a sick newborn. Hypo- or hyperglycemia can both occur.

3. **(E)** Babies with surfactant deficiency have stiff lungs with decreased compliance; compliance of the chest wall in premature babies is high. In surfactant deficiency, a higher pressure is needed to open the alveoli; this manifests as retractions. In a premature baby, RDS or surfactant deficiency is the most likely cause of respiratory distress. Sepsis should always be considered in a baby with respiratory distress. Hypoglycemia can also present as respiratory distress.

4. **(E)** Surfactant is 90% lipid and 10% protein. Surfactant proteins A, B, C, and D are important

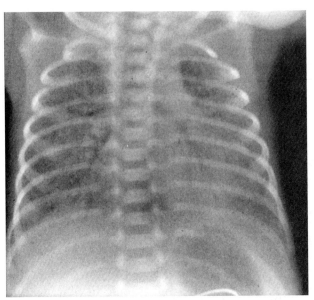

Figure 109-3A. **Reticulogranular pattern with air-bronchograms**

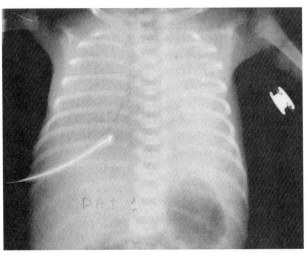

Figure 109-3B. **Chest radiograph showing "white out" in severe respiratory distress syndrome**

for dispersion of surfactant. Exogenous surfactant is administered via an endotracheal tube. Synthetic and natural surfactants are available.

Two different strategies are used for administration of exogenous surfactant. Prophylactic surfactant may be given within 30 minutes after birth; rescue surfactant is given once the diagnosis of respiratory distress syndrome is made by radiologic and clinical criteria. Umbilical lines are placed in premature babies for monitoring blood gases and for IV access. The chest radiograph in the respiratory distress syndrome shows a reticulogranular pattern with air bronchograms (Figure 109-3A). Severe respiratory distress appears as a "white out" (Figure 109-3B). Since the chest radiograph appearance of group B streptococcal pneumonia and surfactant deficiency are similar, any premature baby with respiratory distress should have a work-up for possible sepsis and antibiotic therapy should be initiated.

5. **(E)** A normal ABG determination for a premature baby on day 1 of life would be pH >7.25, $PaCO_2$ of 45 to 55 mm Hg and a PaO_2 >50 mm Hg. The normal cord blood glucose is 80% of the mother's glucose but reaches a nadir at about 2 hours of age. A normal Dextrostix is >45 mg/dL. A general rule of thumb is that the mean BP is roughly the same as the gestational age. For this baby, a mean BP >26 mm Hg is normal. Insensible water loss is inversely proportional to gestational age, i.e., the more immature the baby, the higher the insensible water loss. Since premature babies <750 g have very high insensible water losses, the serum Na should be monitored closely and the fluid administration adjusted accordingly. The serum calcium of a neonate on day 1 of life is higher than that of the mother. Therefore, the patient does not need any calcium added to the IV fluids on day 1 of life. Babies <750 or 1000 g are sometimes placed on prophylactic phototherapy on day 1 of life. An O_2 saturation in the high 80% to the low 90% range is acceptable on day 1 of life. Every NICU has different standards for acceptable O_2 saturation at different times of a premature baby's life and, thus, these concepts may very slightly.

6. **(A)** The serum Na of 150 mEq/mL indicates that we underestimated the insensible water loss and should increase the volume of administered fluids and continue to monitor serum electrolytes. The baby's weight also should be monitored. It is necessary to monitor the serum glucose since the fluid volume being administered is increased. If the serum glucose is normal, D10W can be given. But if the serum glucose is high, a change to D5W should be made as you increase the administered fluid volume. The baby should lose weight in the first couple of days. A weight loss

of 1% to 3% per day is called physiologic dehydration and is desirable.

7. **(E)** The Serum Na concentration is now 152 mEq/mL, so it would be appropriate to increase the total fluids being administered. Since the serum calcium is low, it would be appropriate to add calcium. Blood gases suggest overventilation, so it would be appropriate to adjust the ventilatory settings. Hyperalimentation is usually started in extremely low-birth-weight babies on days 1 to 2 of life.

8. **(A)** Urine is the main avenue of potassium excretion. Once the urine output is good, potassium can be added to the IV fluids if the serum potassium is not high. Since the serum Na is still high, the rate of fluid administration should be increased. In premature babies <750 grams non-oliguric, hyperkalemia can occur. If a patient's serum K is 7.5 to 8, take it seriously. Don't dismiss it as laboratory error or hemolysis.

9. **(A)** The clinical signs of PDA are widened pulse pressure, an active precordium, full or bounding pulses and a pansystolic murmur. An echocardiogram and a chest radiograph should be obtained.

10. **(D)** Excessive fluid administration has been associated with an increased incidence of patent ductus arteriosus. A low hematocrit may aggravate left-to-right shunting by lowering the resistance to blood flow through the pulmonary vascular bed. Higher hematocrits diminish excessive shunting through the PDA. Indomethacin, a prostaglandin inhibitor, is an effective treatment of PDA.

11. **(D)** Indomethacin is associated with vasoconstriction of other vessels including the cerebral, mesenteric, and renal vasculature. Renal function should be assessed before giving indomethacin. Urine output <1 mL/kg/hr or a serum creatinine >1.8 mg/dL is a contraindication to the use of indomethacin. Dilutional hyponatremia has also been reported.

12. **(E)** Abdominal distention and increased gastric residuals prior to feeding are signs of necrotizing enterocolitis (NEC). The diagnosis of NEC is made by abdominal radiograph. Since infection is considered to play a role in pathogenesis of NEC, a sepsis work-up should be done and the patient should be started on antibiotics if you suspect NEC.

13. **(E)** The abdominal radiograph is suggestive of pneumatosis intestinalis. There is no free air and no portal air. NEC is predominately a disease of premature babies although 10% of cases occur in term infants. Signs and symptoms of NEC vary and may include apnea and bradycardia, vomiting, increased residuals, abdominal distention, and heme-positive stools. The diagnostic hallmark of NEC is pneumatosis intestinalis or submucosal air on abdominal radiograph. Once the radiographic diagnosis of NEC is made, serial abdominal radiographs should be done looking for free air. The platelet count should be monitored. A drastic drop in the platelet count is an ominous sign. Since patients can lose a large amount of fluid into the abdominal cavity (third spacing), urine output should be monitored closely. A patient with NEC may require large amounts of IV fluids. It is important to monitor ABGs. Intractable acidosis is an ominous sign.

14. **(A)** The patient in Figure 109-2 has free air in the abdomen. The only absolute indication for surgery is the presence of free air. Other findings such as the fixed loop sign, intractable thrombocytopenia, intractable acidosis, and signs of peritonitis are relative indicators used by surgeons for laparotomy. All these relative signs point to the possibility of necrotic intestine in the abdomen.

15. **(D)** Strictures happen in about 10% of patients following NEC. Sepsis at this point is related to physician-interventions such as indwelling vascular catheters placed for prolonged hyperalimentation.

16. **(A)** Periventricular or intraventricular hemorrhage can occur in 20% to 30% of premature babies. 90% of the hemorrhages occur in the first 72 hours of life. Fifty percent of the hemorrhages are clinically silent; others may present with subtle clinical change. A catastrophic presentation with a bulging anterior fontanel, drop in hematocrit, metabolic acidosis and hyperglycemia can also occur. All premature babies <1500 g or <32- to 34-weeks gestation should have a

first ultrasound of the head at days 3 to 5 of life, the second at days 7 to 10 of life and subsequent ultrasounds based on these early results.

Intraventricular hemorrhages are classified as:

Grade I   Subependymal bleed with no intraventricular extension
Grade II   Intraventricular hemorrhage with no ventricular dilatation
Grade III Intraventricular hemorrhage with ventricular dilatation
Grade IV   Intraparenchymal bleed

Retinopathy of prematurity (ROP) is a disorder of developing retinal blood vessels that continues to be a cause of major visual morbidity in premature infants. All premature infants should have an eye exam for ROP at about 4 weeks of age and continued examinations until the retina is completely vascularized.

SUGGESTED READING

Henry MCW, Moss RL: Current issues in the management of necrotizing enterocolitis. *Semin Perinatol* 28; 221–233, 2004

CASE 110: A TERM BABY WITH HISTORY OF MATERNAL POLYHYDRAMNIOS

A 2800-g baby girl is born to a 20-year-old primigravida by normal, spontaneous, vaginal delivery. There is a history of possible polyhydramnios at birth. The baby's Apgar scores are 8 and 9 at 1 and 5 minutes, respectively. The baby looks good, is pink on room air, in no distress, and is sent to the regular nursery.

SELECT THE ONE BEST ANSWER TO THE FOLLOWING QUESTIONS

1. What primarily controls the volume of amniotic fluid?

    (A) fetal urine output
    (B) swallowing ability of the baby
    (C) placental factors
    (D) A and B
    (E) all of the above

2. All of the conditions listed below are associated with polyhydramnios *except:*

    (A) duodenal atresia
    (B) anencephaly
    (C) hydrops
    (D) postterm gestation
    (E) maternal diabetes

3. In the nursery, the baby is noted to have excessive oral secretions. She requires suctioning with a bulb syringe every 10 to 15 minutes and at times is reported to be choking on these secretions. You are called to assess the situation. The baby looks comfortable and pink on room air but has large amounts of secretions coming out of the mouth. The lungs are clear with good air entry. What is the next step in your evaluation?

    (A) chest radiograph
    (B) blood gas
    (C) placement of a nasogastric or orogastric tube
    (D) sepsis work-up
    (E) antibiotic therapy

4. The nasogastric tube can not be advanced beyond 10 cm. The tube is taped at this position and chest and abdominal radiographs are ordered. What is the most likely diagnosis?

    (A) transient tachypnea
    (B) choanal atresia
    (C) esophageal atresia
    (D) duodenal atresia
    (E) cleft palate

5. Based on the radiographic findings of Figure 110-1, what is the diagnosis?

    (A) esophageal atresia with distal tracheoesophageal fistula
    (B) esophageal atresia without a distal fistula
    (C) "H" type tracheoesophageal fistula
    (D) choanal atresia
    (E) tracheal stenosis

6. What are appropriate steps in the management of this newborn?

    (A) Connect NG tube to a Salem sump or suction
    (B) IV maintenance fluids
    (C) Pediatric surgery consult
    (D) Consider starting antibiotics
    (E) All of the above

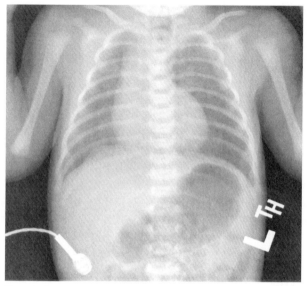

Figure 110-1.

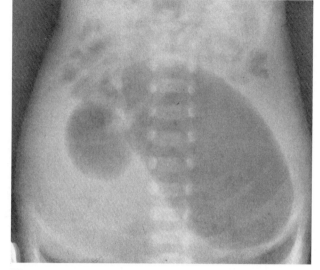

Figure 110-2.

7. What other organ systems or specific anomalies are associated with tracheoesophageal fistula?

   (A) cardiac
   (B) renal
   (C) imperforate anus
   (D) duodenal atresia
   (E) all of the above

8. What are the radiograph findings of duodenal atresia (Figure 110-2)?

   (A) double bubble
   (B) multiple air fluid levels
   (C) non-specific bowel gas pattern
   (D) thumb printing
   (E) all of the above

9. What chromosomal anomaly is associated with duodenal atresia?

   (A) Trisomy 13
   (B) Turner syndrome
   (C) Trisomy 21
   (D none of the above
   (E) A, B, and C

10. Duodenal atresia is the most common intestinal atresia.

    (A) True
    (B) False

11. Abdominal distention is a common presentation of duodenal atresia.

    (A) True
    (B) False

12. Of the intestinal atresias, which is more likely to have associated anomalies?

    (A) jejunal
    (B) ileal
    (C) colonic
    (D) duodenal
    (E) all are about equal in incidence.

13. Which contrast study is indicated emergently in a baby with bilious vomiting?

    (A) upper GI series
    (B) lower GI series
    (C) esophagram
    (D) A and B
    (E) None; all of the above studies would be too dangerous in this situation.

14. A baby does not pass meconium in 36 hours. The baby is vomiting and the abdomen is distended. The differential diagnosis includes:

    (A) meconium plug
    (B) Hirschsprung's disease
    (C) meconium ileus

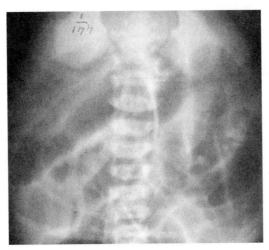

Figure 110-3.

(D) A and B

(E) all of the above

15. What is the most likely diagnosis in a newborn baby with abdominal distention and an abdomen radiograph as pictured in Figure 110-3?

(A) intrauterine TORCH infection

(B) meconium peritonitis

(C) constipation

(D) renal tubular disease

(E) renal tumor

16. What inherited disorder do you want to rule out in a newborn with meconium peritonitis?

(A) galactosemia

(B) G6PD deficiency

(C) cystic fibrosis

(D) B and D

(E) all of the above

17. A 3.5-kg baby is born by normal, spontaneous, vaginal delivery. An abdominal wall defect is noted at birth as seen in Figure 110-4. What is the diagnosis?

(A) gastroschisis

(B) omphalocele

(C) umbilical hernia

(D) prune belly syndrome

(E) renal cell tumor

18. All of the following are important in the immediate management of the baby mentioned in question 17 *except:*

(A) Cover the intestine with gauze soaked in warm saline and keep the gauze wet.

(B) Intravenous fluids, $1\frac{1}{2}$–2 times normal maintenance fluid (normal maintenance is 80 cc/kg. In this case, this would be 120–150 cc/kg).

(C) Nasogastric tube/Salem sump connected to suction

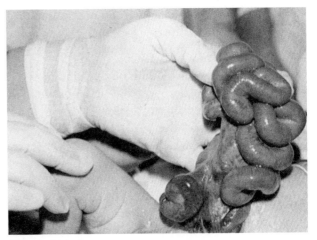

Figure 110-4.

(D) Strict latex precautions

(E) No exception, all of the above are important

19. Is this baby in Figure 110-3 likely to have chromosomal anomalies?

(A) Yes

(B) No

Answers

1. **(D)** The normal amount of amniotic fluid at birth is 0.5 to 2 L. The volume is determined by fetal urine output and swallowing ability of the fetus. Oligohydramnios is defined as an amniotic fluid volume <500 mL. Polyhydramnios is an amniotic fluid volume >2 L at birth. Oligo- and polyhydramnios are both associated with fetal anomalies and poor perinatal outcome.

   Assessment of amniotic fluid volume is done ultrasonographically by calculation of an amniotic fluid index (AFI), a summation of amniotic fluid volume in each of the four quadrants of the uterus. Oligohydramnios is defined as an AFI <5 cm and polyhydramnios is defined as an AFI >24 cm.

2. **(D)** Conditions associated with polyhydramnios:
   - Two-thirds are idiopathic
   - Fetal anomalies
     - GI anomalies → duodenal and esophageal atresia
     - CNS anomalies → anencephaly, primary muscle disease
     - Hydrops → immune and non-immune
   - Maternal diabetes
   - Multiple gestation

   Conditions associated with oligohydramnios:
   - Fetal anomalies → renal-developmental or obstructive malformations
   - Postterm gestation
   - Chronic fetal hypoxia associated with severe preeclampsia
   - Premature rupture of membranes
   - Maternal dehydration
   - Monochorionic twin gestation

3. **(C).**

4. **(C)** Since the nasogastric tube cannot be advanced beyond 10 cm, the most likely diagnosis is esophageal atresia.

5. **(A)** The chest radiograph shows the nasogastric tube coiled in a blind pouch in the neck. The cardiothymic shadow is normal and the lung fields are clear. There is a non-specific bowel gas pattern in the abdomen. The nasogastric tube coiling in a blind pouch indicates esophageal atresia and the air seen in the gastrointestinal tract indicates a distal tracheoesophageal fistula (TEF). If there was no abdominal gas, that would indicate esophageal atresia without a distal TEF. TEF occurs in 1:3000 to 1:4500 live births. Polyhydramnios is present in about one-third of cases with esophageal atresia. Babies with TEF present with excessive oral secretions shortly after birth that may lead to coughing, choking and respiratory distress. Infants with an "H" type TEF generally do not present in the newborn period. Figure 110-5 shows the various types of TEF. The most common is esophageal atresia with distal TEF, the one present in this patient (see Figure 110-1).

6. **(E)** The nasogastric tube or Salem sump should be connected to suction to keep the blind pouch empty to prevent aspiration of secretions. Maintenance intravenous fluids should be started. Since these babies are at high risk for aspiration, antibiotic therapy should be considered.

7. **(E)** Other anomalies may occur in as many as 40% of infants with TEF. These anomalies are generally GI and cardiac.

8. **(A)** The classic radiographic sign of duodenal atresia is the "double bubble" seen in Figure 110-2.

9. **(C)** Infants with duodenal atresia have about a 30% incidence of Down syndrome (Trisomy 21).

10. **(B)** Atresias account for about one-third of intestinal obstructions in the newborn period occurring in about 1:1500 live births. Of the intestinal atresias, jejunoileal atresia is most common (55%), followed by duodenal atresia (30%), and colonic atresia (10%). Failure of the gut to recanalize during the eighth to tenth week of ges-

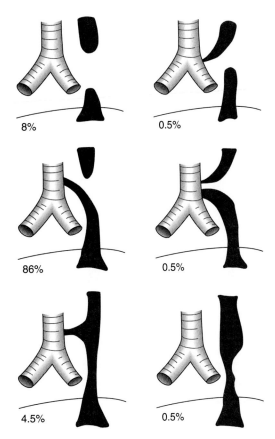

Classification of T.E. Fistula

Figure 110-5.

tation seems to be the most likely cause of duodenal atresia. In the jejunum, ileum and colon, vascular compromise in early gestation may be responsible for bowel atresia.

11. **(B)** A common presentation of duodenal atresia is bilious vomiting. A history of polyhydramnios and abdominal distention is usually absent. Abdominal distention is generally present with jejunal, ileal and colonic atresias and is more pronounced with distal atresias.

12. **(D)** Seventy percent of infants with duodenal atresia have other associated anomalies. These are, in order of frequency, Down syndrome, cardiovascular anomalies, malrotation of the intestine, and esophageal atresia. Extraintestinal anomalies are uncommon with jejunoileal atresias.

13. **(A)** Bilious vomiting in an infant suggests a diagnosis requiring surgical therapy until proven otherwise. Immediate evaluation for malrotation

should be done. The procedure of choice for malrotation is an upper GI series looking for the position of the duodenojejunal junction.

14. **(E)** Failure to pass meconium in the first 24 hours of life can occur in all the conditions listed. A lower GI series will be diagnostic and therapeutic for meconium-related obstruction. A lower GI series in a patient with Hirschsprung's will show a "transition zone," a narrowed rectosigmoid segment distal to a dilated sigmoid segment. The presence of barium in the gut 24 hours after barium enema is suggestive of Hirschsprung's disease. However, the diagnosis of Hirschsprung's disease is confirmed only by rectal biopsy demonstrating an absence of ganglion cells. Meconium ileus is intestinal obstruction produced by thick inspissated meconium.

15. **(B)** Figure 110-3 shows intraabdominal calcifications. The presence of intraabdominal calcifications is indicative of meconium peritonitis. In meconium peritonitis there is in utero intestinal perforation with meconium spillage into the peritoneal cavity.

16. **(C)** About 10% to 20% of neonates with cystic fibrosis have intraluminal obstruction of the terminal ileum from viscid meconium. The meconium in these neonates has a 5 to 10 times higher albumin concentration compared with meconium from unaffected babies.

17. **(A)** Gastroschisis is a right paraumbilical defect in the abdominal wall with the intestine herniating through this defect. An omphalocele is a defect of the umbilical ring. An omphalocele generally has a sac, but it can sometimes be ruptured. If the omphalocele is ruptured, it can be differentiated from gastroschisis by the content of the defect. Gastroschisis contains intestine and sometimes ovaries and Fallopian tubes but never liver. An omphalocele, in contrast, contains intestine and liver. An omphalocele is more common in males.

18. **(D)** The exposed intestine should be covered with gauze soaked in warm saline to control evaporative water loss. The maintenance fluid requirement in this baby is high because of evaporative

losses and third-spacing. The urine output should be monitored closely to assess the adequacy of fluid intake. The stomach is decompressed by nasogastric tube suction.

19. **(B)** Chromosomal anomalies are generally not associated with gastroschisis while 40% to 50% of patients with an omphalocele have a chromosomal anomaly such as a trisomy.

SUGGESTED READING

Gleason PF, Eddleman KA, Stone JL: Gastrointestinal disorders of the fetus. *Clin Perinatol* 27;901–920, 2000.

CASE 111: A NEWBORN WITH A HISTORY OF MATERNAL GROUP B STREPTOCOCCAL COLONIZATION AND A REACTIVE RPR TEST FOR SYPHILIS

A 3230-g infant was born to a 25-year-old G1P1 woman who had prenatal care starting in the third trimester. She had a history of having had syphilis 2 years before, which according to her, had been treated with "shots." Her screening test for syphilis (rapid plasma reagin, RPR) was positive at a titer of 1:4 during this pregnancy. No other problems were identified during her clinic visits except for a history of cocaine abuse. She was found to be a vaginal carrier of group B β-hemolytic streptococcus. On admission, she was in active labor and delivered before receiving prophylactic intrapartum penicillin. The Apgar scores were 8 and 9 at 1 and 5 minutes of life, respectively.

1. How do you know that this woman had, or has, syphilis?

   (A) She has a positive RPR titer.
   (B) You order a fluorescent treponemal antibody test that is positive.
   (C) She says she received penicillin for her past infection.
   (D) A or B.
   (E) None of the above.

2. What additional information would you most like to have from the mother?

   (A) clinic records from 2 years ago
   (B) RPR titers before and after her alleged penicillin treatment

   (C) RPR titer at the beginning of this pregnancy
   (D) a blood smear
   (E) a CRP or ESR

3. Two years ago, her RPR was 1:64; it fell after the penicillin shots. What RPR titer would be indicative of a sufficient response to penicillin treatment?

   (A) ≤1:4
   (B) 1:8
   (C) 1:16
   (D) 1:32
   (E) 1:128

4. Over what period of time would you expect the RPR titer to change significantly in order to confirm adequacy of therapy?

   (A) 1 month
   (B) 2 months
   (C) 3 months
   (D) 6 months
   (E) 12 months

5. Does a current RPR titer of 1:4 confirm the adequacy of the prior treatment?

   (A) Yes
   (B) No

6. If primary or secondary syphilis in an adult is untreated, what will happen over the course of a year or two?

   (A) The RPR will fall over time.
   (B) The RPR will rise over time.
   (C) The symptoms will be proportional to the RPR.
   (D) The RPR will cycle over time.
   (E) A and C

7. In this case, the infant had a normal physical examination. Does this rule out congenital syphilis?

   (A) Yes
   (B) No

8. In addition to serology, which of the tests below are required to confirm a diagnosis of syphilis?

   (A) long bone radiographs
   (B) lumbar puncture
   (C) complete blood count

(D) liver function tests
(E) none of the above

9. Would an RPR of 1:4 on the cord blood diagnose congenital syphilis?

(A) Yes
(B) No

10. Would a positive fluorescent treponemal antibody test (FTA-ABS) on the cord blood diagnose congenital syphilis?

(A) Yes
(B) No

11. Would a negative RPR titer on the cord blood rule out congenital syphilis?

(A) Yes
(B) No

12. In this case, can you rule out the possibility that the mother has been reinfected with syphilis since her treatment 2 years ago?

(A) Yes
(B) No

13. What would be the most conservative approach to the management of this newborn?

(A) Follow the baby's RPR titers over the next 6 months.
(B) Treat the baby with one IM Bicillin injection.
(C) Treat the baby with 10 days of IM aqueous procaine penicillin or IV aqueous penicillin.
(D) Follow the RPR over the next 12 months.
(E) Do an LP to obtain CSF for analysis and serologic testing.

14. If the mother had received adequate intrapartum penicillin prophylaxis for GBBS, would that eliminate the concern over the possibility of congenital syphilis in the newborn?

(A) Yes
(B) No

15. Of the following choices, what should be done with a term newborn whose mother did not receive intrapartum penicillin prophylaxis for her group B streptococcal colonization?

(A) Admit the infant to the NICU and observe.
(B) Draw a blood culture and leukocyte count and admit the infant to the well-baby nursery and observe.
(C) Begin the baby on oral penicillin.
(D) Begin the baby on ampicillin and gentamicin after a leukocyte count and a blood culture.
(E) Give the baby 50 mg/kg IM of ceftriaxone.

16. How long will it likely take for the blood culture to be reported positive, if it is?

(A) within 24 to 36 hours
(B) 48 to 72 hours
(C) greater than 72 hours
(D) there is patient to patient variation
(E) this information is not known

17. If the baby develops symptomatic early onset GBS disease, this will most likely present at:

(A) less than 24 hours of age
(B) after 24 to 48 hours of age

18. How long should the baby in question 15 remain in the hospital for observation for GBS disease assuming she/he is asymptomatic?

(A) 24 hours
(B) 48 hours
(C) 72 hours
(D) >72 hours
(E) No observation is needed if parents have available transportation and a working phone.

Answers

1. **(B)** A treponemal test, usually the fluorescent treponemal antibody absorption test (FTA-ABS), remains reactive for life even after adequate therapy. RPR (rapid plasma reagin) and VDRL (Venereal Disease Research Laboratory) test are non-treponemal tests used to screen patients for syphilis. The non-treponemal tests have high sensitivity but relatively low specificity in the diagnosis of syphilis. They provide quantitative results that can be used to monitor response to therapy and define disease activity. The RPR can be falsely negative in late congenital syphilis. A positive RPR or VDRL must be confirmed with a treponemal test like the FTA-ABS test. A false-positive RPR can

be associated with viral infections, e.g., infectious mononucleosis, varicella, measles, and hepatitis, as well as lymphoma, tuberculosis, malaria, connective tissue disorders, and pregnancy.

2. **(C)** To assess success of therapy, the current RPR titer needs to be compared with previous titers. If this mother was RPR negative at the beginning of this pregnancy, a titer of 1:4 at delivery could be a result of a new infection. If her titer at the beginning was 1:64, the same titer of 1:4 suggests successful therapy.

3. **(A)** A fourfold or higher decrease in RPR titer is probably indicative of adequate therapy although ideally, the test should be non-reactive or minimally reactive 2 years after adequate therapy.

4. **(C)** The RPR titer should decrease significantly by 3 months after therapy and should be non-reactive by 6 to 18 months after therapy. Unfortunately, a similar decline will occur in an infant whose RPR antibody was passively acquired from the mother.

5. **(B)** The RPR generally becomes negative within 1 year after successful treatment if the initial titer was low, e.g., ≤1:8. If the initial titer is high as in this patient, she should have become RPR negative by 2 years. To comment on adequacy of therapy, one needs to know what the titer was when treatment was initiated.

6. **(B)** In the course of a few years, the RPR will continue to increase. Eventually, however, it will fall, even if untreated and it becomes a relatively insensitive test for tertiary syphilis.

7. **(B)** Two-thirds of infants with congenital syphilis are asymptomatic at birth.

8. **(E)** Although all the test options listed may be abnormal in congenital syphilis, it is important to reiterate that most newborns with congenital syphilis are asymptomatic.

9. **(B)** Many experts say that an infant's titer fourfold higher than the mother's titer can be relied on for the diagnosis of congenital syphilis. However, few factual data actually support this idea.

Any positive test for syphilis in a newborn should be viewed with suspicion.

10. **(B)** A positive FTA-ABS test can be secondary to passively acquired IgG antibody and may take 1 year or longer to become negative.

11. **(B)** Serologic tests such as RPR and VDRL may be falsely negative in very early congenital syphilis with infection within 4 to 6 weeks of term.

12. **(B)** This mother, if she was adequately treated 2 years ago, should have become non-reactive by now. Her titer of 1:4 could represent new infection. There is no immunity believed to protect against reinfection.

13. **(C)** This baby should be treated for congenital syphilis. The mother's titer of 1:4 at delivery might represent reinfection. Benzathine penicillin (Bicillin) delivers inadequate levels of penicillin to reliably deal with CNS disease. There is no test available to exclude the possibility of CNS syphilis with certainty although many mistakenly believe that a normal LP excludes neurosyphilis.

14. **(B)** If a mother is treated for syphilis less than 1 month before delivery with any antibiotic regimen, her baby should be evaluated and treated for congenital syphilis.

15. **(B)** Although intrapartum penicillin was not administered, the risk for GBS infection is still low. Observation after a minimal investigative evaluation is acceptable.

16. **(A)** Modern technology in use in clinical microbiology laboratories monitors blood culture bottles continuously for CO_2 production. A blood culture specimen in which bacteria are growing may turn positive at any time. However, most cultures "turn positive" very quickly and will yield positive results in 1 to 2 days.

17. **(A)** Even in the era of intrapartum antimicrobial prophylaxis that has greatly decreased the rate of occurrence of early onset (<7 days) GBS disease, most cases are still recognized in the first day of life.

18. (B) Even though the mother was known to be a carrier, the risk of GBS disease overall is still relatively low in a term baby and most cases are recognized in the first day of life. Taken together with the U.S. health system that does not generally support prolonged observation of asymptomatic term babies, 48 hours of observation is believed by most to be sufficient.

SUGGESTED READING

American Academy of Pediatrics Red Book. 2006 Report of the Committee on Infectious Diseases, 27th Ed; 620–627, 631–644.

CASE 112: A NEWBORN WITH AMBIGUOUS GENITALIA

A full-term 2620-g infant is born to a 28-year-old G2P2 mother who had regular prenatal care. You were asked to attend the delivery because of meconium stained amniotic fluid. The baby is born in good condition with Apgar scores of 9 and 9. No special interventions are required. You and the obstetrician notice that it is unclear whether the newborn is a male or a female. The mother keeps asking "what did I have?"

SELECT THE ONE BEST ANSWER TO THE FOLLOWING QUESTIONS

1. After you quickly examine the baby, you can't decide if there is a small penis or a large clitoris. You answer the mother:

   (A) "The baby is abnormal, I'm not sure."
   (B) "The baby has ambiguous genitalia."
   (C) "The baby's genitalia are incompletely developed."
   (D) "The baby is probably a boy."
   (E) "I have to review the prenatal ultrasound."

2. What is the key diagnostic element of the physical examination?

   (A) presence or absence of palpable gonads in the inguinal canal or scrotum
   (B) length of the phallus
   (C) degree of hypospadias
   (D) degree of posterior labial fusion
   (E) There is no key physical element. This is a laboratory driven diagnosis.

3. What is the most important first laboratory examination to help with gender assignment evaluation?

   (A) karyotype
   (B) Barr body analysis
   (C) blood test for 17-OH progesterone
   (D) serum electrolytes
   (E) head ultrasound

4. In the delivery room, when the genitalia are ambiguous, it is best to announce the probable sex of the infant.

   (A) Yes
   (B) No

5. Assignment of sex in the newborn with ambiguous genitalia is ultimately best made on:

   (A) adequacy of the phallus in the male
   (B) potential fertility in the female
   (C) cosmetic appearance after reconstruction
   (D) desire of parents
   (E) none of the above

6. In female neonates, withdrawal vaginal bleeding typically occurs:

   (A) within the first 3 days of life
   (B) at the end of the first week of life
   (C) at a month of life
   (D) at 2 months of life
   (E) never under normal circumstance

7. In the male neonate, congenital adrenal hyperplasia should be apparent by careful physical examination.

   (A) Yes
   (B) No

8. Male circumcision in the neonate does not require anesthesia.

   (A) True
   (B) False

9. A male neonate who has undergone circumcision must not be discharged home until:

   (A) He has voided after the circumcision
   (B) He has been observed for several hours for bleeding

(C) 12 hours' observation

(D) 6 hours' observation if acetaminophen is used

(E) First dressing change is completed

10. The first clinical test you would perform for a male with a non-tender mass in one hemiscrotum should be:

(A) transillumination

(B) ultrasound

(C) Doppler exam of the scrotal contents

(D) KUB radiograph

(E) B and D

Answers

1. **(C)** The incidence of ambiguous genitalia that results in a child's gender being uncertain is 1:4500. Some degree of male undervirilization or female virilization may be seen in up to 2% of live births.

2. **(A)** In females there should be absence of gonads in the labia majora or the inguinal region. In males there should be palpable gonads in the inguinal canal or scrotum. Only a gonad containing testicular tissue can descend to a palpable position.

3. **(A)** In cases where gender assignment is an issue, karyotype is the most important laboratory test. Most laboratories will give preliminary results in 2 to 3 days.

4. **(B)**.

5. **(E)**. In general, assignment of sex for the purpose of rearing is made as soon as possible based on the internal and external genital phenotype and the results of appropriate investigations. Assignment of sex of rearing can be difficult, particularly in very undervirilized males where results of investigations and multidisciplinary discussions with parents, urologist, endocrinologist, geneticist, and psychologist are needed. Gender assignment may be postponed until laboratory results are available and the effects of exogenous androgens have been evaluated. In the case of a virilized female, there is potential for fertility and these patients are usually raised as girls.

6. **(A)** As a result of maternal estrogen levels in the fetus and there is sudden withdrawal, physiologic bleeding from the uterine mucosa is common.

7. **(B)** Congenital adrenal hyperplasia (CAH) is the most common cause of ambiguous genitalia in females. In CAH, there is a deficiency of cortisol and an increase in cortisol precursors that have androgenic effects leading to masculinization in females. In males, since the testes produce testosterone, normal masculinization occurs.

8. **(B)**.

9. **(B)** While there are no written guidelines for this situation, ensuring that there was no underlying bleeding disorder and that surgical hemostasis has been achieved are the major priorities. Voiding difficulties are rare and would not arise until scarring of a damaged urethra has occurred.

10. **(A)** Transillumination should be the first intervention since it gives prompt feedback as to the nature of the clinical problem. A hydrocele could be diagnosed in this fashion at minimal cost and risk. If transillumination is not definitive, an ultrasound would be the next step.

SUGGESTED READING

American Academy of Pediatrics. Committee on Genetics. Evaluation of the newborn with developmental anomalies of the external genitalia. *Pediatrics* 106; 138–142, 2000.

Ogilvy-Stuart AL, Brain CE: Early assessment of ambiguous genitalia. *Arch Dis Child* 89;401–407, 2004.

CASE 113: A TERM NEWBORN NEEDS AN INITIAL EXAMINATION

A healthy term African-American baby girl is born vaginally without instrumentation after a 12-hour labor. You examine her at 2 hours of life.

SELECT THE ONE BEST ANSWER TO THE FOLLOWING QUESTIONS:

1. You note that her head is "cone-shaped" and there is an ecchymosis and swelling of the scalp at the vertex; when you apply pressure with your finger, an imprint is left. This condition is most likely a:

(A) cephalhematoma
(B) subgaleal hematoma
(C) caput succedaneum
(D) A or B
(E) none of the above

2. The following day, you note a swelling over the right parietal area of the scalp that feels fluctuant. This is most likely a:

(A) cephalhematoma
(B) subgaleal hematoma
(C) caput succedaneum
(D) A or B
(E) none of the above

3. Later on, the mother calls the nurse because the baby has developed a rash. It is red, macular, papular/pustular and is most prominent over the face and trunk. The mother wonders if the baby is allergic to her milk. You explain:

(A) "This is erythema toxicum."
(B) "You will change the baby to soy formula."
(C) "The baby is allergic to the baby lotio.n"
(D) "This is a staphylococcal infection."
(E) "I must perform some laboratory tests to determine the cause."

4. You make a Wright's stain of material from a pustule. You will likely see:

(A) sheets of eosinophils
(B) many bacteria
(C) many neutrophiles
(D) a dendritic pattern
(E) only cellular debris

5. If there had been shoulder dystocia at delivery and the baby was holding one arm limply at her side, but had a good palmar grasp on that side, you would diagnose a probable:

(A) upper brachial plexus injury (Erb's palsy)
(B) lower brachial plexus injury (Klumpke's palsy)
(C) fractured clavicle
(D) A and B
(E) none of the above

6. Within the gluteal fold, at the tip of the coccyx, you find a deep dimple. You should:

(A) get an ultrasound of the spine
(B) get an MRI of the spine
(C) get a neurosurgical consult
(D) do nothing
(E) B and C

7. Just in front of the top part of her ear, you note a pin-hole opening. This is called an ear pit and could be associated with congenital deafness.

(A) True
(B) False

8. You find a minor anomaly on your exam of the baby, namely, bilateral single palmer creases. Should you suspect Down syndrome?

(A) Yes
(B) No

9. The mother asks about the red spots in the white of the baby's eyes. You explain that:

(A) They are small hemorrhages from the pressure of labor on the baby.
(B) They may represent brain injury and you will order tests.
(C) They are from the ointment put in the eyes.
(D) You suspect *Chlamydia*.
(E) You suspect gonorrhea.

10. The mother express concern about a white vaginal discharge. You explain to the mother:

(A) This is normal.
(B) You will do tests for an infection on the baby.
(C) You will obtain an estradiol level on the baby.
(D) You will obtain LH and FSH level on the baby.
(E) You will need to obtain lab work on the mother.

11. There are multiple tiny yellow papules on the baby's nose. These are:

(A) prominent sebaceous glands
(B) epithelial inclusion cysts (milia)
(C) neonatal acne
(D) dermoid cysts
(E) scabies

12. You feel a sharp liver edge 2 to 3 cm below the right costal margin. This represents hepatomegaly.

(A) Yes

(B) No

13. On examination of the hips, you find instability on one side with a palpable "clunk" on the Ortolani maneuver. You should:

(A) Immediately put the baby in a harness.

(B) Order triple diapers for the baby.

(C) Repeat the examination (if the clicks are still apparent, an ultrasound examination is the next step).

(D) Order an MRI.

(E) Order a technetium triple phase bone scan.

14. During your discharge examination on day 2, you hear a grade 2 to 3 systolic murmur. You tell the parents that:

(A) "It is nothing; all babies have murmurs."

(B) "I am going to check an oxygen saturation."

(C) "I am going to order an EKG."

(D) "I am going to call a pediatric cardiologist."

Answers

1. **(C)** Caput succedaneum is a diffuse, sometimes ecchymotic soft tissue swelling of the presenting part in a vertex delivery.

2. **(A)** Cephalhematoma is a subperiosteal hemorrhage. Therefore, it does not cross suture lines but can be bilateral. There is no discoloration of the overlying scalp. Subgaleal hemorrhage occurs as a consequence of subaponeurotic bleeding. It crosses suture lines and is not usually associated with a skull fracture. Since a subgaleal hemorrhage can be large, it can lead to a drop in the hematocrit and resultant hyperbilirubinemia.

3. **(A)** A maculopapular rash on an erythematous base seen 1 to 3 days after birth is most likely erythema toxicum. It has no known allergic component and requires no laboratory investigation.

4. **(A)** Wright's stain of material from pustules will show eosinophils.

5. **(A)** Forty-five percent of brachial plexus injuries are associated with shoulder dystocia. Erb's palsy is an upper brachial plexus injury involving the 5th and 6th cervical nerves. The arm is adducted and pronated. In Erb's palsy, hand grasp is present. In Klumpke's palsy the 7th and 8th cervical and 1st thoracic nerves are affected and the hand grasp is absent.

6. **(D)** Most dimples that fall within the gluteal fold are normal. Dimples that are large and located above the gluteal fold such as a sacral dimple or are associated with other midline skin lesions like hemangiomas, lipomas or skin tags should be further investigated.

7. **(A)** Preauricular pits are common and have been associated with deafness.

8. **(B)** A single palmer crease is a nonspecific finding in an otherwise normal infant. A unilateral single palmer crease is present in 4% of normal people and bilateral single palmer creases occur in about 1% of normal people.

9. **(A)** Small subconjunctival hemorrhages are common and of no clinical significance. No further work-up is necessary.

10. **(A)** This is a result of a maternal hormone effect that will resolve with time.

11. **(B)** Milia are tiny inclusion cysts within the epidermis. Sebaceous hyperplasia occurs in large plaques.

12. **(B)** The liver is usually palpable sometimes 2 to 3 cm below the costal margin.

13. **(C)** The diagnosis is most likely laxity of the ligaments, a benign disorder, but investigation for hip dislocation should occur.

14. **(D)** Any murmur ≥ grade 2 after the first 24 hours of life warrants a cardiology evaluation to check for the presence of an atrial septal defect (ASD) or a ventricular septal defect (VSD) and to evaluate the baby's hematologic status. If the murmur is < grade 2, a follow-up examination suffices as an initial approach because this is most likely a flow or benign murmur.

SUGGESTED READING

Martin R, Fanaroff AA, Walsh M: *Fanaroff and Martin's Neonatal-Perinatal Medicine Diseases of the Fetus and Infant*. Chicago: Elsevier Mosby, 8th Edition 2006.

CASE 114: A TERM BABY FOUND TO BE LOW BIRTH WEIGHT AFTER DELIVERY

A full-term baby is born to a 16-year-old mother. The prenatal course was notable for suspected intrauterine growth retardation. The birth weight is 2325 g, small for gestational age.

SELECT THE ONE BEST ANSWER TO THE FOLLOWING QUESTIONS:

1. In the evaluation of a low-birth-weight, term, small for gestational age (SGA) newborn, which of the following should be considered?

   (A) maternal vascular disease
   (B) fetal chromosomal disorder
   (C) in utero infection
   (D) maternal fibroids
   (E) all of the above should be considered

2. The presence of how many minor anomalies would suggest to you the possibility of a major chromosomal defect?

   (A) 1
   (B) 2
   (C) 3
   (D) 4
   (E) 5

3. An SGA (small for gestational age) baby born to a teenage mother has some petechiae on the face and trunk. You do the following:

   (A) send off titers for cytomegalovirus
   (B) send off titers for rubella virus
   (C) send a urine culture for rubella virus
   (D) all of the above
   (E) none of the above

4. All are risk factors for congenital toxoplasmosis *except:*

   (A) eating steak tartare
   (B) having a cat who lives indoors
   (C) gardening
   (D) exposure of a pregnant woman to an infant with toxoplasmosis
   (E) all of the above

5. The differential diagnosis of a newborn who is SGA with a normal physical examination includes:

   (A) cytomegalovirus (CMV)
   (B) rubella
   (C) toxoplasmosis
   (D) varicella
   (E) A and C

6. Neonatal herpes skin lesions are most likely to be seen on day:

   (A) 1
   (B) 3
   (C) 5
   (D) 8
   (E) 21

7. What percentage of women with neonates who develop herpes simplex virus (HSV) are asymptomatic or have no history of ever having herpes?

   (A) <1%
   (B) 1% to 5%
   (C) 5% to 20%
   (D) 60% to 80%
   (E) >95%

8. Congenital toxoplasmosis has a prevalence in the United States of about:

   (A) 1:100
   (B) 1:1000
   (C) 1:10,000
   (D) 1:100,000
   (E) 1:1,000,000

9. With regard to treatment of congenital toxoplasmosis, all of the following statements are true *except:*

   (A) Prenatal treatment decreases transmission rate.
   (B) Prenatal treatment for a fetus already infected decreases fetal effects.
   (C) Postnatal treatment for one year is needed for infected and symptomatic children.
   (D) Postnatal treatment for one month is needed for infected and asymptomatic children.
   (E) All of the above statements are true.

10. A baby in whom you diagnosed congenital CMV infection passes the hearing screening test. Which of the following statements are true?

    (A) The baby is lucky; there will be no hearing loss.

(B) The baby is still at risk for progressive hearing loss and will require repeat testing in the future.

(C) The baby needs to see an audiologist now for more advance testing.

(D) The auditory brainstem response (ABR) must have been done incorrectly.

(E) All of the above statements are false.

11. An SGA term baby is at risk for:

(A) hypoglycemia
(B) polycythemia
(C) hypothermia
(D) all of the above
(E) none of above

12. SGA neonates should have glucose levels followed for up to:

(A) 2 hours after birth
(B) 12 hours after birth
(C) 24 hours after birth
(D) 3 days after birth
(E) 1 week after birth

13. In SGA infants, the most important predictor of future growth and development is:

(A) weight at birth
(B) head size at birth
(C) length at birth
(D) body mass index (BMI)
(E) body surface area (BSA)

Answers:

1. **(E)** The causes of intrauterine growth retardation can be considered in three main categories:

- Systemic disease or causes in the mother that affect the uteroplacental function. Examples include chronic hypertension, severe diabetes, lupus, and preeclampsia.
- Fetal causes, i.e., those that inhibit the genetic growth potential of the fetus. Examples include chromosomal disorders like Trisomy 18 or TORCH infections.
- Local uterine causes such as large fibroids, bicornuate uterus, or a multiple gestation that impairs the growth of the fetus secondary to space constraints.

2. **(B)** An infant that has two minor anomalies and ≥ one major anomaly is more likely to have an underlying genetic diagnosis.

3. **(E)** Petechiae on the face, trunk and in the groin area can occur in normal infants. Obviously, the platelet count should be checked. If the rest of the examination is normal, there is no need to do any titers or cultures. On the other hand, if there are petechiae in an SGA baby who also has hepatosplenomegaly, this infant should be evaluated further for intrauterine infections such as CMV or rubella. In this instance, there should be associated thrombocytopenia.

4. **(D)** *Toxoplasma gondii* is a protozoan that is acquired through ingestion of undercooked or raw meat containing tissue cyst stage of the parasite or exposure to other food materials that are contaminated by oocysts excreted in the feces of infected cats.

5. **(E)** Ninety percent of newborns congenitally infected with CMV are asymptomatic at delivery and 10% will have signs and symptoms. Affected infants may be small for gestational age. They may also have microcephaly, intracranial calcifications, hepatosplenomegaly, petechiae, thrombocytopenia, hearing loss, etc. So, in this baby, the examination is normal although the baby is SGA. The diagnosis of congenital CMV can be made by viral culture of urine obtained within the first 3 weeks of life. Infants with congenital toxoplasmosis are asymptomatic in 70% to 90% of cases.

6. **(D)** The incidence of neonatal HSV infection is approximately 1:3000 to 1:7000 live births. HSV infection may occur transplacentally, intrapartum or postpartum. Most infected neonates acquire the virus at delivery. Only 30% to 50% of babies present with skin lesions that commonly appear around 7 to 10 days.

7. **(D)** Sixty percent to eighty percent of women with neonates who develop HSV are asymptomatic or have no history of ever having herpes.

8. **(C)**.

9. (**D**) Treatment of mother during pregnancy decreases transmission rate to fetus. If mother and fetus are both infected, treatment of mother with pyrimethamine and sulfadiazine decreases fetal effects. Symptomatic or asymptomatic infected babies should be treated with pyrimethamine and sulfadiazine for 1 year.

10. (**B**) Ninety percent of babies with congenital CMV are asymptomatic at birth. Sensorineural hearing loss is the most common late sequelae.

11. (**D**) SGA babies are at risk for hypoglycemia secondary to decreased glycogen stores, decreased gluconeogenesis and increased sensitivity to insulin. They are at risk for hypothermia secondary to decreased subcutaneous fat and large surface area to body weight ratio. They are at risk for polycythemia secondary to chronic hypoxia.

12. (**D**) Blood sugar should be monitored in an SGA baby for up to 3 days. Glycogen stores generally take 2 to 3 days to develop.

13. (**B**).

SUGGESTED READING

Martin R, Fanaroff AA, Walsh M: *Fanaroff and Martin's Neonatal-Perinatal Medicine Diseases of the Fetus and Infant.* Chicago: Elsevier Mosby, 8th Edition 2006.

CASE 115: A 36-WEEK GESTATION BABY'S MOTHER WANTS AN EARLY DISCHARGE

A 2300-g birth weight, 36-week gestation baby is now 40 hours old. The mother is all set to take him home.

SELECT THE ONE BEST ANSWER TO THE FOLLOWING QUESTIONS:

1. The American Academy of Pediatrics (AAP) guidelines for consideration of early discharge (<48 hours) of the healthy neonate specify that:

   (A) Baby must be at least 34 weeks' gestation.
   (B) Baby must be at least 36 weeks' gestation.
   (C) Baby must be at least 38 weeks' gestation.
   (D) Baby must be at least 40 weeks' gestation.
   (E) Gestational age is not a consideration.

2. The guidelines for early discharge also specify that the newborn must have a birth weight of:

   (A) at least 1800 g
   (B) at least 2000 g
   (C) at least 2500 g
   (D) at least 3000 g
   (E) a birth weight ≥1800 g and AGA

3. All of the following information would be needed for assessment of discharge readiness for this baby *except:*

   (A) serum bilirubin either normal or unlikely to be on a trajectory requiring phototherapy
   (B) feeding ability
   (C) follow-up care arrangements in place
   (D) he has achieved hemostasis after circumcision
   (E) all of the above would be needed information

4. What would be considered the most reliable information for establishing the gestational age in this small baby?

   (A) Ballard score
   (B) prenatal ultrasound before 18 weeks' gestation
   (C) last menstrual period
   (D) bone age, left wrist
   (E) bone age, left foot

5. After your assessment of risk in sending this baby home at 40 hours, what would be the most appropriate thing to tell the parents?

   (A) They should watch for jaundice and call with any concerns.
   (B) They should observe his weight.
   (C) You are concerned enough not to send the baby home.
   (D) They should follow up in 3 days or less with the pediatrician.
   (E) They should watch for jaundice, keep the child in front of a sunny window and call with any concerns.

6. The parents of a term, normal birth weight girl ask to be discharged at 12 hours. The mother is an experienced breast feeder and feedings are going fairly well so far. The baby has not passed any stool. You tell them:

   (A) Your admission examination is normal so the baby can go home.
   (B) You want the baby to have passed meconium before you write an order for discharge.

(C) Baby has no jaundice and therefore can go home.

(D) Child cannot be discharged prior to 36 hours age.

(E) If the discharge examination is normal, she can go home.

7. In order for a baby to be discharged, it is important that:

(A) Baby has completed at least 2 successful feedings.

(B) Baby has coordinated suck and swallow.

(C) Breastfeeding baby latches at the breast without pain to the mother.

(D) Baby has urinated and passed at least one stool.

(E) All of the above.

8. All infants having a short hospital stay must be examined by experienced health personnel within:

(A) 24 hours of discharge

(B) 48 hours of discharge

(C) 72 hours of discharge

(D) within a week of discharge

(E) within the first 2 weeks of life

9. Ductal dependent cardiac lesions may not be apparent until:

(A) 2 hours of life

(B) 6 hours of life

(C) 12 hours of life

(D) 24 hours of life

(E) more than 24 hours of life

10. Contraindications to early discharge are:

(A) low birth weight

(B) congenital anomalies

(C) prematurity

(D) teenage mother

(E) all of the above

11. Prior to early discharge, cord blood type and a Coombs test should be performed on:

(A) all babies

(B) babies whose mothers are group O

(C) all babies with a family history of jaundice

(D) babies whose mothers are Rh negative

(E) B and D

Answers

1. **(C)** Premature babies <38 weeks can have feeding problems and temperature instability. They should be observed for more than 48 hours to establish PO feedings, monitor bilirubin and monitor temperature stability in an open crib.

2. **(E)** Babies that are small for gestational age (SGA) and babies <1800 g have problems maintaining their temperature in an open crib.

3. **(E)** Babies at discharge should be feeding well, have a serum bilirubin level in the low-risk zone of the Bhutani nomogram, should have achieved bleeding hemostasis postcircumcision and have a follow-up appointment.

4. **(B)** The most accurate assessment of gestational age is by first trimester ultrasound measurement of crown-rump length.

5. **(C)**.

6. **(B)** Ninety percent of newborn babies pass meconium in the first 24 hours of life. Babies should be observed long enough to make sure feedings are established nicely, the baby has passed urine and stool, and the bilirubin is in the range of the Bhutani nomogram low-risk zone.

7. **(E)**.

8. **(B)** The American Academy of Pediatrics (AAP) recommends a follow-up visit within 48 hours after early discharge.

9. **(E)**.

10. **(E)** Low-birth-weight babies, premature babies and babies with congenital abnormalities may have feeding problems, temperature instability, hyperbilirubinemia, or metabolic problems like hypoglycemia or hypocalcemia. They should not be discharged home early. Teenage mothers should be evaluated by social workers to make sure that there is an adequate support system at home.

11. (E) Babies born to O-positive mothers or Rh-negative mothers have the possibility of blood group incompatibility if the baby is blood group A or B or Rh positive. Therefore, cord blood type determination and a direct Coombs test should be done in mothers with blood group O or Rh negative.

SUGGESTED READING

American Academy of Pediatrics: Committee on fetus and newborn. hospital stay for healthy term newborns. *Pediatrics* 96:788–790, 1995.

CASE 116: A TERM NEWBORN REQUIRES ROUTINE CARE IN THE NURSERY

A full-term, 3500-g baby girl is born after a normal vaginal delivery following 4 hours rupture of membranes. The mother kept all her prenatal visits and had no complications. Family history is noncontributory.

On examination the baby has normal vital signs and is pink and vigorous.

SELECT THE ONE BEST ANSWER TO THE FOLLOWING QUESTIONS:

1. Are there any procedures that should be done in the birth room?

   (A) administer hepatitis B vaccine
   (B) administer vitamin K IM
   (C) administer vitamin K orally
   (D) apply ophthalmic ointment
   (E) B and D

2. Upon admission to the nursery, are there procedures that should be done?

   (A) glucose screen
   (B) hematocrit screen
   (C) glucose water feeding
   (D) all of the above
   (E) none of the above

3. If the mother's lower vaginal and rectal culture results for group B β-hemolytic streptococcus are unknown, what would you have done for the baby if no prophylactic penicillin had been given to the mother intrapartum?

   (A) Start oral amoxicillin.
   (B) Draw a blood culture and complete blood count, and start intravenous penicillin.
   (C) Do an LP.
   (D) Observe.
   (E) Draw a blood culture and a CBC.

4. If the mother is GBS positive and had received prophylactic intrapartum penicillin for more than 4 hours prior to delivery, what would be your best course?

   (A) obtain blood culture
   (B) obtain CBC
   (C) A and B
   (D) administer IM antibiotics
   (E) none of the above

5. If a mother has a positive cervical culture for gonococcus and was not treated before delivery, what will you do?

   (A) Take a culture of the baby's conjunctivae and wait for results.
   (B) Take a blood culture.
   (C) Observe for illness.
   (D) Give IM ceftriaxone.
   (E) B and D.

6. If a mother has untreated *Chlamydia* at the time of delivery, what will you do?

   (A) Give a double dose of erythromycin ophthalmic ointment.
   (B) Do a nasopharyngeal culture and wait for results.
   (C) Start oral erythromycin.
   (D) Monitor for signs and symptoms of infection.
   (E) A and B.

7. At the end of the first day of life, you see that no urine output has been recorded by the nurse for an otherwise well newborn with a normal examination. Your best course of action should be:

   (A) Catheterize the bladder
   (B) Give 4 ounces of glucose water
   (C) Order a renal ultrasound
   (D) Do nothing
   (E) Give 20 mL/kg bolus IV fluids

8. An 18-hour-old breastfeeding newborn spits yellow material after a feed. You should:

   (A) order an upper GI series

(B) observe
(C) order a lower GI series
(D) order a flat plate of the abdomen
(E) hold all feeds

9. A 40-hour formula fed newborn has had no stools recorded in the nurses' notes. The best course of action includes:

(A) Ask mother if the baby has passed any stools
(B) Order a glycerin suppository
(C) Perform a rectal examination
(D) B and C
(E) Order a suction rectal biopsy

10. The mother of a 10-hour-old newborn wants the formula changed to soy because the baby has vomited the regular formula after taking 40 mL. The best course of action includes:

(A) Agree that the baby cannot tolerate the cow milk based formula.
(B) Take a family history for lactose intolerance.
(C) Suggest that the baby may have been over-fed.
(D) Suggest that more elemental formula be used.
(E) Suggest that a nurse do the next feed.

11. The parents of a breast-fed baby girl tell you on day 2 that the baby is voiding blood. The best course of action includes:

(A) Order STAT prothrombin time (PT) and partial thromboplastin time (PTT) determinations
(B) Explain to the parents that this is vaginal withdrawal bleeding and is normal
(C) Order a renal ultrasound to look for renal vein thrombosis or tumor
(D) Consult hematology/oncology
(E) Consult urology

12. The mother of a 12-hour-old breast-fed baby is worried that the baby is sleepy and has had only one successful feeding. You should:

(A) Order a glucose screen
(B) Order the nurse to feed formula
(C) Ask the mother to put the baby skin to skin with her
(D) Order a glucose water feeding
(E) Turn the heat up in the mother's room

13. On admission physical examination in the nursery, you note a grade 2/6 ejection systolic murmur at the upper left sternal border of an otherwise healthy newborn. The best course of action includes:

(A) Tell the parents that the baby might have congenital heart disease
(B) Request a cardiac consult
(C) Observe
(D) Transfer to the NICU
(E) Obtain a blood gas

14. On discharge physical examination at 50 hours, you find a grade 3/6 systolic murmur at the lower left sternal border. The best course of action includes:

(A) Discharge the baby with instructions to follow up with a pediatrician in 48 hours.
(B) Tell the parents the baby might have congenital heart disease.
(C) Request a cardiac consult.
(D) Order an EKG and oxygen saturation test.
(E) Obtain a blood gas.

15. At the time of discharge of a 2-day-old term baby, you tell the parents to:

(A) Make an appointment with their pediatrician for a 2-week visit.
(B) See how things go, and call the pediatrician as needed.
(C) Establish a pediatric visit prior to leaving the hospital for 1 to 2 days after discharge.
(D) Establish a pediatric visit prior to leaving the hospital for 3 to 4 days after discharge.
(E) A and B.

Answers

1. (**E**) In most hospitals, vitamin K IM and prophylaxis for conjunctivitis are administered in the birth room. Oral vitamin K is not absorbed. The hepatitis B vaccine series is ideally initiated at birth but seldom in the delivery room.

2. (**E**) A term appropriate for gestational age (AGA) baby is not at risk for hypoglycemia. Babies at risk for hypoglycemia are SGA babies, large for gestational age (LGA) babies, infants of diabetic moms and premature babies. Routine hematocrit

is not required. Hematocrit should only be done if the baby looks pale or ruddy.

3. **(D)** Since the baby is born at term gestation and there are no other risk factors such as prolonged rupture of membranes >18 hours, maternal fever, H/O sibling with early onset GBS disease or urine culture positive for GBS during this pregnancy, no work-up or treatment is indicated.

4. **(E)** Baby is term, there are no other risk factors except mother's colonization and she has received adequate intrapartum antibiotic treatment.

5. **(E)** One dose of ceftriaxone IM should be given to babies born to mothers with untreated gonococcal infection. A conjunctival and blood culture are indicated prior to treatment.

6. **(D)** Until recently, AAP Red Book recommended that babies born to mothers with untreated *Chlamydia* infection should be treated with erythromycin for 14 days. Since efficacy of prophylactic treatment is not known and there are reports linking erythromycin use in neonates to hypertrophic pyloric stenosis, the AAP now recommends that only infected infants should be treated. So nothing should be done at birth.

7. **(D)** If baby has been feeding well, looks good, well-hydrated, and examination is normal, chances are that baby had passed urine but was not recorded.

8. **(B)** A small amount of spitting is common. The color of the vomitus is very important. If there is history of the baby vomiting bile or blood, then further investigation should be done. In this patient who is breastfed, yellow spit-up is more than likely breast milk and if abdominal examination is normal, then no work-up is indicated at this time.

9. **(A)** Majority of newborn babies (98%) pass meconium in the first 24 hours of life. Delayed meconium passage beyond 48 hours in an otherwise healthy full-term infant strongly suggests Hirschsprung's disease.

10. **(C)** Generally a 10-hour-old baby will take anywhere from 15- to 30-mL per feeding.

11. **(B)** Pseudomenses or withdrawal bleeding can be seen in normal newborn baby girls in the first couple days of life.

12. **(C)**.

13. **(C)** A grade II/VI murmur on first day of life is most likely secondary to transition from in utero to extrauterine life and is a result of patent ductus arteriosus or tricuspid regurgitation.

14. **(C)** Grade III/VI or higher murmur on day 3 needs to be evaluated by a cardiologist.

15. **(C)** Babies discharged early should be seen by a physician within 2 days of going home to assess bilirubin problems or feeding issues.

SUGGESTED READING

Martin R, Fanaroff AA, Walsh M: *Fanaroff and Martin's Neonatal-Perinatal Medicine Diseases of the Fetus and Infant.* Chicago: Elsevier Mosby, 8th Edition 2006.

15

Nephrology

CASE 119: A 4-DAY-OLD WITH FEEDING PROBLEMS

A 4-day-old boy has become anorexic and comes to your office for evaluation. Mom reports that he had begun to breast-feed avidly but seems much less interested in feeding today and last night. He was the product of a 38-week pregnancy. His mom is 24 years old and had prenatal care. By serology, she had no antibodies to *Treponema pallidum*, rubella, or HIV. She lacked the hepatitis B surface antigen. The baby had an uneventful hospital course. The Apgar scores were 8 and 9 at 1 and 5 minutes. His birth weight was 3100 g. The physical examination reveals a generally healthy looking male infant, with somewhat decreased spontaneous activity. His vital signs and physical examination are entirely normal. You decide to be on the safe side and perform some laboratory tests.

SELECT THE ONE BEST ANSWER TO THE FOLLOWING QUESTIONS:

1. Which of the following statements is correct regarding evaluation for sepsis in this patient?

   (A) A blood culture is not indicated; the patient is afebrile and fever almost always accompanies bacteremia.
   (B) A urine culture need not be performed unless the patient is shown to be bacteremic.
   (C) An LP need not be part of an initial sepsis evaluation since all patients with neonatal meningitis are bacteremic.

   (D) The incidence of neonatal urinary tract infection is roughly equal when stratified by gender.
   (E) A blood leukocyte count has a strong negative predictive value for neonatal bacteremia.

2. Which statement is true regarding evaluation of the urine in a neonate?

   (A) Urine obtained in a sterile plastic bag can be sent for a clinically useful culture provided the genital area is carefully cleaned in advance.
   (B) A specimen should be obtained by bladder puncture or catheterization to minimize the likelihood of contamination.
   (C) $>10^5$ bacteria per mL of urine in a "bagged" specimen is diagnostic of a UTI.
   (D) A and C.
   (E) B and C.

3. Assume that the laboratory tests in the patient in the vignette allowed the diagnosis of a UTI. Which of the following statement(s) is/are correct?

   (A) An ultrasound of the kidneys and a VCUG should be performed on all patients with proven neonatal UTI.
   (B) Patients with neonatal UTI should be treated with a 14-day course of an oral sulfonamide.
   (C) Intravenous pyelography (IVP) should be performed at the time of diagnosis since Wilms' tumor is a common concomitant to UTI.

(D) An ultrasound of the kidneys will allow adequate assessment of a MALE child with a UTI (but not a female).

(E) B and C.

4. Which of the following is (are) true regarding uncomplicated cystitis in school-age children?

(A) Fever is usually absent or low grade.

(B) Uncircumcised males are at risk roughly equal to girls, although circumcised males are at lower incidence compared with girls.

(C) Dysuria is often absent.

(D) A and C.

(E) A, B, and C.

5. Which of the following is true regarding asymptomatic bacteriuria in school-age children?

(A) occurs in about 13% of healthy girls

(B) is a known predictor of end stage pyelonephritis in later life

(C) should be managed with oral antibiotics once identified

(D) is usually cleared spontaneously

(E) none of the above

6. Which of the following is incorrect about pyuria?

(A) It is defined by >5 WBC/high-power field on urinalysis.

(B) It is a sensitive marker for UTI.

(C) It is nonspecific and often absent in a UTI.

(D) It often occurs in Kawasaki disease.

(E) It often occurs during measles infection and after intense exercise.

7. The nitrite dip-stick detection test is

(A) nonspecific even when positive

(B) a sensitive test for UTI

(C) never positive when the cause of the UTI is a gram-positive bacterium

(D) A and C

(E) all of the above

8. The leukocyte esterase (LE) dip-stick detection test is

(A) about 95% sensitive in detection of UTI

(B) has relatively low specificity of about 75%

(C) positive only when gram-negative bacteria are the etiologic agents

(D) is performed on the blood of patients with true pyelonephritis

(E) detects mercury when this metal is in high concentrations in the urine

9. You diagnose an *Escherichia coli* UTI in a 6-year-old girl with dysuria and a low-grade temperature. You decide that she is not clinically toxic, nor has high fever, so you will manage her as an outpatient on oral antimicrobial therapy. You tell the parents which of the following:

(A) This infection is contagious; other children living in the same house as the index patient are at risk for infection.

(B) Amoxicillin is appropriate initial therapy since nearly all *E. coli* isolates are susceptible to it.

(C) Trimethoprim-sulfamethoxazole in a single dose will sterilize her urinary tract and thus is now usually used for initial therapy.

(D) Radiologic studies are an important part of the ongoing evaluation for UTI and should be scheduled.

(E) C and D.

10. The mother of a 3-year-old patient with grade III reflux demonstrated by VCUG comes to you for advice. You tell her that:

(A) Vesicular endoscopic injection of autologous chondrocytes produces a cure in more than half of selected patients.

(B) There is no convincing relationship between reflux and renal scarring; wait and watch is the best plan.

(C) Most pediatricians advise prophylactic antimicrobials in this situation aimed at urinary antisepsis; amoxicillin is a good choice.

(D) Most children will grow out of this condition; reflux will usually cease within a few years.

(E) A and D.

11. Which of the following is (are) known to increase the incidence of UTIs in childhood?

(A) constipation

(B) routine bath exposure

(C) public swimming pool exposure

(D) wiping after urination from back to front

(E) all of the above

12. All of the following can cause cystitis except:

(A) pinworms

(B) ibuprofen

(C) insertion of foreign bodies into the urethra

(D) cyclophosphamide therapy for cancer

(E) all of the above

13. Management of acute pyelonephritis

(A) usually includes a third-generation antimicrobial such as cefotaxime

(B) usually includes a first-generation antimicrobial such as cefazolin

(C) initial therapy should include ceftazidime because *Pseudomonas* spp. is a common etiology

(D) can be accomplished with oral cefixime

(E) A or D are acceptable

14. Which of the following is true regarding the interpretation of a urine culture performed on urine from a school-age child?

(A) The bladder is normally sterile. Any bacteria grown from a specimen of bladder urine is diagnostic of a UTI.

(B) Recovery of several species from a clean catch urine is suggestive of a renal abscess.

(C) Growth of >100,000 bacteria per mL of urine is predictive of bacteria in the bladder.

(D) A and C.

(E) All of the above.

15. Which of the following are risk factors for UTI among adolescents?

(A) ingestion of chocolate

(B) infectious mononucleosis

(C) ingestion of bladder irritants like spicy foods

(D) use of a diaphragm with a spermicide

(E) B and D

Answers

1. (**D**) Neonates who are septic will most often be afebrile. A physician who waits for fever before initiating a septic workup has often waited too long. A urine culture should be part of the evaluation for sepsis in this age group. Meningitis can occur in the absence of bacteremia that may have been cleared by the host without therapy. Although girls of nearly every age group have UTIs at a higher frequency than boys, the singular exception is the neonate where the gender prevalence is roughly equal. The blood leukocyte count in a septic neonate may occasionally be abnormally high or low and may provide a clue as to the presence of a septic process. Most often, however, it is normal.

2. (**B**) Urine obtained in a sterile plastic bag is often contaminated with minute amounts of stool. Since there are large amounts of bacteria in stool, it takes only minuscule contamination of the bagged specimen to yield a "positive" culture result. Any positive culture from this bag must be confirmed by obtaining a specimen of bladder urine before a diagnosis of UTI can be made. The best specimens are those obtained by bladder puncture or catheterization. Bladder urine should be sterile.

3. (**A**) The frequency of anatomic abnormalities of the urinary tract that may require urologic intervention or long-term antimicrobial prophylaxis is sufficiently high to warrant radiologic assessment after even the first well-documented UTI. Oral therapy in the neonatal period is generally avoided because of the few data available regarding absorption or outcomes. Sulfonamides may promote hyperbilirubinemia and are to be avoided in this age group. IVP has been replaced by the less invasive ultrasound evaluation for the upper urinary tract but offers no gender-specific advantage.

4. (**A**) Dysuria is frequent, perhaps the most frequent, clinical symptom. Uncircumcised males are at increased risk compared with circumcised males but all males are at substantially less risk than females in this age group. Fever is usually absent or low grade. High fever accompanied by symptoms and signs of UTI implies pyelonephritis.

5. (**D**) Asymptomatic bacteriuria occurs in about 1% of healthy school girls. The link between it and end-stage pyelonephritis has never been convincingly established. Most experts do not

believe antimicrobials should be routinely prescribed when asymptomatic bacteriuria is discovered. Careful questioning should be performed, however, to ensure that the patient is truly asymptomatic. Asymptomatic bacteriuria is often cleared spontaneously.

6. **(C)** The traditional definition of pyuria has been >5 WBC/high-power field, although modifications have been suggested recently. Most children with symptomatic UTI have pyuria. Pyuria is frequent in patients with Kawasaki disease, measles, and after exercise.

7. **(C)** The nitrate test is highly specific for UTI although not reliably sensitive. It depends on bacteria converting dietary nitrates to nitrites in the urine specimen and requires a >4-hour incubation for the reaction to occur. Gram-positive bacteria do not perform the chemical reaction and thus the test will never be positive when a gram-positive species is the cause.

8. **(B)** LE has about 80% sensitivity depending on the clinical setting. The specificity is lower, however, because pyuria may yield a positive test. The test is performed only on urine and has no value in the detection of mercury.

9. **(D)** There is no reason to believe that anyone else in the house is at risk from the patient's *E. coli* UTI. Amoxicillin is a poor choice as about half of *E. coli* isolates may be resistant. Single-dose therapy of UTI in children has been largely abandoned despite a flurry of one-time interest because the rate of recurrence is unacceptably high. Radiologic studies should be performed in children with a first well-proven UTI.

10. **(E)** Initial success with the relatively noninvasive injection of autologous chondrocytes has been encouraging although relapses occur. There is no convincing relationship between reflux and renal scarring, but most experts advocate antimicrobial prophylaxis for patients like this. Amoxicillin is a poor choice because enteric organisms have unacceptably high rates of resistance. Thus failures are too common. Nitrofurantoin, sulfisoxazole, and trimethoprim-sulfamethoxazole are acceptable choices; no choice will prevent all breakthroughs. Most children with mild to moderate reflux do spontaneously remit, usually within a few years.

11. **(A)** Despite the widely held views that all of the choices increase the incidence of UTI, evidence-based data exist to support the relationship between constipation and increased UTI incidence only. While the other items are frequently advocated by pediatricians, convincing data to support their etiologic relationship are lacking.

12. **(B)** Either by mechanical irritation or by other less well understood mechanisms, pinworms, insertion of foreign bodies into the urethra, and cyclophosphamide can all cause cystitis with symptoms of urgency, frequency, and dysuria. Ibuprofen is the exception. Although a wide variety of toxicities are associated with ibuprofen, cystitis has not been described.

13. **(E)** Although some experts point to the modest in vitro activity of cefazolin against gram-negatives, most experts do not rely on this activity for effective therapy for serious infections such as pyelonephritis that are likely to be caused by gram-negatives. *Pseudomonas* is an unusual cause of UTI and generally not included as an initial target for pyelonephritis. Thus, there is no need for ceftazidime. Oral cefixime fared well in head-to-head evaluation against the parenteral third-generation compound cefotaxime and is probably acceptable therapy unless a patient is quite ill and compliance with any oral regimen in the short term is questionable.

14. **(D)** In theory, no bacteria should be recoverable from urine from a bladder catheterization obtained by sterile technique or from a bladder aspiration. Some clinical microbiology laboratories have introduced a margin of error and use a cutoff of <10,000 bacteria/mL as a negative culture on bladder urine. Traditionally, >100,000 bacteria per mL is used as a predictor of bladder infection, although this value was derived from studies done among healthy, asymptomatic adult women. Some have argued that in a symptomatic person, i.e., one with dysuria for example, a lower bacterial density, e.g., 10,000 to 100,000, may reflect bladder colonization. Mixed bacterial

cultures generally reflect urethral contamination and not any specific disease process.

15. **(D)** Sexual intercourse and use of a diaphragm with spermicide both increase the risk of UTIs among sexually active females. Neither ingestion of any particular food nor infectious mononucleosis have any demonstrated association with UTIs.

SUGGESTED READINGS

Gorelick MH, Shaw KN: Screening tests for urinary tract infection in children: a meta-analysis. *Pediatrics* 104: E54, 1999.

Practice parameter. The diagnosis, treatment, and evaluation of the initial urinary tract infection in febrile infants and young children. American Academy of Pediatrics. Committee on Quality Improvement. Subcommittee on Urinary Tract Infection. [published corrections appear in *Pediatrics* 105:141, 2000, 103:1052, 1999, and 104:118, 1999]. *Pediatrics* 103(Pt 4 1):843–852, 1999.

Hoberman A, Charron M, Hickey RW, et al: Imaging studies after a first febrile urinary tract infection in your children. *N Engl J Med* 348:195–202, 2003.

CASE 120: A 4-MONTH-OLD BOY WITH POOR WEIGHT GAIN, IRRITABILITY, AND LOW URINE OSMOLALITY

A 4-month-old male infant presents with a history of poor weight gain and irritability. He was born at term by vaginal delivery with a birth weight of 3.5 kg. He was breast-fed for 3 months and appeared to have satisfactory weight gain initially. He was then switched to formula feeds, which he has been taking well. Mom says his diapers are always soaking wet. His development has been normal and his immunizations are up to date.

On examination you find an infant who is thin with weight below the 5th percentile and height on the 25th percentile. He appears to be irritable. He has a mildly sunken anterior fontanel, an umbilical hernia, and mild bilateral tibial curvature.

Laboratory studies show:

Hemoglobin	10.8 g/dL
Hematocrit	32.9%
BUN	17 mg/dL
Serum creatinine	0.5 mg/dL
Serum sodium	148 mEq/L
Serum potassium	3.7 mEq/L
Serum chloride	114 mEq/dL
Serum bicarbonate	20 mEq/dL
Serum calcium	9.8 mg/dL
Serum phosphorus	5.5 mg/dL
Serum alkaline phosphatase	360 U/L
Serum magnesium	1.9 mg/dL
Serum glucose	72 mg/dL
Urine specific gravity	1005
Urine pH	6.8
Urine osmolality	198 mOsm/kg of H_2O

SELECT THE ONE BEST ANSWER

1. The serum osmolality in this patient is:

   (A) 296
   (B) 302
   (C) 306
   (D) 300
   (E) none of the above

2. The most likely cause for this infant's failure to thrive is:

   (A) metabolic acidosis because of renal tubular acidosis and urinary concentration defect
   (B) nephrogenic diabetes insipidus
   (C) Bartter's syndrome with polyuria
   (D) Gitelman syndrome
   (E) Liddle's disease

3. Other laboratory investigations that may be helpful include:

   (A) spot urine calcium/creatinine ratio
   (B) serum vasopressin levels
   (C) nasal vasopressin (DDAVP) test
   (D) B and C
   (E) A, B, and C

4. This disease is most commonly inherited as:

   (A) an autosomal recessive disorder
   (B) an autosomal dominant disorder
   (C) an X-linked recessive disorder
   (D) an X-linked dominant disorder
   (E) none of the above

5. This condition is most appropriately treated with:

   (A) low-solute diet

(B) thiazide diuretics with amiloride and prostaglandin-synthesis inhibitors such as indomethacin

(C) thiazide diuretics and prostaglandin-synthesis inhibitors such as indomethacin

(D) all of the above

(E) A and C

6. Urine osmolality *in this patient* is measured to determine:

(A) urine osmolal gap

(B) urine anion gap

(C) urine concentration defect

(D) none of the above

(E) A and B

7. Urine osmolality should be measured in the urine:

(A) in all patients on a routine basis

(B) if a urinary concentration defect is suspected

(C) to measure the urine osmolal gap

(D) all of the above

(E) B and C

8. Normal range of urine osmolality in a child is:

(A) 200 to 1200 mOsm/kg of H_2O

(B) 100 to 1000 mOsm/kg of H_2O

(C) 50 to 1400 mOsm/kg of H_2O

(D) 400 to 800 mOsm/kg of H_2O

(E) 300 to 900 mOsm/kg of H_2O

9. In acquired or secondary nephrogenic diabetes insipidus:

(A) aquaporin 5 expression is decreased

(B) aquaporin 2 expression is decreased

(C) aquaporin 6 expression is decreased

(D) aquaporin 1 expression is decreased

(E) aquaporin 4 expression is decreased

10. Secondary diabetes insipidus can be caused by:

(A) analgesic nephropathy

(B) amoxicillin

(C) lithium therapy

(D) all of the above

(E) A and C

11. Secondary diabetes insipidus occurs with:

(A) obstructive uropathy

(B) chronic renal failure

(C) chronic pyelonephritis

(D) all of the above

(E) A and C

12. Secondary diabetes insipidus can occur in:

(A) hypokalemia

(B) hyponatremia

(C) hypercalcemia

(D) A and C

(E) B only

13. Acquired nephrogenic diabetes insipidus can be caused by all of the following except:

(A) sarcoidosis

(B) iron deficiency anemia

(C) renal dysplasia

(D) nephrocalcinosis

(E) sickle cell anemia and trait

14. Nephrogenic diabetes insipidus can be all of the following except:

(A) caused by unresponsiveness of renal tubules to vasopressin

(B) caused by a vasopressin deficiency

(C) a familial disorder

(D) an acquired disorder

(E) caused by decreased aquaporin expression

15. Infants with nephrogenic diabetes insipidus can present with all of the following except:

(A) failure to thrive

(B) seizures

(C) polyphagia

(D) constipation

(E) dilated ureters

16. Nephrogenic diabetes insipidus in children can cause all of the following except:

(A) short stature

(B) mental retardation

(C) hydronephrosis

(D) microcystis

(E) hyperactivity

17. Children with nephrogenic diabetes insipidus are at risk of developing dehydration with all of the following except:

(A) gastroenteritis
(B) low salt intake
(C) hot weather
(D) exercise
(E) fever

Answers

1. **(C)** Sodium is the major cation in extracellular water and accounts for most of the plasma osmolality. However under pathologic conditions, serum urea nitrogen (as in acute renal failure) and glucose (as in diabetic ketoacidosis) can also contribute significantly to the serum osmolality. Therefore the serum osmolality is calculated as $2 \times$ [Serum sodium] (mEq/L) + [Glucose]/18 (mg/dL) + [BUN]/2.8 (mg/dL). Serum osmolality in this patient is $2 \times 148 + 72/18 + 17/2.8 = 306$ (normal range, 285 to 295).

2. **(B)** This infant does not have renal tubular acidosis and metabolic acidosis as a serum bicarbonate of 20 mEq/L is in normal range for infants (20 to 24 mEq/L). This is one of the typical presentations of congenital nephrogenic diabetes insipidus. Urine specific gravity and osmolality are low with borderline high serum sodium. An initial diagnosis of diabetes insipidus can be made with measurement of paired urine and plasma osmolality. A high serum osmolality with low urinary osmolality (<200 mOsm/kg H_2O) provides evidence for a renal urinary concentration defect. This infant was initially breast-fed. The infant would have received enough free water, therefore, to continue to gain weight since human breast milk has low salt and protein content and, therefore, there is less osmolar load in the glomerular filtrate requiring less obligate water loss in the urine. When switched to formula feeds, however, the baby was on a fixed volume of feeds at 120 to 150 mL/kg/day. Cow's milk has a higher solute and protein load that would lead to greater urinary osmolar load and greater free water losses. Weight loss and failure to thrive are the result.

   Bartter's syndrome is characterized by a defect in Na-K-2Cl cotransporter in the ascending limb of the loop of Henle, leading to loss of sodium, potassium, and chloride in the urine and hy-pokalemic hypochloremic metabolic alkalosis. This infant does not have metabolic alkalosis.

   Gitelman syndrome occurs in older children and is a result of a defect in Na-Cl cotransporter in the distal convoluted tubule, leading to a loss of sodium, potassium, and chloride in the urine and hypokalemic hypochloremic metabolic alkalosis as well as hypomagnesemia a result of increased urinary magnesium loss.

   Liddle's syndrome occurs in adolescents and adults and is caused by upregulation of epithelial sodium channel ENaC in the principal cell of the cortical-collecting duct. It leads to excessive sodium absorption with hypokalemia and hypertension as a result of volume expansion.

3. **(D)** Nephrogenic diabetes insipidus is characterized by renal tubular insensitivity to antidiuretic hormone (ADH) or arginine vasopressin (AVP); therefore vasopressin levels are normal or may be slightly increased in these patients. A vasopressin test may be performed and consists of intranasal administration of a single dose of DDAVP (1-desamino-8-D-arginine vasopressin) followed by urine collection over the next $5\frac{1}{2}$ hours. Patients with nephrogenic diabetes insipidus fail to concentrate their urine and the urine osmolality remains low, usually ≤ 200 mOsm/kg H_2O.

4. **(C)** Congenital nephrogenic diabetes insipidus (NDI) is inherited, most commonly (about 90%) as an X-linked recessive disorder and, therefore, unaffected female carriers transmit the disease to their sons. This usually results in episodes of hypernatremic dehydration during infancy. One common presentation is "failure to thrive" when an infant is switched from breast milk to formula feeds. Rare cases (about 10%) have been described that are a result of mutations in the aquaporin water channel gene as an autosomal recessive or autosomal dominant disorder. Patients with this mutation present with hypokalemia. Associated conditions include renal dysplasia, obstructive uropathy, chronic renal failure, chronic pyelonephritis, sickle cell anemia and trait, analgesic nephropathy, and persons taking lithium therapy.

5. **(D)** Free water replacement is the most important part of the treatment of NDI. As this can be

difficult in infants, a low-solute diet to decrease obligate free water losses in the urine by decreasing the urine osmolar load is prudent.

Thiazide diuretics and dietary salt restriction can decrease the urine volume up to 50% but need supplementation of diet with potassium as they can cause hypokalemia. A combination of a thiazide diuretic with another diuretic like amiloride that acts on epithelial sodium channels (ENaC), the principal cell in the cortical collecting duct, is potassium sparing and effective. Thiazide diuretics have also been used in combination with prostaglandin synthesis inhibitors such as indomethacin as an effective regimen in decreasing the urine output in NDI.

6. **(C)** In this patient, hypernatremia with low urine specific gravity is suggestive of a urinary concentration defect and therefore a simultaneous plasma and urine osmolality would be necessary to make the diagnosis of diabetes insipidus. Urine osmolality can also be measured to determine the urine osmolal gap. This is the measured urine osmolality minus the calculated urine osmolality (based on the formula: $2 \times$ [Urine sodium] (mEq/L) + [Glucose]/18 (mg/dL) + [Urea/2.8] (mg/dL)]. The difference should be a positive number (because the measured osmolality is higher than the calculated osmolality) and represents the amount of ammonium chloride being excreted in the urine. Thus, this calculation measures the amount of ammonium excreted in the urine in patients who are suspected to have renal tubular acidosis. However, in this patient, we are suspecting diabetes insipidus, not renal tubular acidosis.

7. **(E)** Routine urinalysis does not include a urine osmolality. Indications for measuring osmolality are a suspected urinary concentration defect as in diabetes insipidus or a need to calculate the urine osmolar gap as described in the answer to question 6.

8. **(C)** The normal range of urine osmolality in a child is 50 to1400 mOsm/kg and in an infant it is 50 to 600 mOsm/kg H_2O.

9. **(B)** The aquaporin 2 (water channel) is normally present in the principal cell of the cortical collecting duct and leads to water reabsorption under the effect of vasopressin. In secondary NDI, the expression of aquaporin 2 is decreased and leads to impaired water absorption.

10. **(E)** Secondary NDI can be caused by lithium, colchicine, radiocontrast agents, vinblastine, analgesic nephropathy, and tetracyclines.

11. **(D)** Secondary NDI can occur in chronic renal disease such as chronic renal failure, chronic pyelonephritis, polycystic kidney disease, medullary cystic disease, uric acid, or calcium nephropathy.

12. **(D)** Acquired or secondary NDI occurs with electrolyte disorders such as hypokalemia and hypercalcemia and is a common metabolic abnormality associated with a urinary concentration defect.

13. **(B)** Acquired NDI can be caused by diseases such as sickle cell anemia, adrenal insufficiency, sarcoidosis, amyloidosis, and nephrocalcinosis. It can also occur with protein starvation.

14. **(B)** NDI can be familial or acquired. There are two types of familial NDI. The most common is a mutation in the gene encoding vasopressin receptor V2 in the renal tubular cells, an X-linked recessive disorder. Less common is a mutation in the gene encoding the vasopressin-sensitive water channel aquaporin 2 (AQP 2) in the cells of the renal cortical collecting duct and can be an autosomal dominant or recessive disorder. In acquired NDI, there is usually a decrease in AQP2 abundance. Vasopressin deficiency would be a central and not a nephrogenic cause of DI.

15. **(C)** Symptoms of NDI include poor feeding, irritability, eagerness to suck, dehydration, failure to thrive, rarely seizures because of electrolyte imbalance, and constipation. Hydronephrosis and dilated ureters because of polyuria and consequently increased urine flow may be present.

16. **(D)** NDI in children can cause poor growth with short stature. Mental retardation has been reported

because of recurrent episodes of dehydration with intracranial calcifications. Polyuria leading to frequent trips to the washroom with consequent interference with learning has been associated with short attention span, distractibility, and hyperactivity. Increased urine flow in NDI can lead to a large bladder (megacystis), not a small bladder (microcystis).

17. **(B)** All of these can lead to increased fluid and free water losses except for low salt intake, which is a therapeutic option for NDI. A high salt intake would lead to increased obligatory free water losses and, therefore, worsening of the symptoms.

SUGGESTED READING
Knoers NVAM, Monnens LAH: Nephrogenic diabetes insipidus. In: Anver ED, Harmon WE, Niaudet P, (eds): *Pediatric Nephrology*, 5th ed. Philadelphia PA: Lippincott, Williams & Wilkins, 2004, pp 777–788.

CASE 121: AN 8-MONTH-OLD MALE INFANT WITH VOMITING AND WEIGHT LOSS

An 8-month-old male infant presents to the emergency room with vomiting and weight loss of several days' duration. He has also had some loose stools. There is no history of fever. A systematic inquiry is noncontributory. He was born at term by normal vaginal delivery with a birth weight of 3.6 kg (50th percentile) and a length of 51 cm (>50th percentile). His development has been normal and his immunizations are reported to be up to date.

On examination you find a thin infant with mild dehydration. He is irritable. His weight now is 7.8 kg (on 5th percentile) and his height is 68 cm (just below the 25th percentile). The remainder of the examination is unremarkable.

Laboratory results are as follows:

Hemoglobin	10.8 g/dL
Hematocrit	32.5%
BUN	8 mg/dL
Serum creatinine	0.3 mg/dL
Serum sodium	137 mEq/L
Serum potassium	3.2 mEq/L
Serum chloride	110 mEq/L
Serum bicarbonate	16 mEq/L
Serum calcium	8.9 mg/dL
Serum phosphorus	4.6 mg/dL

Serum magnesium	1.9 mg/dL
Urine pH	5.4
Urine specific gravity	1.020
Urine sodium	44 mEq/L
Urine potassium	23 mEq/L
Urine chloride	47 mEq/L
Urine glucose	Negative

Arterial blood gas results:

pH	7.32
P_{CO_2}	38
P_{O_2}	96
BE	2
HCO_3	16

SELECT THE ONE BEST ANSWER

1. This infant has a:

    (A) high anion gap metabolic acidosis
    (B) non–anion gap metabolic acidosis
    (C) hypokalemic hypochloremic metabolic alkalosis
    (D) mixed metabolic and respiratory acidosis
    (E) none of the above

2. The urine anion gap is calculated as follows:

    (A) Urine sodium (mEq/L) + Urine potassium (mEq/L) – Urine chloride (mEq/L)
    (B) Urine sodium (mEq/L) – Urine chloride (mEq/L)
    (C) Urine sodium (mEq/L) – Urine chloride and bicarbonate (mEq/L)
    (D) Urine sodium (mEq/L) + Urine potassium (mEq/L) – Urine chloride and bicarbonate (mEq/L)
    (E) There is no such thing as a urine anion gap

3. The urine anion gap in this case is:

    (A) positive and abnormal
    (B) negative and normal
    (C) normal
    (D) not possible to calculate because of insufficient data
    (E) none of the above

4. This infant has:

    (A) non–anion gap metabolic acidosis because of gastroenteritis and dehydration (the urine anion gap is suggestive of increased ammonium excretion)

(B) non–anion gap metabolic acidosis because of proximal renal tubular acidosis (the urine anion gap is suggestive of increased ammonium excretion)

(C) proximal renal tubular acidosis as the urine anion gap is suggestive of decreased ammonium excretion

(D) non–anion gap metabolic acidosis because of gastroenteritis and dehydration as the urine anion gap is suggestive of decreased ammonium excretion

(E) none of the above

5. Other investigations that may be helpful are:

(A) spot urine protein/creatinine ratio
(B) radiograph of the long bones
(C) renal ultrasound
(D) CT scan of the head
(E) MRI scan of the brain

6. This condition can present as:

(A) an autosomal dominant disorder inheritance pattern
(B) an autosomal recessive disorder inheritance pattern
(C) primary or secondary to an underlying problem
(D) all of the above
(E) none of the above

7. The long-term treatment of this child should consist of:

(A) dietary sodium restriction
(B) oral sodium citrate or bicarbonate with or without potassium citrate
(C) prostaglandin synthesis inhibitors
(D) all of the above
(E) A and B

8. All of the following are recognized types of renal tubular acidosis (RTA) except:

(A) type I RTA
(B) type II RTA
(C) type III RTA
(D) type IV RTA

(E) none of the above (all of the above are recognized types of RTA)

9. Which type(s) of renal tubular acidosis cause(s) hyperkalemia:

(A) type I RTA
(B) type II RTA
(C) type III RTA
(D) type IV RTA
(E) none of the above

10. Which type(s) of renal tubular acidosis cause(s) hypokalemia:

(A) type I RTA
(B) type II RTA
(C) type III RTA
(D) type IV RTA
(E) A and B only

11. Rickets can be present in:

(A) type I RTA
(B) type IV RTA
(C) type II RTA
(D) B only
(E) A and C only

12. Nephrocalcinosis occurs:

(A) more commonly in type I RTA
(B) more commonly in type II RTA
(C) more commonly in type IV RTA
(D) only in type I RTA
(E) commonly in type II and IV, but never in type I RTA

13. All of the following can cause type II or proximal RTA except:

(A) valproic acid
(B) penicillin
(C) ifosfamide
(D) mercaptopurine
(E) sulfonamides

14. All of the following can cause type I or distal RTA except:

(A) analgesic abuse
(B) amphotericin B
(C) lithium

(D) amoxicillin
(E) vitamin D intoxication

15. Type I or distal RTA can be caused by:

(A) a bicarbonate reabsorption defect
(B) a proton pump failure in the cortical collecting duct
(C) a proton back leak into the cortical collecting duct cells
(D) all of the above
(E) B and C only

16. Type II or proximal RTA can be caused by:

(A) a bicarbonate reabsorption defect
(B) an aldosterone deficiency
(C) a proton back leak into the cortical collecting duct cells
(D) insensitivity of the renal cortical collecting duct to aldosterone
(E) proton pump failure in the cortical collecting duct

17. Type IV RTA can be caused by:

(A) aldosterone deficiency
(B) a bicarbonate reabsorption defect
(C) insensitivity of cortical collecting duct to aldosterone
(D) all of the above
(E) A and C only

18. Type IV RTA in children that caused by pseudo-hypoaldosteronism is best treated with:

(A) mineralocorticoid-like fludrocortisone
(B) alkali supplementation
(C) vitamin D supplementation
(D) diuretics such as thiazides or furosemide
(E) none of the above

19. Type IV RTA caused by hyporeninemic hypoaldosteronism is best treated with:

(A) vitamin D and alkali supplements
(B) mineralocorticoids
(C) angiotensin-converting enzyme inhibitors
(D) angiotensin receptor-blocking agents
(E) none of the above

Answers

1. **(B)** The serum anion gap is calculated as: Serum sodium (cation; mEq/L) − Serum chloride (anion; mEq/L) + Serum bicarbonate (anion; mEq/L). The anion gap is this case is [137 − (110 + 16)] = 11. Usually, the anion gap is 10, with a normal range of 8 to 15. The serum chloride concentrate is also high. Therefore, this patient has a normal anion gap or hyperchloremic metabolic acidosis.

2. **(A)** The urine anion gap (UAG) is calculated as: Urine sodium concentration (mEq/L) + Urine potassium concentration (mEq/L) − Urine chloride concentration (mEq/L).

3. **(A)** The UAG is an indirect measure of ammonium excretion in the urine, employed because ammonium is difficult to measure. Ammonium excretion in the urine is one of the ways kidneys excrete protons (H^+) to maintain acid-base homeostasis. Under normal circumstances, the UAG is a negative number that represents the unmeasured ammonium cation (NH_4^+, i.e., ammonium ion). Ammonium ions constitute almost all of the cations in the urine after sodium and potassium are excluded. In this patient, the UAG is a positive number (+20). This is abnormally high and indicates no ammonium ion or the presence of another anion such as bicarbonate. The latter is present in excess in the urine in proximal RTA and is also not measured routinely in the urine. A positive UAG is therefore a result of decreased or impaired production of ammonium and an increased concentration of bicarbonate. Both changes occur in proximal RTA. Once the serum bicarbonate falls below the renal threshold, bicarbonaturia ceases. The urine pH can then decrease to <5.5 as distal acidification in the cortical collecting duct continues to be normal in proximal RTA, which is characterized by bicarbonate loss in the urine.

   In gastroenteritis, a hyperchloremic metabolic acidosis can also occur and there is no increased serum anion gap (SAG). As a compensatory mechanism, the kidneys, if normal, would excrete more ammonium to excrete the proton (H^+). In this instance, one would expect the UAG to be more negative than normal. For example, the UAG may be more negative, e.g., 60 or higher, suggesting increased ammonium excretion.

4. **(C)** The UAG in this patient is positive (+20), suggesting decreased or absent ammonium in the urine. This suggests proximal RTA in this case as the urine pH is also <5.5, lower than that occurring in distal RTA. Patients with distal RTA have a proton pump disorder in the cortical collecting duct with inability to excrete hydrogen ions and therefore are not able to acidify urine to a pH of <5.5.

    If this normal anion-gap metabolic acidosis were a result of gastroenteritis with normal renal function, one would expect a more negative than normal UAG. Such a finding suggests increased urinary ammonium excretion by the kidneys as a compensatory mechanism to maintain acid-base homeostasis.

5. **(C)** Nephrocalcinosis occurs commonly with distal RTA and rarely with proximal RTA. In distal RTA caused by persistent metabolic acidosis and buffering of the acidosis by bones, calcium is released into the serum leading to hypercalciuria. There is also decreased citrate excretion in distal RTA. Citrate in urine inhibits stone formation. These changes in distal RTA make nephrocalcinosis and renal calculus formation more likely in distal RTA. As mentioned, nephrocalcinosis can occur in proximal RTA as well and, therefore, a renal ultrasound may be useful in detecting nephrocalcinosis.

6. **(D)** Proximal RTA can be primary, which includes genetically determined proximal RTA, which can be autosomal recessive or dominant. Proximal RTA can also be secondary to several disorders, including metabolic disorders such as cystinosis, galactosemia, glycogen storage disease, and carbonic anhydrase deficiency. It can also be associated with drugs and toxins and heavy metal poisoning including lead toxicity. It can also occur as an isolated bicarbonate reabsorption defect with consequent bicarbonate loss in the urine or as a part of Fanconi's syndrome, a generalized disorder of proximal tubules leading

to not only bicarbonaturia but also glycosuria, aminoaciduria, and phosphaturia.

7. **(E)** Treatment of both proximal and distal RTA consists of alkali supplementation with either oral sodium bicarbonate or sodium citrate. As both types of RTA can be associated with hypokalemia, supplementation with potassium citrate or potassium chloride may also be needed. Dietary sodium restriction helps to enhance proximal tubular reabsorption of sodium and bicarbonate and decreases the alkali supplementation requirements. Prostaglandin synthesis inhibitors are not known to play a role in the treatment of RTA.

8. **(C)** Type III RTA, originally described as mixed type I and type II RTA, is no longer recognized. In young infants and premature infants there can be a transient physiologic proximal tubular immaturity leading to increased urinary bicarbonate losses. Therefore children with type I RTA resulting from a hydrogen ion secretion defect also have increased urinary bicarbonate losses. Therefore, the term mixed or type III RTA was used. However, this bicarbonaturia tends to resolve as the tubules mature but the distal acidification defect persists. Therefore the patients who were first described as having mixed RTA were actually children with distal RTA and physiologic proximal tubular immaturity that resolved with time.

9. **(D)** Only type IV RTA causes hyperkalemia. In children, this could be the result of pseudohypoaldosteronism (with normal or high serum aldosterone levels) and in adults because of mineralocorticoid deficiency as a result of hyporeninemic hypoaldosteronism. Other causes of hypoaldosteronism leading to type IV RTA include Addison's disease, congenital adrenal hyperplasia, and effects of drugs such as ACE inhibitors, heparin, and cyclosporine.

10. **(E)** Hypokalemia occurs with type I and II RTA. In type I RTA there is a proton pump disorder with failure of hydrogen ion excretion. Therefore, another cation must be excreted with the anions delivered in the filtrate to the cortical collecting duct; this cation is usually potassium. In type II RTA

there is an excess of anions (bicarbonate in this case) that have to be excreted in combination with cations like potassium. This leads to increased excretion of potassium (cation) in the cortical collecting duct and hypokalemia. Both primary type I and II RTA can have autosomal recessive or autosomal dominant inheritance. Patients with both type I and II RTA can present with vomiting, anorexia, constipation, polyuria, polydipsia, or growth retardation. Both conditions have associated hypokalemia with muscle weakness.

11. (E) Rickets can occur in both type I and type II RTA. It is not seen in type IV RTA.

12. (A) Although nephrocalcinosis can occur in both type I and type II RTA, it is much more common in type I RTA (distal RTA). This is because of the following:

    1. persistent metabolic acidosis, which is seen in type I RTA compared with type II (Proximal RTA) where blood pH tends to fluctuate more often than type I RTA.
    2. increased serum calcium because of calcium released from the bone as a result of buffering of persistent metabolic acidosis by the bones.
    3. decreased citrate excretion in the urine or hypocitraturia because of the distal tubular defect in type I RTA. Citrate and magnesium in the urine are known inhibitors of stone formation. In type I RTA, the above-mentioned factors lead to increased incidence of nephrocalcinosis.

13. (B) Penicillin does not cause type II or proximal RTA.

14. (D) All of the mentioned drugs except for amoxicillin can cause type I or distal RTA.

15. (E) A bicarbonate reabsorption defect occurs in type II or proximal RTA, whereas type I or distal RTA can be caused by proton pump failure or back-leak of excreted proton (hydrogen ion) into the cells of the cortical collecting duct. This back-leak phenomenon typically occurs in RTA because of amphotericin.

16. (A) Type II or proximal RTA can be a result of an isolated defect in proximal tubular bicarbonate

absorption, or it can be caused by a bicarbonate reabsorption defect as a part of generalized proximal tubular disorder with aminoaciduria, glycosuria, and phosphaturia (seen in Fanconi syndrome).

17. (E) Type IV or hyperkalemic RTA can be as a result of pseudohypoaldosteronism (because of insensitivity of renal tubular cells to aldosterone) as commonly seen in children, or as a result of aldosterone deficiency from various causes in children and adults. A common associate in adults is with hyporeninemic hypoaldosteronism seen in elderly diabetic patients as a result of hypofunction of the juxtaglomerular apparatus and consequent hyporeninemia and hypoaldosteronism. An example of hypoaldosteronism in children is congenital adrenal hyperplasia.

18. (D) In type IV RTA because of pseudohypoaldosteronism, there is insensitivity of the cortical collecting duct cells to aldosterone. Serum aldosterone levels are normal or high. Therefore mineralocorticoid therapy would not help. These patients are best treated with diuretics such as loop diuretics like furosemide and/or distal tubular diuretics like thiazides. These diuretics help improve hyperkalemia by delivering an excess of sodium in the filtrate to the cortical collecting duct. This increased sodium concentration in the filtrate with a consequent increase in the sodium gradient leads to potassium-sodium exchange in the cortical collecting duct with consequent increased potassium excretion in the urine.

19. (B) Hyporeninemic hypoaldosteronism occurs in elderly diabetic patients as a result of the dysfunction of juxtaglomerular apparatus and is best treated with mineralocorticoids like fludrocortisone.

SUGGESTED READING

Abelow B, ed: *Understanding Acid-Base*, 1st ed. Baltimore, MD: Williams and Wilkins, 1998.

Gennari FJ, ed: *Medical Management of Kidney and Electrolyte Disorders*, 1st ed. New York: Marcel Dekker, 2001, pp 201–202.

Herrin JT: Renal tubular acidosis. In: Anver ED, Harmon WE, Niaudet P, (eds): *Pediatric Nephrology*, 5th ed. Philadelphia: Lippincott, Williams & Wilkins, 2004, pp 757–776.

CASE 122: A 7-YEAR-OLD WITH ENURESIS

A 7-year-old Caucasian girl has a history of bed-wetting. According to mom her daughter was born by normal vaginal delivery at term and had an uneventful neonatal period. She was out of pull-ups during the day at 2 years of age. She currently wets the bed almost every night. However, she did have a 3-month period of dry nights with occasional wettings between 5 and 6 years of age. In the daytime she tends to have urgency and frequency of micturition with occasional dribbling of urine on the way to the washroom. She tends to have increased fluid intake on occasions. Mom has also noticed small round stains of urine on her underwear. There is no history of UTIs. The child's school performance has been satisfactory. The family moved to Chicago 6 months ago and there are no other recent significant events in the family. The family history is negative apart from a history of bed-wetting in the father as a child.

Her physical examination apart from palpable fecal masses in the left iliac fossa and suprapubic areas is unremarkable. There is a sacral dimple with no hairy patch. Her deep tendon reflexes are normal and there is no leg length discrepancy or wasting of muscles in either lower extremity.

The results of laboratory tests are as follows:

Urinalysis:

Specific gravity	1025
pH	5.0
Protein	negative
Blood	negative
Glucose	negative
Urine C & S	negative
Hemoglobin	12.5 g/dL
Hematocrit	37%
BUN	10 mg/dL
Creatinine	0.6 mg/dL
Serum sodium	145 mEq/L
Serum potassium	4.3 mEq/L
Serum chloride	110 mEq/L
Serum bicarbonate	23 mEq/L
Serum glucose	95 mg/dL

SELECT THE ONE BEST ANSWER

1. This girl has enuresis by definition because:

   (A) daytime bladder control is usually achieved at 5 years of age and night-time control at 6 years of age for a girl

   (B) daytime bladder control is usually achieved at 2 years of age and night-time control at 5 years of age for a girl

   (C) daytime bladder control is usually achieved at 4 years of age and night-time control at 8 years of age for a girl

   (D) daytime bladder control is usually achieved at 6 years of age and night-time control at 8 years of age for a girl

   (E) daytime bladder control is usually achieved at 6 years of age and night-time control at 2 years of age for a girl

2. This girl most likely has which of the following:

   (A) secondary daytime and night-time enuresis and constipation

   (B) primary nocturnal enuresis with daytime detrusor hyperactivity and constipation

   (C) secondary nocturnal enuresis with daytime detrusor hyperactivity

   (D) nephrogenic diabetes insipidus

   (E) central diabetes insipidus

3. The prevalence of this condition at this age is:

   (A) 5%
   (B) 10% to 15%
   (C) 25% to 30%
   (D) 40%
   (E) 1% to 5%

4. The differential diagnosis of this condition in this girl includes all except:

   (A) new-onset diabetes mellitus
   (B) obstructive sleep apnea
   (C) urinary tract infection
   (D) posterior urethral valves
   (E) spina bifida occulta

5. Further investigations that must be performed in this patient at this point include:

   (A) renal ultrasound
   (B) voiding cystourethrogram
   (C) urodynamic studies
   (D) all of the above
   (E) none of the above

6. The risk of occurrence of enuresis in a child is:

(A) 44% if one parent had the condition or 77% if both parents had the condition as a child

(B) 15% if one parent had the condition or 25% if both parents had the condition as a child

(C) 5% if one parent had the condition or 10% if both parents had the condition as a child

(D) 0% if one parent had the condition or 15% if both parents had the condition as a child

(E) 0% if one parent had the condition or 50% if both parents had the condition as a child

7. Which of the following pharmacologic agents would most likely help this child's symptoms?

(A) oxybutynin chloride
(B) imipramine
(C) tolterodine tartrate
(D) A and C only
(E) none of the above

8. All of the following nonpharmacologic methods can also be tried in this child except:

(A) fluid restriction in the evenings
(B) regular punishment for every wet night
(C) enuresis alarm program
(D) voiding before bed time
(E) demystification

9. The most effective treatment for primary nocturnal enuresis with a pure arousal mechanism problem or monosymptomatic nocturnal enuresis is:

(A) intranasal or oral 1-desamino-8-D-arginine vasopressin (DDAVP)
(B) imipramine
(C) acupuncture
(D) enuresis alarm program
(E) chiropractic manipulation

10. Primary nocturnal enuresis can be associated with:

(A) abnormal arousal-from-sleep mechanism
(B) night-time wetting with daytime detrusor hyperactivity or uninhibited bladder contractions
(C) night-time polyuria
(D) A and B only
(E) all of the above

11. Nocturnal enuresis can be inherited as an:

(A) autosomal recessive disorder
(B) autosomal dominant disorder
(C) X-linked recessive disorder
(D) all of the above
(E) none of the above

12. An enuresis gene has been identified on:

(A) chromosome 12
(B) chromosome 13
(C) chromosomes 8 and 22
(D) all of the above
(E) none of the above

13. Primary nocturnal enuresis can be associated with:

(A) nocturnal detrusor hyperactivity
(B) nocturnal polyuria
(C) poor arousal-from-sleep mechanism
(D) all of the above
(E) A and B

14. The spontaneous annual resolution rate of monosymptomatic nocturnal enuresis is:

(A) 25%
(B) 30%
(C) 15%
(D) 35%
(E) 40%

15. Functional bladder capacity in a normal child is usually:

(A) age + 2 in ounces
(B) age + 8 in ounces
(C) age + 6 in ounces
(D) age + 4 in ounces
(E) age + 9 in ounces

16. Nocturnal detrusor hyperactivity occurs in:

(A) 50% of all children with nocturnal enuresis
(B) 10% of all children with nocturnal enuresis
(C) 60% of all children with nocturnal enuresis
(D) 30% of all children with nocturnal enuresis
(E) 5% of all children with nocturnal enuresis

17. Enuresis may be associated with all of the following except:

(A) food allergies

(B) constipation
(C) obstructive sleep apnea
(D) ADHD (attention deficit hyperactivity disorder)
(E) asthma

Answers

1. **(B)** Daytime bladder control is usually achieved by 2 years when the child learns to inhibit unwanted detrusor contractions during the day. Night-time bladder control is achieved by 5 years in girls and 6 years in boys. Late achievement of night-time control in boys is attributed to mild developmental lag in boys. Enuresis needs to be differentiated from urinary incontinence. Enuresis is defined as involuntary discharge of urine without any underlying anatomic abnormality, whereas urinary incontinence is involuntary discharge of urine associated with an underlying structural abnormality.

2. **(B)** Three groups of patients with primary nocturnal enuresis are now described.

   1. Patients with pure arousal mechanism problem.
   2. Patients with night-time arousal problem and daytime detrusor hyperactivity.
   3. Patients with night-time arousal problem with night-time polyuria or nocturia.

   Monosymptomatic nocturnal enuresis with arousal mechanism problem is a result of failure of the locus ceruleus in the rostral pons to awaken the child in response to a full bladder. These children have normal voiding otherwise.

   The term non–monosymptomatic nocturnal enuresis refers to these same children who in addition to arousal mechanism problems have coexistent daytime symptoms of urgency or voiding dysfunction because of detrusor hyperactivity and/or nocturnal polyuria.

   Enuresis is "primary" if the child has never had a >6-month period of dry nights and "secondary" if the child, after being dry for >6-month period, starts to have bed-wetting again.

3. **(B)** The prevalence of primary nocturnal enuresis is 10% to 15% at 6 years of age. There is a 10% to 15% spontaneous remission rate annually every year leading to a prevalence of 5% at 10 years of age and 1% at 15 years of age and beyond. Thus, it is important to remember that 1% of adults continue to have the problem.

4. **(D)** All of these conditions can cause bed-wetting in a child. However, this patient is a girl and posterior urethral valves are seen almost exclusively in boys.

   Differential diagnosis includes new-onset diabetes mellitus, diabetes insipidus, spina bifida occulta, obstructive sleep apnea, urinary tract infection, vulvovaginitis, posterior urethral valves in boys, chronic renal failure, and CNS tumors.

   Clinical examination and history should be specifically focused on looking for evidence of constipation, abdominal masses, palpable bladder, high plantar arch, or hammer toes with asymmetric atrophy of lower extremities suggestive of spina bifida occulta, as well as examination of spine and genitalia.

5. **(E)** In this patient the history is very suggestive of primary nocturnal enuresis with daytime detrusor hyperactivity and there is no history of any UTIs. Therefore none of these investigations are indicated. Generally a urinalysis, urine culture, complete blood count, and assessment of renal function with serum BUN, creatinine, and an electrolyte determination is sufficient to rule out UTI and renal functional impairment. The sacral dimple without a hairy patch may be a normal finding in such a patient. However, a sacral dimple with a hairy patch may also be associated with spina bifida occulta, which could potentially cause bladder dysfunction as a result of a tethering of the spinal cord with consequent enuresis. A sacral dimple with a hairy patch should be investigated with an MRI to look for spina bifida occulta.

6. **(A)** In primary enuresis, if one parent had enuresis as a child, the risk of the offspring having enuresis is 43% if the father was affected or 44% if the mother was affected as a child. The risk is 77% if both parents were affected during childhood. Enuresis is more common in boys and first-born children.

   Multiple factors including genetic factors may be responsible for primary nocturnal enuresis. Evidence of genetic susceptibility comes from studies of familial incidence, twin studies, and molecular genetics with linkage analysis. Twin studies show 70% concordance for monozygotic twins and 31% concordance for dizygotic twins. Molecular genetics with linkage analysis has revealed a polymorphism with localization of genes for enuresis on several different chromosomes. Earlier studies localized the gene to the long arm of chromosome 13 (D13S 291 and D13S 263) and the long arm of chromosome 12 (D12S 80 and D12S 43) in two different families.

7. **(D)** Both oxybutynin and tolterodine are anticholinergic drugs that help to inhibit unwanted detrusor contractions and increase urethral sphincter tone. Therefore they can potentially help this child's symptoms. It is important to keep in mind that this child's constipation should also be treated as both oxybutynin and tolterodine because of their anticholinergic effect can make constipation worse. Imipramine has been used to treat primary nocturnal enuresis. It is reported to work through its effect on the arousal mechanism, a decrease in night-time urinary sodium excretion, a consequent decrease in nocturia, and a weak anticholinergic effect. However its use is limited because of possible significant side effects and a high relapse rate of enuresis once the treatment is stopped. In this patient who has symptoms of detrusor hyperactivity, imipramine would not be a treatment of choice.

8. **(B)** Surprisingly, punishment is still used by a fair number of parents on children for wetting the bed and has obvious negative consequences. Demystification in the presence of the child with the explanation to the parents that the child is not intentionally wetting the bed itself has a 15% to 25% therapeutic effect on the child's enuresis. Fluid restriction and voiding prior to going to bed may help augment the effect of other therapeutic modalities. In this patient an enuresis alarm in combination with oxybutynin could prove to be very effective provided the child and the parents are motivated to try the enuresis alarm program, which consists of a behavioral program used with the alarm.

9. **(D)** The enuresis alarm program is the most effective treatment for a child with primary nocturnal enuresis caused by pure arousal mechanism problem with a success rate of >90% and a low incidence of relapse compared with pharmacologic therapies. Imipramine, which is seldom used now, has a response rate of 50% with a relapse rate of almost 100% after discontinuation of the drug; 1-desamino-8-D-arginine vasopressin (DDAVP) has a response rate of 76% but a relapse rate of 60% to 100% after discontinuation.

10. **(E)** As mentioned, primary nocturnal enuresis can be divided into these three groups.

11. **(B)** Primary nocturnal enuresis can be inherited as an autosomal dominant disorder.

12. **(D)** Genes mediating enuresis have been reported to be heterogeneous. Initial molecular genetic methods such as linkage analysis showed foci on chromosomes 13 and 12 in different families. Other studies subsequently showed enuresis gene loci on chromosomes 8 and 22 in other families.

13. **(D)** Primary nocturnal enuresis is now classified into monosymptomatic nocturnal enuresis with isolated arousal disorder or non–monosymptomatic nocturnal enuresis where arousal disorder may be associated with reduced bladder capacity or nocturnal detrusor hyperactivity and or nocturnal polyuria.

14. **(C)** Monosymptomatic nocturnal enuresis has an annual spontaneous resolution rate of 15%. Therefore, for any treatment to be proven effective for enuresis, the rate of resolution of symptoms with the treatment must be more than this background rate.

15. **(A)** One formula to estimate bladder capacity in children described by Berger and co-workers and Koff is: Bladder capacity (in oz) = Age (yr) + 2 up to 15 years of age when the adult bladder capacity is achieved.

16. **(D)** Nocturnal detrusor hyperactivity is reported to occur in 30% of patients with nocturnal enuresis and is one reason for failure to respond to vasopressin. These patients may need other pharmacologic agents such as oxybutynin or

tolterodine to treat detrusor hyperactivity and to improve bladder capacity.

17. **(E)** Food allergies have been reported to lead to enuresis in 10% of affected patients. Some of these children are reported to benefit from elimination of certain foods from the diet, such as citrus fruit, juices, foods high in caffeine and sugar, dairy products, artificially colored drinks, and chocolate. Constipation can potentially interfere with the bladder function as a result of pressure from constipated stools in the sigmoid colon. Obstructive sleep apnea can cause enuresis (hypoxia and increased atrial natriuretic peptide secretion, leading to nocturia, are the proposed mechanisms). There is a higher incidence of enuresis in children with attention deficit hyperactivity disorder.

SUGGESTED READING

Schmitt BD: Nocturnal enuresis. *Pediatr Rev* 18:183–190, 1997.

Cendron M: Primary nocturnal enuresis: Current concepts. *J Am Fam Physician* 59:1205–1214, 1219–1220, 1999.

Husmann D: Enuresis. *Urology* 48:184–193, 1996.

CASE 123: A 6-YEAR-OLD WITH PUFFY EYELIDS AND SWOLLEN LEGS

A 6-year-old Asian-American male is admitted for puffiness of the eyelids and swelling of both lower extremities. The illness started 2 weeks prior to admission with mild puffiness of the eyelids. The eyelids became progressively puffier and, 1 week prior to admission, the patient developed swelling of both lower extremities. The abdomen became protuberant subsequently. There is no history of gross hematuria, fever, or anyone in the family receiving regular medications. On physical examination he was in no acute distress. The temperature was 98.6°F (37°C), heart rate 110/min, respiratory rate 20/min, and blood pressure 120/80 mm Hg. The child had anasarca with pitting edema of both lower extremities. The rest of the physical examination was unremarkable.

The urinalysis revealed a specific gravity of 1.030, pH 5, protein 4+, 5 to 10 RBC/HPF, 1 to 2 WBC/HPF, and an occasional coarse granular cast. The BUN was 29 mg/dL. The serum creatinine 1.0 mg/dL, and the creatinine clearance was 90 mL/min/1.73 m². The streptolysin O antibody was <200 IU/mL, C_3 124 mg/dL (88 to 155 for age 6 to 8). The

ANA was negative and the 24-hour urinary protein was 5.6 g/24 h. The blood cholesterol was 520 mg/dL; the total protein was 4.6 g/dL and the serum albumin was 1.2 g/dL.

SELECT THE BEST ANSWER

1. The urinalysis and blood test data suggest the diagnosis of:

   (A) acute postinfectious glomerulonephritis
   (B) focal segmental glomerulosclerosis
   (C) membranoproliferative glomerulonephritis
   (D) minimal change nephrotic syndrome
   (E) B and D

2. The specific gravity of the urine is very high because of:

   (A) heavy proteinuria
   (B) intravascular volume depletion
   (C) azotemia and increased fractional excretion sodium
   (D) A and C
   (E) A and B

3. Which of the following treatments is definitely not indicated at this time?

   (A) pneumococcal vaccine
   (B) steroids
   (C) HMG-CoA reductase inhibitor
   (D) aspirin
   (E) all are indicated at this time

4. After 14 days of daily prednisone the proteinuria resolved and the patient lost all evidence of edema. Over the next 12 months four relapses of the nephrotic syndrome occurred. This patient is:

   (A) likely to become steroid resistant
   (B) likely to outgrow the disease
   (C) at risk of developing chronic renal insufficiency
   (D) likely to develop premature atherosclerotic heart disease

Answers

1. **(E)** This patient has nephrotic syndrome. The two most common causes in childhood are minimal change nephrotic syndrome (MCNS) and

focal segmental glomerulosclerosis (FSGS). They are clinically indistinguishable at presentation but MCNS responds to steroids and FSGS rarely does. Patients with acute postinfectious GN rarely develop nephrotic syndrome and MPGN is usually associated with depressed C$_3$. Twenty percent of patients with MCNS and FSGS have microscopic hematuria.

2. **(B)** Proteins, especially albumin, have very high molecular weights. Therefore, heavy proteinuria does not contribute significantly to specific gravity, which is a reflection of osmolality and the contribution of osmotic particles. Patients with nephrotic syndrome are edematous but because they have low oncotic pressure, fluid moves from the intravascular space to the extravascular space. Intravascular volume is depleted. Since these patients may have prerenal azotemia (volume depletion), the fractional excretion of sodium is low and the urinary sodium concentration is low.

3. **(C)** Prednisone is the cornerstone of treatment in MCNS. If a patient becomes proteinuria-free after 2 to 4 weeks of daily prednisone, the long-term prognosis is excellent. The two most serious complications are infectious, especially with *Streptococcus pneumoniae* because of defective opsonization of bacteria and thromboembolic phenomena because of loss of thrombinolytic proteins in urine. So, immunization with a pneumococcal vaccine is indicated. Some nephrologists might consider daily low-dose aspirin, but this is usually reserved for patients with chronic nephrotic syndrome who fail to respond to prednisone and most likely have FSGS. Hyperlipidemia and its association with cardiovascular disease is a concern but HMG-CoA reductase inhibitors are not part of the initial treatment of nephrotic syndrome.

4. **(B)** Patients with steroid-responsive nephrotic syndrome (MCNS) have one of three clinical courses. One-third have one episode of nephrotic syndrome, one-third have less than four relapses per year, and one-third have more than four episodes per year. All three groups have the same favorable outcome; they all "outgrow" the disease.

SUGGESTED READING

The primary nephrotic syndrome in children. Identification of patients with minimal change nephrotic syndrome from initial response to prednisone. A report of the International Study of Kidney Disease in Children. *J Pediatr* 98:561–564, 1981.

Sewell RF, Short CD: Minimal-change nephropathy: How does the immune system affect that glomerulus? *Nephrol Dial Transplant* 8:108–112, 1993.

Koyama A, Fujisaki M, Kobayashi M, et al: A glomerular permeability factor produced human T cell hybridomas. *Kidney Int* 40:453–460, 1991.

Brodehl J: The treatment of minimal change nephrotic syndrome: Lessons learned from multicentre cooperative studies. *Eur J Pediatr* 150:380–387, 1991.

Fakhouri F, Bocquet N, Taupin P, et al: Steroid-sensitive nephrotic syndrome: From childhood to adulthood. *Am J Kidney Dis* 41:550–557, 2003.

CASE 124: A 12-YEAR-OLD GIRL WITH SMOKY COLORED URINE

A 12-year-old girl was treated for a sore throat. Two weeks later, the patient developed fever, smoky colored urine, diffuse abdominal pain, and muscle pain. Her urine volume was about a cup for 24 hours.

On physical examination, the blood pressure was 210/130 mm Hg. There was mild facial edema, trace peripheral edema, and marked pallor. The lungs were clear to auscultation and examination of the heart revealed normal sinus rhythm without any murmur. There was no rash.

The urinalysis revealed a grossly reddish smoky color, specific gravity 1.010, protein 4+, serum creatinine was 6.2 mg/dL, Na 135 mEq/L, K 6.5 mEq/L, Cl 105 mEq/L, and total bicarbonate 19 mmol/L. The anti-streptolysin O antibody was >1000 IU/mL. The C$_3$ level was 30 mg/dL (normal >90 mg/dL), and the ANA was negative.

SELECT THE ONE BEST ANSWER

1. The differential diagnosis includes all except:

   (A) MPGN
   (B) acute poststreptococcal glomerulonephritis
   (C) diffuse proliferative lupus nephritis
   (D) SBE with immune complex glomerulonephritis
   (E) IgA nephropathy

2. Treatment at this time consists of all except:

   (A) volume reduction
   (B) vasodilation

(C) penicillin

(D) dialysis

(E) none of the above are needed for treatment at this time

3. Once blood pressure is adequately controlled and renal function improves, outpatient management includes all except:

(A) repeat C_3 levels in 6 weeks

(B) penicillin prophylaxis

(C) yearly urinalysis and blood pressure determination for 2 to 4 years

(D) avoid processed and fast foods

(E) all are needed for outpatient management

Answers

1. **(E)** MPGN, APSGN, DPLN, and SBE are glomerulopathies associated with low C_3 levels. In ASPGN, C_3 levels normalize without specific treatment within 6 weeks. In MPGN, DPLN, and SBE, C_3 levels do not improve without treatment. In IgA nephropathy, C_3 levels are normal.

2. **(D)** If one assumes that a patient with suspected APSGN was normotensive (119/76, 50th percentile 12-year-old female) before the illness, then blood pressure acutely rising to 210/130 represents a medical emergency. Blood pressure is determined by cardiac output and vascular resistance. In APSGN, glomerular filtration is reduced and patients are hypervolemic. Rational treatment is volume reduction with diuretics and fluid restriction but this patient needs urgent reduction in blood pressure. There is a considerable lag period between volume reduction and a decrease in the blood pressure. Therefore, vasodilation is also necessary acutely. If the patient has evidence of active streptococcal infection, penicillin is indicated. Penicillin treatment will not alter the natural history of APSGN. Dialysis at this point is not indicated. Most minor electrolyte imbalances can be managed conservatively. But should this patient have intractable hypervolemia with pulmonary edema or uncontrollable hypertension, acute dialysis is indicated.

3. **(B)** It is important to document that the C_3 level returns to normal. This confirms the diagnosis of APSGN and rules out MPGN, DPLN, and SBE. Penicillin prophylaxis is unnecessary in APSGN. Since only a few strains of group A β-hemolytic streptococci are nephritogenic and the patient now has immunity to one of these strains, prophylaxis is not given. Most cases of APSGN have an excellent prognosis. However, in rare instances, if the presentation is associated with severe renal failure, there may be long-term renal sequelae. Therefore, yearly urinalysis and blood pressure determination should be preferred. Avoidance of processed foods and fast foods that contain preservatives is indicated for all children including those who have had APSGN.

SUGGESTED READING

Lewy JE, Salinas-Madrigal L, Herdson PB, et al: Clinicopathologic correlations in acute poststreptococcal glomerulonephritis: A correlation between renal functions, morphologic damage, and clinical course of 46 children with acute poststreptococcal glomerulonephritis. *Medicine* (*Baltimore*) 50:453–501, 1971.

Tejani A, Ingulli E: Poststreptococcal glomerulonephritis. Current clinical and pathologic concepts. 1990; 55:1–5, 1990.

Potter EV, Lipschultz SA, Abidh S, et al: Twelve to seventeen-year follow-up of patients with poststreptococcal acute glomerulonephritis in Trinidad. *N Engl J Med* 307:725–729, 1982.

CASE 125: A 5-YEAR-OLD BOY WITH BLOODY DIARRHEA AND OLIGURIA

A 5-year-old male from Houston is vacationing with his parents and two siblings in Colorado. They have visited a water slide park. Two days later, the patient developed diarrhea, which turned bloody. The bloody diarrhea was associated with crampy abdominal pain and vomiting. When the vomiting started, the patient was taken to a local emergency department where he was given intravenous fluids and prescribed loperamide for diarrhea. One day later, the patient returned to the emergency department because he looked pale, became somnolent, and had not urinated for 24 hours.

On physical examination this lethargic and pale appearing 5-year-old had a temperature of 100.4°F (38°C), a pulse of 100 beats/min, a respiratory rate of 24/min, and a blood pressure of 128/85 mm Hg. The chest was clear to auscultation and there was mild pretibial edema. The abdominal examination was remarkable for moderate diffuse tenderness without rebound; the liver measured 3 cm below the right costal margin.

The initial laboratory investigations revealed a hemoglobin of 8 g/dL, leukocyte count 17,500 μL, and a platelet count of 19,000/μL; the peripheral blood smear showed 12% schistocytes. The BUN was 35 mg/dL and the serum creatinine was 2.5 mg/dL. The serum sodium was 141 mEq/L, potassium 5.6 mEq/L, chloride 105 mEq/L and total bicarbonate 18 mmol/L. The serum calcium was 8.2 mg/dL, inorganic phosphorus 7.0 mg/dL, and glucose 310 mg/dL.

During the next 24 hours, the patient's urinary output decreased to 55 mL/24 hr, with an increase in the serum creatinine to 3.8 mg/dL. Because the patient remained severely oliguric and uremic with symptoms of nausea and vomiting, peritoneal dialysis was began. After 3 weeks of peritoneal dialysis, the urine output rose to 200 mL/24 hr and platelet count increased to 95,000/μL.

SELECT THE ONE BEST ANSWER

1. The prognosis for recovery of renal function is generally favorable. Mortality during the acute illness is <5% but increases with risk factors. This patient's major risk factor was:

   (A) leukocytosis
   (B) pancreatic involvement with glucose intolerance
   (C) oliguria for 22 days
   (D) initial platelet count 19,000/μL
   (E) B and D

2. Although found in other animals, the main vector of *E. coli* O157:H7 is:

   (A) chicken
   (B) dogs
   (C) pigs
   (D) cattle
   (E) humans

3. Early treatment of diarrhea with antibiotics in this case:

   (A) decreases the likelihood that siblings will develop *E. coli* O157:H7 diarrhea
   (B) decreases the likelihood that the patient will develop hemolytic-uremic syndrome (HUS)
   (C) increases the likelihood that the patient will develop HUS

   (D) exacerbates diarrheal symptoms
   (E) A and B

4. In the present case, which treatment has been shown to be most efficacious?

   (A) supportive treatment
   (B) plasma infusion and/or plasma exchange
   (C) intravenous immune globulin
   (D) tissue-type plasminogen activator
   (E) oral Shiga toxin–binding agent

Answers

1. **(C)** Those children who do not do well during the acute episode often have one or more risk factors. Initial anuria lasting >8 days is associated with poor long-term renal function. A leukocyte count >20,000/mm^3 at presentation reflects neutrophil activation resulting from toxin-induced release from monocytes of the neutrophil chemoattractant interleukin 8; these neutrophils may then contribute to tissue damage. Older age at onset of the disease is a risk factor; up to 70% of children ≥3 years of age progress to terminal renal failure. Atypical HUS occurs at all ages, without GI symptoms, and often with an insidious onset. A high proportion of these patients have permanent renal sequelae.

2. **(D)** Although found in other animals, cattle are the main vector of *E. coli* O157:H7, with the bacteria being present in the intestine and feces. Infection in humans occurs following ingestion of contaminated, undercooked meat, non-pasteurized milk or milk products, water, fruits, and vegetables.

3. **(C)** Early administration of antibiotics to children with diarrhea caused by *E. coli* O157:H7 may promote the development of HUS, perhaps by enhancing release of Shiga toxin as the bacteria are killed. A prospective study of 71 children younger than the age of 10 years with *E. coli* O157:H7 isolated from stool found that those receiving antibiotics were more likely to develop HUS (5 of 9 [56%] versus 5 of 62 who were untreated [8%], P = 0.002).

4. **(A)** Three treatment modalities have been tried in the treatment of HUS: antithrombotic agents

based on the histological evidence of thrombus formation have not been shown to influence duration of renal failure, hemolysis, thrombocytopenia, or long-term outcome. Furthermore, hemorrhagic complications are more common in treated patients. The use of plasma infusion (to supply a missing anticoagulant factor) or plasma exchange (to also remove procoagulant factors) has been successful in many adults with TTP-HUS but in children with typical HUS, plasma infusion has not been shown to be beneficial in the long term.

It is difficult to evaluate the efficacy of such treatment in a disease with such a good long-term prognosis, 90% with normal GFR. Finally, intravenous immunoglobulin, possibly to neutralize antibodies against Shiga-like toxins, has not been shown to influence the duration of hemolysis, thrombocytopenia, or acute renal failure. Oral Shiga toxin–binding agents have been tried in 145 children with HUS and were not effective.

SUGGESTED READING

Remuzzi G, Ruggenenti P: The hemolytic uremic syndrome. *Kidney Int* 48:2–19, 1995.

Repetto HA: Epidemic hemolytic uremic syndrome in children. *Kidney Int* 52:1708–1719, 1997.

Neuhaus TJ, Calonder S, Leumann EP: Heterogeneity of atypical hemolytic uremic syndromes. *Arch Dis Child* 76:518–521, 1997.

Verweyen HM, Karch H, Brandis M, et al: Enterohemorrhagic *Escherichia coli* infections: Following transmission routes. *Pediatr Nephrol* 14:73–83, 2000.

Gerber A, Karch H, Allerberger F, et al: Clinical course and the role of the Shiga toxin-producing *Escherichia coli* infection in the hemolytic-uremic syndrome in pediatric patients, 1997–2000, in Germany and Austria: A prospective study. *J Infect Dis* 186:493–500, 2002.

Georgaki-Angelaki HN, Steed DB, Chantler C, et al: Renal function following acute renal failure in childhood: A long-term follow-up study. *Kidney Int* 35:84–89, 1989.

Bergstein JM, Riley M, Bang NU: Role of plasminogen-activator inhibitor type 1 in the pathogenesis and outcome of the hemolytic uremic syndrome. *N Engl J Med* 327:755–759, 1992.

CASE 126: A 4-YEAR-OLD GIRL WITH A PURPURIC RASH ON THE BUTTOCKS

A 4-year-old girl presents to the emergency department with erythematous maculopapular lesions on the buttocks that extend to the lower extremities and trunk. Initially the lesions blanched on pressure but later became purpuric. As her lower extremities became swollen and painful, her parents brought her to their primary care physician. By the time she was seen by the pediatrician, her most important complaint was severe abdominal pain.

On examination, the temperature was 99.5°F (37.5°C), the pulse was 100 beats/min, the respiratory rate was 20/min, and the blood pressure was 110/83 mm Hg. The patient was in moderate distress because of abdominal pain, which was diffuse and intermittent. Palpation of the abdomen revealed a slightly tender, sausage-shaped mass in the right upper abdomen. The chest was clear to auscultation and examination of the heart revealed normal sinus rhythm without a murmur. Examination of the skin over the trunk and buttocks revealed many (10 to 12) 0.5- to 1-cm purpuric lesions. The patient had mildly swollen ankles and knees with pain on passive movements in all directions.

The urinalysis revealed: specific gravity 1.018, pH 5, protein 3+, 10 to 20 RBC/HPF, and 5 to 6 WBC/HPF. The urinary protein/creatinine ratio was 1.8. The BUN was 31 mg/dL, the serum creatinine was 0.6 mg/dL, and the Hgb was 11.4 gm/dL. The total protein was 6.4 gm/dL, the albumin was 3.7 gm/dL, and the cholesterol was 151 mg/dL. The C_3 was 115 mg/dL, the anti-streptolysin O antibody <200 IU/mL, and the ANA 1:40.

SELECT THE ONE BEST ANSWER

1. The first consults to be requested are:

   (A) ICU team
   (B) surgery
   (C) dermatology
   (D) oncology
   (E) consult is not needed

2. The renal prognosis in this case:

   (A) is indeterminate at this time
   (B) is excellent since renal function is normal
   (C) depends on the magnitude and persistence of proteinuria
   (D) is guarded because of the presence of hematuria/proteinuria
   (E) is extremely poor (the patient will likely require a kidney transplant)

3. The renal histopathology in Henoch-Schönlein purpura (HSP) resembles:

(A) membranoproliferative glomerulonephritis
(B) acute poststreptococcal glomerulonephritis
(C) IgA nephropathy
(D) diffuse proliferative lupus nephritis
(E) none of the above

Answers

1. **(A)** Henoch-Schönlein purpura is a systemic vasculitis with a prominent cutaneous component. The clinical manifestations include a classic tetrad that can occur in any order and at any time over a period of several days to several weeks: rash, arthralgias, abdominal pain, and renal disease. Gastrointestinal symptoms are present in the majority of patients with HSP.

    Most concerning is the sausage shaped-mass in the RUQ that could represent an intussusception. Intussusception, usually ilio-ilial, is a medical emergency that requires a surgical consult before a diagnostic/therapeutic corrective attempt is performed, if possible, by radiology.

2. **(C)** Renal disease is usually noted within a few days to 4 weeks after onset of systemic symptoms. The urinalysis in affected patients reveals mild proteinuria with an active urinary sediment characterized by microscopic (or macroscopic) hematuria with red cell and other cellular casts. Most patients have relatively mild disease characterized by asymptomatic hematuria and proteinuria with a normal or only slightly elevated creatinine level. However, more marked findings may occur including the nephrotic syndrome, hypertension, and acute renal failure. There is a general but not absolute correlation between the severity of the clinical manifestations and the findings on renal biopsy. Patients with asymptomatic hematuria usually have only focal mesangial proliferation and, if protein excretion is in the nephrotic range, frequent crescent formation. The percent of glomeruli showing crescents seems to be the most important prognostic finding.

3. **(A)** Henoch-Schönlein purpura is characterized by tissue deposition of IgA-containing immune complexes. The pathogenesis of this disorder may be similar to that of IgA nephropathy which is associated with identical histological findings in the kidney. The description of the simultaneous occurrence of HSP and IgA nephropathy in twins after an adenoviral infection is further evidence in support of a common pathogenesis. IgA deposition is prominent in both HSP and IgA nephropathy.

SUGGESTED READING

Kauffmann RH, Herrmann WA, Meyer CJ, et al: Circulating IgA-immune complexes in Henoch-Schönlein purpura. A longitudinal study of their relationship to disease activity and vascular deposition of IgA. *Am J Med* 69:859–866, 1980.

Gardner-Medwin JM, Dolezalova P, Cummins C, Southwood TR: Incidence of Henoch-Schönlein purpura, Kawasaki disease, and rare vasculitides in children of different ethnic origins. *Lancet* 360:1197–1202, 2002.

Meadow SR. Henoch-Schönlein syndrome. In: Edelmann, CM (ed): *Pediatric Nephrology*, 2nd ed. Boston: Little, Brown, 1992, p 1525.

Blanco R, Martinez-Taboada VM, Rodriguez-Valverde V, et al: Henoch-Schönlein purpura in adulthood and childhood: Two different expressions of the same syndrome. *Arthritis Rheum* 40:859–864, 1997.

Cameron JS: Henoch-Schönlein purpura: Clinical presentation. *Contrib Nephrol* 40:246–249, 1984.

Saulsbury FT: Henoch-Schönlein purpura in children. Report of 100 patients and review of the literature. *Medicine (Baltimore)* 78:395–409, 1999.

Levy M, Broyer M, Arsan et al: Anaphylactoid purpura nephritis in childhood: Natural history and immunopathology. *Adv Nephrol Necker Hosp* 6:183–228, 1976.

Habib R, Niaudet P, Levy M: Henoch-Schönlein purpura nephritis and IgA nephropathy. In: Tisher, CC, Brenner, BM (eds): *Renal Pathology with Clinical and Functional Correlations*. Philadelphia: Lippincott, 1993, p 472.

CASE 127: A 10-YEAR-OLD GIRL WITH BED WETTING AND PROTEINURIA

A 10-year-old African-American female is being evaluated for bedwetting. She had been dry during the day since age 2 years but is wet every night. A urinalysis was performed as part of the evaluation for enuresis. It demonstrated 3+ proteinuria with an occasional RBC/HPF.

She denied symptoms of preseptal, pedal or pretibial edema; there was no history of arthralgias, headaches, dizziness, or rash. Her father was known to have proteinuria and is being evaluated for it.

On physical examination this healthy-appearing 10-year-old weighed 46.3 kg, measured 61.3 cm in length, and had blood pressure 122/78 mm Hg. The chest was clear to auscultation and there was no evidence of peripheral edema. The abdominal evaluation was normal. There was no rash.

The laboratory examination reveals a urinalysis with specific gravity 1.018, pH 6.5, protein 3+, 3 to 5 WBC/HPF, and occasional RBC/HPF. The urinary protein/creatinine ratio is 3.5. The BUN is 10 mg/dL, serum creatinine 0.7 mg/dL, total protein 6.7 g/dL, albumen 3.7 g/dL, and cholesterol 158 mg/dL. The C_3 level is 110 mg/dL and the ANA is <1:40.

SELECT THE ONE BEST ANSWER

1. The next test that should be ordered is:

   (A) renal ultrasound

   (B) creatinine clearance

   (C) 24-hr urinary protein excretion

   (D) first voided sample for protein/creatinine ratio

2. The morning urinary protein/creatinine ratio was 3.0 (normal is <2). A likely cause of asymptomatic fixed proteinuria in a 9- to 10-year-old girl with enuresis is:

   (A) minimal change nephrotic syndrome

   (B) reflux nephropathy

   (C) focal segmental glomerulosclerosis

   (D) membranoproliferative glomerulonephritis

3. The renal ultrasound and voiding cystourethrogram are normal. The pediatric nephrologist performs a percutaneous renal biopsy. The most likely tissue diagnosis is:

   (A) focal segmental glomerulosclerosis

   (B) minimal change nephrotic syndrome

   (C) membranoproliferative glomerulonephritis

   (D) membranous nephropathy

Answers

1. **(D)** Although this patient with asymptomatic proteinuria had a random protein/creatinine ratio of 3.5, one should always exclude orthostatic proteinuria before proceeding to a more complicated evaluation. The long-term prognosis for orthostatic proteinuria is excellent. The urinary protein/creatinine ratio is commonly used in pediatrics because it is difficult to collect an accurately timed specimen. Since creatinine is a byproduct of muscle metabolism and is produced and excreted at a constant rate, the ratio of total protein (or any other substance)/creatinine is constant and reproducible regardless of whether the urine is concentrated or dilute.

2. **(B)** Reflux nephropathy can be diagnosed with a renal ultrasound that shows irregular contours and thinned cortex. A voiding cystourethrogram most likely will demonstrate vesicoureteral reflux. The natural history of reflux is that it improves with time, but if reflux is severe enough to cause nephropathy then it would likely still be present. Hypertension is often present with reflux nephropathy. Minimal change, focal segmental glomerulosclerosis, and membranoproliferative glomerulonephritis all require percutaneous renal biopsy for diagnosis.

3. **(A)** Focal segmental glomerulosclerosis is the most common finding on biopsy in patients, especially African-Americans, who have asymptomatic, isolated, fixed proteinuria. Minimal change and membranous nephropathy present with symptomatic nephrotic syndrome. Membranoproliferative glomerulonephritis may or may not be associated with nephrotic syndrome but is always associated with hematuria. FSGS in the context of asymptomatic proteinuria has a much better prognosis than in patients who have steroid-resistant nephrotic syndrome and biopsy-proven FSGS. However, even this patient with only moderate proteinuria and FSGS was successfully treated with cyclosporine and the protein/creatinine decreased to 0.56.

SUGGESTED READING

Hogg RJ, Portman RJ, Milliner D, et al: Evaluation and management of proteinuria and nephrotic syndrome in children: Recommendations from a pediatric nephrology panel established at the National Kidney Foundation Conference on Proteinuria, Albuminuria, Risk, Assessment, Detection and Elimination (PARADE). *Pediatrics* 105:1242, 2000.

Houser MT, Jahn MF, Kobayashi A, Walburn J: Assessment of urinary protein excretion in the adolescent:

Effect of body position and exercise. *J Pediatr* 109: 556, 1986.

Vehaskari V, Rapola J: Isolated proteinuria: Analysis of a school-age population. *J Pediatr* 101:661, 1982.

Rytand DA, Spreiter S: Prognosis in postural (orthostatic) proteinuria: Forty to fifty-year follow-up of six patients after diagnosis by Thomas Addis. *N Engl J Med* 305:618, 1981.

Roy S 3rd, Stapleton FB: Focal segmental glomerulosclerosis in children: Comparison of nonedematous and edematous patients. *Pediatr Nephrol* 1:281, 1987.

CASE 128: A 15-YEAR-OLD BOY WITH FLANK PAIN AND BLOODY URINE

A 15-year-old Asian-American male presented to the emergency department with right flank pain and otherwise painless gross hematuria. The patient is adopted and his adoptive parents were unaware of any family history of renal disease or nephrolithiasis. The past medical history was unremarkable except for seasonal allergies.

On physical examination this healthy-appearing 15-year-old weighed 61.5 kg, measured 169 cm in height, and had a blood pressure of 144/92 mm Hg. The chest was clear to auscultation and there was no evidence of peripheral edema. The abdominal examination was within normal limits. The laboratory tests revealed a urinalysis with a specific gravity 1.010, pH 8, 3+ proteinuria, 10 to 20 WBC/HPF, and >20 RBC/HPF. The urinary protein/creatinine ratio was 0.23 and the calcium/creatinine ratio was 0.09. The urine culture was negative.

The BUN was 13 mg/dL, serum creatinine 0.9 mg/dL, and Hgb 16.1 gm/dL. The serum C3 level was 131 mg/dL (83 to 177 for adults), C_4 44 mg/dL (15 to 45 for adults), and the anti-streptolysin O antibody <200 IU/mL. The patient was referred to the pediatric renal clinic.

SELECT THE ONE BEST ANSWER

1. In the evaluation of hematuria with minimal proteinuria the most important part of the evaluation is:

   (A) history
   (B) physical examination
   (C) urinary calcium/creatinine ratio
   (D) BUN/creatinine

2. Which is the least common cause of hematuria?

   (A) benign familial hematuria
   (B) idiopathic hypercalciuria
   (C) Alport syndrome
   (D) IgA nephropathy

3. If the urinary calcium/creatinine ratio was 0.45 and reconfirmed, the patient should be:

   (A) encouraged to drink more than 2 L of fluids in 24 hours
   (B) placed on a low-sodium, normal-calcium diet
   (C) treated with thiazides
   (D) none of the above

4. Gross hematuria persisted for 7 days. An abdominal ultrasound was ordered that showed enlargement of both kidneys with multiple cysts bilaterally consistent with autosomal dominant polycystic kidney disease. The next test that should be ordered is:

   (A) MRA brain
   (B) CT of abdomen
   (C) voiding cystourethrogram
   (D) genetic testing for PKD1 and PKD2

5. This 15-year-old male with autosomal dominant polycystic disease will likely demonstrate during childhood all of these clinical manifestations except:

   (A) pain
   (B) hematuria
   (C) hypertension
   (D) renal insufficiency

Answers

1. **(A)** There are many causes of asymptomatic hematuria without significant proteinuria. The most important part of the evaluation is a careful history. The history of present illness should confirm that patient is truly asymptomatic—no history of trauma, lower urinary tract symptoms, no edema, and so on. Also, the family history is important—hematuria, renal failure, deafness, and nephrolithiasis.

2. **(B)** Benign familial hematuria is a common cause of hematuria and is diagnosed by screening first-

degree relatives. Idiopathic hypercalciuria is also a common cause of hematuria. It is diagnosed if the urinary calcium/creatinine is >0.21. IgA nephropathy is a strong consideration. It is characterized by 1 to 2 days of gross hematuria during an upper respiratory tract infection. Between episodes of gross hematuria there is microscopic hematuria. Diagnosis is made by renal biopsy showing deposition of IgA on immunofluorescence. Alport syndrome is a rare condition that consists of hereditary nephritis accompanied by neurosensory hearing loss.

3. **(D)** Idiopathic hypercalciuria is a common cause of microscopic hematuria in childhood. Patients with the disorder are more likely to develop nephrolithiasis. However, treatment is reserved for patients who have previously had nephrolithiasis or patients with a strong family history of hypercalciuria and nephrolithiasis. Increased fluid intake, restricted animal protein and salt, ample intake of calcium (1200 mg/day), and thiazide treatment are helpful in preventing recurrent nephrolithiasis.

4. **(A)** Renal involvement is characterized by cystic dilatations in all parts of the nephron including Bowman's space. In the early stages there may only be a few irregularly distributed macrocysts. Later, both kidneys are enlarged and large cysts are present in the cortex and medulla. Cysts in the liver, pancreas, and other organs are common in ADPKD but congenital hepatic fibrosis is rare. Cerebral vessel malformations have been described. An MRA of the brain should be performed to exclude cerebral aneurysms.

5. **(D)** The manifestations of disease such as pain, hematuria, and hypertension are associated with large or enlarging kidneys. The glomerular filtration rate does not deteriorate in this population of children. This is consistent with the natural history of ADPKD in which renal insufficiency develops after the age of 30 years.

SUGGESTED READING

Dodge WF, West EF, Smith EH, et al: Proteinuria and hematuria in schoolchildren: Epidemiology and early natural history. *J Pediatr* 88:327–347, 1976.

Vehaskari VM, Rapola J, Koskimies O, et al: Microscopic hematuria in school children: Epidemiology and clinicopathologic evaluation. *J Pediatr* 95 (5 Pt 1): 676–684, 1979.

Ingelfinger JR, Davis AE, Grupe WE: Frequency and etiology of gross hematuria in a general pediatric setting. *Pediatrics* 59:557–561, 1977.

Jais PJ, Knebelmann B, Giatras I, et al: X-linked Alport syndrome: Natural history in 195 families and genotype-phenotype correlations in males. *J Am Soc Nephrol* 11:649–657, 2000.

Feld LG, Meyers KE, Kaplan BS, et al: Limited evaluation of microscopic hematuria in pediatrics. *Pediatrics* 102:E42, 1998.

Stapleton FB: Idiopathic hypercalciuria: Association with isolated hematuria and risk for urolithiasis in children. The Southwest Pediatric Nephrology Study Group. *Kidney Int* 37:807–811, 1990.

Kaplan BS, Kaplan P, Rosenberg HK, et al: Polycystic kidney diseases in childhood. *J Pediatr* 115:867–880, 1989.

Shaikewitz ST, Chapman A: Autosomal recessive polycystic kidney disease: Issues regarding the variability of clinical presentation. *J Am Soc Nephrol* 3:1858–1862, 1993.

Kissane JM: Renal cysts in pediatric patients: A classification and overview. *Pediatr Nephrol* 4:69–77, 1990.

Borghi L, Schianchi T, Meschi T, et al: Comparison of two diets for the prevention of recurrent stones in idiopathic hypercalciuria. *N Engl J Med* 346:77–84, 2002.

Neurology

16

CASE 129: A 6-YEAR-OLD GIRL WITH STARING SPELLS

The teacher of a 6-year-old African-American female refers her to your clinic for an evaluation of frequent episodes of staring. The episodes occur daily and are brief, lasting no more than 5 to 8 seconds. She typically has several events per day. Occasionally, when the children are playing during recess, the child will stop what she is doing and exhibit a blank facial expression. She often picks at her clothes during these episodes. Following the event, she resumes her activity. Her mother states that she has not noticed any of these particular spells, but states that the child frequently "daydreams" at home, during which she is unresponsive to verbal stimuli. The child was born at full term without complications. There is no history of bowel or bladder incontinence, headache or emesis. The child states that she is unaware of the episodes, but believes there are times when she has missed things that have been said to her. She denies any aura. There is no history of febrile seizures, CNS infections, or head trauma.

On reviewing her family history, you discover that the child has a maternal great-aunt with "terrible seizures" unresponsive to medications. Her mother recalls having similar "daydreaming episodes" as a child for which she was treated with medication until high school. There is a strong family history of depression.

On physical examination, she has a large café-au-lait spot on her back. On neurologic examination, she has normal intelligence. Her cranial nerve examination is unremarkable. She has normal strength in both the upper and lower extremities. Her deep tendon reflexes are symmetric at 2+ out of 4. Her gait is normal.

SELECT THE ONE BEST ANSWER

1. Based on the clinical history, this child most likely has which of the following diagnoses?

   (A) depression
   (B) absence seizures
   (C) complex partial seizures
   (D) juvenile myoclonic epilepsy
   (E) attention deficit disorder

2. In order to establish the diagnosis in the clinic, which of the following actions would be the most helpful?

   (A) assessment of risk factors for depression
   (B) Connor scales
   (C) visual screening
   (D) hyperventilation
   (E) none of the above

3. Which of the following diagnostic studies would be the most helpful in establishing the diagnosis?

   (A) electroencephalogram (EEG) with hyperventilation and photic stimulation
   (B) MRI of the brain with and without contrast
   (C) urine toxicology screen
   (D) electrolytes
   (E) polysomnogram

4. The drug treatment of choice for this patient would be which of the following medications?

(A) lamotrigine
(B) ethosuximide
(C) carbamazepine
(D) methylphenidate
(E) fluoxetine

5. A child presents to your office with the chief complaint of staring lasting up to 80 seconds. During the event, the child exhibits lip smacking. The child states that on occasion a "strange feeling" precedes the episodes. He has had one generalized tonic-clonic seizure observed by the school nurse. An EEG is most likely to demonstrate which of the following?

(A) bilateral, synchronous 3-Hz spike and wave activity
(B) anterior temporal spikes
(C) high-amplitude slow waves, multifocal spikes, and sharp waves with periods of electrodecrement
(D) high-amplitude sharp waves occurring over the central-temporal regions bilaterally during sleep
(E) diffuse slowing

6. A 5-year-old girl comes to your office because she has started to lose the ability to speak. Her mother states that she was born full-term and developed normally, speaking in full sentences by 3 years of age. Which of the following studies is most likely to yield the diagnosis?

(A) MRI of the brain with and without contrast
(B) routine EEG
(C) 24-hour long-term video EEG monitoring
(D) methyl CpG-binding protein 2 gene mutation analysis (MECP2)
(E) hearing test

7. A 15-year-old male with a history of complex partial seizures recently moves into your practice area. He comes into your office for a general physical examination. During the visit, he states that he has been seizure-free for approximately 2½ years. His spells consisted of staring with automatisms, but occasionally they would progress to generalized tonic-clonic seizures. As

he is concerned about driving next year, he asks you when he can go off his medication. He is currently treated with carbamazepine. The most appropriate response would be which of the following?

(A) "Let's obtain an EEG. If that test is normal, there is an approximately 70% chance you will be seizure-free."
(B) "Never. Epilepsy is a lifelong condition."
(C) "Children with complex partial seizures need to be seizure-free for at least 5 years before a decision can be made."
(D) "It all depends on the epilepsy syndrome or type and complex partial seizures seldom go into remission."
(E) None of the above.

8. Which of the following antiepileptic drugs are generally considered the first- and second-line therapies for neonatal seizures?

(A) diazepam and phenobarbital
(B) phenobarbital and phenytoin
(C) phenytoin and midazolam
(D) phenobarbital and lorazepam
(E) phenobarbital and valproic acid

9. Which of the following is the most common form of childhood seizures?

(A) complex partial seizures
(B) absence seizures
(C) infantile spasms
(D) benign rolandic epilepsy
(E) febrile seizures

10. Which of the following medications is the least likely to lower a patient's seizure threshold?

(A) methylphenidate
(B) fluoxetine
(C) disperidone
(D) haloperidol
(E) atomoxetine

11. Which of the following statements is not true about febrile seizures?

(A) A febrile seizure is considered "complex" if it is prolonged, focal, or occurs multiple times per febrile illness.

(B) A family history of febrile seizures in a first- or second-degree relative is a risk factor for the development of febrile seizures.

(C) Developmental delay is a risk factor for the development of a first febrile seizure.

(D) Up to 10% of patients with febrile seizures develop epilepsy.

(E) Carbamazepine and phenytoin are equally effective in the treatment of febrile seizures should one consider treatment.

12. Which of the following are causes of neonatal seizures?

(A) a hypoxic-ischemic episode
(B) metabolic abnormalities
(C) infection
(D) inborn errors of metabolism
(E) all of the above

MATCH EACH OF THE FOLLOWING ANTI-EPILEPTIC DRUGS WITH ITS COMMONLY REPORTED SIDE EFFECT

13. Lamotrigine

14. Valproic acid

15. Phenytoin

16. Carbamazepine

17. Phenobarbital

18. Topiramate

(A) gingival hyperplasia
(B) Stevens-Johnson Syndrome
(C) hepatotoxicity
(D) weight loss
(E) agranulocytosis
(F) hyperactivity

Answers

1. (**B**) This patient most likely has absence seizures (petit mal). Absence seizures are relatively uncommon, accounting for less than 10% of all seizure types. They tend to be more common in females than males. The average age of onset is approximately 4 years and they are rarely seen prior to the age of 2 years. In typical absence seizures, patients exhibit brief (<30 seconds) staring spells; however, motor, behavioral, and autonomic phenomena are frequently observed. The child can have multiple spells per day. Automatisms, such as chewing, grimacing, or lip licking, may be observed. They are never associated with an aura, bowel or bladder incontinence, or postictal impairment. Most children with typical absence seizures have normal intelligence and physical examination. There is a strong genetic predisposition. An EEG demonstrates generalized 3-Hz spike-wave activity. The prognosis of typical absence seizures is favorable with approximately 80% achieving remission by 10 to 11 years of age. Atypical absence seizures are similar to typical absence seizures, but are more likely to have diminished postural tone and tonic or myoclonic activity as part of their initial clinical presentation. Automatisms are less likely. Many children go on to develop Lennox-Gastaut syndrome. The EEG demonstrates asymmetric <2.5-Hz spike-wave activity with multifocal spikes and sharp waves. In contrast, complex partial seizures tend to last much longer (>1 minute on average), are frequently associated with aura, and can be followed by a postictal state. The EEG usually demonstrates rhythmic focal spikes or sharp waves over the temporal or frontal regions during a seizure. Juvenile myoclonic epilepsy (JME) typically occurs between the ages of 12 and 18 years. Children as young as 8 years have been reported to develop JME. JME is a familial, generalized seizure disorder in which patients demonstrate jerks of the shoulders and arms, typically occurring shortly after awakening. Loss of consciousness is seldom noticeable. Many of these patients respond to valproic acid.

2. (**D**) Hyperventilation is a strong activator of typical absence seizures. The child is asked to hyperventilate for 3 to 5 minutes, during which a seizure is induced. Photic stimulation is also used to induce generalized seizure disorders, but does not appear to be as effective an activator in typical absence seizures as hyperventilation. Connor scales are used to screen for attention deficit disorder.

3. (**A**) The differential diagnosis of absence seizures includes complex partial seizures, daydreaming, and pseudoseizures. The most effective way of es-

tablishing the classification of a seizure or establishing a diagnosis is to capture a spell while performing an EEG. In this case, hyperventilation can be used to precipitate a seizure, enabling the physician to capture the spell while recording. Bilateral, synchronous 3-Hz spike-wave activity would confirm the diagnosis of typical absence seizure. In complex partial seizures, one may observe intermittent spikes or sharp waves over the temporal or frontal regions during the interictal (between seizures) stage, and rhythmic activity over these regions during the seizure. The EEG should be normal in daydreaming and pseudoseizures. MRI of the brain, urine toxicology, and electrolyte analysis can be important in the diagnosis and management of seizures, but given the clinic history, an EEG with hyperventilation has the highest yield. The former studies are normal in typical absence seizures.

4. **(B)** Three drugs are primarily used in the treatment of absence seizures: ethosuximide, valproic acid, and lamotrigine. For typical absence seizures, most neurologists would start therapy with ethosuximide given its side effect profile compared to that of valproic acid. It is not useful for patients who have generalized tonic-clonic seizures with their absence seizures. In this case, valproic acid is preferred. Carbamazepine is used in the treatment of complex partial seizures. In primary generalized seizure disorders, such as absence seizures, it may make the patient worse. Methylphenidate is used in the treatment of attention deficit/hyperactivity disorder, while fluoxetine is used to treat anxiety, depression, and obsessive-compulsive disorders.

5. **(B)** This child most likely has complex partial seizures with secondary generalization given the single generalized tonic-clonic seizure and clinical history. As a result, the EEG will most likely demonstrate anterior temporal spikes in between seizures. Bilateral, synchronous 3-Hz spike-wave activity is seen in absence seizures. High-amplitude slow waves, multifocal spikes, and sharp waves with periods of electrodecrement (flatting of brain electrical activity) defines hypsarrhythmia, seen in patients with infantile spasms. Benign rolandic epilepsy is characterized by high-amplitude sharp waves occurring over the central-temporal regions bilaterally during sleep. Diffuse slowing is ob-

served in toxic-metabolic encephalopathies or during a postictal state.

6. **(C)** This child most likely has an acquired epileptiform aphasia, such as Landau-Kleffner syndrome (LKS). LKS often occurs between the ages of 5 and 7 years. Typically, children afflicted with LKS develop an abrupt or gradual loss of language ability. Expressive and receptive language dysfunction is observed. These children can also have behavioral and psychomotor disturbances, such that they resemble an autistic child. The EEG most commonly demonstrates sharp wave and spike-wave activity over the temporal or parietal-occipital regions bilaterally more commonly observed during sleep. Electrical status of slow-wave sleep is a condition similar to LKS in which spike-wave activity is the dominant pattern observed during sleep. This disorder occurs with a peak age of onset between 4 and 5 years of age. The prognosis for both conditions is variable. Although some may recover fully, others continue to have speech and cognitive impairments. In order to capture slow-wave sleep (stage IV), a 24-hour EEG is usually required. MECP2 gene mutation is associated with Rett syndrome.

7. **(A)** If a child is seizure free for approximately 2 years, there is an approximately 70% chance that the child will go into remission. Generalized seizures, a normal neurological examination, and age of onset prior to approximately 12 years predict a more favorable outcome. Some studies suggest that a normal EEG or resolution of interictal spikes also predicts a favorable outcome.

8. **(B)** It is generally accepted among pediatric neurologists and neonatologists that phenobarbital is the first-line therapy for neonatal seizures, while phenytoin is the second-line therapy. Although many centers prefer to use fosphenytoin, a benzodiazepine is considered third-line therapy. Caution must be exercised when using phenobarbital in conjunction with a benzodiazepine, as respiratory suppression, a potential side effect of both medications, is more likely.

9. **(E)** The most common form of childhood seizures are febrile seizures, occurring in 2% to 4% of the population in the United States.

10. **(E)** Occasionally, children with epilepsy have co-morbid conditions such as attention deficit/hyperactivity disorder, depression, and tics. Many of the medications used to treat these comorbid conditions can lower the seizure threshold. Atomoxetine, a selective norepinephrine reuptake inhibitor used to treat attention deficit/hyperactivity disorder, does not seem to lower the seizure threshold.

11. **(E)** Febrile seizures are considered complex if they are prolonged, lasting more than 10 to 15 minutes, are focal, or occur multiple times per febrile illness. Risk factors for a first febrile seizure include developmental delay, admission to the neonatal intensive care unit for longer than 30 days, attendance at day care, and having a family history of febrile seizures in a first- or second-degree relative. Based on data obtained from several large studies of children with febrile seizures, the risk of developing subsequent epilepsy is approximately 2% to 10%. Although treating febrile seizures remains controversial, daily phenobarbital has been shown effective in reducing the risk of recurrent febrile seizures. Diazepam given orally or rectally at the onset of a febrile illness reduces the probability of a febrile seizure. Carbamazepine and phenytoin are *not* effective in the treatment of febrile seizures.

12. **(E)** The causes of neonatal seizures are diverse and must be investigated to ensure adequate treatment. For example, seizures resulting from hypoglycemia require adequate glucose replacement.

13. **(B)** Stevens-Johnson syndrome secondary to lamotrigine administration occurs in 1% to 2% of children and 0.1% of adults. Other side effects of lamotrigine include dizziness, diplopia, and blurred vision.

14. **(C)** Fatal hepatotoxicity can occur in children treated with valproic acid. Children between the ages of 0 and 2 years are particularly at risk: 1/118,000 for patients on monotherapy and 1/800 on polytherapy. Other side effects include weight gain in some children and thrombocytopenia.

15. **(A)** Long-term administration of phenytoin has been associated with gingival hyperplasia, hirsutism, acne, and rash (Stevens-Johnson syndrome).

Toxic serum levels of phenytoin may result in ataxia, nystagmus, diplopia, and incoordination.

16. **(E)** Although serious hematologic complications with carbamazepine therapy are very rare, thrombocytopenia, aplastic anemia, agranulocytosis, and pancytopenia have been reported. Drowsiness, ataxia, dyskinesia, dizziness, and visual disturbances may also be observed.

17. **(F)** Behavioral side effects, especially hyperactivity and aggressiveness, can be seen in almost half the children taking phenobarbital. Dose-dependent side effects include sedation and respiratory depression.

18. **(D)** Weight loss has been reported as a side effect of topiramate therapy, usually beginning during the first few months of administration and peaking at 12 to 18 months.

SUGGESTED READING

Wyllie E (ed): *The Treatment of Epilepsy: Principles & Practice*, 3rd ed. Philadelphia: Lippincott, Williams & Wilkins, 2001.

Holmes GL: Generalized seizures. In: Swaiman KF, Ashwal S (eds): *Pediatric Neurology: Principles & Practice*, 3rd ed. St. Louis: Mosby, 1999, p 634.

Baram TZ: Myoclonus and myoclonic seizures. In: Swaiman KF, Ashwal S (eds): *Pediatric Neurology: Principles & Practice*, 3rd ed. St. Louis: Mosby, 1999, p 668.

Shinnar S: Febrile seizures. In: Swaiman KF, Ashwal S (eds): *Pediatric Neurology: Principles & Practice*, 3rd ed. St. Louis: Mosby, 1999, p 676.

Kriel RL, Birnbaum AK, Cloyd JC: Antiepileptic drug therapy in children. In: Swaiman KF, Ashwal S (eds): *Pediatric Neurology: Principles & Practice*, 3rd ed. St. Louis: Mosby, 1999, p 692.

CASE 130: A 5-MONTH-OLD BOY WITH SEIZURES AND A BIRTH MARK

You are called to the emergency department to evaluate a 5-month-old infant male who presents with the chief complaint of "unusual leg movements" on awakening. The patient was born at full term by normal spontaneous vaginal delivery. The pregnancy was unremarkable except for spotting in the first trimester. Developmentally, his mother states that he is not yet rolling over. He startles to loud noises and occasionally vocalizes. Although he smiled responsively at 2 months of age, she has noticed he no longer seems to smile. His mother states that he often "spits up" after feeds. There is no family history of seizures.

During the evaluation, you observe a cluster of spells as the baby awakens. The spells consist of flexion of the head and body with extension of the legs. You are unable to stop the movements by applying gentle pressure. The baby was given a bottle feed approximately 1 hour ago.

On physical examination, he has a temperature of 98.2°F (36.8°C), a heart rate of 164, a respiratory rate of 32, and a blood pressure of 78/51 mm Hg. The tympanic membranes are normal bilaterally. He has an irregular heartbeat. His lungs are clear to auscultation. Examination of his skin reveals three hypopigmented lesions over his abdomen and back. On neurological examination, his tone is decreased centrally. He has a poor response to traction with a significant head lag. His reflexes are brisk symmetrically. His plantar reflexes are extensor.

SELECT THE ONE BEST ANSWER

1. Given the history and physical examination, the most appropriate study in the initial management of this patient is which of the following?

   (A) ECG
   (B) echocardiogram
   (C) head CT
   (D) EEG with concurrent administration of pyridoxine
   (E) MRI of the brain with and without contrast

2. The EEG demonstrates hypsarrhythmia, while the head CT reveals periventricular calcifications. A small, mineralized subependymal nodule is also observed. The most likely diagnosis is which of the following?

   (A) Fahr disease
   (B) neurofibromatosis type 1
   (C) tuberous sclerosis complex
   (D) toxoplasmosis
   (E) incontinentia pigmenti achromians (hypomelanosis of Ito)

3. This patient is at risk for developing which of the following complications?

   (A) hydrocephalus
   (B) renal cell carcinoma
   (C) bony involvement

   (D) giant cell astrocytoma
   (E) all of the above

4. Which of the following is considered the most effective in the treatment of this patient's seizure?

   (A) topiramate
   (B) phenobarbital
   (C) primidone
   (D) adrenocorticotropic hormone
   (E) phenytoin

5. Which of the following statements is true regarding the genetics of tuberous sclerosis?

   (A) It is transmitted as an autosomal recessive trait.
   (B) It is transmitted as an autosomal dominant trait with variable penetrance.
   (C) The disorder demonstrates an X-linked mode of inheritance.
   (D) The disorder is the result of triplet repeat expansion.
   (E) Relatively little is known about the mode of transmission of this disorder.

6. Which of the following seizure types is *not* more common in tuberous sclerosis complex?

   (A) infantile spasms
   (B) complex partial seizures
   (C) absence seizures
   (D) simple partial seizures
   (E) atonic seizures

7. When would you most likely expect adenoma sebaceum (facial angiofibromas) to present in this child?

   (A) shortly after birth
   (B) between the ages of 1 and 4 years
   (C) between the ages of 6 and 9 years
   (D) during puberty
   (E) adulthood

8. An 18-month-old female presents to your clinic for continued pediatric care. Her family recently moved to your area and you haven't yet received her medical records. On physical examination, she has a nevus flammeus (port-wine stain) over the left side of her face and a contralateral hemiparesis. This patient is most likely to have which of the following?

(A) ipsilateral leptomeningeal angioma
(B) intracranial calcifications on head CT
(C) glaucoma
(D) A and B
(E) all of the above

9. Which of the following statements is true regarding the genetics of Sturge-Weber Syndrome?

(A) It is transmitted as an autosomal recessive trait.
(B) It is transmitted as an autosomal dominant trait.
(C) The disorder demonstrates an X-linked mode of inheritance.
(D) The disorder is the result of triplet repeat expansion.
(E) Relatively little is known about the mode of transmission of this disorder.

10. Each of the following neurocutaneous disorders is transmitted as an autosomal dominant trait except for:

(A) neurofibromatosis 1
(B) Von Hippel-Lindau Disease
(C) tuberous sclerosis complex
(D) ataxia-telangiectasia
(E) neurofibromatosis 2

11. A 26-month-old male presents to your clinic for an evaluation of multiple café-au-lait spots. On close inspection, you determine that he has six spots greater than 0.8 cm over the trunk. On funduscopic examination, you notice optic disc pallor in the left eye. The most likely cause of the optic disc pallor and atrophy is which of the following?

(A) optic neuritis
(B) papilledema
(C) optic nerve glioma
(D) meningioma
(E) retinal artery infarction

12. The patient's father in question 11 offers that he has similar birthmarks to that of his son. The most likely diagnosis is which of the following?

(A) neurofibromatosis 2
(B) neurofibromatosis 1
(C) ataxia-telangiectasia

(D) neurocutaneous melanosis
(E) linear sebaceous nevus

13. Which of the following is the most common CNS tumor observed in neurofibromatosis 1?

(A) low-grade astrocytoma
(B) meningioma
(C) medulloblastoma
(D) ependymoma
(E) primitive neuroectodermal tumors

14. Which of the following is not a diagnostic criteria of neurofibromatosis 1 (NF1)?

(A) two or more Lisch nodules
(B) optic nerve glioma
(C) five or more café-au-lait spots 1.5 cm or larger in postpubertal individuals
(D) a first-degree relative with NF1
(E) two or more neurofibromas or one or more plexiform neurofibroma

MATCH EACH OF THE FOLLOWING DIAGNOSTIC FEATURES WITH ITS NEUROCUTANEOUS DISORDER

15. Bilateral acoustic neuromas

16. Periungual fibroma

17. Retinal hemangioblastoma

18. Decreased immunoglobulin A and E levels

19. Inguinal freckling

(A) neurofibromatosis 1
(B) Von Hippel-Lindau disease
(C) neurofibromatosis 2
(D) ataxia-telangiectasia
(E) tuberous sclerosis complex

Answers

1. **(A)** This patient most likely has infantile spasms given the clinical history and observations. Infantile spasms typically occur between 3 and 8 months of age. Although there are many causes of infantile spasms, such as intrauterine infections and perinatal asphyxia, it is the most common seizure type

seen in tuberous sclerosis complex (TSC). Patients typically have myoclonic jerks in clusters that usually occur on awakening. The seizures can consist of head and body flexion or extension. The movements observed in this child are the more common presentation. As seen in this child, the loss of milestones and developmental arrest are not uncommon at the onset of infantile spasms. The presence of hypopigmented spots supports the diagnosis of tuberous sclerosis and, to some extent, infantile spasms. Approximately half the patients with TSC can have cardiac rhabdomyomas. The cardiac rhabdomyomas affect the myocardium and can be solitary, multiple, or infiltrative. Cardiac rhabdomyomas can cause arrhythmias, congestive heart failure, obstruction to blood flow, or even sudden death. The arrhythmias include ventricular tachycardia, supraventricular tachycardia (SVT), and Wolff-Parkinson-White syndrome. As a result, it is important to clarify the arrhythmia and begin the necessary treatment. An echocardiogram will probably reveal a cardiac rhabdomyoma. Neuroimaging would reveal periventricular calcifications, seen better on head CT, and subependymal nodules, hamartomas, and tubers. An EEG would reveal the pattern known as hypsarrhythmia, which is necessary for the diagnosis of infantile spasms. The triad of hypsarrhythmia, flexor spasms, and mental retardation is known as West syndrome. The administration of pyridoxine, an important step in the evaluation of infantile seizures, would not result in normalization of the EEG as it would for seizures due to a pyridoxine deficiency.

2. (**C**) In order to make a definite diagnosis of TSC, 2 of 11 major features or 1 major feature plus 2 of 9 minor features must be present. The features are listed below (slightly modified from Kandt, 2002):

Major diagnostic features:
   Cardiac rhabdomyoma
   Renal angiomyolipoma
   Lymphangiomyomatosis
   Facial angiofibromas
   Ungual fibroma
   Shagreen patch
   Cortical tuber
   Three or more hypomelanotic macules
   Multiple retinal nodular hamartomas
   Subependymal giant cell astrocytoma
   Subependymal nodule
Minor diagnostic features:
   Multiple renal cysts
   Retinal achromic patch
   Multiple dental pits
   Bone cysts
   Non-renal hamartoma
   Gingival fibromas
   "Confetti" skin lesions
   Cerebral white matter radial migration lines
   Hamartomatous rectal polyps

In hypomelanosis of Ito patients have hypopigmented skin lesions, which vary from linear streaks following a dermatomic distribution to whorls with irregular margins. Females are more frequently affected than males. Periventricular calcifications, tubers, and subependymal nodules are not observed. Fahr disease (familial basal ganglia calcification) is a hereditary condition in which calcification is particularly observed in the dentate and lenticular nuclei. The disease is not associated with hypopigmented skin lesions. Toxoplasmosis is a disease caused by the protozoan, *Toxoplasma gondii*. The major reservoir for this organism in the United States is the cat, which excretes oocysts in the feces. The disease is associated with cerebral calcification in approximately 60% of affected individuals. Although seizures, hydrocephalus, microcephaly, chorioretinitis, and psychomotor retardation are seen in toxoplasmosis, skin lesions are not described.

3. (**E**) Patients with tuberous sclerosis are at risk for developing all of the complications described. Most renal tumors are renal cysts or renal angiomyolipomas. However, a small percentage of patients (<2%) develop renal carcinoma. For reasons that are unclear, female patients are at risk to develop pulmonary complications. Tubers can obstruct normal cerebral spinal fluid (CSF) flow if located near the foramen of Monro or the Sylvian aqueduct.

4. (**D**) The American Academy of Neurology recently published a practice parameter reviewing the medical treatment of infantile spasms. The recommendation is that adrenocorticotropic hormone is probably effective in the short-term treatment of infantile spasms. Vigabatrin may be useful in the

treatment of infantile spasms, particularly caused by tuberous sclerosis. However, this medication is not FDA approved, as it causes retinal toxicity.

5. **(B)** TSC is transmitted as an autosomal dominant trait with variable penetrance. However, spontaneous mutation rates may be observed in more than 50% of patients.

6. **(C)** Absence seizures cause a primary generalized seizure disorder and are not seen more frequently in TSC.

7. **(B)** Some lesions seen in TSC occur at various developmental stages. Adenoma sebaceum typically develops between 1 and 4 years. It rarely is seen at birth.

8. **(E)** This patient probably has Sturge-Weber syndrome, which is characterized by a facial angioma (nevus flammeus, port-wine stain) and ipsilateral leptomeningeal angioma. The facial angioma typically involves the upper face and occasionally the nasopharynx, mucous membranes, and ocular choroidal membrane. Choroidal membrane involvement can lead to glaucoma in approximately 25% of patients. Neuroimaging studies demonstrate calcium deposits in the walls of some small cerebral vessels and outer cortical layers. This is best observed on head CT. In one study, seizures occurred in three quarters of the cases. Patients can have a contralateral hemiparesis with hemiatrophy. Hemianopsia is also observed.

9. **(E)** No clear evidence of heredity has been discovered for this disorder.

10. **(D)** Ataxia-telangiectasia is a neurocutaneous disorder characterized by progressive cerebellar ataxia, immune defects, oculocutaneous telangiectasis, and a predisposition to malignancy. Patients can have a tendency to develop sinopulmonary infections and skin infections. Cellular and humoral immunity can be impaired. The disease is transmitted in a sporadic or autosomal recessive manner.

11. **(C)** Approximately 50% of children with optic nerve gliomas have neurofibromatosis 1 (NF1). Most of the children present with optic pallor and atrophy, as well as decreased visual acuity.

Depending on the location of the tumor, the child can present with visual field defects.

12. **(B)** In order to make a diagnosis of NF1, two or more of the following criteria are required:

- Two or more neurofibromas of any type or one or more plexiform neurofibromas
- Optic nerve glioma
- Six or more café-au-lait spots 1.5 cm or larger in postpubertal individuals and 0.5 cm or larger in prepubertal children
- A first-degree relative with NF1
- Two or more Lisch nodules
- Axillary or inguinal freckling
- A distinctive osseous lesion (dysplasia of the sphenoid bone or thinning of long bone cortex)

13. **(A)** The most common CNS tumors in NF1 are low-grade astrocytomas, mostly occurring in the optic pathway. Meningiomas, medulloblastomas, ependymomas, and primitive neuroectodermal tumors also occur, but are much less common.

14. **(C)** Six or more café-au-lait spots are required to make the diagnosis. See diagnostic criteria listed for answer 12 above.

15. **(C)** In order to make a diagnosis of neurofibromatosis 2 (NF2), bilateral eighth nerve masses must be seen with neuroimaging. Alternatively, the patient must have a first-degree relative with NF2 and either a unilateral eighth nerve mass or two of the following: meningioma, glioma, neurofibroma, schwannoma, and juvenile posterior subcapsular lenticular opacity.

16. **(E)** Periungual fibromas are seen in TSC. Ungual fibromas are pathologically similar to the facial angiofibromas.

17. **(B)** A rare disorder, transmitted as an autosomal dominant trait, Von Hippel-Lindau disease is characterized by retinal and cerebellar hemangioblastomas. Spinal cord angiomas and cystic tumors of the pancreas, epididymis, and kidney are also observed.

18. **(D)** See explanation for question 10.

19. **(A)** See diagnostic criteria for NF1 listed in answer 12.

SUGGESTED READING

Mackay MT, Weiss SK, Adams-Webber T, et al: Practice parameter: medical treatment of infantile spasms. *Neurology* 62:1668–1681, 2004.

Kandt RS: Tuberous sclerosis complex and neurofibromatosis type 1: the two most common neurocutaneous diseases. *Neurol Clin North Am* 20:941–964, 2002.

Berg BO: Neurocutaneous syndromes: phakomatoses and allied conditions. In: Swaiman KF, Ashwal S (eds): *Pediatric Neurology: Principles & Practice*, 3rd ed. St. Louis: Mosby, 1999, p 530.

CASE 131: A 2-YEAR-OLD GIRL WITH HEADACHE AND FEVER

You are called to the emergency department (ED) to evaluate a 2-year-old girl who presents with headache and confusion. In the emergency room her temperature is 102°F. The patient was in good health until 6 days prior to presentation when she developed malaise and low-grade fevers. Shortly after, her mother states she complained of headaches, which have increased in severity. She states her daughter is usually very pleasant, but recently has become agitated and increasingly irritable. Over the last couple of days, she has become more somnolent. Immunizations are up to date. The ED staff has ordered a head CT, which is reportedly within normal limits. A lumbar puncture, performed by the ED physician, revealed 340 white blood cells/mm³ with a predominance of polymorphonuclear cells, a glucose of 35 mg/dL, and a protein of 55 mg/dL. Although the patient knew her name on arousal, she has become stuporous and cannot abduct her left eye.

On your physical examination, the girl is obtunded, but withdraws appropriately to pain. She is unable to abduct her left eye and her pupils are sluggish. The remainder of her cranial nerve examination is normal, including fundoscopic examination. The deep tendon reflexes are mildly hyperactive and she has bilateral upgoing toes. Her skin examination is unremarkable.

SELECT THE ONE BEST ANSWER

1. A Gram stain of the patient's CSF would most likely reveal which of the following?

   (A) gram-positive or gram-negative diplococci
   (B) gram-negative rods
   (C) mixed bacterial morphology
   (D) gram-positive cocci
   (E) gram-positive bacillus

2. Which of the following antibiotics is the treatment of choice for this patient without known drug allergies?

   (A) penicillin
   (B) ceftriaxone
   (C) vancomycin
   (D) rifampin
   (E) B and C

3. Important causes of bacterial meningitis in this age group include:

   (A) *Streptococcus pneumoniae*
   (B) *Haemophilus influenzae*, type b
   (C) *Listeria monocytogenes*
   (D) *Neisseria meningitidis*
   (E) A and D

4. The most important next step in the management of this patient is which of the following?

   (A) supportive care including intravenous fluids
   (B) intubation
   (C) mannitol 0.25 to 1 g/kg
   (D) MRI of the brain with and without infusion
   (E) B and C

5. Which of the following are complications of bacterial meningitis?

   (A) sensorineural deafness
   (B) hydrocephalus
   (C) syndrome of inappropriate secretion of antidiuretic hormone (SIADH)
   (D) extra-axial fluid collections
   (E) all of the above

6. Prior to discharge, children treated for pneumococcal meningitis routinely require which of the following tests?

   (A) neuropsychological evaluations
   (B) repeat lumbar puncture
   (C) MRI of the brain
   (D) hearing evaluation
   (E) EEG

7. Which of the following organisms is the most common cause of acute bacterial meningitis in the neonatal period?

   (A) group B streptococcus

(B) *Streptococcus pneumoniae*
(C) *H. influenzae*, type b
(D) *L. monocytogenes*
(E) coagulase-negative staphylococci

8. *L. monocytogenes* is treated with which of the following antibiotics?

(A) gentamicin
(B) ampicillin
(C) vancomycin
(D) cefotaxime
(E) A and B

9. You are called to the emergency department to evaluate a 2½-week-old full-term infant who experienced a focal tonic seizure witnessed by the nurse. The infant was initially described as irritable, but now appears lethargic. The child has a slight fever. On careful history taking, you learn that the infant's mother has a history of STDs. She denies any history of vaginal vesicular lesions prior to delivery. Laboratory evaluation reveals a lymphocytic pleocytosis and elevated protein in the CSF. The Gram stain was negative. A head CT was normal. An EEG performed earlier revealed left temporal sharp waves. The most likely cause of this child's symptoms is which of the following?

(A) HSV1
(B) HSV2
(C) cytomegalovirus
(D) human immunodeficiency virus
(E) human herpes virus type 6

10. The action most likely to support your diagnosis for the case presented in question 9 is which of the following?

(A) assay for HSV DNA by polymerase chain reaction
(B) viral culture
(C) MRI of the brain with and without contrast
(D) urine for CMV
(E) non-infused head CT

11. The most appropriate antimicrobial therapy for this infant is which of the following drugs?

(A) ganciclovir
(B) methylprednisolone
(C) acyclovir

(D) zidovudine
(E) no effective therapy known

12. In utero herpes simplex viral infection can cause which of the following clinical features?

(A) intrauterine growth retardation
(B) microcephaly
(C) intracranial calcifications
(D) cataracts
(E) All of the above

13. All of the following are causes of arthropod-transmitted encephalitis except for which of the following?

(A) lymphocytic choriomeningitis virus
(B) West Nile virus
(C) Japanese encephalitis virus
(D) St. Louis encephalitis virus
(E) eastern equine encephalitis virus

14. A 6-year-old boy presents to your clinic with the chief complaint of new-onset headache, fever, and neck stiffness on returning from a camping trip. He has also had a sore throat for 3 days. On physical examination, he has an erythematous rash over the palms of his hands and vesicular lesions and ulcers over the oropharynx. The most likely cause of this child's symptoms is which of the following?

(A) echovirus
(B) herpes simplex virus type 1
(C) human immunodeficiency virus
(D) Chikungunya virus
(E) West Nile virus

15. Which of the following parasites is responsible for cysticercosis?

(A) *Diphyllobothrium latum*
(B) *Taenia multiceps*
(C) *Taenia solium*
(D) *Angiostrongylus cantonensis*
(E) *Plasmodium falciparum*

16. Which of the following anaerobic organisms is responsible for brain abscess formation?

(A) *Actinomyces*
(B) *Bacteroides*

(C) *Peptostreptococcus*

(D) *Propionibacterium*

(E) All of the above

MATCH EACH OF THE FOLLOWING PARASITES WITH THE CORRESPONDING TREATMENT

17. *T. gondii*

18. *P. falciparum*

19. *A. cantonensis*

20. *T. solium*

(A) no specific therapy required

(B) quinidine gluconate

(C) pyrimethamine/sulfadiazine

(D) praziquantel

Answers

1. **(A)** This patient most likely has *S. pneumoniae*, which, along with *N. meningitidis*, has become the most common cause of bacterial meningitis in children and adults since the institution of a vaccine for *H. influenzae*, type b. *S. pneumoniae* is a gram-positive diplococci. Group B streptococci (*Streptococcus agalactiae*) are also gram-positive diplococci, while *N. meningitidis* is a gram-negative diplococcus. *Escherichia coli* is a gram-negative rod, while *L. monocytogenes* is a gram-positive bacillus. Staphylococci are gram-positive cocci appearing in "grape-like" clusters. Mixed bacterial flora rarely cause meningitis.

2. **(E)** Recent concern has been raised regarding the increased prevalence of penicillin-resistant *S. pneumoniae*. As a result, children older than 1 month of age who are suspected of having bacterial meningitis should be treated with vancomycin and ceftriaxone or cefotaxime. If the child is allergic to β-lactam antibiotics, the cephalosporin is replaced with rifampin. The therapy is especially indicated if the Gram stain reveals gram-positive diplococci (see answer 1 above). Of course, susceptibility testing should be performed, and the antimicrobial therapy can be altered based on that laboratory testing.

3. **(E)** As a result of *H. influenzae* and now, *S. pneumoniae* vaccination programs, the epidemiology of meningitis has changed with *H. influenzae*, type b disease virtually absent in the United States and the incidence of pneumococcal meningitis drastically reduced. Importantly, these vaccines are not yet in the routine immunization programs of many nations.

4. **(E)** A serious complication of bacterial meningitis is increased intracranial pressure (ICP). In severe cases, the increased ICP can lead to herniation and immediate action must be taken. Clinically, the first clinical signs of increased ICP in children are headache, lethargy, vomiting, and irritability (in small children or infants). In this vignette, the child is becoming increasingly stuporous. She cannot abduct her left eye, which represents a sixth cranial nerve palsy. This is considered a false localizing sign as the abnormality is not caused by a lesion within the brainstem or from a posterior fossa tumor, which are more common in children. Rather, hydrocephalus results in herniation during which the brainstem is pushed downward, resulting in stretching of the sixth nerve over the petrous tip. The acute treatment of increased ICP includes intubation followed by controlled hyperventilation (maintaining a P_{CO_2} at approximately 30 torr). Mannitol (0.25 to 1 g/kg) can be administered intravenously and repeated every 2 to 4 hours as needed.

5. **(E)** Sensorineural hearing loss, hydrocephalus, SIADH, and extra-axial fluid collections are all complications of bacterial meningitis. In addition, seizures, cranial nerve involvement (as seen in this case), infarction, and disseminated intravascular coagulation are also observed.

6. **(D)** Bacterial meningitis is an extremely important cause of acquired sensorineural deafness. Sensorineural hearing loss can be caused by the infectious agent, especially *S. pneumoniae*, or use of ototoxic antibiotics. Prior to discharge, each child should have audiometry or brainstem auditory-evoked potentials in a younger child. If total deafness is observed, cochlear implants should be considered.

7. **(A)** Group B streptococcus and *L. monocytogenes* can both cause bacterial meningitis in the neo-

nate. *L. monocytogenes*, however, while often considered, does so quite rarely.

8. **(E)** *Listeria monocytogenes* is treated with ampicillin and gentamicin. The gentamicin is added to provide synergy.

9. **(B)** This infant most likely has a neonatal herpes simplex virus 2 infection obtained during passage through an infected birth canal. Although the mother denied a history of vaginal vesicular lesions, in a majority of cases, infection occurs in children of asymptomatic mothers. Outside the neonatal period, HSV2 is a relatively rare cause of viral encephalitis. In older individuals, HSV1 is more likely to cause encephalitis with an estimated annual occurrence of 1 in 250,000 to 500,000 individuals. Most individuals acquire HSV1 through oral transmission. HSV2 infection in neonates can be divided into three categories, each representing roughly a third of the total number of cases: (1) encephalitis (localized disease); (2) skin, eye, mouth disease; and (3) disseminated disease. In the case of localized disease, symptoms typically occur 2 to 3 weeks after birth. HSV2 seems to have a predilection for the insula, temporal cortex, and cingulate gyrus; however, focal abnormalities may be seen in other cortical regions. Unilateral and bilateral lesions can be observed on neuroimaging. In the past, HSV2 infection was more commonly thought of as a hemorrhagic encephalitis. This perception was based on postmortem studies prior to the widespread use of polymerase chain reaction analysis. As a result of the latter, it is now known that HSV encephalitis can occur without the presence of red blood cells in the CSF. In severe cases (those that resulted in the postmortem studies), red blood cells in the CSF are observed. CMV is the most frequent cause of intrauterine viral infection. Affected infants may present asymptomatic or have a petechial skin rash, intrauterine growth retardation, sensorineural hearing loss, hepatosplenomegaly, microcephaly, seizures, and retinitis. Periventricular calcifications can be observed on head CT. Although the clinical manifestations of HIV are highly variable, infants who acquire HIV vertically typically become symptomatic around 3 months of age. These children may present with

failure to thrive, lymphadenopathy, neurologic disease, hepatomegaly, or opportunistic infections. Some children will not manifest symptoms for several years. Human herpes virus 6 causes roseola in children. It has been linked to encephalitis and myelitis in young children and adults. Incidentally, acyclovir seems to be an ineffective treatment, despite the fact that this virus is a member of the herpes viride family.

10. **(A)** Although HSV can be isolated by culture from CSF, the yield is relatively low (25% to 35%). As a result of this low yield, the use of PCR to detect HSV DNA has become routine in laboratory investigation. The sensitivity and specificity of this test are greater than 90%. An MRI of the brain or head CT may reveal destruction of the insular and temporal areas, but is not specific for HSV. A head CT may be helpful in detecting intracranial calcifications seen following CMV infection, toxoplasmosis, or in utero HSV infection.

11. **(C)** Acyclovir treatment of neonatal herpes infection involving the CNS is 60 mg/kg/d in three divided doses given for 21 days, assuming normal renal function.

12. **(E)** HSV virus is acquired in utero in approximately 5% of cases. Under these circumstances, infants experience intrauterine growth retardation, cataracts, microcephaly, and vesicular rash. Intracranial calcifications are also observed.

13. **(A)** Lymphocytic choriomeningitis virus (LCMV) is acquired by inhalation of aerosolized virus or by direct contact with contaminated fomites. The natural host and reservoir is the common house mouse. The virus can be transmitted vertically if a pregnant woman acquires the virus and develops viremia. The virus can also be transmitted to the infant during delivery. Although a third of patients are asymptomatic and many develop a self-limited febrile illness, others may experience symptoms of an aseptic meningitis: fever, headache, nuchal rigidity, photophobia, and malaise. Most patients recover fully, although on rare occasions LCMV can be fatal.

14. **(A)** This patient has an aseptic meningitis due to enterovirus (non-poliovirus) infection, most likely

caused by echovirus. Other members of the enterovirus (non-poliovirus) family include group A coxsackie viruses, group B coxsackie viruses, and enteroviruses. The illness is more common in children and often the patients have a mild pharyngitis or other respiratory symptoms. A rash can commonly occur, but varies with the specific virus involved. Treatment is primarily supportive.

15. **(C)** Cysticercosis is caused by *Taenia solium*, the pork tapeworm. It is the most common parasitic infection of the CNS. Headache, seizures, meningeal signs, neuropsychiatric symptoms, visual loss, and ataxia are common symptoms seen in neurocysticercosis. *D. latum* is a fish tapeworm, which causes vitamin B_{12} deficiency. The neurologic symptoms of this parasite are caused by the vitamin deficiency. *T. multiceps* is a canine tapeworm that results in symptoms similar to cysticercosis with more pronounced ophthalmic involvement. This condition is extremely rare. *A. cantonensis* is a nematode responsible for eosinophilic meningitis. Humans are infected by eating snails or shrimp. *P. falciparum* is the parasite responsible for malaria.

16. **(E)** All of these anaerobic organisms have been isolated from brain abscesses. In addition, aerobic organisms, such as *Staphylococcus*, *Streptococcus*, *Enterobacteriaceae*, and *Haemophilus* have been isolated. Frequently, brain abscesses contain more than one organism. Fungal brain abscesses can occur, primarily in immunocompromised hosts. The causal organism depends on the underlying condition: head injury, postoperative infection, chronic otitis media, and cardiac disease.

17. **(C)**

18. **(B)**

19. **(A)** Usually supportive therapy is sufficient.

20. **(D)**

SUGGESTED READING

American Academy of Pediatrics. In: Pickering LK, Baker CJ, Overturf GD, et al (eds): *Red Book: 2003 Report of the Committee on Infectious Diseases*, 26th ed. Elk Grove Village, IL: American Academy of Pediatrics, 2003

Bonthius DJ, Karacay B: Meningitis and encephalitis in children—an update. *Neurol Clin North Am* 20:1013–1038, 2002.

Snyder RD: Bacterial infections of the nervous system. In: Swaiman KF, Ashwal S (eds): *Pediatric Neurology: Principles & Practice*, 3rd ed. St. Louis: Mosby, 1999, p 981.

Bale JF: Viral infections of the nervous system. In: Swaiman KF, Ashwal S (eds): *Pediatric Neurology: Principles & Practice*, 3rd ed. St. Louis: Mosby, 1999, p 1001.

Meloff KL, Ashwal S: Fungal, rickettsial, and parasitic diseases of the nervous system. In: Swaiman KF, Ashwal S (eds): *Pediatric Neurology: Principles & Practice*, 3rd ed. St. Louis: Mosby, 1999, p 1025.

Volpe JJ: Viral, protozoan, and related intracranial infections. In: Volpe JJ (ed): *Neurology of the Newborn*, 4th ed. Philadelphia: WB Saunders, 2001, p 717.

Whitley RJ, Kimberlin DW: Viral encephalitis. *Pediatr Rev* 20:192–198, 1999.

Cochrane DD: Brain abscess. *Pediatr Rev* 20:209–215, 1999.

CASE 132: A 17-YEAR-OLD FEMALE WITH MUSCLE WEAKNESS

A 17-year-old athletic, right-handed female comes into your clinic with the chief complaint of lower extremity muscle weakness. She states that she first noted the weakness 1 month ago, while playing soccer. At that time, she noted that she was unable to keep up with her teammates. She states that she feels fine for the first 10 to 15 minutes, but after that seems to fatigue. In addition, during routine practices, she falls approximately 10 to 12 times per session. She states that although she can walk well, she has difficulty climbing stairs. She has to rest after two flights and cannot climb without holding onto the railing. In addition to soccer, the patient runs competitively, stating she used to be able to run 400 meters in 65 seconds. She can no longer compete. These symptoms were not present prior to a month ago. She denies any history of muscle pain, myoglobinuria, or previous infectious illness. She denies any history of rash or joint swelling.

On review of her past medical history, she was born at full term without complications. She has a history of bifrontal headaches associated with photophobia and phonophobia. A head CT was reportedly normal. On review of symptoms she has experienced occasional diplopia. She states that her vision is worse in the evening and better in the morning. There is no family history of rheumatological or neuromuscular disorders. She has a maternal aunt with "thyroid problems." On physical exam, she is alert and in no apparent distress. Her general examination is unremarkable. Her cranial nerves are intact. However, on prolonged upward gaze, she developed moderate bilateral ptosis after 20 seconds. When asked to abduct her left arm repetitively, she developed left deltoid weakness after 45 attempts. Her strength returned to normal following a 4-minute rest period. The remainder of her neurological examination was normal.

SELECT THE ONE BEST ANSWER

1. The action least likely to support your diagnosis is which of the following?

   (A) single fiber electromyography
   (B) monospot test
   (C) nerve conduction velocities with repetitive stimulation
   (D) edrophonium test
   (E) antibody testing

2. Nerve conduction studies with repetitive stimulation will most likely demonstrate which of the following in this patient?

   (A) jitter
   (B) incremental response of the compound motor action potential
   (C) decremental response of the compound motor action potential
   (D) conduction block
   (E) normal response

3. You send blood for a creatine kinase (CK) level and antibodies to the acetylcholine receptor. The CK comes back at 89 (45 to 230) U/L. The acetylcholine binding, blocking, and modulating antibody titers are 69 (0 to 0.4) mmol/L, 55% (0 to 15), and 46% (0 to 20), respectively. The most likely diagnosis is which of the following?

   (A) botulism
   (B) congenital myasthenia
   (C) Lambert-Eaton myasthenic syndrome
   (D) juvenile myasthenia gravis
   (E) neonatal myasthenia gravis

4. An important study to obtain in the management of this patient is which of the following?

   (A) muscle biopsy
   (B) pulmonary function tests
   (C) chest CT
   (D) oropharyngeal motility testing
   (E) thyroid function tests

5. Treatment of this patient's condition includes which of the following?

   (A) pyridostigmine
   (B) corticosteroids
   (C) azathioprine
   (D) plasmapheresis
   (E) all of the above

6. A patient with myasthenia presents to the emergency department with the chief complaint of dysphagia. The patient is given a dose of pyridostigmine. Shortly after, the patient complains of nausea and abdominal cramps. The patient has a hard time handling her secretions. The patient soon develops respiratory distress. The most likely cause of this patient's exacerbation is which of the following?

   (A) myasthenic crisis
   (B) cholinergic crisis
   (C) pneumonia
   (D) Guillain-Barré syndrome
   (E) none of the above

7. In counseling this patient, you warn her that certain common medications may make her condition worse. From the following list of medications, which will potentially exacerbate her condition?

   (A) erythromycin
   (B) penicillin
   (C) lidocaine
   (D) phenytoin
   (E) all of the above

8. A 4-year-old boy comes to your clinic with the chief complaint of muscle weakness. During the examination, you notice a waddling gait and hypertrophic calves. He has a high serum CK enzyme level. A muscle biopsy reveals the findings shown below (Figure 132-1). The most likely diagnosis would be which of the following?

   (A) Duchenne muscular dystrophy
   (B) limb-girdle muscular dystrophy
   (C) scapuloperoneal muscular dystrophy

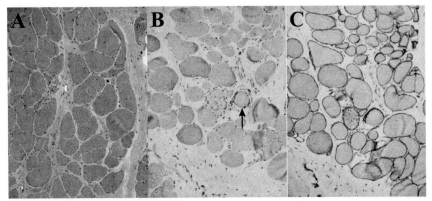

Figure 132-1. ***Muscle biopsy obtained from the 4-year-old patient described in question 8. (A) Muscle stained with hematoxylin and eosin. (B) Immunohistochemical staining for the C-terminus of dystrophin. The arrow indicates a "revertant fiber." (C) Immunohistochemical staining of the same region of muscle for merosin. See color plates. (Photographs courtesy of Dr. Manuel Utset, The University of Chicago.)***

(D) congenital muscular dystrophy
(E) myotonic dystrophy

9. Which of the following statements is true regarding the genetics of Duchenne muscular dystrophy?

(A) It is transmitted as an autosomal recessive trait.
(B) It is transmitted as an autosomal dominant trait with variable penetrance.
(C) The disorder demonstrates an X-linked mode of inheritance.
(D) The disorder is the result of triplet repeat expansion.
(E) Multiple modes of inheritance are possible.

10. Which of the following statements is true regarding the genetics of Becker muscular dystrophy?

(A) It is transmitted as an autosomal recessive trait.
(B) It is transmitted as an autosomal dominant trait.
(C) The disorder demonstrates an X-linked mode of inheritance.
(D) The disorder is the result of triplet repeat expansion.
(E) The disorder is a result of mutations of mitochondrial DNA.

11. Which of the following statements is true regarding the genetics of myotonic dystrophy?

(A) It is transmitted as an autosomal recessive trait.

(B) Little is known regarding the molecular genetics of this disorder.
(C) The disorder demonstrates an X-linked mode of inheritance.
(D) The disorder is the result of triplet repeat expansion.
(E) The disorder is a result of mutations of mitochondrial DNA.

12. Gowers' sign indicates which of the following?

(A) proximal muscle weakness
(B) distal muscle weakness
(C) hypotonia
(D) high riding scapulae and facial weakness
(E) none of the above

13. Children with congenital muscular dystrophy are deficient in which of the following proteins?

(A) dystrophin
(B) α-sarcoglycan
(C) F-actin
(D) dysferlin
(E) merosin

14. You are called to the intensive care nursery to evaluate a 4-day-old male infant who is reportedly "floppy." The infant was born at full term with Apgars of 5 and 7. Shortly after birth, he developed respiratory distress requiring mechanical ventilation. A prenatal ultrasound revealed polyhydramnios. On review of his family history, you learn that a previous child died at 36 hours of

life. His maternal aunt also had a male child who died shortly after birth. On physical examination, the cranial nerves are intact with the exception of slight ptosis and a weak gag. There are no tongue fasciculations. The infant has decreased tone and absent deep tendon reflexes. There is no arthrogryposis (nonprogressive contracture of the joints). This infant most likely has which of the following disorders?

(A) nemaline myopathy
(B) central core disease
(C) spinal muscular atrophy type I
(D) centronuclear (myotubular) myopathy
(E) congenital muscular dystrophy

15. Tongue fasciculations are most commonly seen with which of the following disorders?

(A) spinal muscular atrophy
(B) Duchenne muscular dystrophy
(C) nemaline myopathy
(D) centronuclear myopathy
(E) none of the above

MATCH EACH OF THE FOLLOWING DISEASES WITH ITS CORRESPONDING DEFECT OR DEFICIENCY

16. Myoclonus epilepsy with ragged-red fibers (MERRF)

17. Pompe's disease

18. McArdle's disease

(A) myophosphorylase
(B) acid maltase
(C) tRNA Lys gene
(D) phosphorylase B kinase
(E) lactate dehydrogenase

Answers

1. **(B)** In many cases the clinician can make the diagnosis of myasthenia gravis based on the history and physical examination. Single-fiber electromyography (EMG), nerve conduction studies with repetitive stimulation, antibody testing, and an edrophonium (Tensilon) test can confirm the diagnosis. In nerve conduction studies with re-

petitive stimulation, a motor nerve (such as the ulnar nerve) is given repetitive stimuli at 3 Hz. Documentation of a decremental response of the compound muscle action potential (CMAP) suggests a defect in neuromuscular junction transmission, as occurs in myasthenia gravis. Single-fiber EMG is a more sensitive measure of neuromuscular transmission. Edrophonium testing involves the administration of intravenous drug to patients with suspected myasthenia gravis. The drug is a cholinesterase inhibitor. A positive test consists of clinical improvement following administration of the drug, such as resolution of dysarthria or improved ocular motility. The most specific test for myasthenia gravis is the detection of acetylcholine receptor antibodies in the patient's serum. However, it should be remembered that antibodies are not detected in all patients with myasthenia gravis. In fact, children with myasthenia gravis often do not have serum antibodies.

2. **(C)** Nerve conduction studies help to evaluate a motor nerve's response to a brief stimulus. Distal latency, conduction velocity, and amplitude can be measured. Surface electrodes are used to measure CMAP, which represent the sum of action potentials generated by a single muscle fiber. Decrement of the CMAP to repetitive stimulation is observed in myasthenia gravis. In Lambert-Eaton syndrome (LES), an incremental response of CMAP amplitude is observed following repetitive stimulation. Weakness associated with LES is worse in the morning and improves throughout the day. The syndrome is characterized by the presence of antibodies to voltage-gated calcium channels. "Jitter" is seen with single-fiber EMG and reflects variation in the amount of time in which muscle fibers of the same motor unit fire.

3. **(D)** Nearly a quarter of patients with myasthenia gravis will develop the disease during childhood and adolescence. The condition is characterized by muscles weakness and, importantly, fatigability. Muscles of the eye, oropharynx, and extremities can be involved. In addition, respiration can be affected. Exertion and stress can bring on the symptoms. There are different categories of myasthenia gravis. This patient presents with juvenile myasthenia gravis in which onset is usually

after the age of 10 years. It is more common in girls. Typically, most patients present with ocular findings, such as ptosis. However, extremity weakness can be the initial presenting sign and usually principally involves the proximal muscle groups. Neonatal myasthenia gravis is a transient condition resulting from the placental transfer of acetylcholine receptor antibodies to the fetus. Congenital myasthenic syndromes are a collection of rare diseases that are not autoimmune related. In these patients, antibodies are not found and immunosuppressive therapy is ineffective. Most patients develop symptoms in the first couple of years. Symptoms include limb weakness, ocular findings, respiratory dysfunction, and feeding difficulties. Botulism can result in dysarthria, dysphagia, ptosis, and blurred vision. In infantile botulism, hypotonia is commonly observed. This condition is caused by a toxin produced by *Clostridium botulinum*, which acts on presynaptic nerve terminals to block calcium-dependent acetylcholine release. LES is briefly discussed above.

4. **(C)** Although some debate exists, it is generally accepted that most pubertal patients with juvenile myasthenia gravis will benefit from a thymectomy with or without thymoma. The presence of a thymoma is an absolute indication for thymectomy in patients with juvenile myasthenia gravis. As a result, it is imperative that all newly diagnosed patients with myasthenia gravis undergo a chest CT to evaluate for thymoma.

5. **(E)** The main treatment of myasthenia gravis is the use of acetylcholinesterase inhibitors, such as pyridostigmine. Side effects include diarrhea, nausea, and gastrointestinal cramping. In addition, an immunosuppressive agent is usually employed, such as a corticosteroid. Azathioprine, cyclosporine, and cyclophosphamide have also been used. Azathioprine has been used when patients relapse on corticosteroids or as a steroid-sparing agent. Other forms of therapy that have been tried include plasmapheresis and the administration of intravenous immunoglobulin. Thymectomy has been considered above.

6. **(B)** This patient has developed cholinergic crisis, respiratory failure secondary to an overdose of acetylcholinesterase inhibitors. Overstimulation of the muscarinic and nicotinic cholinergic receptors results in nausea, abdominal cramps, excessive secretions, and bronchospasm. Myasthenic crisis refers to respiratory failure that results from the patient's disease. Treatment of the patient with cholinergic crisis involves intubation and mechanical ventilation. The patient is admitted to the intensive care unit and acetylcholinesterase inhibitors are discontinued.

7. **(E)** Patients with myasthenia gravis can exhibit worsening of their disease should they take medications that interfere with neuromuscular transmission. Antibiotics, such as sulfonamides, clindamycin, fluoroquinolones, and tetracycline can also exacerbate myasthenia gravis with aminoglycosides being the most commonly implicated antimicrobial agent.

8. **(A)** Figure 132-1A demonstrates abnormal muscle characterized by the presence of central nuclei, endomysial fibrosis, degenerating/regenerating fibers, and a split fiber. Figure 132-1B demonstrates the lack of dystrophin staining with the exception of a single "revertant fiber."

   Many patients with Duchenne muscular dystrophy (DMD) will demonstrate a small percentage of dystrophin-positive "revertant fibers," which are believed to be the result of alternative splicing or secondary mutation events that restore an open reading frame. In this case, it serves as a positive control for the dystrophin staining. Figure 132-1C demonstrates normal merosin staining. A subset of children with congenital muscular dystrophy lack merosin. Boys with DMD typically present with muscle weakness of the hip girdle muscles producing a waddling gait. Later in the course, shoulder girdle muscles are affected. Smaller children may demonstrate a Gower's sign (see below) when attempting to stand up from a sitting position on the floor. Calf hypertrophy is also observed. This is best characterized as a pseudohypertrophy as the apparent increase in muscle mass is caused by normal muscle being replaced by collagen and adipose tissue. Although adipose replacement is not seen in this example, endomysial fibrosis is present (Figure 132-1). Limb girdle muscular dystrophies (LGMD) represent a heterogeneous group of muscle disorders that are inherited in an autosomal dominant (LGMD1) or autosomal recessive (LGMD2) fashion. Mutations of calpain 3, α-sarcoglycan, and dysferlin, to name a few, result in this phenotype. This condition should be considered if dystrophin mutations have been excluded. Scapuloperoneal muscular dystrophy is a dominantly inherited condition characterized by leg weakness, foot drop (peroneal and anterior tibial muscle wasting), proximal arm weakness, and scapular winging. The calf muscles are usually unaffected. Myotonic dystrophy is inherited in an autosomal dominant fashion and caused by a trinucleotide repeat expansion mutation of a protein kinase gene. Clinically, patients with myotonic dystrophy demonstrate a high degree of variability. While some patients can be asymptomatic, others can be profoundly affected by the disease. For example, neonates may have severe hypotonia, swallowing difficulties, and respiratory distress requiring ventilatory support. Classically, patients demonstrate elongated facies, myotonia, facial diplegia, ptosis, tented upper lip, and wasting of the temporalis muscles.

9. **(C)** DMD is transmitted as an X-linked recessive disorder with mutations occurring on the short arm of the chromosome (Xp21). Most males with DMD have an absence of dystrophin.

10. **(C)** Becker muscular dystrophy is transmitted as an X-linked recessive disorder with mutations occurring on the short arm of the chromosome (Xp21). In contrast to DMD, dystrophin is present in reduced amounts.

11. **(D)** Myotonic dystrophy is inherited as an autosomal dominant trait (chromosome 19). Expansion of the triplet repeat (CTG) results in decreased expression of a protein kinase gene. This disorder demonstrates the phenomenon of anticipation; the severity of the disease progresses in subsequent generations.

12. **(A)** Gower's sign occurs when a child uses all four limbs to push himself up off the floor from a sitting position. The child then braces his hands on his knees and thighs to push himself into an upright position. The maneuver is necessary as patients with DMD exhibit hip muscle weakness, primarily of the gluteus maximus.

13. **(E)** Congenital muscular dystrophies (CMD) refer to a group of disorders characterized by proximal muscle weakness and hypotonia presenting in early infancy. The diseases can occur with or without major brain malformations. A portion of children with CMD are deficient in merosin (α_2 chain of laminin). Patients with dysferlin and sarcoglycan mutations have limb girdle muscular dystrophies types 2B and 2D, respectively.

14. **(D)** This child has one of the congenital myopathies, which represent a diverse group of skeletal muscle disorders. The group of disorders is represented in this question by central core disease, nemaline myopathy, and centronuclear myopathy. Most patients with congenital myopathy have a benign clinical course with some cases occurring in late childhood or adulthood. The congenital myopathies are differentiated from one another based on characteristic pathological findings of the skeletal muscle, predominantly affecting type 1 myofibers. The congenital myopathies often come to mind in a floppy child without reflexes. The myopathies can have overlapping clinical features with each other, as well as with CMD. As a result, in the absence of a muscle biopsy, it may be difficult to distinguish one from the other. The clinical history presented in this case suggests X-linked recessive transmission. Of the choices listed, only centronuclear (myotubular) myopathy demonstrates X-linked recessive transmission. In fact, the X-linked or neonatal form of centronuclear myopathy is particularly severe. Neonatal onset is associated with a rapidly progressive course in which infants often develop respiratory complications leading to death. Other forms of centronuclear myopathy exist with onset occurring in late infancy and childhood (autosomal recessive transmission) or adulthood (autosomal dominant transmission). The name, myotubular myopathy, is generally used for the severe X-linked form of the disease. As its name implies, centronuclear myopathy is characterized by the presence of centrally located nuclei in small type 1 myofibers on histology. The first congenital myopathy described was central core disease due to

palely stained cores within type 1 myofibers on histology. The disease is inherited as an autosomal dominant trait. Nemaline myopathy was the second congenital myopathy to be defined based on its distinctive morphologic feature of myogranules or "rods," located beneath the sarcolemma, stained reddish/purple on trichrome staining. However, nemaline rods are not entirely specific to nemaline myopathy. Autosomal dominant and recessive inheritance has been observed for this disorder. Spinal muscular atrophy type 1 (Werdnig-Hoffmann disease) is an autosomal recessive disorder characterized by the loss of lower motor neurons in the anterior horn of the spinal cord. It is the most severe of the three types, resulting in death by 2 years of age from respiratory failure or infection. Infants demonstrate severe weakness of the intercostal muscles and limbs, tongue fasciculations, and polyminimyoclonus (a fine tremor) of the hands. Deep tendon reflexes are usually absent.

15. **(C)** Fasciculation of the tongue, as well as atrophy, occurs with injury to the ipsilateral hypoglossal nucleus or hypoglossal nerve (cranial nerve XII). Fasciculations are commonly seen in spinal muscular atrophy type 1.

16. **(C)** Many cases of MERRF are caused by mutations to the tRNA Lys gene of mitochondrial DNA. However, there does appear to be genetic heterogeneity, as not all patients with MERRF have this mutation. Any patient with seizures, myoclonus, and a myopathy should raise the suspicion of a mitochondrial disorder such as MERRF.

17. **(B)** As muscle is a highly energy-dependent tissue, any disruption of energy metabolism can result in a myopathy. Pompe's disease (type II glycogenosis), a disorder of glycogen metabolism, is caused by an acid maltase deficiency and refers to the more severe generalized disease of infancy. A more benign form, with onset in childhood or adulthood, also exists. Patients with Pompe's disease present with weakness, hypotonia, macroglossia, hepatomegaly, and cardiomegaly.

18. **(A)** McArdle's disease (type V glycogenosis), a cause of recurrent myoglobinuria, is caused by a

myophosphorylase deficiency. Patients experience myoglobinuria following exercise. Resting serum creatine kinase levels are increased.

SUGGESTED READING

Wolfe GI, Barohn RJ: Neuromuscular junction disorders in childhood. In: Swaiman KF, Ashwal S (eds): *Pediatric Neurology: Principles & Practice*, 3rd ed. St. Louis: Mosby, 1999, p 1216.

Smith SA, Swaiman KF: Muscular dystrophies. In: Swaiman KF, Ashwal S (eds): *Pediatric Neurology: Principles & Practice*, 3rd ed. St. Louis: Mosby, 1999, p 1235.

Riggs JE, Bodensteiner JB, Schochet Jr SS: Congenital myopathies/dystrophies. *Neurol Clin North Am* 21: 779–794, 2003.

Mathews KD: Muscular dystrophy overview: genetics and diagnosis. *Neurol Clin North Am* 21:795–816, 2003.

CASE 133: A 7-YEAR-OLD MALE WITH HEAD JERKS

A 7-year-old boy with attention deficit disorder comes to your clinic for a routine follow-up examination. During the examination, you notice occasional eye blinking and right-sided head jerks. His mother states that she has noticed these movements for approximately 6 months. A year ago, the patient would repetitively open his mouth wide open, as if to "stretch his jaw." The movements seem to come and go, but never disappear for more than 2 months. The movements are infrequent and she always assumed they were behavioral or "part of his allergies." The child states that the movements are involuntary. On questioning his mother further about the allergies, you learn that he has periods of sniffing and throat clearing. Her previous pediatrician stated these were symptoms of seasonal allergies. The movements never occur during sleep and are exacerbated by stress. The patient states that if he tries hard enough, he can suppress the behaviors for brief periods of time. There is no history of seizure-like activity. There is a family history of psychiatric illness on both sides of the family. On review of his past medical history, you note that he has not had any history of strep throat infections. His physical examination is normal.

SELECT THE ONE BEST ANSWER

1. In further evaluating this child it is important to ask which of the following questions?

(A) "What medications does you child currently take?"

(B) "Does your child suffer from any sleep disorders?"

(C) "Are the movements bothersome to the child or do his friends comment on the movements?"

(D) "Does your child suffer from any psychiatric conditions, such as obsessive-compulsive disorder, depression, or anxiety?"

(E) All of the above

2. His mother states that he is currently taking an antihistamine for his allergies and denies any history of psychiatric illness. The most likely diagnosis of this child's medical problem is which of the following?

(A) seizure disorder
(B) Wilson's disease
(C) Tourette's syndrome
(D) allergic rhinitis
(E) anxiety disorder

3. His mother states that she was given a prescription for methylphenidate to treat his attention deficit-hyperactivity disorder (ADHD), but that he hasn't started taking it yet. In counseling the mother regarding the use of this medication, which of the following statements is appropriate?

(A) "Methylphenidate is best given before the patient goes to bed."

(B) "Methylphenidate will also help control the motor movements."

(C) "There is a chance that the methylphenidate will exacerbate the movements and, as a result, she should consider a medication that treats both the tics and ADHD, such as clonidine."

(D) "An EEG should be obtained prior to starting the medication."

(E) None of the above

4. The *Diagnostic and Statistical Manual of Mental Disorders, 4th edition*, diagnostic criteria for Tourette syndrome include all of the following except?

(A) Onset must have occurred before the age of 18 years.

(B) The patient demonstrates multiple motor tics.

(C) The duration of symptoms must be longer than 6 months.

(D) Vocal tics must be present.

(E) The disorder is not the result of a medical condition.

5. Which of the following neuropsychological problems are associated with Tourette's syndrome?

(A) obsessive-compulsive disorder
(B) attention deficit-hyperactivity disorder
(C) depression
(D) behavioral problems
(E) all of the above

6. On further questioning, you learn that the patient frequently washes his hands, as he believes they are contaminated with harmful germs. He frequently checks to make sure that the windows are locked to the point that he cannot leave the house until he has checked each window. The most appropriate treatment for this disorder is which of the following medications?

(A) clonazepam
(B) dextroamphetamine
(C) risperidone
(D) desipramine
(E) fluoxetine

7. Which of the following statements is false regarding Tourette's syndrome?

(A) Females are more commonly affected than males.

(B) The mean age of onset is between 6 and 7 years of age.

(C) An MRI of the brain is most often normal in these patients.

(D) Treatment of tics should be reserved for those patients who have failed nonpharmacological treatments and in whom the movements are disturbing or functionally disabling.

(E) In terms of prognosis, tics will remain stable or increase in approximately a quarter of the patients, while most will show at least some improvement into adulthood.

8. All of the following have been used in the treatment of tic disorders except for which of the following medications?

(A) pimozide
(B) clonazepam
(C) haloperidol
(D) baclofen
(E) fluphenazine

9. A 12-year-old girl comes to your office with the chief complaint of writhing movements involving the hands and feet. In addition, the patient experiences random muscle jerks that prevent her from using eating utensils. She was referred to a child psychiatrist as she has had periods of inappropriate laughter mixed with periods of extreme sadness. Her past medical history is significant for a severe pharyngitis she experienced approximately 3 months ago. There is no family history of Huntington's disease. On general examination, the patient is a thin female who has a hard time sitting still. Her vital signs are within normal limits. She has a new cardiac murmur, which you confirmed with her previous pediatrician. You note the movements described above, but her neurological examination is otherwise within normal limits. This patient most likely has which of the following diagnoses?

(A) restless legs syndrome
(B) Sydenham's chorea
(C) rheumatic heart disease
(D) Wilson's disease
(E) both B and C

10. The next most important action/study in the evaluation of the patient from question 9 is which of the following?

(A) an electroencephalogram
(B) MRI of the brain with and without contrast
(C) referral to a pediatric cardiologist for an echocardiogram and ECG
(D) enteroviral titers
(E) ceruloplasmin

11. Opsoclonus myoclonus is associated with which of the following disorders?

(A) Wilm's tumor
(B) neuroblastoma
(C) epilepsy
(D) benign myoclonus of early infancy
(E) Pelizaeus-Merzbacher disease

12. You are asked to see an 8-year-old girl who recently developed torticollis and dystonic posturing of her upper limb 30 minutes after an oral dose of medication. The medication most likely to cause these symptoms is which of the following?

(A) baclofen
(B) acetaminophen
(C) diphendydramine
(D) prochlorperazine
(E) phenobarbital

13. An almost 18-year-old female presents to your clinic for evaluation of bilateral hand tremor. On physical examination you notice a coarse, resting tremor that increases with volitional movement. You also note subtle side-to-side head movements. The tremors never occur during sleep. On obtaining a substance abuse history, the patient reluctantly admits to occasional alcohol use. Interestingly, she states that her tremors are better following an alcoholic beverage. Her father, a recovering alcoholic, developed similar symptoms when he was in his early 20s. This patient most likely has which of the following conditions?

(A) juvenile Parkinson's disease
(B) delirium tremens
(C) physiologic tremor
(D) essential familial tremor
(E) drug-induced Parkinson's disease

14. For the patient above (question 13), which of the following treatments would be the most beneficial?

(A) abstinence
(B) propranolol
(C) valproic acid
(D) carbidopa/levodopa
(E) diazepam

15. Brown, copper deposits occurring on the iris (Kaiser-Fleischer rings) are seen in which of the following disorders?

(A) tuberous sclerosis
(B) neurofibromatosis, type 1
(C) Wilson's disease
(D) Tay-Sachs disease
(E) Sturge-Weber syndrome

MATCH EACH OF THE FOLLOWING MOVEMENTS WITH ITS DEFINITION

16. Tremor

17. Dystonia

18. Myoclonus

19. Chorea

20. Ballismus

(A) violent, flinging movements typically involving the shoulder

(B) very rapid, involuntary, repetitive contractions of a muscle or group of muscles

(C) continuous, rhythmic, oscillatory movement of a body part occurring at rest or with movement

(D) sustained simultaneous contraction of agonist and antagonist muscles

(E) smooth, "dance-like" movements of the extremities involving several body parts

Answers

1. **(E)** This child most likely has a tic disorder, which range in severity from a transient tic disorder to Tourette's syndrome. In the evaluation of tic disorders, the physician must determine if the disorder is primary (Tourette's syndrome) or secondary (Tourette-like disorder). Certain medications, such as stimulants, used in the treatment of ADHD, have been shown to "unmask" tics in patients who may subsequently develop Tourette's syndrome. Neuropsychological problems are often seen in patients with Tourette's syndrome and include obsessive-compulsive behaviors, anxiety, depression, aggressive behaviors, ADHD, and sleep disturbances. In terms of deciding on a treatment course, it is important to know if the movements are functionally disabling to the child or psychologically bothersome.

2. **(C)** This child most likely has Tourette's syndrome given the presence of multiple motor tics, at least one vocal tic, and symptoms occurring for longer than 1 year with an age of onset before the age of 18 years. In addition, the child has not been symptom free for longer than 3 months, which is a *DSM-IV* criteria. The differential diagnosis of tic disorders includes seizure disorders, Wilson's disease, juvenile Huntington's disease, and PANDAS (*p*ediatric *a*utoimmune *n*europsychiatric *d*isorders *a*ssociated with *s*treptococcal infection). Many of these disorders can be excluded with an accurate history and physical examination. Ultimately, as there is no specific diagnostic test for Tourette's syndrome, the diagnosis is made clinically.

3. **(C)** Methylphenidate is a stimulant used in the treatment of ADHD. The use of stimulants in patients with ADHD and tic disorders is controversial, as some of the medications used in the treatment of ADHD, such as methylphenidate, can exacerbate the movements. Clonidine has been used to treat both ADHD, as well as, tic disorder and may be tried in this setting. As methylphenidate is a stimulant, when used, it is best given in the morning, as patients who take it later in the day or evening may have difficulty falling asleep. Motor and vocal tics are not associated with electrographic changes on EEG, hence, the study would not add anything to the decision-making process.

4. **(C)** The *DSM-IV* diagnostic criteria for Tourette's disorder require that the patient experience symptoms for at least 1 year. The course is gradual in which certain types of tics may come and go. At least one vocal tic must be present. In order to be considered Tourette's disorder, the patient cannot have more than 3 consecutive months without symptoms. The disorder cannot be a side effect of drugs or caused by a medical condition.

5. **(E)** Children with Tourette's syndrome can have a number of neuropsychological problems including obsessive-compulsive disorder (OCD), ADHD, depression and behavioral problems. Obsessions include intrusive, unwelcome thoughts or ideas. The obsessions (for example, feeling that one's hands are covered with bacteria) may result in a compulsion, a purposeful repetitive behavior designed to relieve the obsession (for example, hand washing). The incidence of OCD in patients with Tourette's syndrome ranges from approxi-

mately 30% to 60% depending on the study. ADHD is comorbid in approximately 50% of patients with Tourette's syndrome. ADHD may precede the diagnosis of tics by a few years. Although children with Tourette's syndrome can have significant difficulties in school, the presence of comorbid ADHD is probably the most important contributing factor. Psychosocial factors, behavioral problems, and depression are also important contributing factors to poor school performance.

6. **(E)** This patient most likely has an OCD in addition to Tourette's syndrome. OCD can be treated with selective serotonin reuptake inhibitors (SSRIs), such as fluoxetine, or a serotonin/norepinephrine reuptake inhibitor, such as clomipramine.

7. **(A)** Tourette's syndrome (TS) is more common in males than females with a mean age of onset of 6 to 7 years. As there is no diagnostic test specific for TS, neuroimaging, as well as routine blood work, is typically normal. Over the course of the illness, most tics will change in quality and even severity. The tics are exacerbated by stress, fear, fatigue, and excitement. Treatment is generally reserved for those patients in whom the tics become troublesome, either by causing impairment of function or by harming the child on a psychosocial level. In this circumstance, the child has also failed nonpharmacological modes of treatment.

8. **(D)** Pimozide, clonazepam, haloperidol, and fluphenazine have all been used in the treatment of tic disorders. Baclofen has been used in the treatment of chorea and spasticity.

9. **(E)** This patient is experiencing chorea and emotional lability, two of three classical characteristics of Sydenham's chorea, a condition that occurs after a group A streptococcal infection of the tonsils and pharynx. The third classical characteristic is hypotonia. In addition to the symptoms above, the patient now has a new cardiac murmur suggestive of a rheumatic myocarditis. Rheumatic myocarditis is almost always associated with a heart murmur due to valvulitis. The hallmark heart murmur of rheumatic myocarditis is that of mitral regurgitation. As a result of the chorea and carditis, the patient meets crite-

ria for a diagnosis of rheumatic fever given that she has two major manifestations of the Jones criteria. The other three major manifestations are polyarthritis, erythema marginatum, and subcutaneous nodules. There are also minor manifestations such as fever, arthralgia, elevated acute phase reactants (erythrocyte sedimentation rate and C-reactive protein), and prolonged PR interval. Rheumatic heart disease is seen in approximately one-third of patients with Sydenham's chorea. Several medications have been tried to control the choreiform movements, including diazepam, phenothiazines, valproic acid, and butyrophenones.

10. **(C)** The severity of rheumatic myocarditis can vary from mild cases to cardiac failure resulting in death. Under the circumstances this patient should be referred to a pediatric cardiologist, who based on his/her physical examination, may obtain an echocardiogram to confirm the type of murmur heard on auscultation. In addition, the cardiologist may order an electrocardiograph as a baseline study or to assess the PR interval. An EEG and MRI of the brain would most likely be normal in patients with Sydenham's chorea. Enteroviruses cause protean manifestations in children but not illness similar to this girl's. Serum concentrations of ceruloplasmin are decreased in Wilson's disease.

11. **(B)** Opsoclonus myoclonus ("dancing eyes") is a paraneoplastic or postinfectious movement disorder characterized by ataxia, myoclonus, and oscillopsia, which is multidirectional, chaotic eye movements. The syndrome typically presents in infancy or early childhood (6 to 36 months of age). When observed, the clinician should begin an investigation for a neural crest tumor, most commonly neuroblastoma, as 50% of patients with opsoclonus myoclonus will have such a tumor. The pathogenesis of this syndrome is poorly understood, but is most likely immune mediated. This is supported by the observation that treatment with steroids and other immunotherapies, such as intravenous immunoglobulin (IVIG) and azathioprine, are of some benefit.

12. **(D)** A number of prescription medications can result in neurological morbidity, including acute

dystonia, parkinsonism, tardive dyskinesia, acute akathisia, and neuroleptic malignant syndrome. Some of the more common medications that can cause an acute dystonia include phenothiazines, butyrophenones, levothyroxine, and some antiepileptics (carbamazepine and phenytoin). Prochlorperazine is a phenothiazine used commonly as an antiemetic. Patients can develop an acute dystonia following a single dose of a neuroleptic. The acute dystonic reactions are usually self-limited and can be quite diverse in presentation. Some patients may present with oculogyric crisis, torticollis, or opisthotonic posturing. Anticholinergic agents, such as diphenhydramine or benztropine, can provide immediate relief in most patients.

13. (D) Essential familial tremor is a common form of tremor. It is inherited as an autosomal dominant trait with a typical onset in the patient's teens. The diagnosis is usually evident by the time the patient is in his or her 20s or 30s. Patients typically manifest a coarse, resting tremor in the upper extremities that worsens with volitional movement. The tremor is not present during sleep. Head and face may also be involved, often resembling titubation (shaking or tremor of the head due to cerebellar dysfunction). Interestingly, essential tremors get better with alcohol ingestion. The clinical characteristics of Parkinson's disease include rigidity, bradykinesia, tremor, and postural instability. The tremor in Parkinson's disease is in fact a resting tremor; however, voluntary movement suppresses the tremor. Physiologic tremor occurs when the patient extends their arms forward. Certain drugs, such as valproic acid, can exacerbate a physiologic tremor.

14. (B) Provided there are no contraindications, propranolol (β-blockers) has been found to be useful in the treatment of essential familial tremor.

15. (C) Wilson's disease constitutes the clinical findings of tremor, rigidity, drooling, and Kayser-Fleischer rings in the setting of liver dysfunction. The disease is caused by an impairment of copper metabolism, which results in the deposition and accumulation of copper in various tissues, including the liver. On ingestion, copper binds to albumin and is transferred to the liver where it will be incorporated into ceruloplasmin. The concentration of this protein is decreased in patients with Wilson's disease. Kayser-Fleischer rings are pathognomonic for Wilson's disease. The rings form as a result of copper granule deposition in Descemet's membrane. The disease is transmitted in an autosomal recessive trait. The disease is treated by restricting copper from the diet and chelation therapy with D-penicillamine.

16. (C)

17. (D)

18. (B)

19. (E)

20. (A)

SUGGESTED READING

Swaiman KF: Movement disorders and disorders of the basal ganglia. In: Swaiman KF, Ashwal S (eds): *Pediatric Neurology: Principles & Practice*, 3rd ed. St. Louis: Mosby, 1999, p 801.
Pranzatelli MR: Movement disorders in childhood. *Pediatr Rev* 17:388–394, 1996.

CASE 134: A 16-YEAR-OLD GIRL WITH HEADACHES AND BLURRED VISION

A 16-year-old female presents to your clinic with the chief complaint of headaches and blurred vision. The patient was in her usual state of health until approximately 2 months ago when she started to experience headaches over the "top of her head." The headaches occur daily and are exacerbated by coughing or exercise. The headaches seem to be worse in the morning. She states that she has been treating the headaches with acetaminophen with little, if any, benefit despite taking the medication daily. Recently, she started experiencing blurred vision and vertigo. She denies any history of nausea, vomiting, or photophobia. There is no family history of migraines. Her paternal grandfather died of "brain cancer."

On physical examination, she is a well-nourished female in mild distress. Her body mass index is 28. She is afebrile and her vital signs are stable. On examination of her fundi, you note bilateral papilledema. Examination of her visual fields with bedside testing reveals bilateral enlarged blind spots. Her pupils are round, reactive, and equal to light. Extraocular eye movements are intact without pain on lateral or upward gaze. The remainder of her cranial nerve examination is normal. On motor examination, her muscle tone, bulk, and strength are normal in the upper and lower extremities bilaterally. Her deep tendon reflexes, gait, and sensory examination are normal.

SELECT THE ONE BEST ANSWER

1. The next appropriate action in the evaluation of this patient is which of the following?

   (A) neuroimaging with head CT or MRI of the brain
   (B) lumbar puncture
   (C) visual field testing
   (D) tonometry
   (E) no further action is necessary for diagnosis

2. Which of the following medical conditions or prescription drugs can cause papilledema?

   (A) tetracycline
   (B) primary CNS tumors
   (C) Guillain-Barré syndrome
   (D) lupus erythematosus
   (E) all of the above

3. This patient has papilledema of the optic nerve. What other cranial nerve abnormality is this patient at most risk for developing?

   (A) cranial nerve III
   (B) cranial nerve IV
   (C) cranial nerve VI
   (D) cranial nerve VII
   (E) none of the above

4. You were able to obtain an MRI of the brain with and without contrast that same day. The radiologist calls you to tell you that the study is completely normal. At this point, the highest yield diagnostic study is which of the following?

   (A) static Humphrey perimetry (visual field testing)
   (B) vitamin A level
   (C) cerebral angiography
   (D) lumbar puncture
   (E) erythrocyte sedimentation rate

5. Intraocular pressure as measured by tonometry was within normal limits. Assuming the patient has an elevated opening pressure on lumbar puncture (280 mm H_2O), which of the following is the most likely diagnosis of this patient's medical problem?

   (A) glaucoma
   (B) pseudotumor cerebri
   (C) migraine without aura
   (D) Arnold-Chiari type I malformation
   (E) chronic daily headache

6. In terms of counseling this patient, which of the following statements are especially important in this case?

   (A) "The patient should reduce her intake of nonsteroidal anti-inflammatory drugs to no more than 2 to 3 times per week as she is at risk for medication overuse headaches."
   (B) "A decrease in body weight of at least 15% will help reduce or alleviate her headaches."
   (C) "Certain drugs and vitamins, such as oral contraceptives and vitamin A, are risk factors for her condition."
   (D) "She should not drive."
   (E) All of the above are correct.

7. Following the spinal tap, the patient's headaches and visual symptoms dramatically improve. You decide to start the patient on a daily medication to help manage her headaches. Which of the following medications is most likely to benefit the patient?

   (A) valproic acid
   (B) propranolol
   (C) acetazolamide
   (D) ibuprofen
   (E) dihydroergotamine

8. A 10-year-old boy comes to your office for evaluation of headaches. He states he first experienced headaches at the age of 8 years. The pain is localized to the frontal regions bilaterally. He describes a pulsating quality to the headaches and cites that they are extremely severe. The headaches are associated with nausea, photophobia, and phonophobia. They are aggravated by routine physical activity. He has averaged approxi-

mately one headache per month, but states that last summer he did not experience any head pain. His physical examination is normal. A head CT was performed in the emergency department and is reportedly normal. This patient's headache is most likely due to which of the following?

(A) migraine headache with aura (classic migraine)
(B) episodic tension-type headaches
(C) migraine headache without aura (common migraine)
(D) complicated migraine
(E) basilar artery migraine

9. An 8-year-old boy complains of unilateral headache, photophobia, nausea, and vomiting. He has had symptoms on and off for approximately 15 months. On occasion, the headaches are so severe he needs to stay home from school. Prior to many of the headaches, he sees brightly colored lights for approximately 12 minutes. This patient's headache is most likely due to which of the following disorders?

(A) migraine with aura (classic migraine)
(B) complex partial seizure
(C) basilar artery migraine
(D) ophthalmoplegic migraine
(E) complicated migraine

10. An 18-year-old male presents to the emergency room with the chief complaint of headache. He has had occasional headaches before this one, but states "this is the worst headache of my life." On the way to the emergency room, the patient complained of nausea and vomited. He now complains of pain on flexing his head forward. The patient is afebrile. The next most appropriate action is which of the following?

(A) Order a head CT.
(B) Perform a lumbar puncture.
(C) Administer an opiate analgesic agent, such as morphine.
(D) Order a urine toxicology screen.
(E) Assure the patient that this is probably a migraine, which will get better.

11. The radiology resident for the patient in question 10 calls you to tell you that the head CT is probably normal. With this information, you next decide

to perform a spinal tap, which reveals a yellow fluid with occasional red blood cells. This patient most likely has which of the following diagnoses?

(A) complicated migraine
(B) herpes simplex hemorrhagic meningoencephalitis
(C) acute subdural hematoma
(D) subarachnoid hemorrhage
(E) glioblastoma multiforme

12. Which of the following drugs are used as prophylactic agents in the treatment of migraine headaches?

(A) cyproheptadine
(B) valproic acid
(C) amitriptyline
(D) propranolol
(E) all of the above

13. Hemicrania continua is especially responsive to which of the following medications?

(A) ibuprofen
(B) sumatriptan
(C) cyproheptadine
(D) indomethacin
(E) none of the above

14. Sumatriptan is an example of which of the following categories of medications used in the treatment of migraines?

(A) antidepressant
(B) β-blocker
(C) 5-HT receptor agonist
(D) antiepileptic drug
(E) nonsteroidal anti-inflammatory agent

15. Which of the following are typical triggers of migraine headaches?

(A) menstruation
(B) stress
(C) cheese
(D) fatigue
(E) all of the above

16. Which of the following primary brain tumors is the most common type encountered in children younger than 15 years of age?

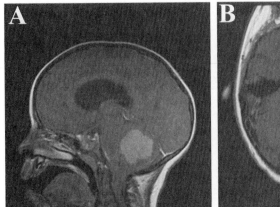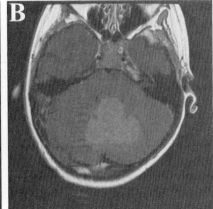

Figure 134-1. *A brain MRI of a 3-year-old boy presenting with headache, nausea, and vomiting from question 17.* *(A) Sagittal T1-weighted image following contrast administration. (B) Axial T1-weighted image. (Photographs courtesy of Dr. Daniel Curry, The University of Chicago.)*

(A) meningioma
(B) supratentorial low-grade astrocytoma
(C) medulloblastoma
(D) ependymoma
(E) cerebellar astrocytoma

17. A 3-year-old boy presents to the emergency department with a 3-month history of headache, nausea, and vomiting. The patient has progressively gotten worse and now is ataxic. Figure 134-1 demonstrates an MRI of his brain. Based on this information, this patient most likely has which of the following posterior fossa brain tumors?

(A) cerebellar astrocytoma
(B) medulloblastoma
(C) ependymoma
(D) brainstem glioma
(E) meningioma

18. On the same night you see the patient presented above, a 4-year-old boy presents to the emergency department with similar symptoms. He has a 3-month history of progressive headaches, nausea, vomiting, and ataxia. His ataxia is so severe that he no longer is able to walk. He was recently seen by his primary physician who treated him with antibiotics for an otitis media without resolution of his symptoms. His MRI of the brain is shown in Figure 134-2. This patient most likely has which of the following diagnoses?

(A) cerebellar astrocytoma
(B) medulloblastoma

(C) ependymoma
(D) brainstem glioma
(E) meningioma

19. A 2-year-old girl presents to the emergency room with inconsolable crying and vomiting. An MRI of the brain and a head CT are shown in Figure 134-3. The most likely cause of this patient's symptoms is which of the following?

(A) choroid plexus papilloma
(B) subependymal giant cell astrocytoma
(C) hydrocephalus
(D) colloid cyst
(E) A and C are correct

Answers

1. **(A)** In a patient who presents with headache and papilledema, it is important to rule out hydrocephalus or a mass lesion given the potential of developing a herniation syndrome. In fact, in this case neuroimaging is mandatory prior to performing a lumbar puncture. Although an MRI of the brain with and without contrast is the preferred study, especially if the practitioner suspects meningeal disease, a head CT with contrast can be used. In fact, the head CT may be more readily available and the only option if the patient is extremely obese (other than an open MRI). In addition, a head CT would be very helpful in evaluating an intracerebral hemorrhage. For postpartum patients or those on oral contraceptives, MRI has

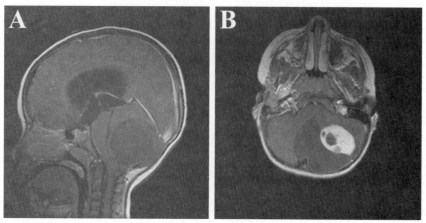

Figure 134-2. A brain MRI of a 4-year-old boy presenting with headache, nausea, and vomiting from question 18. (A) Sagittal T1-weighted image following contrast administration. (B) Axial T1-weighted image following contrast administration. (Photographs courtesy of Dr. Daniel Curry, The University of Chicago.)

the added advantage of being able to perform a magnetic resonance venogram (MRV) to rule out cerebral venous thrombosis. Once a structural lesion and hydrocephalus are ruled out, a lumbar puncture can be performed. Tonometry is used to measure intraocular pressure as in an evaluation for glaucoma. Although visual field testing is a sensitive tool in assessing optic nerve involvement, the test would be performed following a neuroimaging study done to define the cause of the papilledema.

2. **(E)** In evaluating a patient with papilledema, it is important to look for an underlying cause. Several medical conditions are associated with papilledema. These medical conditions include neurological conditions, such as CNS tumors (primary and metastatic); infectious conditions; medications and toxins, such as tetracycline, vitamin A, and lead; certain endocrine diseases; autoimmune diseases, such as lupus erythematosus; vascular diseases, and hematologic diseases.

3. **(C)** As a result of raised intracranial pressure, patients can develop unilateral or bilateral abducens nerve paresis as a false localizing sign. Frequently, these patients complain of diplopia. Examination of eye motility may unmask a cranial nerve VI palsy.

4. **(D)** The study most likely to yield the diagnosis in this patient is the lumbar puncture. In order to ac-

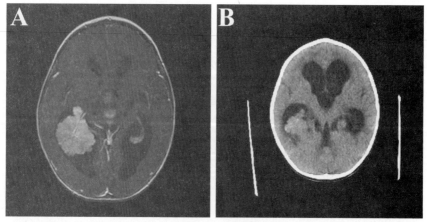

Figure 134-3. A brain MRI and head CT of a 2-year-old girl presenting with inconsolable crying and vomiting from question 19. (A) Sagittal T1-weighted image following contrast administration. (B) Head CT. (Photographs courtesy of Dr. Daniel Curry, The University of Chicago.)

curately assess visual function in patients with papilledema, perimetry, either by Goldmann field testing or by the static Humphrey method, should be performed. In the case of papilledema, an enlargement of the blind spot is typically seen. Although perimetry is the most useful test for evaluating visual function, it does not provide us with the etiology for the papilledema. Vitamin A toxicity has been associated with diplopia and pseudotumor cerebri. However, one should be able to assess for vitamin A toxicity with good history-taking skills. Erythrocyte sedimentation rate is a nonspecific test for inflammation and may be elevated in patients with autoimmune conditions. If cerebral vasculitis is clinically suspected, a cerebral angiogram should be performed to assess for narrowing of the blood vessels. If a venous sinus thrombosis is clinically suspected, then conventional cerebral angiography should be performed, especially if noninvasive methods, such as magnetic resonance angiography and computed tomography angiography, are not available.

5. **(B)** The normal range of CSF pressure is 100 to 200 mm H_2O. Hence, a pressure of 280 mm H_2O is elevated. Given the papilledema, normal MRI of the brain, and raised intracranial pressure as measured by lumbar puncture, this patient most likely has pseudotumor cerebri. Glaucoma, an elevation in intraocular pressure, can mimic the visual field deficit seen in pseudotumor cerebri, as it can cause optic nerve damage. The normal intraocular pressure measured by tonometry rules out this diagnosis. An Arnold-Chiari type I malformation refers to cerebellum and cerebellar tonsillar displacement greater than or equal to 5 mm beyond the foramen magnum line. Patients may also have syringomyelia. Clinically, patients with Arnold-Chiari type I malformation complain of recurrent headaches, primarily over the frontal and occipital regions, neck pain, difficulty swallowing, and ataxia. The headaches can be exacerbated by exertion. In patients with syringomyelia, upper limb sensory changes and weakness are sometimes also observed. Arnold-Chiari type II malformations are similar to type I, but are associated with myelomeningocele. A type III Arnold-Chiari malformation consists of the cerebellar displacement defined above and an encephalocervical meningocele. Type IV consists of hypoplasia of the cerebellum and may actually represent a variation of a Dandy-Walker malformation. The normal MRI of the brain rules out the Arnold-Chiari malformations. Finally, migraines and chronic daily headaches are not associated with abnormal physical findings, such as papilledema or elevated intracranial pressure.

6. **(E)** Pseudotumor cerebri, or idiopathic intracranial hypertension, is characterized by increased intracranial pressure without evidence of a brain tumor or mass lesion as the cause of elevated pressure. Patients typically present with headaches, papilledema, visual field defects (typically an enlarged blind spot), and occasionally diplopia. There is no gender predilection in early childhood. An important risk factor for pseudotumor cerebri is obesity. Other risk factors include various drugs, such as oral contraceptives, high levels of vitamin A, and corticosteroids, which the patient should avoid if possible. Steroid use can also play a role in weight gain. In terms of treatment, weight reduction is strongly recommended in those patients who are obese. A drop in body weight by 15% may even lead to resolution of symptoms, including elevated intracranial pressure. Given this patient's visual symptoms she should not drive until her vision has been restored. Finally, given the daily use of analgesics, this patient is at risk for developing a medication overuse headache, formerly known as rebound headaches. Patients with medication overuse headaches usually see their primary headache disorder (for example, migraines or pseudotumor cerebri) transformed into chronic daily headaches. Once medication overuse headaches develop, they can be very difficult to treat and patients may also develop a comorbid depression. Patients usually need to be detoxified for approximately 2 weeks. As the headaches may be severe, some patients may require hospitalization. Other treatment strategies have been reported.

7. **(C)** Each of the drugs listed in this question have been used in the treatment of migraines. However, acetazolamide has been shown to decrease the formation of CSF. For those patients who are allergic to sulfa drugs, furosemide may be used for similar purpose. Side effects of acetazolamide include drowsiness, numbness, renal calculi, and

anorexia. Incidentally, patients with pseudotumor cerebri and obesity should avoid valproic acid (if clinically possible), as this medication may also cause weight gain.

8. **(C)** Migraines without aura are the most common type of migraine in children and adolescents. When evaluating a patient with headaches it is important to note the temporal pattern to the headache. The examiner should ascertain whether the headache is acute versus chronic, single versus recurrent, or progressive versus nonprogressive. At times, the physician may observe a mixed pattern. This question gives an example of an acute recurrent headache. Typically, acute recurrent headaches, separated by pain-free intervals, and associated with nausea, vomiting, photophobia, or phonophobia are a result of migraines. As this patient does not have an aura prior to the headache it would be classified as migraine without aura. Patients with complicated migraine typically have a transient neurologic deficit associated with their headache. This deficit could include weakness or sensory loss. However, complicated migraine is a diagnosis of exclusion and, as a result, a structural lesion should be ruled out by neuroimaging. Basilar migraines typically present with symptoms referable to the brainstem, cerebellar, or other posterior circulation territories. These symptoms include blurred vision, vertigo, ataxia, dizziness, paresis, dysarthria, nausea, and vomiting. It is more common in adolescent females.

9. **(A)** This is an example of classic migraines or migraines with aura. The headaches are acute and recurrent with pain-free intervals. The patient can describe the aura as brightly colored lights and does not appear to lose consciousness during the episode, thus ruling out complex partial seizures. Patients with ophthalmoplegic migraines complain of severe pain located behind the eye. They also present with a complete or incomplete third cranial nerve palsy (for example, ptosis, diplopia, lateral eye deviation, and mydriasis), which may persist for several days even after the headache has subsided.

10. **(A)** When a patient without a history of severe headaches complains of the "worst headache of

his/her life" in the setting of meningismus and emesis, the clinician should consider a diagnosis of subarachnoid hemorrhage. In this case, a head CT can be performed relatively quickly to evaluate for blood. Certainly, a neuroimaging study would be performed prior to lumbar puncture. Intracranial hemorrhage, stroke, and seizures have been reported following cocaine use. As a result, a urine toxicology screen may be an appropriate study in the evaluation of this patient. In terms of the next appropriate action, a neuroimaging study would enable the physician to not only confirm the diagnosis, but also assist in further managing the patient should he or she need a neurosurgical consultation or neuro-intensive care.

11. **(D)** Subarachnoid hemorrhages may be difficult to appreciate on head CT. A more definitive test may be the lumbar puncture. In patients with subarachnoid hemorrhage, the CSF may contain red blood cells that do not clear in subsequent samples. In addition, xanthochromia may be seen as early as 4 hours after the bleed. Subarachnoid hemorrhages can be seen following head trauma, meningitis, birth trauma, and coagulopathies. However, the most likely etiology is vascular malformations, although exceedingly rare in very young children. Patients with complicated migraine should not have red blood cells or xanthochromia on lumbar puncture. Subdural hematoma, hemorrhagic herpes meningoencephalitis, and glioblastoma multiforme are typically observed with head CT.

12. **(E)** Treatment of migraines involves both pharmacologic and nonpharmacologic methods. The patient first needs to be assured that he/she does not have a serious or life-threatening condition. The clinician should always start with nonpharmacologic methods in the treatment of migraines. This includes recognition and elimination of triggering factors, such as relaxation methods to reduce stress, adequate sleep, and a regular diet. In terms of pharmacologic therapy, prophylactic agents can be used should nonpharmacologic methods fail and the patient continue to experience frequent headaches. Typically, this type of patient has severe headaches and misses several days of school. Some commonly used

prophylactic drugs include amitriptyline, valproic acid, propranolol, and cyproheptadine.

13. **(D)** Hemicrania continua is an example of an indomethacin-responsive headache. This headache consists of severe, steady pain localized to one side of the head. The patients are usually female without a family history of such headaches.

14. **(C)** This question highlights several of the classes of medications used in the prophylactic treatment of migraine headaches. Sumatriptan is an example of a 5-HT receptor agonist.

15. **(E)** Menstruation, certain foods, fatigue, and stress are common triggers of migraines. Other triggers include oral contraceptive pills, anxiety, physical exertion, alcohol, sleep deprivation, and weather changes.

16. **(B)** The three most common primary brain tumors in children are, in order of decreasing frequency, supratentorial low-grade astrocytoma, medulloblastoma, and cerebellar astrocytoma.

17. **(B)** Medulloblastomas are posterior fossa tumors typically occurring in the midline. They tend to be well-demarcated tumors. Cyst formation, hemorrhage, and calcifications are rare in comparison to cerebellar astrocytomas. Some studies have suggested that the presence of the *c*-myc oncogene is associated with a poorer prognosis. Brainstem gliomas tend to occupy the region of the brainstem near the fourth ventricle and aqueduct of Sylvius. Often, thickening of the pons is observed. Ependymomas can occur anywhere along the ventricular system. Most of the tumors (two-thirds) are infratentorial. Ependymomas are well-defined and can be very cystic. Meningiomas are relatively uncommon tumors in children. When they are observed in children, they tend to occur in the posterior fossa or in the ventricular system, often causing obstructive hydrocephalus. This question highlights the importance of recognizing chronic progressive headaches, which usually imply some pathologic process, such as brain tumor, pseudotumor cerebri, subdural hematoma, or hydrocephalus, to name a few. In general, migraine headaches are rare in patients younger than the age of 5 years.

18. **(A)** In contrast to medulloblastomas, cerebellar astrocytomas can occur anywhere in the cerebellum. The majority of these tumors are cystic, as shown in this example. In some cases, a solid mural nodule is associated with a large cyst. Calcifications are seen in a quarter of the patients. Cerebellar astrocytomas can be separated into two groups: diffuse astrocytoma and juvenile cerebellar astrocytoma. Most of the astrocytomas fall into the latter category. Juvenile cerebellar astrocytoma, shown in this example, is cystic and associated with better survival rates than the diffuse type.

19. **(E)** Choroid plexus tumors, colloid cysts, giant cell astrocytomas, and meningiomas are all examples of ventricular tumors. This figure demonstrates a choroid plexus papilloma involving the lateral ventricle, a typical site for this tumor in older children. These tumors are usually found in the fourth ventricle in very young children and adults. Unlike colloid cysts, which are found in the third ventricle, choroid plexus tumors are rarely seen in the third ventricle. Patients with choroid plexus tumors often present with signs of increased intracranial pressure, such as vomiting and headache. Subependymal giant cell astrocytomas occur in the region of the ventricles and are often associated with tuberous sclerosis. They are commonly seen in the area around the foramen of Monro.

SUGGESTED READING
Cohen ME, Duffner PK: Tumors of the brain and spinal cord including leukemic involvement. In: Swaiman KF, Ashwal S (eds): *Pediatric Neurology: Principles & Practice*, 3rd ed. St. Louis: Mosby, 1999, p 1049.
Evans RW (ed): Secondary headache disorders. *Neurol Clin North Am* 22(1), 237–249, 2004.
Mathews MK, Sergott RC, Savino PJ: Pseudotumor cerebri. *Curr Opin Ophthalmol* 14:364–370, 2003.
Winner P, Rothner AD: *Headache in Children and Adolescents*. Hamilton, Ontario: BC Decker, 2001.

CASE 135: AN 8-YEAR-OLD BOY WITH DIFFICULTY IN SCHOOL

An 8-year-old boy is referred to your clinic for evaluation of a learning disability. His mother states that her son was born at full term and met all of the developmental milestones at the appropriate ages. A week ago, she attended a meeting with his schoolteacher who expressed concerns about his grades and inability to pay attention in class. When asked about his behavior at home, she describes her son as very active. She admits that it is probably beyond what most would consider "normal boy behavior." For example, he recently took a set of markers and scribbled all over the kitchen walls. She states that she has to keep an eye on him every minute of the day to ensure that he doesn't get into any mischief. He has a hard time sitting still and jumps from task to task. As a result, very few of the neighborhood children will play with him, as he never seems to complete any of the games and is very disruptive. When she tries to talk to him, he doesn't seem to want to listen.

During the examination, the child has a hard time sitting still. He empties all the equipment from the drawers, despite his mother's objections. When asked to write the alphabet, he gets to the letter "E" before running out the door. His mother has an exasperated look on her face as she chases him into the waiting room. While she is gone, his father states that he had similar problems in school. On the child returning to the examination room, you manage to complete the physical examination with difficulty and find that it is within normal limits.

SELECT THE ONE BEST ANSWER

1. In order to make a diagnosis and begin therapy, you will need which of the following pieces of information?

   (A) a letter from the schoolteacher delineating some of the observed behaviors and academic difficulties
   (B) an MRI of the brain looking for frontal lobe injury
   (C) completion of behavior rating scales by the parents and schoolteachers
   (D) psychiatric evaluation
   (E) A and C

2. You obtain the appropriate information and it confirms your initial hypothesis. The most likely diagnosis in this patient is which of the following?

   (A) conduct disorder
   (B) attention-deficit hyperactivity disorder (ADHD)

   (C) mental retardation
   (D) bipolar disorder
   (E) oppositional defiant disorder

3. His father asks if he could have passed on these symptoms to his son. In fact, he has wondered about treatment for himself. Which of the following is the most appropriate response?

   (A) "The likelihood is small as ADHD is probably not a genetic disorder."
   (B) "Probably not, as ADHD is an X-linked disorder."
   (C) "Possibly, however, environmental factors, such as upbringing and maternal drug use, are much more important."
   (D) "ADHD is probably a genetic disorder, as a child born to a parent with ADHD has a greater than 50% risk of developing symptoms."
   (E) "Not much is known about the genetics of ADHD as concordance for monozygotic twins is low."

4. Which of the following is not a *DSM-IV* diagnostic criteria for ADHD?

   (A) Symptoms of hyperactivity and/or inattention are present for at least 6 months.
   (B) Impairment from the symptoms occurs in two or more settings.
   (C) Hyperactive or inattentive symptoms must be present after the age of 7 years.
   (D) The patient must have at least six symptoms of either inattention or hyperactivity-impulsivity to be considered for that specific type of ADHD or six from each to be considered for the combined type.
   (E) The symptoms cannot be due to another condition, such as pervasive developmental delay or a psychotic disorder.

5. You decide to start the patient on therapy. Which of the following treatment options could be considered in patients with ADHD?

   (A) behavioral therapy
   (B) dextroamphetamine
   (C) methylphenidate
   (D) all of the above
   (E) only B and C are correct

6. You decide to start the patient on a stimulant. You inform his parents that you will need to see him in the clinic every 1 to 3 months to assess for which of the following?

(A) growth progress
(B) academic progress
(C) cardiovascular side effects
(D) psychological well-being
(E) all of the above

7. Although the patient demonstrates significant improvement following initiation of therapy, he continues to have some academic difficulty despite several medication adjustments. At this point, the most appropriate action would be which of the following choices?

(A) a second opinion
(B) request for a child psychiatry consultation
(C) neuropsychological or psychoeducational testing
(D) an electroencephalogram
(E) treatment with nonstimulant medications, such as bupropion or tricyclic antidepressants

8. Which of the following medications used in the treatment of ADHD is associated with chemical hepatitis and rarely, fulminant liver failure?

(A) methylphenidate
(B) dextroamphetamine
(C) pemoline
(D) clonidine
(E) bupropion

9. Which of the following is the most frequently observed learning disorder?

(A) mathematics disorder
(B) disorder of written expression
(C) reading disorder
(D) atypical learning disorder
(E) none of the above

10. A child in the third grade presents to your clinic for evaluation of a learning disorder. His mother states that although he has a good memory and does well with rote learning, he has problems with comprehension, organization of information, and concept formation. He initially did well in math, but now struggles to finish his homework, despite a significant amount of effort. She states that he doesn't seem to have good reasoning skills. Which of the following learning disorders is most likely in this child?

(A) dyslexia
(B) mental retardation
(C) mathematics disorder
(D) nonverbal learning disability
(E) disorder of written expression

11. A 7-year-old girl comes to your clinic with a letter from her teacher. The letter states that the child is having problems with reading, especially with phonologic processing. In particular, she has a problem identifying phonemes. Her father states that he had reading difficulties as a child. You ask the child to read a short paragraph and she has a hard time associating sounds with letters and often mispronounces words. When asked to write the alphabet, she demonstrates a tendency to reverse certain letters. She has a hard time spelling simple words. Her physical examination is unremarkable. This patient most likely has which of the following diagnoses?

(A) mental retardation
(B) reading disorder
(C) attention-deficit hyperactivity disorder
(D) disorder of written expression
(E) nonverbal learning disability

12. In terms of evaluating the patient from question 11 further, which of the following would be helpful in making the diagnosis?

(A) chromosome karyotyping
(B) MRI of the brain pre- and post-contrast
(C) EEG
(D) behavior rating scales
(E) no further studies

13. In the *DSM-IV*, the category "Pervasive Developmental Disorders" has five subgroups. Which of the following is not a subgroup of this category?

(A) autistic disorder
(B) Asperger syndrome
(C) childhood disintegrative disorder
(D) Angelman syndrome
(E) Rett syndrome

14. A 3-year-old female presents to your clinic for an evaluation of profound language delay. Although the child is capable of vocalizing, mostly in the form of screaming, she has no words and cannot communicate her needs. Her mother states that her verbal development has never been normal. She does not make eye contact and seems oblivious to your presence. Her mother states that she is not very affectionate and has been unable to make friends with the child next door who is her same age. During the examination, the child repetitively opens and closes a drawer containing medical supplies without removing them. A hearing test was reportedly normal. You try to perform your physical examination, but the child cries and floridly flaps her arms. Her head circumference has been stable at the 97th percentile for the last year. The most likely diagnosis of this patient's symptoms is which of the following?

    (A) childhood disintegrative disorder
    (B) autism
    (C) Rett syndrome
    (D) Asperger syndrome
    (E) Landau-Kleffner syndrome

15. Which of the following statements is true regarding the association of autism and seizures?

    (A) Approximately a third of patients with autism will develop epilepsy by adulthood.
    (B) Studies have suggested that up to 80% of patients with autism can have abnormal EEGs.
    (C) A family history of seizures is a risk factor for the development of seizures in a patient with autism.
    (D) Patients with autism and seizures are more likely to have complex partial seizures, although all seizure types can occur.
    (E) All of the above statements are true regarding autism and seizures.

16. In evaluating a child with speech and language disorders, the only test considered mandatory in the evaluation is which of the following studies?

    (A) EEG
    (B) MRI of the brain
    (C) audiometry
    (D) chromosome analysis
    (E) serum amino acids

17. An 18-month-old girl presents to your clinic for evaluation of language delay and poor social skills. The patient was born at full term and developed normally until a couple of months ago. Recently, she has developed frequent bouts of screaming fits. Her mother states that there has been a regression in speech and language skills. She has lost the ability to use her hands purposefully. On examination, she has truncal ataxia and an apraxic gait. She demonstrates stereotyped hand movements in the form of hand-wringing. This patient most likely has which of the following diagnoses?

    (A) Angelman syndrome
    (B) autism
    (C) pervasive developmental delay
    (D) Rett syndrome
    (E) childhood disintegrative disorder

18. A 7-year-old boy presents to your clinic for an evaluation of behavior problems. The patient gets very angry when he does not "get his way." His mother states that her son has a hard time making friends, even though he has a strong desire to be with other children. She states that the other children often refuse to play with him, as he "only wants to play by his rules." He is not very empathetic. Recently, he has started collecting bottle caps. He exhibits hand-flapping behavior. His language development was normal. This patient most likely has which of the following diagnoses?

    (A) autism
    (B) Asperger syndrome
    (C) childhood disintegrative disorder
    (D) oppositional defiant disorder
    (E) pervasive developmental delay

Answers

1. (E) This child most likely has ADHD, the combined type. However, in order to make the diagnosis, *DSM-IV* criteria require that the patient have symptoms that occur in at least two different settings, such as home and school. Hence, the diagnosis is based on information obtained from both parents and school reports. Several behavioral rating scales have been created to al-

low for a more systematic approach to documenting the symptoms of inattention, hyperactivity, and impulsivity. Although the diagnosis of ADHD can be made based on the compilation of findings from the clinical history, school reports, and physical examination, behavior rating scales are useful adjuncts not only in the diagnosis, but also in serving as baseline measures of ADHD symptoms, which can then be used to monitor therapy efficacy. Laboratory studies in the diagnosis of ADHD are typically not very helpful and routine neuroimaging in the setting of a normal physical examination is not indicated. Laboratory studies, such as electroencephalography or blood work looking for systemic disease (for example, thyroid function tests) should be performed only if clinically indicated. As patients with ADHD can develop symptoms of depression and low self-esteem, it is important to monitor for these symptoms. However, in the absence of these symptoms a psychiatric evaluation is not necessary to make the diagnosis. It should be stressed, however, that clinically depressed patients can have symptoms consistent with a diagnosis of ADHD. As a result, a *DSM-IV* diagnostic criterion for ADHD is that the symptoms cannot be better accounted for by another mental disorder, such as a mood disorder. One can have devastating consequences should a diagnosis of major depression be attributed to ADHD.

2. **(B)** This child has ADHD, combined type, which is approximately two to four times more common in males than females. In order to be diagnosed with ADHD, combined type, patients must have at least six symptoms of inattention plus six or more symptoms of hyperactivity and impulsivity. The symptoms should be present for at least 6 months and present before the age of 7 years. Symptoms of inattention include difficulty paying attention, making frequent careless mistakes in school work, reluctance to engage in tasks, forgetfulness, distractibility, difficulty organizing activities, inability to listen while others are speaking, and a tendency to lose objects. Symptoms of hyperactivity and impulsivity include talking excessively, difficulty playing quietly, fidgeting, abruptly leaving the classroom seat, difficulty waiting one's turn, blurting out answers before being called on, and interrupting others during con-

versations or games. If patients meet criteria for only the inattentive symptoms, then a diagnosis of ADHD, predominantly inattentive type is given. This type is more common in girls. If the patient only has symptoms of hyperactivity, then the diagnosis of ADHD, predominantly hyperactive-impulsive type is given. This type of ADHD is rare. The differential diagnosis of ADHD includes disruptive behavioral disorders, such as conduct disorder and oppositional defiant disorder; mental retardation; bipolar disorder; schizophrenia; anxiety disorder; and certain drugs, such as phenobarbital in the older child.

3. **(D)** Assuming the patient's father truly had ADHD, the correct response is D, as children born to a parent with ADHD have an almost 60% chance of developing symptoms. In addition, concordance for monozygotic twins is high. Having a sibling with ADHD imposes a 30% risk. Given the mechanism of action of the pharmacologic agents used to treat ADHD and recent research, the dopamine receptor and transporter have been implicated in the pathogenesis. However, it is likely that several genes may be involved.

4. **(C)** Some symptoms of hyperactivity/impulsivity or inattention should be present before the age of 7 years.

5. **(D)** Treatment of ADHD includes nonpharmacologic and pharmacologic approaches. Nonpharmacologic approaches include educational counseling and cognitive-behavioral therapies. Educational counseling may include providing one-on-one tutoring in the classroom, minimizing distractions by rearranging the classroom seating arrangement, and teaching organizational skills. Educational counseling can be provided by a number of individuals, including pediatricians, nurses, social workers, psychologists, and mental health professionals. The counseling can occur on an individual basis or in groups. Cognitive-behavioral therapies employ techniques such as positive and negative reinforcement to modify self-control problems and encourage active participation in learning activities. Parents of a child with ADHD often experience feelings of incompetence or social isolation. Indeed, the difficulties in raising a child with ADHD can lead to problems in the

marriage. As a result, parents may benefit from a consultation with a mental health professional or social worker. Some families have benefited from family therapy to assess for family dysfunction and help with behavior management. In addition, support groups are available to further assist parents.

6. **(E)** Once a decision is made to start a child on medication, follow-up is arranged to assess for patient growth (height and weight), academic progress, cardiovascular side effects, and psychological well-being. Studies have shown that stimulants have significant short-term benefits in most children (up to 80%) with ADHD. With dose adjustments and perhaps trials with other stimulant medications, response rates can be nearly 90%. Hence, it is important to monitor the child for dose adequacy and academic progress. It may be helpful to have the parents and schoolteachers repeat behavior rating scales to quantitate improvement. Stimulant medications have side effects, most of which are transient and manageable with close monitoring. The more common side effects include anorexia, insomnia, irritability, and headaches. It is important to monitor the patient's weight and height, as stimulants can cause weight loss and reduced height velocity. Exacerbation of tics with concurrent stimulant use is observed in some children. Stimulants may cause slight elevations in heart rate and blood pressure and, as a result, these parameters should be monitored. Finally, children with ADHD are at risk for developing psychiatric comorbidity. They can have feelings of low self-esteem and depression. In addition, approximately one-third of children with ADHD will experience an anxiety disorder during the course of their life. Hence, it is important to monitor for psychiatric symptoms.

7. **(C)** If a child continues to have academic difficulties, despite pharmacologic and nonpharmacologic interventions, it is important to perform psychoeducational or neuropsychological testing, if not already done, to evaluate for a learning disability. The association of learning disabilities, especially reading disorders (dyslexia), and ADHD is significant and probably, quite common. Some studies have found that up to 90% of children with ADHD may also have a reading disorder. Other studies have not seen as dramatic an association.

8. **(C)** Pemoline has been associated with chemical hepatitis and rarely, fulminant liver failure. Although the onset of hepatitis is unpredictable, many clinicians will monitor liver function at least every 6 months following baseline liver function tests at initiation of the drug.

9. **(C)** Learning disorders are seen in approximately 10% of the population. Roughly half of the patients with learning disorders have a reading disorder (dyslexia). The remaining half are due to mathematics disorder, atypical learning disorders, and disorder of written expression. Most children with learning disorders are diagnosed in preschool through the second grade when it becomes clear that the child is not keeping up with his/her peers or grades start to fall. Boys are twice to four times as likely as girls to have a learning disorder.

10. **(D)** This patient most likely has a nonverbal learning disability (NVLD). Patients with NVLD tend to do well with rote learning. They have simple verbal skills and strengths in nonvisual memory. Weaknesses include problems with motor skills, problem solving, concept formation, and comprehension. Initially, these children tend to do well in math, given the rote nature of beginning lessons. However, as the child with NVLD progresses through school, he struggles with nonverbal reasoning and more advanced math concepts. Social difficulty develops as social skills depend on the child's ability to perform nonverbal processing. Written expression and reading comprehension are often problematic. In mathematics disorder, patients have a hard time performing calculations. At times, patients with NVLD may appear to have a mathematics disorder, but the weaknesses listed above often give an indication that the mathematics disability is part of the larger learning disability that is NVLD. Patients with disorder of written expression have a decreased ability to present information in writing compared to verbal expression.

11. **(B)** This patient has a reading disorder (dyslexia), the most common type of learning disorder. Pa-

tients with reading disorder have a hard time processing sound units and sound-symbol relationships. They often have difficulty with phonologic processing. Although dyslexia has been characterized by frequent letter reversals in the lay literature, this feature is not required to make the diagnosis. Another myth is that dyslexia is primarily a disorder of males. More recent population-based studies did not demonstrate a difference in prevalence rates between males and females.

12. **(E)** This patient most likely has a reading disorder (dyslexia). In patients with reading disorders, a thorough history and physical examination, including an assessment of reading, are sufficient to make the diagnosis. Laboratory evaluations, such chromosome karyotyping, electroencephalography, and neuroimaging studies, are performed when clinically indicated. Behavior rating scales are helpful adjuncts in the evaluation for ADHD. Although patients with ADHD can have underlying learning disabilities, dyslexia and ADHD are separate conditions. Should a patient with reading disorder manifest signs and symptoms of ADHD, an evaluation would be warranted.

13. **(D)** Autism and pervasive developmental disorders (PDD) represent a spectrum of disorders associated with cognitive and neurobehavioral problems. Patients demonstrate impairments in verbal and nonverbal communication and social interaction. In addition, they can demonstrate repetitive and restricted patterns of behavior. The five subgroups listed under the pervasive developmental (autistic spectrum) disorders category in the *DSM-IV* are autistic disorder; Asperger syndrome; pervasive developmental disorder, not otherwise specified; childhood disintegrative disorder; and Rett syndrome. Angelman syndrome is not listed as a subtype of the autistic spectrum disorders, although there seems to be a high comorbidity between this disorder and autism.

14. **(B)** This patient probably has autism. Patients with autism often demonstrate impairment in social interaction manifested by decreased eye contact, failure to develop peer relationships, lack of awareness of others, and failure to participate in groups. These patients are often described as not being very affectionate. Patients with autism also demonstrate impairment in communication, which can be quite variable. Some patients have no spoken language, while other demonstrate immature forms of language, such as echolalia. There may be a stereotyped or repetitive use of language. Those with adequate speech may be unable to sustain a conversation. Finally, patients with autism typically demonstrate restrictive repetitive and stereotypic behaviors, such as hand-flapping. They may be fascinated with parts and movements of an object, such as the opening and closing of drawers. Children with autism are usually inflexible in their adherence to certain routines. Onset is before the age of 3 years. Patients with childhood disintegrative disorder demonstrate significant regression in two or more areas of functioning after at least 24 months of normal early development. It is a relatively rare disorder that usually occurs between the ages of 3 and 4 years of age, but can occur up to approximately 10 years of age.

15. **(E)** Depending on the study, approximately 80% of the children with autistic spectrum disorder will have an abnormal EEG. The abnormalities can range from slowing of the background activity to overt epileptiform activity. As children with autism approach adulthood, the cumulative prevalence of developing a seizure disorder is approximately 35%. Although patients with autism can experience all types of seizures, the type most frequently encountered seems to be complex partial seizures. Patients with autism can exhibit unusual behaviors, and, as a result, it may be difficult to determine if a behavior is truly epileptiform. Home monitoring video EEG has been useful in assessing if a behavior is associated with epileptiform activity. A family history of seizures and mental retardation are significant risk factors for the development of seizures.

16. **(C)** Of all the tests available for the evaluation of a patient with speech and language disorder, the only one that is mandatory is audiometry. Routine testing with neuroimaging, chromosome analysis, serum amino acids, or other metabolic tests are usually not helpful in the absence of historical or physical findings warranting these tests. Likewise, electroencephalography should be performed if the clinical suspicion of seizures is high. If a patient demonstrates regression of

language skills, a prolonged EEG capturing sleep should be performed to rule out disorders such as Landau-Kleffner syndrome.

17. **(D)** This patient most likely has the neurodegenerative disorder, Rett syndrome. This disorder mainly occurs in females who develop symptoms following a period of normal development. The birth history is typically normal. Patients have normal head circumferences. At some point between 6 and 18 months of age, patients start to manifest symptoms characterized by deterioration of behavior, regression of speech and language skills, truncal ataxia, loss of purposeful hand movements, stereotyped hand movements (hand wringing), autistic behavior, seizures, and acquired microcephaly. The key features in this case are the regression of skills, loss of purposeful hand movements, stereotyped hand movements, and ataxia. Patients with Angelman syndrome can also exhibit developmental delay, seizures, ataxia, and acquired microcephaly. Patients with Angelman syndrome typically do not demonstrate the stereotyped hand movements. They have characteristic facial features such as prognathism, a protruding tongue, and wide mouth. Most cases of Angelman syndrome are due to deletions of chromosome 15q11-q13.

18. **(B)** This patient most likely has Asperger syndrome. Patients with Asperger syndrome demonstrate sustained impairments in social interaction, especially among their peers. Similar to autism, patients with Asperger syndrome demonstrate repetitive, restricted, and stereotypic behaviors. In contrast to patients with autism, language development is typically normal, although they may demonstrate pragmatic abnormalities in language. IQ tends to be in the normal or borderline range. Boys tend to be affected more than girls. Some clinicians believe Asperger syndrome is a milder form of autism.

SUGGESTED READING

Dunn DW, Kronenberger WG: Attention-deficit/hyperactivity disorder in children and adolescents. *Neurol Clin North Am* 21:933–940, 2003.

Filipek PA: Autistic spectrum disorders. In: Swaiman KF, Ashwal S (eds): Pediatric *Neurology: Principles & Practice*, 3rd ed. St. Louis: Mosby, 1999, p 606.

Kronenberger WG, Dunn DW: Learning disorders. *Neurol Clin North Am* 21:941–952, 2003.

Miller KJ, Castellanos FX: Attention deficit/hyperactivity disorders. *Pediatr Rev* 19:373–384, 1998.

Shaywitz BA, Fletcher JM, Shaywitz SE: Attention-deficit hyperactivity disorder. In: Swaiman KF, Ashwal S (eds): Pediatric *Neurology: Principles & Practice*, 3rd ed. St. Louis: Mosby, 1999, p 585.

Tuchman R: Autism. *Neurol Clin North Am* 21:915–932, 2003.

CASE 136: A 2-YEAR-OLD BOY WITH DEVELOPMENTAL DELAY AND SPASTICITY

A 2-year-old boy presents to your clinic with the chief complaint of developmental delay. His mother states that he was born at 34 weeks' gestational age. The pregnancy was complicated by premature rupture of membranes 5 weeks prior to delivery. His mother was hospitalized and received a 7-day course of ampicillin and two doses of betamethasone. At the time of delivery, she developed a fever of 102°F. The baby was delivered by cesarean section secondary to fetal tachycardia and arrest of descent. As the baby was found to have a poor heart rate and respiratory effort, CPR was initiated. His Apgar scores were 1, 2, and 5 at 1, 5, and 10 minutes, respectively. He was admitted to the NICU for management of sepsis. A head ultrasound revealed a "hemorrhage" according to his mother.

At 7 months of age, his mother states that she became concerned, as her son was not able to sit without support. By 15 months of age, he was still not walking. His language development is normal. She presented to her primary pediatrician who referred her to an Early Intervention program. As a result of occupational and physical therapies, he is now able to use a spoon and a sippy cup. He developed the ability to crawl and in fact, is now able to cruise around furniture. Although his mother is pleased by his developmental progress, she notes that he still has a tendency to use his left hand more than his right.

On physical examination, he is a very happy and active child. His head circumference is at the 50th percentile. His cranial nerve examination is normal. On motor examination, he is able to reach for a block, but clearly favors his left hand. His right thumb is persistently adducted. He was unable to perform a pincer grasp with his right hand. His muscle tone is increased over the right side of his body. His heel cord on the right is tight. His deep tendon reflexes are asymmetric with the right side of his body slightly brisker than the left side. He is able to bear weight on his legs, but stands on his tiptoe on the right. Examination of his skin reveals a small café-au-lait spot on his back.

SELECT THE ONE BEST ANSWER

1. Intraventricular hemorrhages are most likely to affect which of the following brain structures in the premature infant?

   (A) cortex
   (B) middle cerebral artery
   (C) germinal matrix
   (D) basal ganglia
   (E) lenticulostriate arteries

2. You were able to review the patient's head ultrasound, which demonstrated blood within the ventricular system. The ventricle was not distended. What grade intraventricular hemorrhage does this patient have based on the head ultrasound?

   (A) grade I
   (B) grade II
   (C) grade III
   (D) grade IV
   (E) none of the above

3. This child most likely has which of the following diagnoses?

   (A) mental retardation
   (B) spastic hemiplegic cerebral palsy
   (C) ataxic cerebral palsy
   (D) spastic diplegic cerebral palsy
   (E) mixed cerebral palsy

4. Which of the following are risk factors for the development of cerebral palsy?

   (A) low birth weight
   (B) hyperbilirubinemia
   (C) maternal antenatal methyl mercury ingestion
   (D) preterm delivery
   (E) all of the above

5. Which of the following are classifications of cerebral palsy?

   (A) spastic
   (B) choreoathetotic
   (C) ballismic
   (D) A and C
   (E) all of the above

6. A 4-year-old boy born to immigrant parents comes to your clinic. He presents with the following symptoms: sensorineural hearing loss, supernuclear ophthalmoplegia, enamel hypoplasia, and choreoathetosis. The most likely cause of his symptoms is which of the following?

   (A) stroke
   (B) congenital infection with cytomegalovirus
   (C) congenital infection with rubella
   (D) kernicterus
   (E) lissencephaly

7. A preterm infant is most likely to have which of the following forms of cerebral palsy?

   (A) spastic diplegia
   (B) spastic quadriplegia
   (C) spastic hemiplegia
   (D) choreoathetotic
   (E) atonic or hypotonic

8. Which of the following statements regarding the spastic hemiplegic form of cerebral palsy is false?

   (A) For unknown reasons, the left hemisphere is more often affected than the right hemisphere.
   (B) The arm is usually more affected than the leg.
   (C) Facial involvement is typical.
   (D) Provided the child has no other major problems, he or she will most likely walk by 2 years of age.
   (E) All of the above statements are false.

9. Which form of cerebral palsy is most often associated with birth asphyxia?

   (A) spastic diplegia
   (B) spastic quadriplegia
   (C) spastic hemiplegia
   (D) choreoathetotic
   (E) atonic or hypotonic

10. The patient's mother asks you what treatment options are available for her son should his spasticity get worse. Which of the following interventions have been used in the treatment of cerebral palsy?

    (A) selective dorsal rhizotomy
    (B) botulinum toxin injections

(C) physical therapy

(D) baclofen

(E) all of the above

11. A 7-year-old male presents to your clinic for an evaluation of behavioral problems and new-onset seizures. In addition, during the last 3 months, he has received poor grades, especially in writing. His mother states that until recently he was a completely normal child. She is concerned as her estranged sister had a male child with similar symptoms before he died. Over the next couple of months, the patient rapidly deteriorates. He now has a spastic paraparesis and visual loss. The study most likely to help make the diagnosis is which of the following?

(A) electroencephalogram

(B) galactocerebroside beta-galactosidase levels

(C) MRI of the brain

(D) plasma very long chain fatty acids

(E) C and D

12. An MRI of the brain demonstrates bilateral parieto-occipital white matter lesions. The most likely diagnosis in this patient is which of the following?

(A) Alexander disease

(B) X-linked adrenoleukodystrophy

(C) metachromatic leukodystrophy

(D) Canavan disease

(E) Pelizaeus-Merzbacher disease

13. All of the following are consider lipidoses except which of the following diseases?

(A) Niemann-Pick disease

(B) Krabbe disease

(C) Tay-Sachs disease

(D) X-linked adrenoleukodystrophy

(E) Gaucher disease

14. Which of the following statements is true regarding the genetics of Niemann-Pick disease?

(A) It is transmitted as an autosomal recessive trait.

(B) It is transmitted as an autosomal dominant trait.

(C) The disorder demonstrates an X-linked mode of inheritance.

(D) The disorder is the result of triplet repeat expansion.

(E) The disorder is the result of mutations of mitochondrial DNA.

MATCH EACH OF THE FOLLOWING DISEASES WITH ITS CORRESPONDING DEFECT OR DEFICIENCY.

15. Gaucher disease

16. Tay-Sachs disease

17. Metachromatic leukodystrophy

18. Rett Syndrome

19. Krabbe disease

(A) β-glucocerebrosidase

(B) methyl-CpG-binding protein

(C) galactocerebroside beta-galactosidase

(D) arylsulfatase A

(E) hexosaminidase A

Answers

1. (C) Intraventricular hemorrhages occur within the germinal matrix. The germinal matrix, along with the germinal ventricular zone, is the site of neuronal and glial precursor cell proliferation. This structure remains relatively intact until approximately 34 weeks' gestational age, after which it starts to involute, a process completed by term. Preterm infants are most likely to experience intraventricular hemorrhages within the first 3 to 4 days following birth.

2. (B) There are four grades of intraventricular hemorrhages (IVH). A grade I IVH consists of bleeding within the germinal matrix. In a grade II IVH, blood is found within the ventricular system, but does not cause distension. If there is bleeding within the ventricle with concomitant distension, then the IVH is considered grade III. In a grade IV IVH, there is parenchymal involvement of the hemorrhage.

3. (B) This case is an example of a nonprogressive encephalopathy. This child most likely has the spastic hemiplegic form of cerebral palsy given that the

right side of his body is weak and spastic with increased reflexes (signs of upper motor neuron involvement). Cerebral palsy is a nonspecific term, which describes a disability of motor function seen in early infancy. The patients usually demonstrate problems with muscle tone (typically spasticity), ataxia, or involuntary movements. Although cognitive, behavioral, and sensory problems can be observed in children with cerebral palsy, these symptoms are not necessary to make the diagnosis. Patients with spastic hemiplegia can exhibit difficulties with gross and fine motor coordination. The child is usually unable to perform a pincer grasp with the affected hand, as was the case in this child. Facial involvement is unusual in the spastic hemiplegic form of cerebral palsy. Over time the affected limbs usually demonstrate growth retardation. This is often best demonstrated by comparing the affected limb with the opposite normal limb. This needs to be monitored closely, as a growth discrepancy of the leg may cause problems with ambulation and lead to further orthopedic difficulties. An older study looking at patients with spastic hemiplegia suggested that up to a third might have mental retardation and/or seizures. A wide range of medical conditions may lead to the spastic hemiplegic form of cerebral palsy including infarction and hemorrhage.

4. **(E)** Low birth weight and preterm delivery are significant risk factors for the development of cerebral palsy. Twin gestation also may predispose to cerebral palsy as the infants are at risk for low birth weight. Marked hyperbilirubinemia was once a common cause of choreoathetotic cerebral palsy in the setting of kernicterus. Finally, ingestion of certain toxins, such as methyl mercury, during pregnancy has been associated with the subsequent development of cerebral palsy. Intrauterine and neonatal infections can also lead to the development of cerebral palsy. It should be noted that although birth trauma and asphyxia can result in cerebral palsy, they are not the leading causes.

5. **(E)** Cerebral palsy is classified based on neurologic signs and symptoms. These include the following: spastic, choreoathetotic, dystonic, ballismic, ataxic, and mixed. Based on the limb involvement, the classes can be further subdivided. Hence, a patient with spasticity and bilateral lower extremity involvement would have spastic diplegia, while an individual with four-extremity involvement would have spastic quadriplegia.

6. **(D)** This patient presents with the classical clinical tetrad observed in kernicterus: sensorineural hearing loss, supernuclear ophthalmoplegia, enamel hypoplasia, and choreoathetosis. However, rarely does one observe all four symptoms in a single affected patient. Kernicterus is caused by the deposition of bile pigments in various nuclei of the brain (brainstem, cerebellum, and basal ganglia) and spinal cord. Infants with marked hyperbilirubinemia may manifest symptoms as early as the second or third day of life. Sensorineural hearing loss is common and results from degeneration of the cochlear nuclei.

7. **(A)** Approximately 80% of preterm infants with the spastic form of cerebral palsy will have the diplegic form. These patients demonstrate periventricular leukomalacia at the germinal matrix. Porencephalic cysts may also be observed.

8. **(C)** As stated above, facial involvement is rare in patients with spastic hemiplegia. Approximately two-thirds of patients will have left hemispheric involvement for unclear reasons. The arm is usually more affected than the leg. Most children with spastic hemiplegia walk by the age of 2 years compared to spastic diplegia where a little more than half walk by 3 years of age. Spastic hemiplegic patients who learn to walk may have a circumductive gait.

9. **(B)** Birth asphyxia typically leads to the spastic quadriplegic form of cerebral palsy. In this form of cerebral palsy the legs are more involved than the arms. Approximately half of the children with spastic quadriplegia have seizures of the generalized tonic-clonic type.

10. **(E)** A major goal in the treatment of cerebral palsy is to maximize function so that the patient will be able to satisfy his/her daily needs. To that extent, all of the interventions listed in this question have been used in the treatment of cerebral palsy. As every patient's needs are different, the treatment is tailored to the individual patient. Physical and occupational therapy programs are almost always employed in the overall treatment plan of cerebral palsy. These

therapies help increase range of motion and prevent contractures. In addition, patients are taught normal movement patterns and methods of compensation. Orthotic devices, such as braces, are employed to prevent contractures. Surgical techniques, such as selective dorsal rhizotomy, which involves cutting half of the dorsal roots, can be employed with the goal of decreasing muscle tone in the affected limb. A number of medications have been tried to reduce hypertonicity. These medications include diazepam, baclofen, and dantrolene. Baclofen can be given orally or intrathecally via an infusion pump. These medications are especially useful if the spasticity is generalized. Botulinum toxin injections offer the advantage of isolating specific muscles. The toxin inhibits the release of acetylcholine from the presynaptic terminal. The benefits of the injection typically last around 3 months.

11. **(E)** Based on the clinical history, this child has a progressive neurological disorder as evident by the regression of skills and rapid clinical deterioration. Although the electroencephalogram would be helpful in confirming the clinical suspicion of seizures, and in fact, may help to classify seizure type, it is unlikely in this case to yield the diagnosis. An MRI of the brain would be helpful given the rapid development of spastic paraparesis and clinical seizures. The MRI would be able to determine whether the underlying disease process affects primarily grey matter, as would be suspected given the history of seizures, white matter, or both. A primarily white matter process would suggest a leukodystrophy, while grey and white matter lesions would be suggestive of a mitochondrial process. Two disorders, globoid cell leukodystrophy (Krabbe disease) and X-linked adrenoleukodystrophy can present with visual loss. Given the possibility that the mother's nephew died of the same condition, an X-linked disorder should be suspected. In the early stages, involvement of the parieto-occipital white matter is seen in Krabbe disease, possibly resembling X-linked adrenoleukodystrophy. As the latter is a peroxisomal disorder, plasma very long chain fatty acids will be increased.

12. **(B)** Given the clinical history and MRI findings, this patient most likely has X-linked adrenoleukodystrophy. Male children are usually normal until 4 to 8 years of age when symptoms begin. This disorder is rapidly progressive. In approximately 85% of the cases, the MRI of the brain demonstrates hyperintensity of the parieto-occipital white matter. Alexander and Canavan disease are two leukodystrophies associated with macrocephaly. Alexander disease has a predilection for the frontal white matter, while the MRI findings in Canavan disease demonstrate diffuse white matter involvement with prominent involvement of the subcortical U fibers. The MRI of a patient with Pelizaeus-Merzbacher disease demonstrates heterogeneous hyperintense lesions in the white matter with scattered small foci of normal areas, lending the name "tigroid" pattern.

13. **(D)** The term lipidoses refers to a group of inherited disorders in which lipid metabolism is abnormal. Lysosomal enzymes are affected. Niemann-Pick disease (sphingomyelin lipidosis), Krabbe disease (galactosylceramide lipidosis), Tay-Sachs disease (GM_2 gangliosidosis), and Gaucher disease (glucosylceramide lipidosis) are all examples of lipidoses. X-linked adrenoleukodystrophy is an example of a peroxisomal disorder.

14. **(A)** All types of Niemann-Pick disease (A to D) are transmitted as an autosomal recessive inheritance pattern.

15. **(A)** Gaucher disease is the most common among Ashkenazi Jews, and, in fact is one of the most frequent lysosomal disorders. The deficient enzyme is β-glucocerebrosidase. Glucosylceramide accumulates in various tissues: brain, spleen, bone marrow, and liver.

16. **(E)** Children with Tay-Sachs disease present with hyperacusis and a propensity to startle with noise. Patients can have myoclonic seizures and a "cherry red spot" on fundoscopic examination. The disorder is transmitted in an autosomal recessive fashion, especially in those of Ashkenazi Jewish decent. The deficient enzyme is hexosaminidase A.

17. **(D)** Approximately 80% of patients with metachromatic leukodystrophy generally develop symptoms in the first 2 years of life. Symptoms include ataxia, neuropathy, optic atrophy, seizures, and spasticity. Loss of speech, intellect, and coordination are also observed. The enzyme deficiency is arylsulfatase A.

18. **(B)** Methyl-CpG-binding protein 2 (MeCP2) most likely regulates gene expression and chromatin structure by binding to methylated DNA. This gene is mutated in the majority of cases of sporadic Rett syndrome.

19. **(C)** Krabbe disease or globoid cell leukodystrophy is caused by a deficiency of the lysosomal hydrolase, galactocerebroside β-galactosidase.

SUGGESTED READING

Crumrine PK: Degenerative disorders of the central nervous system. *Pediatr Rev* 22:370–379, 2001.

Neul JL, Zoghbi HY: Rett syndrome: A prototypical neurodevelopmental disorder. *Neuroscientist* 10:118–128, 2004.

Osborn AG: Inherited metabolic, white matter and degenerative diseases of the brain. In: Osborn AG (ed): *Diagnostic Neuroradiology*. St. Louis: Mosby, 1994, p 716.

Swaiman KF, Russman BS: Cerebral palsy. In: Swaiman KF, Ashwal S (eds): *Pediatric Neurology: Principles & Practice*, 3rd ed. St. Louis: Mosby, 1999, p 312.

CASE 137: A 17-YEAR-OLD BOY WITH WEAKNESS AND PARESTHESIAS

You are called to the emergency department to evaluate a 17-year-old young man who presents with upper and lower extremity weakness and back pain. The patient states that he was in his usual state of health until approximately 2½ weeks ago when he developed an upper respiratory tract infection. His primary doctor felt that the infection was most likely due to a virus. Yesterday, the patient states he experienced tingling over the soles of his feet. His gait became unsteady and his legs "felt weak." On awakening this morning, the patient states that the weakness had spread to his arms. His lower extremities are also weaker compared to the previous day and he cannot walk 5 meters without support. There is no history of trauma. The patient states that he has had a hard time urinating.

On physical examination, the patient is an athletic-appearing young man in mild distress. He is afebrile with a heart rate of 124 bpm. His blood pressure seems to fluctuate. His mental status and cranial nerve examination are normal. On motor examination, he has normal tone and bulk. He is barely able to lift his legs from the bed and cannot move his toes. He is barely able to move his arms against gravity. His deep tendon reflexes are absent bilaterally in the lower ex-

tremities and 1+ out of 4+ in the upper extremities. Sensation to vibration and pinprick are slightly diminished in the lower extremities.

SELECT THE ONE BEST ANSWER

1. In evaluating this patient further, which of the following studies could help in confirming the diagnosis?

   (A) MRI of the spine
   (B) lumbar puncture
   (C) nerve conduction velocities
   (D) electromyography
   (E) all of the above

2. An MRI of the spine is performed with and without contrast. The study is unremarkable. CSF examination in this patient is most likely to reveal which of the following?

   (A) elevated opening pressure, elevated protein, normal glucose, and a cell count of 300 lymphocytes/mm^3
   (B) normal opening pressure, normal protein and glucose, and a cell count of 10 leukocytes/mm^3
   (C) normal opening pressure, elevated protein, normal glucose, and a cell count of 10 mononuclear cells/mm^3
   (D) elevated opening pressure, elevated protein, decreased glucose, and 1000 polymorphonuclear cells
   (E) no abnormal CSF findings

3. This patient most likely has which of the following diagnoses?

   (A) transverse myelitis
   (B) Guillain-Barré syndrome (GBS)
   (C) chronic inflammatory demyelinating polyneuropathy
   (D) tick paralysis
   (E) myasthenia gravis

4. Nerve conduction studies will most likely demonstrate which of the following results if performed in this patient?

   (A) no abnormalities
   (B) reduction of the compound motor action potential (CMAP) amplitudes evoked by stimulation of the median and posterior tibial nerves

(C) prolonged motor nerve conduction velocities
(D) conduction block
(E) B, C, and D

5. If the patient presented with ophthalmoplegia, facial/bulbar weakness, ataxia, and areflexia, he would be considered to have which of the following disorders?

(A) axonal GBS
(B) polyneuritis cranialis
(C) Miller-Fischer syndrome
(D) GBS with central nervous system manifestations
(E) none of the above

6. Miller-Fischer syndrome is associated with which of the following antecedent infections?

(A) *Borrelia burgdorferi*
(B) *Mycoplasma pneumoniae*
(C) *Campylobacter jejuni*
(D) CMV
(E) EBV

7. The serological test most likely to be abnormal in the Miller-Fischer syndrome is which of the following?

(A) anti-GM-1 antibody titers
(B) anti-GQ1b antibody titers
(C) anti-myelin antibody
(D) anti-Hu
(E) anti-Ri

8. Which of the following therapies are used in the treatment of GBS?

(A) plasmapheresis
(B) intravenous immunoglobulin
(C) high-dose corticosteroids
(D) A and B
(E) A, B, and C

9. The differential diagnosis of GBS includes all of the following diagnoses except which of the following?

(A) porphyria
(B) botulism
(C) HIV infection
(D) hysteria

(E) all of the above

10. Which of the following statements regarding GBS is false?

(A) In children, acquired inflammatory neuropathy is the most frequent cause of peripheral nerve disease.
(B) For the most part, males and females are equally affected.
(C) Surgery has been shown to be a cause of GBS.
(D) Sensory symptoms are more common than weakness.
(E) GBS occurs in all parts of the world.

11. Which of the following are complications of plasmapheresis?

(A) hypocalcemia
(B) hemorrhage
(C) transfusion reactions
(D) septicemia
(E) all of the above

12. Which of the following heavy metals is associated with neuropathy, alopecia, and GI symptoms?

(A) lead
(B) mercury
(C) thallium
(D) arsenic
(E) none of the above

13. A 15-year-old girl comes to your clinic with the chief complaint of right facial weakness. The patient is unable to close her right eye. She was healthy until a couple of weeks ago when she developed an upper respiratory tract infection. She is otherwise fine. On physical examination, there is no other sign of weakness. She does not demonstrate fatigue on sustained motor testing. Her deep tendon reflexes are normal. A head CT performed in the emergency room is reportedly normal. Which of the following is the most likely cause of her symptoms?

(A) Möbius syndrome
(B) GBS
(C) Bell's palsy
(D) myasthenia gravis
(E) cerebellar tumor

14. Which of the following cervical nerves are injured in an Erb's palsy?

(A) C5, C6
(B) C6, C7
(C) C7, C8
(D) C8, T1
(E) C5, C6, C7

15. Which of the following cervical nerves are injured in a Klumpke paralysis?

(A) C5, C6
(B) C6, C7
(C) C7, C8
(D) C8, T1
(E) C5, C6, C7

16. A 12-year-old girl presents to your clinic with the chief complaint of left foot weakness and mild sensory loss. Her mother states that both she and the patient's maternal grandfather have the same condition. On physical examination, the patient has a pes cavus deformity with permanently flexed toes. Proprioception and pinprick are mildly decreased in the toes. Deep tendon reflexes are absent bilaterally in the lower extremities. The peripheral nerve in the affected extremity is easily palpated. There is no autonomic involvement. Electrophysiologic testing reveals a marked reduction in motor nerve conduction velocities. This patient is most likely to have which of the following conditions?

(A) hereditary motor and sensory neuropathy, type I (autosomal dominant form)
(B) hereditary motor and sensory neuropathy, type II (autosomal dominant form)
(C) hereditary motor and sensory neuropathy, type I (autosomal recessive form)
(D) hereditary motor and sensory neuropathy, type II (autosomal recessive form)
(E) Dejerine-Sottas disease

17. Which of the following vitamins can result in a sensory neuropathy if taken in large doses?

(A) vitamin A
(B) pyridoxine
(C) cobalamin
(D) vitamin C
(E) vitamin E

18. Friedreich ataxia is transmitted by which mode of inheritance?

(A) It is transmitted as an autosomal recessive trait.
(B) It is transmitted as an autosomal dominant trait.
(C) The disorder demonstrates an X-linked mode of inheritance.
(D) The disorder is the result of mutations of mitochondrial DNA.
(E) Not much is known about the genetics of Friedreich ataxia.

Answers

1. **(E)** This patient most likely has GBS, the diagnosis of which can be made by the history and physical examination. However, a number of confirmatory studies can be performed to support the diagnosis. These include MRI of the spine, lumbar puncture, and electrophysiological studies, such as nerve conduction velocities and electromyography. Enhancement of the cauda equine and lumbar roots following contrast administration is sometimes observed in GBS, indicating that an inflammatory process is indeed involved. An additional reason to perform an MRI of the spine with and without contrast is to exclude or confirm a transverse myelitis, which is in the differential diagnosis.

2. **(C)** The characteristic CSF finding in GBS is elevation of protein without significant pleocytosis (albuminocytologic dissociation). Approximately 10% of patients will have 10 to 50 cells/mm^3. Most of these cells are lymphocytes. A cell count greater than 50 cells/mm^3 should cause the practitioner to consider an alternative diagnosis. The protein level may be normal in the first few days, but subsequently elevates to a peak in 4 to 6 weeks. Opening pressure and glucose are usually normal.

3. **(B)** GBS or acute inflammatory demyelinating polyradiculoneuropathy is a disorder in which patients experience progressive motor weakness, areflexia, paresthesias, and elevated CSF protein levels typically following an upper respiratory tract infection. In 1990, Asbury and Cornblath

proposed a set of diagnostic criteria. The criteria are listed below.

Features required for diagnosis:

Progressive weakness of both arms and legs or more than 1 limb

Areflexia

Clinical features supportive of diagnosis:

Progression up to 4 weeks

Relative symmetry of signs

Cranial nerve involvement

Autonomic dysfunction

Recovery usually beginning 2 to 4 weeks after progression ceases

Absence of fever at onset

Laboratory features supportive of diagnosis:

Elevated CSF protein with less than 10 cells/μL

Electrodiagnostic features of conduction block or nerve conduction slowing

Autonomic dysfunction consists of sinus tachycardia, supraventricular tachycardia, bradycardia, fluctuations in blood pressure, sphincter dysfunction, anhidrosis, and postural hypotension. Patients can experience respiratory difficulty requiring mechanical ventilation. Weakness usually starts in the lower extremities and ascends in a distal to proximal fashion. Cranial nerves can be affected with facial diplegia as the most common presentation. Paresthesias are a frequent, early symptom and involve mild sensory loss and pain. Low back pain and myalgias are common. The pathogenesis of GBS involves immune-mediated segmental demyelination of peripheral nerves. By definition, the progression of symptoms ends by 4 weeks into the illness. If the progression lasts 4 to 10 weeks, then the term subacute inflammatory demyelinating polyradiculoneuropathy is used. If the progression is chronic or the patient experiences multiple relapses, then the condition is termed chronic inflammatory demyelinating polyradiculoneuropathy.

4. (E) Approximately 90% of GBS cases will have abnormalities on electrophysiological testing as the multifocal demyelination evolves with secondary axonal injury. The most common abnormalities seen are conduction block, prolonged motor conduction velocities, decreased CMAP amplitudes, and prolonged F-wave latencies. An F-wave results when stimulation of any motor nerve results in antidromic conduction to the an-

terior horn cells followed by orthodromic propagation of the impulse back to the innervated muscle (reflected impulse). Prolonged F-wave latencies are a very early finding in GBS.

5. (C) There are many clinical variants of GBS, including axonal GBS, polyneuritis cranialis, GBS with CNS manifestations, and Miller-Fischer syndrome. The clinical features of Miller-Fischer syndrome include ophthalmoplegia, facial/bulbar weakness, ataxia, and areflexia. In the axonal form of GBS, an acute axonal neuropathy is observed. Polyneuritis cranialis presents with the acute onset of multiple cranial nerve abnormalities. Patients can present with dysphagia, bilateral facial weakness, and dysphonia. GBS with CNS manifestations is rare. Patients have an encephalopathy in addition to the peripheral nerve symptoms of GBS.

6. (C) All of the infections listed in this question have been associated with the development of GBS. However, *Campylobacter jejuni* has been associated with the Miller-Fischer variant.

7. (B) Antibodies against the ganglioside GQ1b are elevated in approximately 90% of the patients with this variant. The antibodies recognize similar epitopes from certain *C. jejuni* strains. Anti-Hu and anti-Ri antibodies are found in paraneoplastic syndromes. Anti-Hu antibodies can cause a sensory neuropathy and are associated with neuroblastoma and small cell lung cancer.

8. (D) Plasmapheresis and intravenous immunoglobulin appear to be equally effective in the treatment of GBS or acute inflammatory demyelinating polyneuropathy. Corticosteroids are not effective in the treatment of GBS. Corticosteroids, however, have been shown to be effective in the treatment of chronic inflammatory demyelinating polyneuropathy.

9. (E) The differential diagnosis of GBS is broad. The differential includes porphyria, transverse myelitis, acute myasthenia gravis, diphtheria, botulism, tick paralysis, hexane inhalation, Lyme disease, HIV infection, poliomyelitis, and hysteria. A good history and physical examination can help to exclude some of these possibilities.

10. **(D)** GBS is regarded as a predominantly motor neuropathy with occasional sensory symptoms. Approximately three-fourths of the patients present with weakness. Pain and paresthesias are observed, but to a lesser degree than the motor symptoms.

11. **(E)** Although plasmapheresis appears to be safe in children, there are a number of potential complications, including hypocalcemia, hemorrhage, hypotension, transfusion reactions, arrhythmias, and infection.

12. **(C)** Ingestion of certain heavy metals can result in a neurotoxic neuropathy. The heavy metals include lead, mercury, and thallium. Certain rat poisons and insecticides contain thallium. Ingestion may cause a sensory and motor peripheral neuropathy, nausea, vomiting, abdominal pain, and alopecia. Alopecia typically occurs 2 to 3 weeks after intoxication.

13. **(C)** This patient most likely has a Bell's palsy or facial nerve paralysis. Bell's palsy often follows an upper respiratory tract infection. Patients are unable to close the eyelid. Facial weakness develops over several hours to a few days. Lacrimation and taste may also be affected. Males and females are equally affected. Although approximately two-thirds of children recover fully without therapy, steroids have been used in the treatment of Bell's palsy. Supportive eye care, including placement of an eye patch for protection and eye drops to prevent corneal dryness, is usually needed. The prognosis for recovery is good.

14. **(A)** Erb's palsy is the most common brachial plexus injury in newborns. In Erb's palsy, damage to the upper trunk of the brachial plexus (C5 and C6 nerves) results in weakness of the upper arm. The patient presents with the humerus internally rotated and adducted. The elbow is extended and the wrist flexed.

15. **(D)** Klumpke's palsy is a rare cause of brachial plexus injury in newborns. It results from damage to the lower brachial plexus (C8 and T1 nerves). Patients demonstrate weakness of the forearm extensors, wrist flexors, finger flexors, and intrinsic hand muscles. Horner's syndrome can be present.

16. **(A)** This patient most likely has hereditary motor and sensory neuropathy (HMSN) type I or Charcot-Marie-Tooth disease given the family history, clinical presentation, and nerve conduction findings. Motor nerve conduction velocities in type II would probably be normal to slightly reduced. Type I hereditary neuropathy is much more common than type II. The hereditary neuropathies consist of several different types. Type I HMSN is the demyelinating or hypertrophic form, while Type II HMSN is the neuronal form (axonal defect) of the disease. Autosomal dominant and recessive modes of inheritance exist for both types. In addition, there is an X-linked form of type I. Dejerine-Sottas disease (HMSN type III) is a hypomyelinating neuropathy in which the Schwann cells are unable to produce normal myelin. The disease typically presents in the first year of life with hypotonia and developmental delay. In HMSN type I, patients typically present in the first or second decade of life. A pes cavus deformity due to progressive weakness of the anterior tibialis muscle is observed. Lower extremity muscle wasting and a hammer toe deformity are also observed. Sensory loss, especially proprioception, is noted. The deep tendon reflexes are absent in the affected extremity. The peripheral nerves are hypertrophied and, as a result, easily palpated. The hypertrophy results from increased Schwann and fibroblast cells. The treatment is supportive. Patients with HMSN type II tend to manifest symptoms later than patients with type I. Muscle weakness and atrophy tend to be milder than that found in type I. Axonal degeneration is observed on biopsy and the nerves are not hypertrophied.

17. **(B)** Large doses of pyridoxine can result in a sensory neuropathy with intact muscle strength. Paresthesias, autonomic dysfunction, diffuse sensory loss, and sensory ataxia are observed.

18. **(A)** Friedreich ataxia is transmitted as an autosomal recessive trait. It is also one of the triplet repeat disorders. Patients with Friedreich ataxia develop a slowly progressive ataxia, cardiomyopathy, and sensory neuropathy. Deformities, such as pes cavus and hammer toes, are also observed.

SUGGESTED READING

Asbury AK, Cornblath DR: Assessment of current diagnostic criteria for Guillain-Barré syndrome. *Ann Neurol* 27:S21–S24, 1990.

Sladky JT, Ashwal S: Inflammatory neuropathies in childhood. In: Swaiman KF, Ashwal S (eds): *Pediatric Neurology: Principles & Practice*, 3rd ed. St. Louis: Mosby, 1999, p 1202.

Smith AS, Ouvrier R: Peripheral neuropathies in children. In: Swaiman KF, Ashwal S (eds): *Pediatric Neurology: Principles & Practice*, 3rd ed. St. Louis: Mosby, 1999, p 1178.

Rheumatology

CASE 138: A 5-YEAR-OLD BOY WITH FEVERS AND JOINT SWELLING

A 5-year-old, previously healthy boy has had a daily spiking fever up to 104°F (40°C) in the evenings for 4 weeks. His temperature is normal between spikes. When febrile, the child is irritable, has malaise and does not want to play or move. He is often active and playful when afebrile. He appears stiff in the morning. His mother is concerned that his finger and knee joints appear swollen.

SELECT THE ONE BEST ANSWER

1. This child's diagnosis is most likely:

    (A) rheumatic fever
    (B) systemic arthritis
    (C) periodic fever syndrome
    (D) Kawasaki disease
    (E) systemic lupus erythematosus

2. All of the following laboratory abnormalities are expected in this disease except:

    (A) decreased platelets
    (B) increased white blood cell count
    (C) decreased hemoglobin
    (D) increased sedimentation rate
    (E) negative antinuclear antibody (ANA)

3. Which of the following is/are true about the skin rash in this entity?

    (A) It is evanescent, macular, salmon-colored, and often accompanies the fever.

    (B) Biopsy shows a leukocytoclastic vasculitis.
    (C) Skin lesions may be elicited by scratching (Koebner phenomenon).
    (D) A and C
    (E) All of the above

4. Multisystem extra-articular involvement in this disease may include the following:

    (A) eye inflammation
    (B) polyserositis
    (C) hepatosplenomegaly and lymphadenopathy
    (D) B and C
    (E) all of the above

5. The first medication usually given to treat the fevers and joint symptoms of this disease is:

    (A) a systemic corticosteroid
    (B) acetaminophen
    (C) a non-steroidal anti-inflammatory drug
    (D) methotrexate
    (E) an antitumor necrosis factor drug

6. Systemic corticosteroids should not be expected to:

    (A) stop the progression of joint disease
    (B) improve the anemia
    (C) help control fevers
    (D) decrease symptoms of pericarditis
    (E) decrease joint pain and swelling

7. Complications of methotrexate therapy include all except:

(A) liver enzyme elevation

(B) leukopenia

(C) oral ulcers

(D) hematuria

(E) nausea

8. Potential long-term complications of this disease include:

(A) growth delay, short stature, and osteoporosis

(B) micrognathia

(C) functional disabilities with fine and gross motor skill limitations

(D) risk of neurologic problems related to cervical spine arthritis

(E) all of the above

9. A 7-year-old girl was well until 3 months ago when she developed pain in her left knee. Her mother notes that she occasionally limps. There is no history of trauma or fevers. Her physical examination reveals mild left knee swelling and approximately a 5-degree loss of extension and 10-degree loss of flexion. She is mildly tender to knee palpation and guarded on ranging. She has mild left quadriceps atrophy. Her other joints are normal. Which of the following should be considered in the differential diagnosis?

(A) pauciarticular arthritis

(B) osteosarcoma

(C) psoriatic arthritis

(D) Lyme disease

(E) all of the above

10. Diagnostic work-up in the patient from question 9 should include:

(A) rheumatoid factor

(B) plain film radiograph

(C) joint aspiration for synovial fluid culture

(D) A and B

(E) all of the above

11. Which is a true statement about laboratory results in children with pauciarticular arthritis?

(A) CBC and sedimentation rate may be normal.

(B) ANA is positive in all patients.

(C) C-reactive protein is always elevated when active joint disease is present.

(D) Leukocyte and complement levels are often decreased.

(E) Rheumatoid factor is present in 25% of these patients.

12. The best way to detect early uveitis in children with arthritis is to:

(A) assess visual acuity

(B) perform visual field testing

(C) do a funduscopic examination

(D) perform a slit lamp examination

(E) refer patients to ophthalmology immediately if they develop eye symptoms

13. All of the following statements are true about special school needs and children with chronic arthritis except:

(A) A school district can transfer the child to another district if it is unable to provide the requested special services.

(B) A public school must evaluate the child for special services if the parent requests them for the child.

(C) Services which may be requested if needed by the child to ensure proper education within the public school system include: transportation between home and school, an extra set of books for home use, homebound instruction if unable to attend school, consultation by physical and occupational therapy services, and adaptive physical education.

(D) Congress has passed legislation requiring that public school districts provide services to children with special needs.

14. Potential long-term problems in a child with pauciarticular disease include:

(A) flexion contracture of the involved joint

(B) blindness secondary to uveitis

(C) leg-length discrepancy secondary to accelerated bone growth if a knee joint is involved

(D) progression to polyarticular disease in a small percent of these children

(E) all of the above

15. When evaluating a child in your office who has complaints of unilateral hip pain for the past several weeks, your differential diagnosis should include:

(A) Legg-Calvé-Perthes
(B) tumor
(C) transient (or toxic) synovitis
(D) early juvenile ankylosing spondylitis
(E) all of the above

16. All are true regarding juvenile ankylosing spondylitis except:

(A) Peripheral arthritis may precede axial (spine and sacroiliac) inflammation.
(B) Males are affected more frequently than females.
(C) Rheumatoid factor is usually negative.
(D) HLA-B27 must be present.
(E) Enthesitis (inflammation at tendon insertion sites) is often present.

17. Benign hypermobility syndrome is a common cause of joint pain in children. Which statement below is not true regarding this syndrome?

(A) It is most common in children 3 to 10 years of age, and decreases with age.
(B) A criterion for diagnosis is hyperextension at elbows and knees by ≥10 degrees.
(C) Joint pain secondary to benign hypermobility syndrome is unrelated to physical activity.
(D) A criterion for diagnosis is the ability to touch the thumb to the volar forearm.
(E) It is seen more often in girls than boys.

Match each entity that is associated with joint symptoms in questions 18 through 29 with one descriptive characteristic A through L.

18. Psoriatic arthritis
19. Rheumatoid factor positive arthritis
20. Ankylosing spondylitis
21. Gonococcal arthritis
22. Lyme disease
23. Familial Mediterranean fever
24. Reiter's syndrome
25. Postinfectious arthritis

(A) Enthesitis
(B) Night pain without objective findings; well in a.m.
(C) Mutation of gene encoding for pyrin
(D) Conjunctivitis and urethritis
(E) Scattered vesiculopustular lesions on extremities
(F) Increased pain after activity and sometimes at night

26. Growing pains
27. Rheumatic fever
28. Hypermobility syndrome
29. Inflammatory bowel disease arthritis

(G) Resolves by 6–12 weeks
(H) Nail pitting
(I) Erythema chronicum migrans
(J) Arthritis may precede abdominal symptoms
(K) Erythema marginatum
(L) Rheumatoid nodules, scleritis and vasculitis

Answers

1. **(B)** Systemic arthritis is the most likely diagnosis in a child with a daily spiking fever. Known as a quotidian fever, this fever pattern is characterized by one or two daily spikes >102.2°F (39°C) with a rapid return to baseline (98.6°F [37°C]) or below for the rest of the day. The fever spike classically occurs in the late afternoon or evening hours, but can occur any time of day. The child often appears well when afebrile.

  Systemic arthritis is one of three types of arthritis included in the juvenile rheumatoid arthritis (JRA) classification system:

- Systemic onset
- Pauciarticular (or oligoarticular) – ≤4 joints involved
- Polyarticular – ≥5 joints involved
  - rheumatoid factor negative
  - rheumatoid factor positive

  In 1998, a new classification was proposed for chronic childhood arthritis. It also includes systemic arthritis as one of the categories, along with several other types of childhood arthritis which were not included in the JRA classification. This new nomenclature is juvenile idiopathic arthritis (JIA), and the new classification is:

- Systemic arthritis
- Oligoarthritis – persistent
- Oligoarthritis – extended (patient develops >4 joint involvements more than 6 months after diagnosis)
- Polyarticular – rheumatoid factor negative
- Polyarticular – rheumatoid factor positive
- Psoriatic arthritis
  - presence of arthritis and psoriasis **or**

○ presence of arthritis and at least 2 of the following 3: dactylitis, nail abnormalities, psoriasis in a first-degree relative
- Enthesitis-related arthritis:
  ○ Presence of arthritis and enthesitis **or**
  ○ Presence of either arthritis or enthesitis with at least two of the following: + HLA B27; onset of arthritis in male >8 years of age; sacroiliac or inflammatory back pain; + family history (ankylosing spondylitis, enthesitis-related arthritis; sacroiliitis with inflammatory bowel disease; reactive arthritis or acute anterior uveitis in a first- or second-degree relative)
- Unable to be categorized

This newer classification system includes the spondyloarthropathies, such as enthesitis-related and psoriatic arthritis. This system should increase the homogeneity of the subgroups of childhood arthritis patients. This may promote improved recognition of the disease presentation and course, response to treatment and long-term outcomes of each arthritis subgroup. Research projects, such as studies on disease pathogenesis or genetic markers, may yield more information. Literature published after 1998 often refers to JIA instead of JRA.

2. **(A)** The CBC in active systemic arthritis usually has a marked elevation of the leukocyte count (can be >30,000/mm^3) and platelets (often >500,000/mm^3), as well as anemia (hemoglobin usually <10 g/dL). Low normal or below normal platelet counts should raise concern of malignancy, especially leukemia, which can present with clinical and laboratory features (e.g., hepatosplenomegaly, lymphadenopathy, joint pain, fevers, anemia, increased erythrocyte sedimentation rate) similar to those seen in systemic arthritis. Children with systemic arthritis have a negative ANA. (Note: A very rare complication of systemic arthritis, macrophage activation syndrome (MAS), is associated with depressed platelet levels. This acute illness is characterized by disseminated intravascular coagulation, purpura, hepatic failure, encephalopathy and other features. MAS has a high mortality rate if not treated rapidly and aggressively. High-dose in-

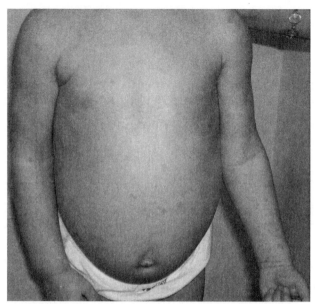

Figure 138-1. **Evanescent salmon-colored, macular or maculopapular rash of systemic arthritis. See color plates.**

travenous corticosteroids are the first line of treatment.)

3. **(D)** The classic systemic rash is migratory and so evanescent that it resolves within a few hours or less (Figure 138-1). There is no need (nor time!) to biopsy it. This precipitous and complete resolution of the rash would not be expected in a leukocytoclastic vasculitis lesion. The rash usually occurs during the fever spikes. It appears most often on the trunk and extremities, but may be present also on the face, palms and soles. It may occasionally be pruritic.

4. **(D)** Eye involvement, so common in other types of childhood arthritis, is typically absent in systemic arthritis.

5. **(C)** The first-line medication for systemic arthritis is a non-steroidal anti-inflammatory drug (NSAID), such as ibuprofen (35 to 40 mg/kg/day; maximum dose of 2400 mg/d) and naproxen (15 to 20 mg/kg/d; maximum dose of 1000 mg/d), both of which are approved for children and available in liquid form. Note that anti-inflammatory doses are higher than those recommended for analgesia and antipyrexia. Other NSAIDs approved for children include tolmetin,

diclofenac and sulindac, as well as indomethacin which may control fevers and polyserositis symptoms better than other NSAIDs, but frequently causes epigastric pain and headaches. Corticosteroids are used to treat systemic features not responding to NSAIDs. Prior to starting corticosteroid treatment, the physician must be certain that no other diagnosis, such as leukemia, is being overlooked. Methotrexate may help decrease systemic symptoms, but is generally used to treat active joint inflammation that does not quiet down despite use of NSAIDs. Antitumor necrosis factor α (antiTNF α) drugs are used to treat active joint disease which has not responded adequately to methotrexate. Three antiTNF α medications are available: etanercept, infliximab and adalimumab. This class of medication may be less efficacious in systemic arthritis compared with other subtypes of childhood arthritis. Currently, only etanercept is approved for use in childhood arthritis.

6. **(A)** Although systemic steroids may help decrease joint pain and possibly swelling, they do not halt the progression of the joint disease and destruction in childhood arthritis.

7. **(D)** Complications of low-dose weekly methotrexate include liver and bone marrow toxicity, which is generally mild and reversible, as well as mouth sores and nausea. Supplementation with folic acid may decrease these side effects. The concern for significant hepatotoxicity in patients with high cumulative methotrexate doses after years of treatment does exist, but has yet to be substantiated in studies evaluating liver biopsies in these patients. Alcohol consumption is contraindicated in patients on methotrexate. Immunosuppression tends to be mild at the low methotrexate doses given for childhood arthritis, so severe or opportunistic infections rarely occur. The infection risk may be increased if the child is also receiving corticosteroids. It is recommended that children on methotrexate not be immunized with live attenuated vaccines. Methotrexate is highly teratogenic; therefore, it is essential that patients who are sexually active use effective birth control methods while on this medication.

8. **(E)** Delayed growth, short stature, and osteoporosis are attributable to chronic illness, corticosteroid treatment and poor nutrition. Decreased weight bearing and limited participation in physical activities contribute further to the osteoporosis. Micrognathia develops in many patients, and may cause chewing difficulties, orthodontic problems, and even obstructive sleep apnea. Patients with significant cervical spine arthritis, which results in C1-C2 instability or ankylosis of posterior vertebral processes, are at risk for spinal cord injury (Figure 138-2). Functional disabilities historically occurred in 15% to 30% of children; with early aggressive treatment, this can be decreased.

9. **(E)** The differential diagnosis of monoarticular arthritis is broad, and is influenced by several factors, including the duration of joint symptoms, severity of symptoms, and the patient's age and gender. The differential can be divided into five main categories: rheumatologic; orthopedic; infectious; tumor; miscellaneous entities. Rheumatologic diseases include pauciarticular arthritis (which involves ≤4 joints), psoriatic arthritis, juvenile ankylosing spondylitis and sarcoidosis, with the first two diagnoses being more likely in this patient. Orthopedic problems affecting the knee include Osgood-Schlatter disease and patellofemoral syndrome, both of which are unlikely in a child this young. The main infectious cause to consider in a patient with a three-month history of knee swelling is Lyme disease. A septic joint or osteomyelitis is unlikely, considering the duration of symptoms. Possible tumors are osteosarcoma, Ewing's sarcoma, and pigmented villonodular synovitis. Although these tumors tend to occur in an older child, the clinician must always maintain a level of suspicion when the patient's complaints are unifocal. Concern for a malignant bone tumor increases if the child has pain that is out of proportion to findings on physical examination and/or has a history of frequent focal bone pain that occurs at night.

10. **(B)** A plain film radiograph is essential in a monoarticular presentation to rule out a bone tumor. Rheumatoid factor is negative in >90% of patients with childhood arthritis. When present, it is usually found in older children with poly-

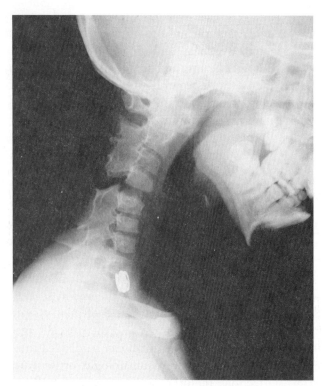
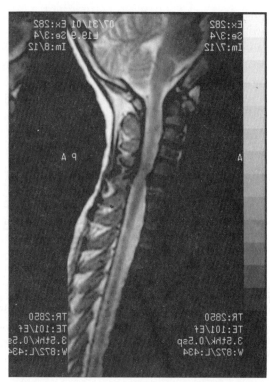

Figure 138-2.   (left) Cervical spine radiograph showing fusion of the spinous processes of C2-C4 and C5-C7 in 9-year-old boy with systemic arthritis since 18 months of age. (right) MRI of the same patient showing cervical cord impingement at the C4-C5 level; note that impingement is only at the cervical level which is not fused and where all neck flexion and extension takes place.

articular disease. Furthermore, false-positive results can occur, making rheumatoid factor a very poor screening test for childhood arthritis. A joint aspiration for synovial fluid culture is not indicated in this child. The main reason to perform a joint aspiration is to rule out an acute bacterial infection, which is not expected in this case based on the long duration of relatively mild symptoms. Synovial fluid cultures for *Borrelia burgdorferi* are usually unsuccessful. Polymerase chain reaction of synovial fluid has a much higher yield for identifying the presence of the Lyme-causing spirochete. Furthermore, if Lyme disease is suspected because the patient resides in or has traveled to a Lyme-endemic region, serologic studies (Lyme titers/Western blot) are usually performed, rather than joint aspiration.

11. **(A)** The CBC, erythrocyte sedimentation rate and C-reactive protein are often normal in pauciarticular arthritis. The ANA is positive in 40% to 60% of these children, usually in relatively low titers (≤1:320).

12. **(D)** By performing a slit lamp examination, the ophthalmologist can detect inflammatory cells in the aqueous humor of the anterior chamber of the eye. This is the best examination to detect early uveitis, an insidious eye disease in which most young patients lack eye symptoms. Later complications, such as cataracts, band keratopathy, and synechiae can be seen by examination with an ophthalmoscope. However, by then, irreversible injury to the eye may have already taken place. High risk factors associated with chronic uveitis in childhood arthritis are: female gender, young age (<6 years), positive ANA, disease duration <4 years, pauciarticular arthritis and, less commonly, polyarticular (rheumatoid factor negative) arthritis. Children at high risk for uveitis should have a slit lamp examination performed every 3 months. Initial treatment for children with uveitis includes topical steroids and mydriatics. If inflammation persists, treatment with systemic corticosteroids, methotrexate or even antiTNF α medications may be indicated.

13. **(A)** The local public school district is required by Congress (Individuals with Disabilities Education Act 1975, amended in 1997, and the Disabilities Act Section 504) to provide special services to children with disabilities, including arthritis. It may not transfer this responsibility to other school districts.

14. **(E)** Although pauciarticular arthritis has a good to excellent outcome in the majority of patients, a significant percentage of patients may have long-term morbidity secondary to this disease. Appropriate management during periods of active disease can minimize morbidity.

15. **(E)** Tumor should always be included in the differential of focal bone or joint pain. Orthopedic conditions involving the hip include Legg-Calvé-Perthes (idiopathic avascular necrosis) in younger children and slipped capital femoral epiphysis in older children. Hip arthritis occurs commonly in spondyloarthropathy. It is extremely rare in pauciarticular arthritis. Transient or toxic synovitis of the hip is a self-limited process (<2 weeks' duration), often noted to follow a respiratory infection. The child with toxic synovitis is generally 3 to 10 years of age, may limp, complain of pain in the hip, thigh or knee, and may have limited hip range of motion. If there is any clinical suspicion that the patient may have septic arthritis, the hip joint must be aspirated immediately.

16. **(D)** The presence of HLA-B27 is associated with increased risk of developing ankylosing spondylitis, but it need not be positive to make this diagnosis. It is present in approximately 90% of Caucasians but only 60% of African-Americans with ankylosing spondylitis. Juvenile ankylosing spondylitis falls under the category of enthesitis-related arthritis in the JIA classification system. Enthesitis is inflammation at tendon insertion sites, for example, the Achilles insertion. Ankylosing spondylitis is considered one of the spondyloarthropathies. The term spondyloarthropathy has historically referred to a group of entities that have certain clinical and laboratory characteristics in common: inflammation of spine and sacroiliac joints, frequent positive family history for diseases (including ankylosing spondylitis, inflammatory bowel disease, psoriatic arthritis, and Reiter's syndrome), association with HLA-B27, extra-articular features such as acute iritis, and absence of rheumatoid factor.

17. **(C)** The diagnosis of benign hypermobility syndrome is made by the presence of certain physical findings. These include answers B and D, as well as the ability to hyperextend at the metacarpophalangeal joints when the wrist is in extension so that the fingers are parallel to the forearm and also able to touch the floor with the palms of the hands with knees straight. Look for these physical findings in young children (especially between the ages of 3–10 years) who have increased pain after activity, as well as intermittent night pain, The incidence of benign hypermobility syndrome is increased in girls (female-to-male ratio is 2:1). It is more common in Asians and West Africans than in Caucasians. Rarely, a small joint effusion at ankles or knees may be observed; otherwise, there is absence of any clinical or laboratory signs of inflammation. Treatment includes: parental and patient reassurance and education about this entity, avoidance of high-impact activities which increase joint symptoms, physical therapy to work on muscle strengthening and joint protection education, supportive footwear, and evening acetaminophen or ibuprofen on occasion.

18. **(H)** nail pitting

19. **(L)** rheumatoid nodules, scleritis and vasculitis

20. **(A)** enthesitis (inflammation at tendon insertion sites)

21. **(E)** scattered vesiculopustular lesions on extremities

22. **(I)** erythema chronicum migrans

23. **(C)** mutation of gene encoding for pyrin

24. **(D)** conjunctivitis and urethritis

25. **(G)** resolves by 6–12 weeks

26. **(B)** night pain without objective findings; well in a.m.

27. **(K)** erythema marginatum

28. **(F)** increased pain after activity and sometimes at night

29. **(J)** arthritis may precede abdominal symptoms

SUGGESTED READING

Petty RE, Cassidy JT: Chronic arthritis. In: Cassidy JT, Petty RE Laxer RM, Lindsley CB (eds): *Textbook of Pediatric Rheumatology*, 5th ed. Philadelphia: Elsevier Saunders, 2005, p 206–323.

Schaller JG: Juvenile rheumatoid arthritis. *Pediatr Rev* 18: 337–349, 1997.

Petty RE, Southwood TR, Baum J, et al: Revision of the proposed classification criteria for juvenile idiopathic arthritis: Durban 1997. *J Rheumatol* 25:1991–1994, 1998.

Olsen NJ, Stein CM: New drugs for rheumatoid arthritis. *N Engl J Med* 350:2167–79, 2004.

CASE 139: A 15-YEAR-OLD GIRL WITH FATIGUE, FEVER AND ARTHRITIS

A previously healthy 15-year-old girl has had fatigue, low-grade fevers, sore throat and joint pain and stiffness for the past few weeks. On physical examination, she has cervical adenopathy and mild swelling of her finger joints. Her throat culture is negative for group A streptococcus. CBC: leukocyte count 3.9/mm^3 with a normal differential; the platelets are 165,000/mm^3 and the hemoglobin is 10.5 g/dL.

SELECT THE ONE BEST ANSWER

1. The differential diagnosis for this patient includes:

(A) Epstein-Barr virus infection
(B) leukemia
(C) systemic lupus erythematosus (SLE)
(D) all of the above
(E) none of the above

2. Her antinuclear antibody (ANA) titer is 1:320. In addition to being present in SLE, ANAs can be found in which of the following?

(A) patients taking phenytoin
(B) healthy individuals
(C) patients with an Epstein-Barr virus infection
(D) A and C
(E) all of the above

3. Autoantibodies that are specific for SLE include:

(A) antidouble stranded DNA (anti-dsDNA) and antiribonuclear protein (antiRNP)
(B) anti-dsDNA and anti-Smith
(C) anti-SS-A and anti-Smith
(D) anti-histone antibodies and anti-dsDNA
(E) anti-SS-A and antiRNP

4. Classification criteria used for the diagnosis of SLE include all the skin findings below except:

(A) Erythema marginatum
(B) photosensitivity
(C) malar rash
(D) discoid lesions
(E) mucocutaneous ulcerations (oral and/or nasal)

5. Complications which may occur in SLE include all except:

(A) platelet counts less than 5000/mm^3
(B) psychosis, seizures, or cognitive dysfunction
(C) interstitial pneumonitis, interstitial fibrosis or pleuritis
(D) progressive, erosive arthritis in the majority of patients who have joint swelling
(E) pericarditis, myocarditis, or valvular dysfunction

6. Which statement regarding renal disease in pediatric SLE is true?

(A) A normal urinalysis rules out lupus nephritis.
(B) Lupus nephritis usually recurs in a transplanted kidney.
(C) Lupus nephritis occurs in >75% of children with SLE.
(D) Patients with mesangial disease on biopsy are at increased risk for progression to renal failure compared with those with proliferative lesions.
(E) The presence of anti-Smith antibodies increases risk of lupus nephritis.

7. All of the following are true regarding laboratory evaluation in SLE except:

(A) Sedimentation rate and C-reactive protein are good markers for following SLE disease activity.

(B) An elevated leukocyte count is often secondary to infection or is associated with the use of high-dose corticosteroids.

(C) C3 and C4 complement levels may be helpful in following disease activity.

(D) Increases in anti-dsDNA levels may indicate impending exacerbation of disease.

(E) Patients with SLE may have a combination of a Coombs positive hemolytic anemia and thrombocytopenia, known as Evan's syndrome.

8. Which statement is false regarding antiphospholipid antibodies (APLA)?

(A) Risk of both venous and arterial thrombosis is increased in patients with APLA.

(B) All patients with SLE should be checked for the presence of APLA.

(C) Examples of APLA include: lupus anticoagulant, anticardiolipin antibodies, anti-β_2-glycoprotein.

(D) The presence of APLA increases the risk of miscarriage.

(E) More than 90% of patients with APLA have an underlying rheumatic disease.

9. Which statement regarding treatment of SLE in children is not true?

(A) Hydroxychloroquine is often used to treat skin, joint and muscle inflammation.

(B) Complications of corticosteroid treatment include avascular necrosis, osteoporosis, hypertension and diabetes.

(C) Long-term prednisone doses of < 8 mg/day in children will not cause growth suppression.

(D) Cyclophosphamide treatment may cause gonadal injury and increase risk of oncogenesis.

(E) Stress doses of corticosteroids may be necessary up to 12 months after cessation of chronic corticosteroid treatment.

10. The following statement(s) is/are true about the outcomes in childhood SLE:

(A) Infection is a major cause of mortality in children with SLE.

(B) Cardiovascular disease, including myocardial infarction and stroke, is a major long-term cause of morbidity and mortality.

(C) Most children are able to discontinue all medications after 5 years of treatment.

(D) A and B.

(E) All of the above.

11. All are true about neonatal lupus except:

(A) The risk of having a baby with neonatal lupus increases if the mother has active lupus during pregnancy.

(B) The majority of children with congenital atrioventricular heart block will require a pacemaker.

(C) Neonatal lupus rash, thrombocytopenia and hepatitis usually resolve spontaneously by six months of age.

(D) Neonatal lupus is strongly associated with the presence of anti-Ro (SS-A) and anti-La (SS-B).

(E) A mother may have a baby with neonatal lupus even if she has never had a diagnosis or symptoms of a rheumatic illness.

12. Which statement is correct regarding drug-induced lupus?

(A) All patients require treatment with corticosteroids to control symptoms.

(B) Renal involvement is common.

(C) Anti-dsDNA is usually positive.

(D) Minocycline is one of several drugs known to cause drug-induced lupus.

(E) Complement levels are usually depressed in drug-induced lupus.

13. The following is/are true about Raynaud's:

(A) The order of the triphasic color change is: red → white → blue.

(B) Primary Raynaud's, which is not associated with any underlying rheumatic disease, is more common in children than adults.

(C) Raynaud's phenomenon occurs in approximately one-third of children with SLE and in >90% of children with systemic sclerosis (diffuse scleroderma).

(D) A and C.

(E) All of the above.

14. Approximately 4 weeks ago, a mother noticed that her 7-year-old son had a rash on his face and

knuckles. A few weeks later, she noted that he had decreased endurance, and was having difficulty running and climbing at the playground. His school teacher reported to his mother that he was having problems ascending two flights of stairs to go to music class. Physical examination of this child may reveal all the following except:

(A) dystrophic calcification
(B) violaceous discoloration of the upper eyelids
(C) Gowers' sign
(D) muscle tenderness
(E) diffuse cutaneous vasculitis

15. All of the following are helpful in diagnosing juvenile dermatomyositis (JDM) except:

(A) presence of Gottron's papules and a heliotrope rash over the eyelids
(B) presence of ANA and an elevated sedimentation rate
(C) elevated serum muscle enzymes
(D) proximal muscle weakness
(E) muscle biopsy showing inflammatory cell infiltrate, and perifascicular atrophy and necrosis

16. All are true about the complications and outcome of JDM except:

(A) calcinosis may cause limitation in joint range and cosmetic problems
(B) more than two-thirds of patients have good to excellent functional outcomes
(C) mortality is usually secondary to respiratory failure or gastrointestinal vasculitis
(D) dysphagia and reflux are secondary to lower esophageal sphincter dysfunction
(E) in severe cases, dysphonia may be present

17. For the past few days a 5-year-old child has been complaining of intermittent abdominal pain. No emesis or diarrhea was reported. Then her mother noted a red rash on her legs, and brought her to your office. Your examination reveals a non-toxic child who is afebrile. She has palpable purpuric lesions, coalescing by the ankles, and ascending up to the buttocks. Her abdominal exam reveals mild diffuse tenderness, but no rebound. You suspect that she has Henoch-Schönlein purpura (HSP). All of the following are true about HSP except:

(A) rash frequently recurs over the first 6 weeks after presentation, often increasing after physical activity
(B) arthritis, especially of ankles and knees, is common
(C) in a small percentage of children, the purpuric rash is secondary to thrombocytopenia
(D) edema of the scalp, hands and feet is common in children younger than 4 years old
(E) skin biopsy will show a leukocytoclastic vasculitis with IgA deposition

18. All the following are true about GI involvement in HSP except:

(A) GI hemorrhage is common, and may be occult or gross.
(B) GI symptoms can present before the rash.
(C) A normal barium enema rules out intussusception in HSP.
(D) Complications include intussusception, bowel infarction and perforation.
(E) Ultrasonography may show edema of bowel wall and may identify an intussusception.

19. Which statement is true for renal involvement secondary to HSP?

(A) The majority of children who have hematuria during the acute phase of HSP illness have progression of renal disease.
(B) It is associated with a membranous lesion on renal biopsy.
(C) It usually presents shortly after HSP diagnosis with nephrotic syndrome and hypertension.
(D) It may persist in 1% to 5% of children and may progress to end-stage disease in approximately 1%.
(E) It occurs more commonly in patients <8 years old at the time of HSP diagnosis.

Match each entity in questions 20 through 32 to one descriptive characteristic A through M.

20. Progressive systemic sclerosis
21. Polyarteritis nodosa
22. Sjögren's syndrome

(A) Large vessel vasculitis
(B) + cANCA (antineutrophil cytoplasmic antibodies)
(C) May affect growth of limb

23. En coup de sabre
24. Wegener's granulomatosis
25. Kawasaki disease
26. Linear scleroderma
27. Serum sickness
28. Behçet's disease
29. Sarcoidosis
30. Takayasu's arteritis
31. Erythema nodosum
32. Rheumatic fever

(D) Severe uveitis of anterior and posterior uveal tracts
(E) Esophageal dysmotility
(F) A type of panniculitis
(G) Sicca complaints (dry eyes and ↓ oral secretions)
(H) Vasculitis of small and medium-sized vessels
(I) Presents 7 to 14 days after antigen exposure
(J) Elevated anti-DNase B titers
(K) Linear scleroderma of the face
(L) Non-caseating granulomas
(M) Treatment with intravenous gammaglobulin

Answers

1. **(D)** The patient's clinical complaints, physical findings and CBC results are all non-specific and are not diagnostic for any particular disease. It is important to have a broad differential when first assessing this type of patient. Malignancy, such as leukemia, should be considered in children with this clinical history and depressed cell lines on CBC. Arthralgias and arthritis may be present in children with leukemia. Systemic lupus erythematosus (SLE) should be considered in any patient who presents with multi-system problems. Constitutional complaints, such as fevers, fatigue, and weight loss are common in SLE, as is joint involvement which is present in approximately 75% of patients. Mild cytopenias are common laboratory findings in SLE. Epstein-Barr virus (EBV) infection, especially in the teenager, can present with multisystem complaints similar to those seen in SLE, including constitutional symptoms, arthralgias/arthritis, and adenopathy. Children with EBV infections often have cytopenias and positive antinuclear antibodies (ANAs), which can add to the challenge of differentiating between SLE and EBV. Further laboratory evaluation (EBV antibody profile, complement levels, autoantibodies such as antiSmith and antidouble stranded DNA) may help guide the clinician to the correct diagnosis.

2. **(E)** ANAs are found in many clinical settings, even in healthy individuals (especially in those who have primary relatives with autoimmune disease, or in the elderly). They are detected in infections (e.g., EBV, streptococcal, sub-acute endocarditis, hepatitis C), autoimmune disease (SLE, mixed connective tissue disease, dermatomyositis, scleroderma, juvenile arthritis, Sjögren's syndrome), drug-induced process (e.g., secondary to anticonvulsants, isoniazid, penicillamine, hydralazine, procainamide, certain antibiotics), organ-specific autoimmune disease (autoimmune hepatitis, thyroiditis). ANA is present in almost all patients with SLE (>98%). Titers are variable in SLE, but are usually ≥1:320. It is important to recognize that while virtually all patients with SLE have a +ANA, most people with a +ANA do not have SLE.

3. **(B)** Antidouble stranded DNA (anti-dsDNA) and antiSmith (antiSm) are specific for SLE, and are present in approximately 70% and 20% of SLE patients, respectively. Other autoantibody subtypes may be present, but are not specific for SLE, and may be identified with other autoimmune entities:

Specific Autoantibody	Clinical Associations
Anti-dsDNA	SLE
AntiSmith	SLE
Anti-U1-RNP	Mixed connective tissue disease; SLE
Anti-Ro/SS-A	SLE; Sjögren's syndrome; neonatal lupus; C2 and C4 deficiencies
Anti-La/SS-B	Sjögren's syndrome; SLE; neonatal lupus
Anti-Scl 70	Systemic sclerosis
Anti-Jo-1	Polymyositis, especially with interstitial lung disease
Antihistone	Drug-induced lupus; SLE
Anticentromere	Limited scleroderma (CREST)

4. **(A)** The American College of Rheumatology 1997 criteria for classification of SLE are helpful diagnostic tools for SLE. The criteria are:

- Malar rash (Figure 139-1)
- Discoid rash
- Photosensitivity
- Oral or nasal ulcerations

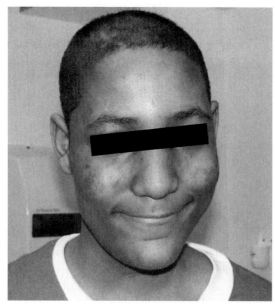

Figure 139-1. **Malar rash in a teenage boy with systemic lupus erythematosus. See color plates.**

- Non-erosive arthritis
- Polyserositis
- Nephritis (proteinuria >0.5 g/day or cellular casts)
- Encephalopathy (seizures or psychosis)
- Cytopenia
- +ANA
- Positive immunoserology: +anti-dsDNA or +antiSm, or presence of antiphospholipid antibodies

The presence in a patient with 4 of these 11 criteria has a sensitivity and a specificity of >95% for the diagnosis of SLE. SLE should be suspected in children who present with multisystem complaints and signs. Although not included in the diagnostic criteria, several other features may be present which may increase suspicion for SLE, such as myalgias/myositis, Raynaud's phenomenon, decreased cognitive function, chorea, cranial nerve palsies, retinopathy, lymphadenopathy, hepatosplenomegaly, myocarditis, endocarditis, and depressed complement levels. (Note: erythema marginatum is a skin finding in acute rheumatic fever.)

5. **(D)** The arthritis in SLE patients is rarely erosive, and joint deformity is uncommon.

6. **(C)** Lupus nephritis occurs in >75% of children. The risk of renal involvement is increased in those with antibodies to dsDNA, but not in those with antiSmith antibodies. Although some patients may present with nephrotic syndrome, hypertension and renal insufficiency, the majority initially have no clinical symptoms. Therefore, it is important to perform frequent urinalyses, assess protein excretion (the easiest way is by performing a protein/creatinine ratio on a spot urine), and follow serum creatinine and albumin. Rarely, patients with a normal urinalysis may have renal involvement. As urine and blood studies are indirect assessments of renal status in SLE patients, a kidney biopsy is often necessary to provide important information to help with treatment decisions. The World Health Organization (WHO) classification, and more recently, the International Society of Nephrology (ISN) classification systems categorize renal lesions based on light (and occasionally electron) microscopy, and immunofluorescence. The ISN classification describes six classes:

- Class I—minimal mesangial lupus nephritis
- Class II—mesangial proliferative lupus nephritis
- Class III—focal proliferative glomerulonephritis
- Class IV—diffuse proliferative glomerulonephritis
- Class V—membranous nephritis
- Class VI—advanced sclerosing lupus nephritis

Patients with class I or II lesions generally respond well to corticosteroid treatment. Class III is potentially a more significant lesion that may improve with immunosuppressive treatment, but may also progress to a more severe renal lesion, such as class IV. Classes IV and V require aggressive medical management to hopefully decrease progression to renal insufficiency and failure. Class VI has marked glomerular sclerosis, suggesting an end-stage kidney. In addition to histological classification, activity (inflammation) and chronicity (scarring) indices are also assessed, which further impact medical treatment decisions and renal prognosis. Lupus nephritis is associated with increased morbidity and decreased long-term survival. The poorer outcome is related to renal complications such as hypertension, nephritic syndrome and renal failure. The treatment (cytotoxic drugs and high corticosteroid doses) further contributes to morbidity. If progression to renal failure occurs, the patient undergoes dialysis until a transplant can be performed. Renal transplantation is generally postponed until the patient's SLE has become quiescent. Fortunately, clinically significant lupus nephritis occurs in <5% of transplanted kidneys.

7. (**A**) The sedimentation rate and C-reactive protein (CRP) are not helpful markers for SLE disease activity. Both are non-specific studies, affected by infection and other inflammatory conditions. The complement levels and anti-dsDNA titers reflect disease activity more reliably.

8. (**E**) The presence of antiphospholipid antibodies (APLA) is associated with venous or arterial thrombosis, recurrent fetal loss, hemolytic anemia, thrombocytopenia and livedo reticularis. Approximately one-half the patients with APLA do not have an underlying rheumatologic disease (primary APLA syndrome), while the rest have secondary APLA syndrome, usually related to a rheumatic disease (especially SLE). It is important to test for the presence of APLA in any individual who presents with an unexplained venous or arterial thrombosis, and also in patients diagnosed with SLE. APLA studies include lupus anticoagulant, anticardiolipin antibodies, and also anti-β_2-glycoprotein.

9. (**C**) Corticosteroid (CS) treatment is necessary to help control multisystem involvement in the vast majority of children with SLE. Unfortunately, prolonged use can lead to multiple complications. These include: growth suppression (starting at doses equivalent to ≥ 3 mg/day in small children), musculoskeletal (osteoporosis, avascular necrosis, muscle wasting, myopathy), cardiovascular (hypertension, hyperlipidemia), ophthalmologic (cataracts, glaucoma), skin (striae, impaired healing), diabetes, secondary adrenocortical insufficiency, and immunosuppression. A major goal of medical therapy is to minimize the CS doses given. This, in part, is accomplished by using combination therapy. Hydroxychloroquine is often effective in treating skin, muscle and joint involvement. It may also decrease the incidence of exacerbations in SLE. Immunosuppressive therapy (including cyclophosphamide, azathioprine, mycophenolate mofetil, methotrexate, or cyclosporine A) is often given to patients whose disease is not controlled by CS, or who have major organ system involvement, especially

the renal and central nervous systems. Unfortunately, current treatment for SLE is not specific, and usually involves general immunosuppressive therapy. Medical management of SLE also includes treatment of hypertension, hyperlipidemia, and osteoporosis.

10. (**D**) Although the prognosis for SLE has improved, most children with SLE are unable to discontinue all medications given to control the disease. Ten-year survival has increased from <50% in the 1950s to >85% in the 1990s. The most common cause of death is infection, followed by renal failure. Mortality occurring more than 10 years after SLE diagnosis is often secondary to cardiovascular complications such as myocardial infarction and stroke.

11. (**A**) Anti-Ro (SS-A) and/or anti-La (SS-B) antibodies are present in virtually all mothers who have babies with neonatal lupus (NLE). These autoantibodies may be present in individuals with SLE, Sjögren's syndrome, and even in women with no rheumatologic symptoms or diagnosis. In women with SLE, only the presence or absence of anti-Ro and anti-La has an impact on the risk of having a baby with NLE, not the status of SLE disease activity. (However, women with active and severe SLE may be at increased risk of premature delivery and other pre- and perinatal complications.) Clinical manifestations of NLE include rash, hepatitis, thrombocytopenia and permanent congenital heart block (CHB). Except for CHB, the NLE manifestations resolve by 6 months of age, corresponding to the disappearance of maternal autoantibodies from the baby's circulation. Some children may have residual scarring from skin lesions. The majority of children with CHB require pacemakers, many during the first few weeks of life.

12. (**D**) The majority of patients with drug-induced lupus (DIL) have milder symptoms and less organ-system involvement than those with idiopathic SLE. The most common clinical manifestations in DIL are arthralgias/arthritis, myalgias, serositis, rash and constitutional symptoms (such as fatigue and fever). Renal and neurologic involvement is very rare. Patients usually have 4 of 11 criteria expected for diagnosis of SLE. Antibodies to his-

tones are generally present, while anti-dsDNA is almost always negative. Complement levels tend to be normal. The most commonly implicated drugs in children include anticonvulsants (especially hydantoins and ethosuximide), isoniazid and minocycline. Reported cases of DIL secondary to minocycline have increased greatly over the past decade, corresponding to its increased use in teenagers for treatment of acne. In adults, hydralazine and procainamide are the most frequent triggers of DIL. Definitive treatment for DIL is discontinuation of the suspected medication. NSAIDs are useful to treat symptoms such as fever, musculoskeletal involvement and serositis. Although the majority of patients do not require corticosteroids, some may require treatment for rare major organ system involvement or persistence of symptoms.

13. **(C)** Raynaud's may occur in patients with rheumatologic disease (secondary Raynaud's or Raynaud's phenomenon), and in individuals without an underlying rheumatologic process (primary Raynaud's or Raynaud's disease). Primary Raynaud's is most common in adult women, usually during their third and fourth decades of life. It may occur in teenage girls, but is rare in prepubertal children and teenage boys. In both primary and secondary Raynaud's, the triphasic color change, in order, is white → blue → red. The pathogenesis is arterial vasoconstriction with subsequent reduction in local blood flow, particularly to the hands, and also the toes, and occasionally to the ears, nose tip and lips. It is usually triggered by cold or emotional stress. It is important to know if a child with Raynaud's has a primary or secondary process. The history, physical examination, and laboratory evaluations are all essential to help determine this. The history may reveal multisystem complaints. The presence of pitting or scarring of the distal digital pulp, finger edema, sclerodactyly, or changes in the nailfold vessels suggest a secondary Raynaud's process, as does the presence of a high +ANA titer. Raynaud's phenomenon occurs in systemic sclerosis (>90% of patients), mixed connective tissue disease (~50%) and SLE (~35%). Treatment includes patient education to keep the extremities warm and the core temperature up, vasodilators (such as calcium channel blockers) and biofeedback.

14. **(A)** Dystrophic calcification, or calcinosis, is a late feature of juvenile dermatomyositis (JDM), usually developing months to years after the initial symptoms of rash and muscle weakness.

15. **(B)** ANA and the erythrocyte sedimentation rate are non-specific laboratory studies which do not help in making a diagnosis of JDM. The diagnosis requires the presence of the classic rash. This rash consists of Gottron's papules which are scaly, erythematous lesions over the dorsal aspects of the metacarpophalangeal and interphalangeal joints (Figure 139-2), and a heliotrope discoloration over the upper eyelids, often with mild periorbital edema. The presence of at least two of the four following criteria are also needed to make the diagnosis: 1) symmetric proximal muscle weakness, 2) elevation in the serum of one or more skeletal muscle enzymes (creatine kinase, aldolase, aspartate aminotransferase, lactic dehydrogenase), 3) electromyography (EMG) demonstrating myopathy and denervation, 4) muscle biopsy showing inflammation and necrosis. If the first two criteria are present, the invasive studies of EMG and muscle biopsy are rarely needed. It may be difficult to evaluate the presence of muscle weakness in a child younger than 7 years of age in whom it is often not possible to perform formal muscle strength grading. Therefore, assessment of gross motor skills (such as ability to squat and arise, balance, jump, hop, get on and off the floor, and ascend stairs) is an essential part of the physical examination. Look for a positive Gower's sign (the

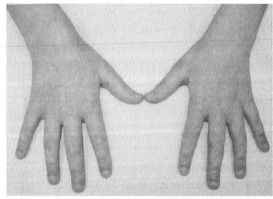

Figure 139-2. **Erythematous, scaly lesions (Gottron's papules) over the dorsal aspects of the metacarpophalangeal and interphalangeal joints in a 10-year-old girl with dermatomyositis. Nailfold telangiectasias can also be seen. See color plates.**

use of the arms to assist in transitioning from a kneeling or prone position to standing, by "walking" the hands up the thighs).

16. **(D)** In JDM, weakness of the skeletal muscles employed in swallowing (palatal, pharyngeal, hypopharyngeal, and proximal esophageal muscles) may lead to dysphagia, regurgitation of liquids through the nose and dysphonia with nasal speech. The risk of aspiration is significant in these patients. These children require aggressive medical management, and may need protection of the airway. Overall, the prognosis of JDM has improved greatly since the availability of corticosteroids (CS), which is the first line of treatment. In the presteroid era, at least one-third of patients died (usually secondary to respiratory failure or gastrointestinal vasculitis) and another third had major morbidity (significant residual weakness and/or severe calcinosis). Currently, CS treatment is given to all JDM patients, with duration of therapy lasting >1 year, often 18 to 24 months, depending on clinical response. A rapid taper of CS or total treatment duration <6 months is often associated with disease exacerbation. Some JDM patients require additional medications (such as methotrexate, cyclophosphamide, cyclosporine, intravenous immunoglobulin) to control the disease. Currently, long-term survival is >95%, and more than two-thirds of patients have good to excellent outcomes. Calcinosis is still a major cause of morbidity, and reflects prolonged periods of poorly controlled disease. Early diagnosis and appropriate treatment of JDM are essential, as they have been shown to reduce mortality and morbidity.

17. **(C)** Henoch-Schönlein purpura (HSP), the most common vasculitic syndrome of childhood, is characterized by the presence of a palpable purpuric rash (Figure 139-3). Distribution is primarily over the dependent areas of legs (especially prominent by the ankles) and buttocks, but may also occur on the hands and arms. Ulceration of the lesions may occasionally occur. Recurrence of the purpuric rash, especially after increased physical activity, is common during the first 6 weeks. Subcutaneous edema may be prominent in younger children, and occurs on the dorsum of hands and feet, periorbital areas, scalp, and scrotum. The

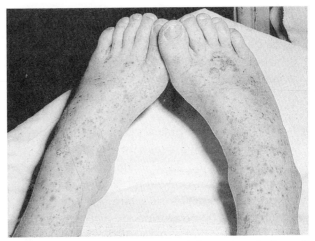

Figure 139-3. **Palpable, purpuric lesions on the legs of a child with Henoch-Schönlein purpura. See color plates.**

rash is never associated with thrombocytopenia. Skin biopsy shows a leukocytoclastic vasculitis with IgA deposition. Arthritis, most commonly involving ankles and knees, occurs in 60% to 80% of children. Treatment of the arthritis is usually not necessary, although NSAIDs may be helpful. However, they should be used with caution because of the possible gastrointestinal and renal involvement seen in HSP.

18. **(C)** GI involvement occurs in more than two-thirds of patients, and can be mild or severe. It is usually characterized by colicky pain, and may be associated with emesis and GI hemorrhage, either occult or gross. Abdominal pain is thought to be secondary to bowel wall edema and hemorrhage. Mucosal ulceration may occur. When the GI symptoms present before the rash (15% to 35% of cases), the diagnosis may be unclear, and an acute surgical abdomen may be suspected. GI complications include intussusception (2% to 4%), and, rarely, bowel infarction, bowel wall perforation, pancreatitis and hydrops of the gallbladder. Intussusception in HSP is usually ileoilial, as opposed to the more common ileocolic location seen in idiopathic intussusception. Therefore, a barium enema will often not detect intussusception in HSP. A much more helpful study to evaluate GI involvement in HSP is ultrasonography, which demonstrates bowel wall edema in children with GI symptoms, as well as complications such as intussusception and perforation. Although placebo-controlled studies are

lacking, children with severe GI manifestations are often given corticosteroids. A reasonable treatment regimen is 1 to 2 mg/kg/day for 1 week, tapering off over the next few weeks. Intravenous corticosteroid administration may be required initially to assure systemic absorption.

19. **(D)** Renal involvement occurs in 20% to 40% of patients, and generally presents within 3 months of the HSP diagnosis with microscopic hematuria. Mild proteinuria may also be present, but nephrotic syndrome, renal insufficiency and hypertension are uncommon. Urinalysis should be performed weekly initially, and then at least monthly for the first 3 months after HSP diagnosis, and perhaps beyond in those with increased risk factors for renal disease: older age (>8 years of age); persistent rash; history of severe abdominal symptoms. Renal involvement progresses in 1% to 5% of patients, and may result in renal failure. Early renal characteristics which are associated with persistent nephropathy or renal failure include proteinuria >1 g/day, nephrotic syndrome and renal insufficiency. Renal biopsy findings range from mild mesangial proliferation in those with mild UA changes to severe crescentic glomerulonephritis in patients with more severe renal involvement. IgA deposition is present on immunofluorescence. Treatment of renal disease in HSP is controversial because of a lack of prospective multicenter trials. However, recent studies suggest improved outcomes of HSP renal disease with corticosteroids, alone or combined with an immunosuppressive medication such as cyclophosphamide, azathioprine, mycophenolate mofetil, or cyclosporine.

20. **(E)** Esophageal dysmotility

21. **(H)** Vasculitis of small and medium-sized vessels

22. **(G)** Sicca complaints (dry eyes and ↓ oral secretions)

23. **(K)** Linear scleroderma of the face

24. **(B)** + cANCA (antineutrophil cytoplasmic antibodies)

25. **(M)** Treatment with intravenous gammaglobulin

26. **(C)** May affect growth of limb

27. **(I)** Presents 7 to 14 days after antigen exposure

28. **(D)** Severe uveitis of anterior and posterior uveal tracts

29. **(L)** Non-caseating granulomas

30. **(A)** Large vessel vasculitis

31. **(F)** A type of panniculitis

32. **(J)** Elevated anti-DNase B titers

SUGGESTED READING

Petty RE, Laxer RM: Systemic lupus erythematosus. In: Cassidy JT, Petty RE, Laxer RM, Lindsley CB (eds): *Textbook of Pediatric Rheumatology*, 5th ed. Philadelphia: Elsevier Saunders, 2005, p 342–391.

Klein-Gitelman M, Reiff A, Silverman E: Systemic lupus erythematosus in childhood. *Rheum Dis Clin North Am* 28:561–577, 2002.

Weening JJ, D'Agati VD, Schwartz MM, et al: The classification of glomerulonephritis is systemic lupus erythematosus revisited. *J Am Soc Nephrol* 15:241–250, 2004.

Pachman LM: Juvenile dermatomyositis. Pathophysiology and disease expression. *Pediatr Clin North Am* 42: 1071–1098, 1995.

Saulsbury FT: Henoch-Schonlein purpura in children. Report of 100 patients and review of the literature. *Medicine (Baltimore)* 78:385–409, 1999.

Wagner-Weiner L: Laboratory evaluation of pediatric rheumatic diseases. *Pediatr Ann* 31:362–371, 2002.

Index

Page numbers followed by *t* and *f* indicate tables and figures, respectively.